AF683794

Laryngeal Cancer

Edited by

Carl E. Silver M.D.

Professor of Surgery,
Professor of Otolaryngology
Albert Einstein College of Medicine

Chief, Head and Neck Surgery
Montefiore Medical Center
Bronx, New York

1991
Thieme Medical Publishers, Inc., New York
Georg Thieme Verlag, Stuttgart • New York

Thieme Medical Publishers, Inc.
381 Park Avenue South
New York, New York 10016

Laryngeal Cancer
Carl E. Silver, M.D.

Library of Congress Cataloging-in-Publication Data

Laryngeal cancer / Carl E. Silver, editor.
p. cm.
Includes bibliographical references and index.
ISBN 0-86577-395-5 (Thieme Medical Publishers). — ISBN 3-13-771901-1 (Georg Thieme Verlag)
1. Larynx—Cancer. I. Silver, Carl E.
[DNLM: 1. Laryngeal Neoplasms—surgery. WV 520 L336]
RC280.T5L37 1991
616.99′422—dc20
DNLM/DLC
for Library of Congress 91-798
CIP

Copyright © 1991 by Thieme Medical Publishers, Inc. This book, including all parts thereof, is legally protected by copyright. Any use, exploitation or commercialization outside the narrow limits set by copyright legislation, without the publisher's consent, is illegal and liable to prosecution. This applies in particular to photostat reproduction, copying, mimeographing or duplication of any kind, translating, preparation of microfilms, and electronic data processing and storage.

Important note: Medicine is an ever-changing science. Research and clinical experience are continually broadening our knowledge, in particular our knowledge of proper treatment and drug therapy. Insofar as this book mentions any dosage or application, readers may rest assured that the authors, editors, and publishers have made every effort to ensure that such references are strictly in accordance with the state of knowledge at the time of production of the book. Nevertheless, every user is requested to carefully examine the manufacturers' leaflets accompanying each drug to check on his own responsibility whether the dosage schedules recommended therein or the contraindications stated by the manufacturers differ from the statements made in the present book. Such examination is particularly important with drugs that are either rarely used or have been newly released on the market.

Some of the product names, patents, and registered designs referred to in this book are in fact registered trademarks or proprietary names even though specific reference to this fact is not always made in the text. Therefore, the appearance of a name without designation as proprietary is not to be construed as a representation by the publisher that it is in the public domain.

Printed in the United States of America.

5 4 3 2 1

TMP ISBN 0-86577-395-5
GTV ISBN 3-13-771901-1

This book is dedicated to the memory of

Max L. Som, M.D.
1904–1990

a pioneer in the treatment of laryngeal cancer;
my teacher, colleague, and friend.

Contents

Charles W. Vaughan, M.D.
Chief, Department of Otolaryngology–Head and Neck Surgery
Boston Veteran's Administration Hospital
Associate Professor
Department of Otolaryngology
Boston University
Boston, Massachusetts

Bhadrasain Vikram, M.D.
Chairman, Department of Radiation Oncology
Beth Israel Medical Center
New York, New York

William I. Wei M.B.B.S., D.L.O.
Senior Lecturer in Surgery
Department of Surgery
University of Hong Kong
Queen Mary Hospital, Hong Kong

Charles D. Wendt, M.D.
Assistant Radiotherapist
Instructor in Radiotherapy
University of Texas
M.D. Anderson Cancer Center
Houston, Texas

Preface

Yes sir. Certainly, it was I who found the body. This morning, as usual, I went to cut my daily quota of cedar, when I found the body in a grove in a hollow in the mountains.

—Ryunosuke Akutagawa,
from Rashomon and Other Stories.*

The above passage begins a series of accounts of a murder and rape, related by several participants and observers. Although ultimately the event is described consistently in each version, the details, motives, and conclusions differ according to the viewpoint of the narrator. The story is a parable whose truth underlies all facets of our life—religion, politics, and, indeed, science.

There are few areas of medical science where such allegory is more relevant than in the field of laryngeal cancer. Surgeons and radiation oncologists have long debated the preferred method of treatment of laryngeal cancer in various stages, and clinicians differ among themselves as to the indications for and applicability of particular treatments and procedures. The significance of certain histopathological findings in malignant and premalignant lesions, the relevance of cellular kinetics to prognosis, the role of modern imaging procedures in staging and choice of therapy, the efficacy of chemotherapy, the place of extended conservation surgery, protocols for treatment of advanced tumors, choice of reconstructive methods after major ablative procedures, and the selection and utility of prosthetic speech devices all constitute spheres of controversy within this discipline.

This volume is based on a search of the literature of the past decade. The contributors were selected because of their investigation and advocacy of various viewpoints, modalities, and techniques, as well as their stature within their respective fields. Thus the editor's purpose has been to compile a representative tableau of the current status of laryngeal cancer. Opinions, techniques, and conclusions discussed by the authors are often in disagreement with each other, and, sometimes, with those of the editor. The reader will not find here a consistent and uniform approach for management of neoplasms of the larynx. It is hoped that he will acquire an accurate approximation of the available techniques and opinions expressed in the contemporary literature, and, possibly, a basis for cultivating his own thoughts.

I would like to express my sincere appreciation to the many distinguished contributors to this volume. The ready cooperation of these notable investigators and authors was most gratifying and has enabled presentation of truly authoritative as well as representative viewpoints.

Carl E. Silver, M.D.

*English translation by Takashi Kojima, Liveright Publishing Corp, New York, 1970.

2

Spread and Barriers to Spread of Cancer within the Larynx

John A. Kirchner

Whole-organ sections of the intact laryngectomy specimen demonstrate its anatomic structure and the pathways by which cancer has infiltrated it. In specimens removed by partial laryngectomy the intralaryngeal barriers that limit the spread of early cancer can be demonstrated. These consist of fibroelastic membranes, ligaments, and perichondrium. Patterns of invasion into the laryngeal muscles and skeleton are seen in later stages, and pathways of spread can be studied. Sections are made in the frontal, sagittal, or transverse plane, according to the tumor's site of origin, so that its path of invasion can be followed from front to back, side to side, or top to bottom.

PREPARATION OF SECTIONS

Sectioning an entire larynx requires that it be mounted in a material that is sufficiently solid to immobilize it during the cutting process. Celloidin fulfills this purpose, as it does for the temporal bone, and allows the advantage of storing unstained sections for future use if needed.[1] Whole organ sections also allow the display of a complete, wrinkle-free section through the larynx in any of three planes, so that its two sides can be viewed simultaneously in the coronal or transverse planes, or from front to back in the sagittal. Despite these advantages, celloidin embedding has serious disadvantages: it is time-consuming, usually requiring 8 months or more from start to finish; the sections are thick, about 20 μm, making cell detail obscure; and celloidin has become almost prohibitively expensive.

Alternate methods are variations of the conventional paraffin-embedding technique and produce thin sections of 6 to 8 μm with details of cellular structure readily identifiable. Paraffin-embedded specimens yield stained sections within a few days after decalcification. Since it is difficult with paraffin embedding to obtain wrinkle-free sections from a large specimen, the extirpated larynx is usually cut into several segments, each one perpendicular to the surface. Although this precludes viewing both sides of the larynx in the same section, the individual segments contain all necessary information about the tumor's pattern of growth and spread. By extrapolation, one can determine the progress of cancer throughout the entire larynx. The technique is aptly described and illustrated in a report by Glanz.[2]

Both celloidin and paraffin embedding allow the study of numerous histopathologic features. These include the tumor's anatomic location, size, depth of invasion, submucosal spread, and relationship to elastic tissue membranes and tendons, as well as its pathways of spread along nerve trunks, blood vessels, and mucous glands and its extension through the laryngeal framework. The thinner paraffin sections are superior for determination of degree of cellular differentiation, peripheral growth pattern, lymphocytic response, and other evidence of tumor-host reaction.

In addition to the information provided for individual tumors, whole-organ sections may form the basis of a more accurate staging system, as well as a more precise interpretation of preoperative computed tomography or magnetic resonance imaging.

SPREAD OF TUMOR WITHIN THE LARYNX

Intralaryngeal Compartments

The endolaryngeal soft tissues are contained within anatomic spaces bounded, to a large extent, by fibroelastic membranes.[3] These structures tend to limit the spread of early cancer to definite compartments, so that small tumors can often be removed by partial laryngectomy, with adequate margins. Once these fibroelastic barriers have been breached, cancer spreads readily into adjacent compartments, or into adjoining soft tissue or laryngeal framework.

Laryngeal cancer may spread from its original site to other parts of the larynx by direct mucosal and submucosal extension, by lymphatic or vascular permeation, by perineural spread or by direct invasion of adjacent structures.[4]

Glottic Cancer

In situ glottic carcinoma is limited by the basement membrane. Invasive carcinoma of the mobile cord is limited, in its early stage, by a fibroelastic membrane that comprises the conus elasticus and the vocal ligament with its extension along the floor of the ventricle, the thyroglottic ligament.[5] Glottic tumors that involve the entire length of the true cord, with normal mobility, or that cross the anterior commissure to the opposite vocal cord (T_{16}) are confined to the loose tissue overlying the vocal ligament and conus elasticus (Reinke's space).

In crossing the anterior commissure, T_{16} glottic cancer has been the source of much misinformation regarding its potential for deep invasion. Whole-organ studies have shown that such lesions, confined to the level of the glottis, with mobile vocal cords, do not invade the underlying thyroid cartilage. Anterior spread is limited by the dense mass of fibroelastic tissue at the anterior attachment of the true cords representing the confluence of the vocal ligament, the thyroepiglottic ligament, the conus elasticus, and the internal perichondrium of the thyroid ala. This "tendon" is virtually avascular[6] and offers a dense barrier to the spread of early glottic cancer[7,8] (Fig. 2–1, p. 9). Invasion of the thyroid cartilage has been observed only in those anterior glottic neoplasms that extend upward to attack the base of the epiglottis. These will be discussed with "transglottic" lesions.

T_3 glottic cancer, characterized by a fixed vocal cord, usually displays infiltration of the thyroarytenoid muscle in whole-organ sections (Fig. 2–2, p. 9). The thyroarytenoid muscle occupies the paraglottic space, a compartment bounded by the conus elasticus medially, thyroglottic ligament superiorly, and perichondrium of the thyroid ala laterally. Because ordinarily only the most advanced lesions are removed by total laryngectomy, it is difficult to follow, by whole-organ section, the progress of T_3 glottic cancer from incipiency to the fixed-cord condition. Two possible routes of invasion into the paraglottic space seem likely; both have been demonstrated in whole-organ serial sections. One route appears to be from an origin on the superior surface of the true cord, or floor of the ventricle. As this lesion continues its lateral spread, it may "outflank" the lateral edge of the thyroglottic ligament and invade the paraglottic space from above (Fig. 2–3, p. 9). An alternate route is by direct invasion into this compartment through the conus elasticus, a structure that gradually loses its functional integrity with advancing age (Fig. 2–4, p. 9).

As cancer advances within the paraglottic space, its downward spread is controlled to a large degree by the conus elasticus medially and the perichondrium of the thyroid ala laterally. As a result, the tumor sometimes escapes the larynx between the thyroid and the cricoid cartilages through the cricothyroid membrane. This type of spread is nearly always accompanied by invasion of the lower, ossified edge of the thyroid ala and often by invasion of the upper edge of the cricoid (Fig. 2–5, p. xxx). The internal perichondrium of the thyroid cartilage acts as an effective barrier to the early spread of cancer. In glottic carcinoma with more than 1 cm subglottic extension, or in transglottic neoplasms 3 cm or larger, the laryngeal framework is usually invaded.[9] It is not clear whether the perichondrium alone, or perichondrium in combination with the underlying cartilage is the real barrier. Reports from Folkmann's laborabory suggest that cartilage itself can resist invasion by cancer.[10] The fact that ossified parts of the laryngeal skeleton are invaded in preference to the cartilaginous portions supports this conclusion. Perichondrium appears to be a more effective barrier when it overlies unossified parts of the same framework.

Supraglottic Cancer

Although the concept of a barrier between the supraglottic and glottic portions of the larynx has been supported by both laboratory and clinical observations, whole-organ sections have failed to demonstrate an anatomic structure within the fundus of the ventricle that could qualify as a barrier to downward spread of cancer from the ventricular band. Nevertheless, cancer that remains confined to the supraglottic larynx on gross examination is usually found, in whole-organ sections, to have spared the ventricle. This fact allows resection of supraglottic cancer by horizontal partial laryngectomy with an oncologically adequate inferior margin of only a few millimeters. Further support for this concept is provided by the fact that recurrences after horizontal supraglottic laryngectomy are situated almost invariably in the base of the tongue and not at the lower margin of resection. Bocca[11] attributes the integrity of these intralaryngeal compartments to their two independent embryologic sources. The supraglottic larynx develops from the buccopharyngeal anlage, the glottic and subglottic portions from the tracheopulmonary. The two units fuse at the laryngeal ventricle. The physical basis for oncologic independence of these two parts of the larynx, however, remains obscure, despite these observations. The anatomic "compartment" becomes less definite with cancer of the aryepiglottic fold, especially when it spreads toward the pyriform sinus.

Cancer of the infrahyoid portion of the epiglottis tends to spread anteriorly into the preepiglottic space. This compartment is bounded posteriorly by the epiglottic cartilage and thyroepiglottic ligament, anteriorly by the thyrohyoid membrane and hyoid bone, and superiorly by the hyoepiglottic ligament. The anterior extension of epiglottic cancer is initially limited by the epiglottic perichondrium and the thyroepiglottic ligament (Fig. 2–6, p. 10). After breaching the epiglottic perichondrium, cancer may grow through the fenestrations within the epiglottic cartilage and infiltrate the fatty areolar tissue of the preepiglottic space itself.

After invading the preepiglottic space, cancer is confined for a time by a fibroelastic membrane that gives to its advancing margin the appearance of a "pushing edge," almost as though it were encapsulated (Fig. 2–7, p. 10). This feature of supraglottic cancer nearly always results in a tumor-free space between the hyoid bone and the advancing edge of the tumor, thus allowing preservation of the hyoid bone at horizontal supraglottic laryngectomy[12] (Fig. 2–8, p. 10). This technique assures more secure reconstruction of the pharynx and, in the opinion of many surgeons, earlier rehabilitation of deglutition. Only large, far-advanced lesions in the preepiglottic space require removal of the hyoid bone. This latter type of behavior was found in only two of 112 supraglottic lesions in our collection. The need for

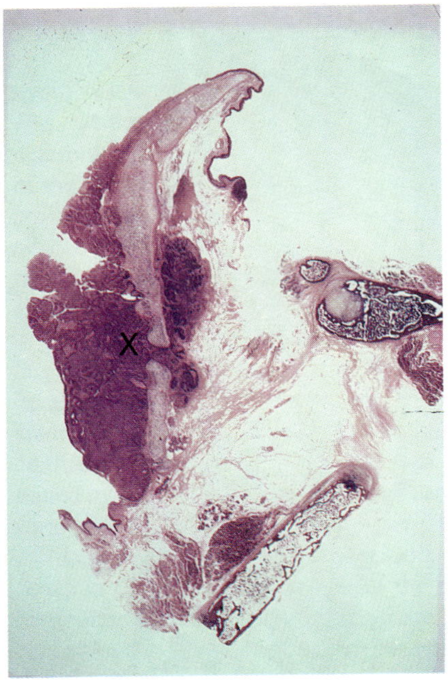

Figure 2–6. The spread of early epiglottic cancer is resisted by the perichondrium, but the tumor may infiltrate the preepiglottic space through a natural fenestra (x). Sagittal section.

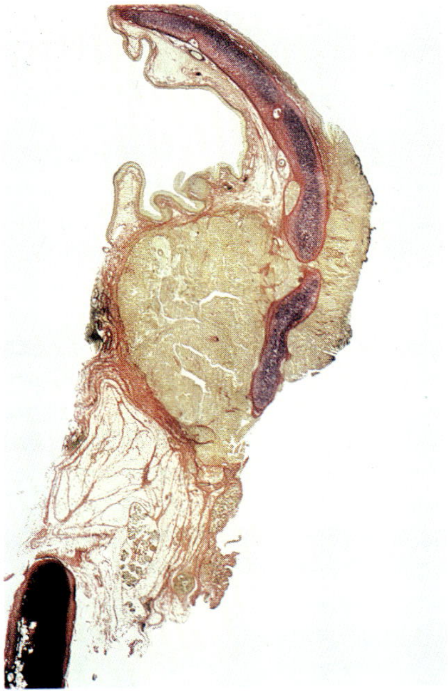

Figure 2–7. A more advanced form of invasion into the preepiglottic space, with the characteristic fibroelastic membrane at its advancing edge. Sagittal section. (Elastic tissue stain.)

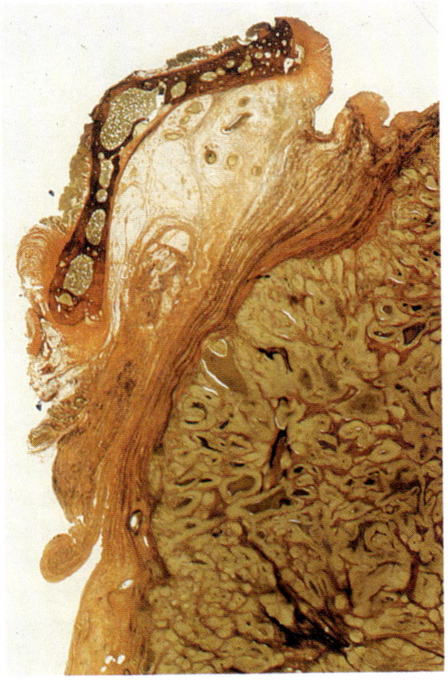

Figure 2–8. Large epiglottic cancer invading the preepiglottic space, showing the usual membrane at its leading edge, and the tumor-free space between it and the hyoid bone. Preservation of the hyoid is oncologically safe in most cases of epiglottic cancer. (Elastic tissue stain.)

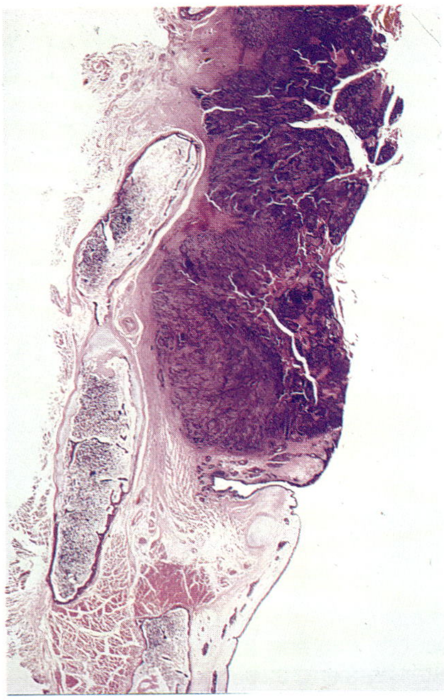

Figure 2–9. Coronal section of a large supraglottic cancer showing the usual tumor-free ventricle and normal vocal cord, despite the size of the lesion. An incipient thyroid foramen and its accompanying blood vessel are seen here as an incidental feature of this specimen.

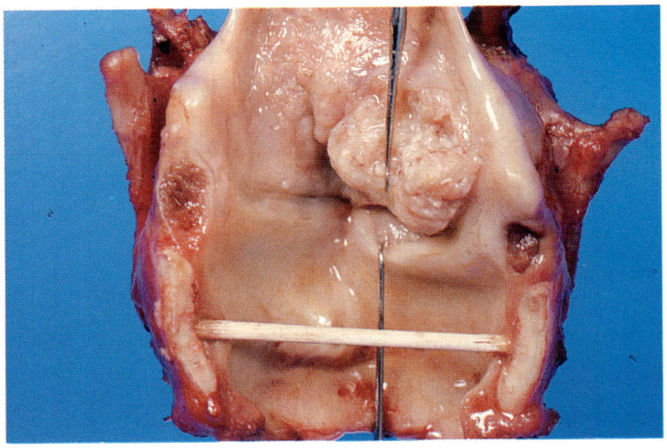

Figure 2–10. Cancer of the ventricular band may hide the true cord, as in this case, suggesting a transglottic rather than supraglottic location.

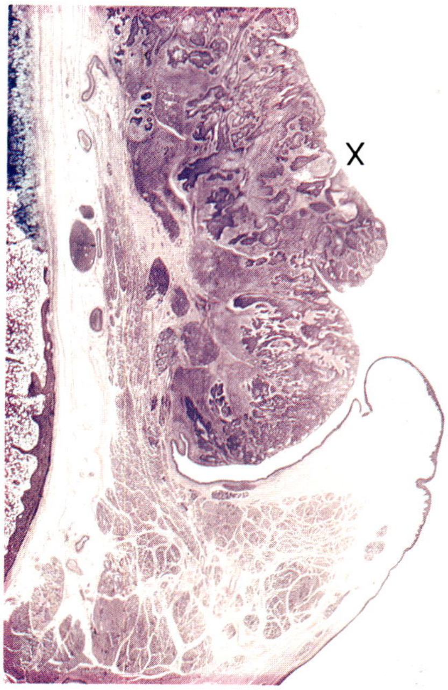

Figure 2–11. Coronal section of the specimen shown in Figure 2–10. The true cord is free of tumor, a fact difficult to ascertain by laryngoscopy or radiography. Large piece of the tumor was removed at (x) for the pathologist's record and originally overhung the true cord and hid it from view.

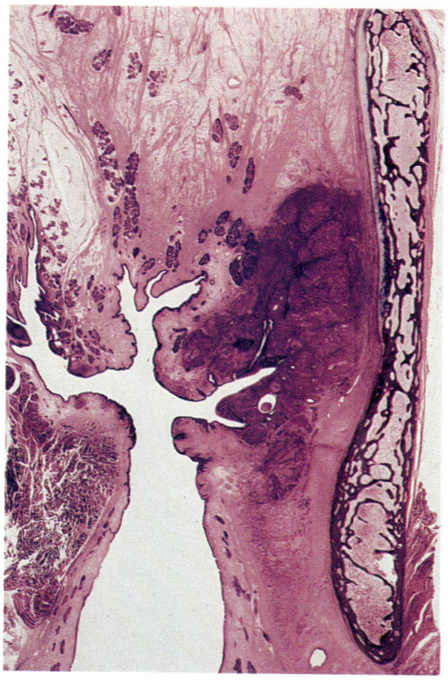

Figure 2–12. Early transglottic cancer originating in the ventricle. The tumor was covered by intact mucosa in this and all other sections in this specimen.

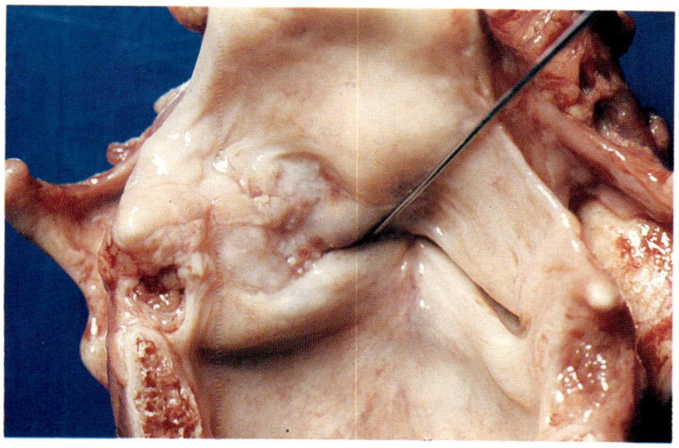

Figure 2–13. Supraglottic cancer extending downward submucosally and invading the substance of the true cord from behind the ventricle. The ventricle itself, shown at the end of the probe, is free of tumor. A sluggish or fixed cord is indicative of this type of spread.

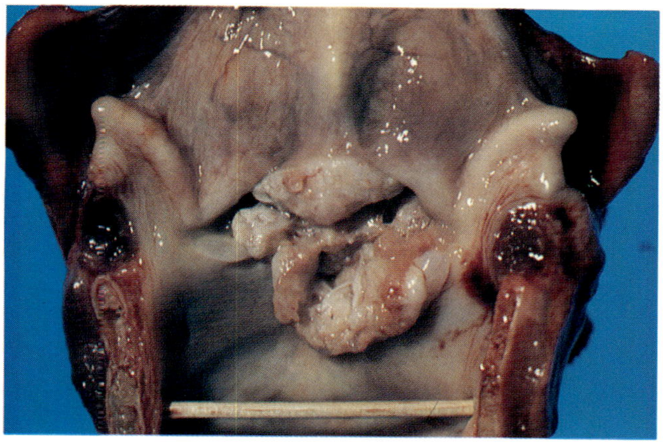

Figure 2–14. Cancer above and below the anterior commissure, as in this specimen, usually invades the adjacent laryngeal framework.

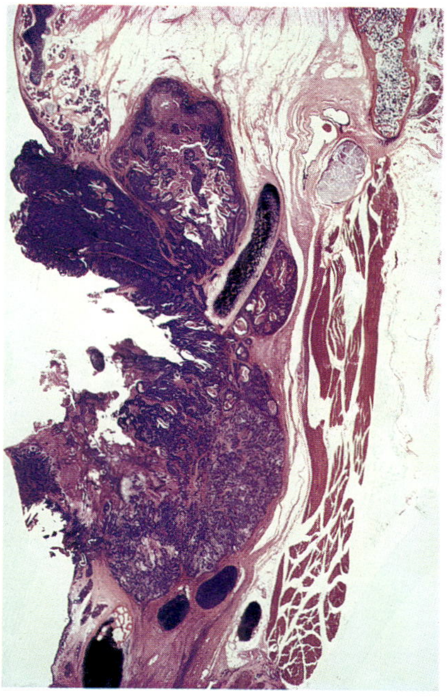

Figure 2–15. Sagittal section of a lesion similar to the one shown in Figure 2–14. Extensive invasion and destruction of thyroid cartilage.

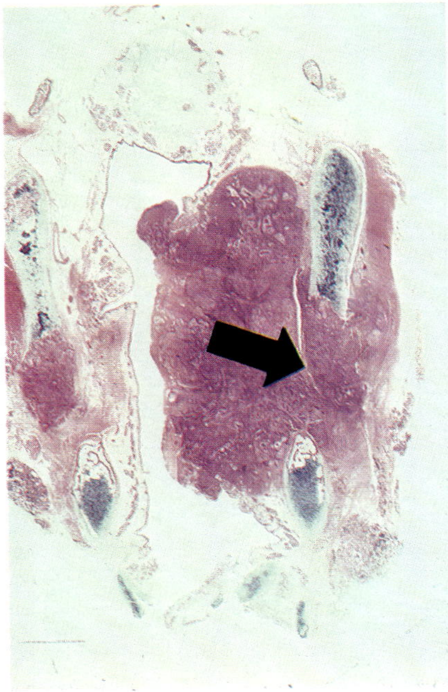

Figure 2–16. Transglottic cancer invading ossified edge of thyroid ala and spreading to the lower edge of the ala on the opposite side of the larynx (arrow), some distance from the visible tumor. This type of spread has been seen only with lesions that have broken through the anterior thyroid cartilage.

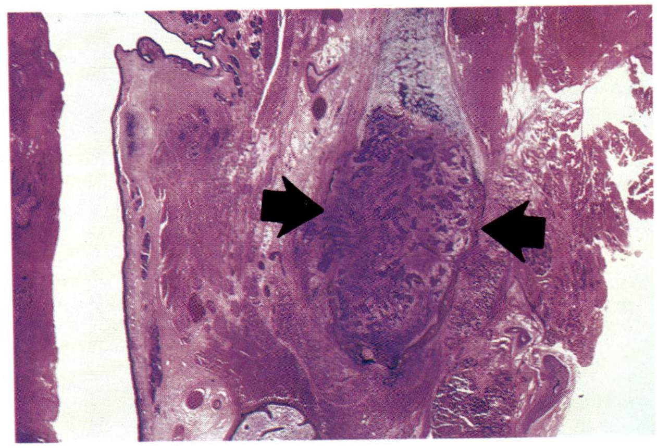

Figure 2–17. Higher power view of the right side of the thyroid ala shown in Figure 2–16. The cancer has spread to this side of the larynx between intact layers of perichondrium (arrows).

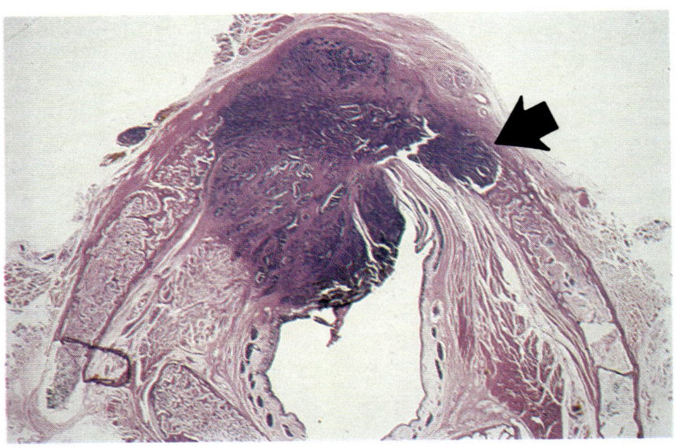

Figure 2–18. Transverse section showing cancer breaking through the anterior laryngeal framework and starting to infiltrate the thyroid ala between the inner and outer layers of perichondrium (arrow).

endolarynx is not present in this or other parts of the hypopharynx. Invasion of the posterior edge of the thyroid ala was found in 38% of our series of 102 pyriform sinus specimens. In each case, there was clinical involvement of the apex and lateral wall of the pyriform sinus.

LYMPHATIC SPREAD OF TUMOR

There are two major groups of laryngeal lymphatic channels: those that drain the areas superior to the fundus of the ventricle and those that drain the areas inferior to it. The supraglottic group leaves the larynx by piercing the thyrohoid membrane along with the superior laryngeal artery and vein. This group drains mainly into the subdigastric and superior jugular group of nodes. The lymphatics draining the glottic and subglottic areas exit through the cricothyroid ligament and drain into the prelaryngeal node, the paratracheal nodes, and the deep cervical nodes along the inferior thyroid artery.

Because of the variations in intercommunication between lymphatic channels, it is impossible to predict the exact location of potential metastases from laryngeal cancer, particularly after radiotherapy or surgery.[13] For example, the practice of sampling the subdigastric node or nodes during surgery for supraglottic cancer to determine the need for radical neck dissection is unreliable in at least 10% of cases.

The lymphatics of the true vocal cord are few and are of small diameter. As a result, T_1 and T_2 glottic cancers rarely produce cervical node metastases (1 to 4% in large series). Metastatic rates of T_3 glottic cancer vary widely, since the current staging system includes tumors varying greatly in size within this category. Thus, a small lesion limited to a fixed cord as well as a fixed cord lesion that crosses the ventricle and involves the epithelial surfaces of both the true and false vocal cords are both classified as "glottic T_3 " The latter "transglottic" lesion, which invades the rich lymphatic bed of the supraglottic larynx, where regional metastases are likely to originate, is more likely to produce lymphatic metastases than the former.

Cervical node metastases have been observed in 48 to 54% of supraglottic cancers reported from other centers. One hundred four (37%) of 282 patients with supraglottic cancer seen at Yale since 1962 had clinically positive nodes on admission. Metastatic nodes appeared subsequently in 30 additional patients, a total incidence of 48%.

In our 91 specimens of transglottic cancer, the incidence of cervical node metastases was directly related to primary tumor size. Metastases were found in 34% of lesions under 4 cm in diameter and 55% of lesions larger than 4 cm. The actual incidence of late postoperative metastases in both groups is probably higher than stated here because many of the patients, in recent years, were not under my follow-up control.

Cancer originating in the subglottis (within the cricoid ring) is rare. Cancer from this area metastasizes to the paratracheal nodes where it may be undetectable by palpation.

CONCLUSIONS

Whole-organ sections of laryngectomy specimens have demonstrated the fibroelastic membranes that form the boundaries of intralaryngeal compartments within which cancer is confined in its early stages. These studies have substantiated the conclusions of previous workers who observed the spread of fluids, dyes, and radioisotopes to be limited to the individual compartments into which these materials had been injected, and that these materials spread diffusely when injected into the ventricle. Observation by whole organ serial section of growth of cancer within a compartment, its extension from one compartment to the one adjoining it, and its pattern of dissemination from within the ventricle correspond closely to these earlier observations.

ACKNOWLEDGMENT

This work was supported by a grant from the National Cancer Institute (2R01-CA22101-10).

REFERENCES

1. Tucker GF, Smith HR. A histological demonstration of the development of laryngeal connective tissue compartments. Trans Am Acad Ophthalmal Otolaryngol 1962;66:308–18.
2. Glanz H. Growth, p-classification and grading of squamous cell carcinoma of the vocal cords. Adv Otorhinolaryngol 1984;32:1–123.
3. Pressman JJ, Simon MB, Monell CM. Anatomic studies related to the dissemination of cancer of the larynx. Cancer 1961;14:1131–1138.
4. Batsakis JG. Neoplasms of the larynx. In: Batsakis JG, ed. *Tumors of the head and neck,* 2nd ed. Baltimore: Williams & Wilkins, 1979:200–25.
5. Kirchner JA. Growth and spread of laryngeal cancer as related to partial laryngectomy. Laryngoscope 1975;85:1516–21.
6. Andrea M. Vasculature of the anterior commissure. Ann Otol Rhinol Laryngol 1981;90(Pt. 1):18–20.
7. Bagatella F, Bignardi L. Behavior of cancer at the anterior commissure of the larynx. Laryngoscope 1983;93:353–6.
8. Kirchner JA, Fischer J. Anterior commissure cancer—a clinical and laboratory study of 39 cases. Can J Otolaryngol 1975;4:637–43.
9. Kirchner JA, Cornog JL, Holmes RE. Transglottic cancer. Arch Otolaryngol 1974;99:247–51.
10. Langer R, Brem H, Falterman K, et al. Isolation of a cartilage factor that inhibits tumor neovascularization. Science 1976;201:70–1.
11. Bocca E. Supraglottic cancer. Laryngoscope 1975;85:1318–1326.
12. Kirchner JA, Carter D. Intralaryngeal barriers to the spread of cancer. Acta Otolaryngol (Stockh) 1987;103:503–13.
13. Johner CM. The lymphatics of the larynx. Otolaryngol Clin North Am 1970;3:349–450.

3

Framework Invasion in Laryngeal Carcinoma

Reinhold Theophilus Gregor

BACKGROUND AND PREVIOUS INVESTIGATIONS

It is well known that ossified cartilage is much more susceptible to cancer invasion than nonossified cartilage.[1–8] The reason for this has not yet been fully explained, but it has been suggested that cartilage releases a substance or substances that inhibit tumor or inhibit tumor substances that enhance invasion.[6]

Olszewski[5] has related the invasion of ossified cartilage to vascularization. Twenty larynges were studied by silicone rubber blood vessel injection. There was evidence that invasion of a neoplasm develops in accordance with the penetration of vessels into the focus of ossification. This evidence, in addition to the discovery of a tumor angiogenic factor,[9] suggests that there may be a relationship between the ossification of cartilage, the production of tumor hormones, and the invasiveness of laryngeal tumors.

Ossification of Cartilage

The ossification of laryngeal cartilages has been studied by Kirchner,[6] Keen and Wainwright,[10] and Harrison and Denny.[11] Although the correlation with age is poor, ossification usually occurs in the third decade of life and not before the age of 21 years. The changes are similar to ordinary endochondral ossification and are preceded by calcification of the cartilage. Although Harrison and Denny discovered no substantial difference in ossification between sexes, Keen and Wainwright found that ossification proceeds at a slower rate in females.

Ossification of the thyroid cartilage invariably begins at the posterior border near the root of the inferior cornu, spreads along the inferior border, and reaches the midline, where there is usually a separate center of ossification. It then extends upward along the posterior border toward the superior cornu, which was ossified in only 20% of Harrison and Denny's specimens. The process continues upward in the thyroid lamina, eventually involving the superior border and usually leaving two unossified islands in each lamina. These islands may produce a radiographic appearance suggestive of cartilage erosion and thus falsely indicate tumor invasion.

Cricoid ossification occurs about the same time as the thyroid and begins at the upper border of the posterior lamina, immediately anterior to each cricoarytenoid joint. From these two points, ossification spreads into the lamina and forward into the arch, the anterior extent of which is usually the last to ossify. Ossification of the arytenoids starts in the muscular processes and spreads forward, but rarely reaches the apex or vocal process. The pattern of ossification in the larynx has been thought to correspond to the insertion of the main intrinsic and extrinsic laryngeal muscles,[12,13] possibly due to increased tension at these sites. Harrison and Denny, having studied various mammalian larynges, believed that this was a tenable explanation for the progression of bony changes.

Pattern of Invasion

The pattern of framework invasion has been studied by Kirchner[6] in 185 larynges. Invasion of the laryngeal framework occurred almost invariably in the lower third of the thyroid cartilage and the upper edge of the cricoid ring in the early stages. The perichondrium appeared to resist tumor invasion. When cancer infiltrated one point and expanded the cartilage, most of the perichondrium remained intact. This phenomenon has been reported by other authors as well.[4,12,13]

Transglottic lesions produced the highest incidence of framework invasion.[1–4] Harrison[7] found no instance of transglottic tumor penetrating external perichondrium in the absence of tumor escape via the lateral cricothyroid space or membrane. None of the pure supraglottic tumors in Kirchner's series showed cartilage invasion.

An explanation for the occurrence of tumor invasion at sites of cartilage ossification has been advanced by Yeager and Archer[12,13] and confirmed the observation of Kirchner and Harrison regarding the sites of cartilage invasion and their identity with areas of ossification, as well as the fact that these are the points of attachment of laryngeal musculature and consequently under the most stress. Yeager and Archer noted that these are also areas that are deficient in perichondrium, because of the attachment of fibrous collagen bundles (Sharpey's fibers). Perichondrium has been shown to present a barrier to cancer, but in the following areas the perichondrium is deficient:

1. The area of the anterior commissure tendon (ligament).
2. The junction of the anterior one fourth and posterior three fourths of the lower thyroid lamina.
3. The medial aspect of the posterior border of the thyroid lamina.
4. The cricoarytenoid joint.
5. The areas of attachment of the cricothyroid and cricotracheal membranes.

Cancer cells have been seen to separate the collagen bundles (which pass through the perichondrium) finding a linear passage to the cartilage. This feature was pointed out by Broyles[14] in 1943 in his study of the anterior commissure tendon. Archer et al[13] believe that the observation of cancer invading ossified cartilage is related to their findings regarding the collagen bundles. They believe that the ossification is related to the attachment of fibers and muscles and lines of stress and that the correlation between tumor invasion and ossification is incidental.

Clinical Significance

The fact that cartilage invasion per se, without invasion of extralaryngeal structures, influences the survival of the patient has been reported by Kirchner[6] but disputed by Harrison.[7] Kirchner found that invasion of the framework reduced the 3-year survival rate for glottic carcinomas from 72 to 38%. A similar effect was observed by Pittam and Carter.[15] Harrison[7] and Ogura[16] attributed this to the high rate of lymph node metastases associated with cartilage invasion, although this finding was not confirmed by McGavran et al[17] in their well-known study correlating certain features of laryngeal cancer with lymph node metastases. Framework invasion, in any case, must be considered an important prognostic finding even though its correlation with morbidity may be a result of an increase in the incidence of lymph node metastases.

Histologic Features of Framework Invasion

This area has been extensively studied by Carter and his group in London.[8,15,18–20] Carter and Tanner,[8] in agreement with other authors,[13] found no histologic pattern that appeared to predispose to framework invasion. Pittam and Carter[15] found that the ossified areas of the laryngeal cartilages were histologically identical to organized bone, containing trabeculae lined with osteoblasts and hemopoietic marrow. Osteoclasts were inconspicuous. In specimens with framework invasion, the invasive process was concentrated in regions of metaplastic ossification. Direct invasion of unchanged cartilage was unusual and was always overshadowed by deeper infiltration into nearby foci of ossification.

The morphologic changes associated with the carcinomatous invasion into metaplastic bone were consistent in all cases studied. Most common was an increase in osteoclasts that accumulated near the edge of spreading tumor cells. The bone was found to be progressively destroyed by characteristic "scalloping" defects produced by the osteoclastic activity. Direct mingling of tumor cells and osteoclasts on the bone surface was rarely seen. Osteoclastic, the predominant type of cell in uninvaded bone, were always outnumbered in the invaded regions. In some cases with extensive destruction of the laryngeal framework, the osteoclastic activity appeared to wane and direct contact between the receding bone and tumor cells occurred. The authors did not think that radiotherapy or infection were responsible for these changes.[8]

In a study of bone invasion in other tumors of the head and neck, Carter et al[18] found similar changes. In some cases, however, there was a combination of osteoclastic and osteoblastic activity in advance of the invading carcinoma. Although the osteoclasts outnumbered the osteoblasts, they usually evoked a measure of osteoid and new bone formation.

Biochemical Factors

The findings given herein indicate that bone invasion is a complex process. Most of the bone destruction is achieved by host cells, which are apparently stimulated by the presence of the tumor. In another study, Bennett et al[20] have demonstrated a prostaglandin-like substance that is produced by carcinomas of the head and neck. Although the cellular origin of these prostaglandins, and other tumor-associated osteoclast-activating products, is unclear, it is thought by these authors that host cells such as macrophages may play a part in their production. The mechanisms responsible for osteoblastic stimulation, apparently linked to the increased osteoclastic activity, are obscure.[18]

Similar mechanisms have been described in skeletal metastases. Galasko[21] has shown in autopsy specimens and in animal experiments that bone is resorbed by osteoclasts and the tumor secretes a diffusable osteoclast activating factor. In many cases an associated osteoblastic reaction and new bone production was taking place independently. There was usually a fibrous reactive stroma in the space between the osteoclasts and the tumor mass. The osteoclasts disappeared when the tumor had grown sufficiently large to envelope residual trabeculae of bone, but bone destruction continued. There appeared to be two mechanisms; one in which a humoral substance was involved and another in which the tumor cells seemed to mediate late bone destruction by a mechanism not involving osteoclasts.

Galasko and Bennett[22] showed that prostaglandin E_2 could be extracted from tumors with bone invasion and could be abolished by treating the experimental animals with indomethacin. In the indomethacin-treated animals bone destruction and osteoclastic activity was markedly diminished.

In previous studies Galasko[23] found skeletal metastases to be associated with new bone formation and destruction that occur simultaneously. The new bone formation and destruction have some relationship, as for example in a fracture. Once destruction has become grossly evident, and malignant cells surround the residual bone, no new bone is formed.

Orr et al[24] determined that during the process of resorption bone releases a factor strongly chemotactic for tumor cells. This factor is released by a variety of agents that induce resorption of bone.

Abramson et al[25] measured collagenase activity in various head and neck carcinomas. These authors cultured cells from biopsies from 14 patients with head and neck malignancies, including eight laryngeal cancers. Oral cavity tumors showed greater activity than did the laryngeal carcinomas, although both sites were more active than uninvolved mucosa from the same patients. At 18 months after diagnosis, four of the six patients with greatest collagenase activity were dead of cancer and one patient was alive with persistent cancer. The authors concluded that high collagenase activity may be a factor in the clinical aggressiveness of epidermoid carcinomas of the head and neck.

The explanation for the fact that cartilage appears resistant to tumor invasion may be related to discovery of the inhibition of tumor angiogenesis mediated by cartilage. Brem and Folkman[26] have shown that cartilage inhibits capillary proliferation induced by tumor. With rabbit cornea employed as an assay medium, neonatal scapular cartilage was found to inhibit capillary proliferation induced by tumor. Inactivation of the cartilage by heat abolished this effect. These results suggest existence of a diffusable material produced by normal cartilage which inhibits capillary proliferation by tumor.

Summary

Framework invasion would appear to depend on many factors in addition to blood supply. Tumors have been found to produce prostaglandin-like substances that activate osteoclasts to erode bone. Cartilage has been found to inhibit tumor angiogenesis. It appears likely that there is a combination of osteoblastic and osteoclastic activity taking place when bone invasion occurs. This may account for some of the computed tomography (CT) appearances that have been found in cancer of the larynx. The agents responsible for an increase in osteoblastic activity are, however, still obscure.

EVALUATION OF THE LARYNGEAL FRAMEWORK BY COMPUTED TOMOGRAPHY

Conventional Radiography

The pattern of the laryngeal cartilage ossification in the living patient has been studied using conventional radiography.[27] Basically, the patterns were the same as those found by Keen and Wainwright[10] and Harrison and Denny[11] (see before) who performed examinations on laryngeal specimens.

Hately et al[27] confirmed the observations that calcification and subsequent ossification occur symmetrically on right and left sides, that ossification of the thyroid cartilage progressed more slowly in females and that the anterior portions of the thyroid laminae and midline area remain cartilagenous to a more advanced age. Radiologic observations of the cricoid also coincided with the earlier specimen studies, revealing ossification beginning at the superior border of the lamina (in front of the cricoarytenoid joint) and spreading forward and downward, the anterior extent of the arch being the last to ossify. The arytenoid cartilages start to calcify and ossify in the muscular processes, then into the base, with spread upward into the body. The ossification never reaches the apex or the vocal process. The only disparity was in Hately's finding that ossification of the arytenoid occurred more often in females, whereas Keen and Wainwright[10] had reported the opposite.

Computed Tomography

CT has allowed a much better assessment of the laryngeal framework, whether or not the cartilage had ossified, although cartilaginous areas, particularly in the thyroid cartilage, may mimic tumor invasion. Several studies have concentrated on the assessment of the laryngeal cartilages.[13,28–36]

An investigation by our group[37] produced the striking and previously unreported revelation that an increase in density of the arytenoid and cricoid on CT had a high correlation with early tumor invasion in the larynges (Fig. 3–1). At first, this feature

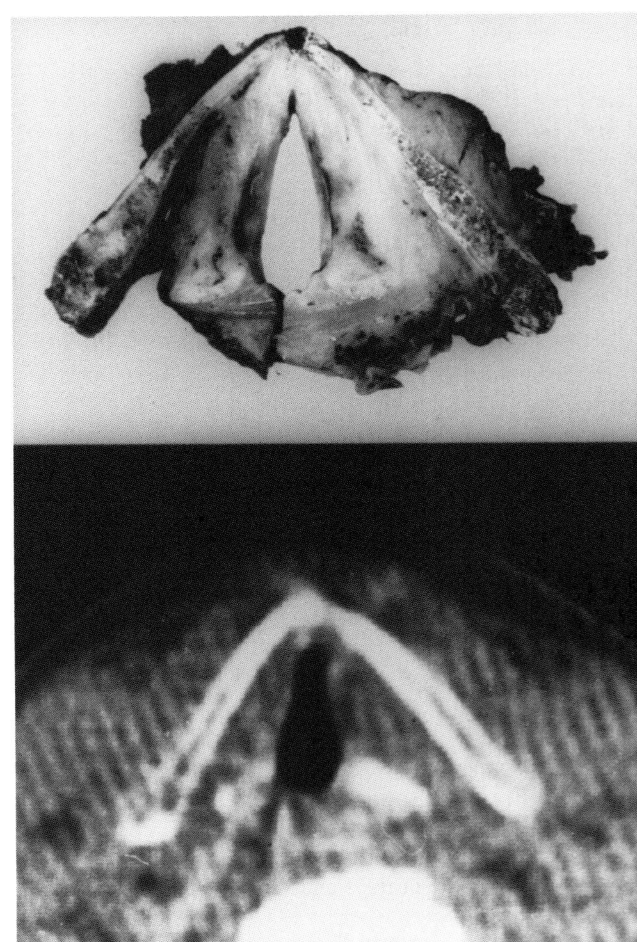

A

B

Figure 3–1. **A:** A macroslice taken from a larynx with tumor in the right paraglottic space. The tumor was invading the right arytenoid. **B:** Preoperative computed tomography showing an equivalent slice level. The right arytenoid appears more dense than the left (scan reversed to conform with tissue section).

was thought to be artefactual, but examination of histologic slides and radiographs of the tissue slices confirmed increased density of the bone, which in most cases was associated with early invasion, or very close microscopic proximity, of cancer. Archer and Yeager[28] had previously demonstrated the same feature, but they made no comment on this phenomenon. Two figures in their article show the previously described appearance affecting the right arytenoid in one of their patients.

Lloyd et al[31] in follow-up on our original observation studied eight patients who showed invasion of cartilage on subsequent histologic examination. Review of CT in these cases led to retrospective diagnosis of 11 of 14 sites of cartilage invasion. Four of these showed erosion of cartilage, and five showed osteosclerosis. The arytenoid was most often affected by the characteristic changes and in five cases showed strong, moderate, or minor degrees of increased density on the side affected by tumor in comparison to its fellow on the normal side. Since most of these patients had undergone previous radiotherapy, the authors concluded that the changes of increased bone formation were related to previous radiation and perichondritis.

Although there has been general disappointment with the ability of CT to demonstrate early framework invasion, several features exhibited by CT scans have clarified our understanding of the invasion of cartilage, both ossified and unossified. The work of Archer and Yeager[12,13] has been valuable in the identification of the sites most commonly invaded, and the histologic correlation of these areas with the attachment of collagen bundles through the perichondrium. The position of the tumor and the level of its maximum dimension related to the arytenoid has reflected the findings of many large pathologic studies showing that it is the transglottic, subglottic, and advanced glottic tumors that show most of the cartilage invasion.

INVESTIGATION OF HISTOLOGIC AND BIOCHEMICAL FEATURES OF FRAMEWORK INVASION

We have employed serial sections to study 154 larynges for framework invasion and other features of tumor spread.[38–40]

Materials and Methods

The majority of the laryngeal specimens were collected from the operating rooms and fixed in 10% buffered formol saline for at least 48 hours. Following decalcification, the larynges were sliced and photographed. Where tissue was required for biochemical assay, the larynges were collected fresh from the patient and immediately deep frozen. The frozen larynges were then sliced in the same manner. Tissue blocks taken from these slices were processed in the standard way.[38] Specimens were taken for biochemical assay of alkaline phosphatase (ALP) from the frozen specimens.[39]

Tetracycline was given preoperatively to two patients in the following manner: Three hundred milligrams of demeclocycline was given twice a day for 2 days, followed by a 12-day drug-free period, after which 300 mg was administered twice daily for 4 days. The larynges of these patients were treated as just described. After sectioning the larynges (without decalcification), sections were prepared and examined in ultraviolet light.[39]

The calcification rate (CR) was measured by obtaining an average distance between the labeled lamellae. Bone formation rate (BFR) could thus be measured by the formula BFR = CR × fraction labeled trabeculae. All histologic sections were carefully examined for invasion of the laryngeal cartilages.

Results

FREQUENCY AND PATTERN OF CARTILAGE INVASION

Most larynges showed at least early calcification or ossification of the cartilages, hence the reference to "framework" invasion. Normal unmodified cartilage was almost never invaded. There was almost equal distribution between larynges showing framework invasion and those that did not; 76 (49.4%) showed no invasion and 78 (50.6%) had some degree of invasion. The pattern of invasion is shown by Figures 3–2 and 3–3. As can be seen, the thyroid cartilage was the most frequently invaded by tumor. Invasion of thyroid cartilage occurred in 37.7% of the 154 cases. Thyroid was also the most frequent site of single cartilage invasion, usually in the midline, either superiorly or inferiorly. In 10.4% of specimens, the thyroid was involved in combination with the arytenoid or cricoid. In these instances the posterior inferior thyroid lamina was invaded by tumor in the posterior cricothyroid space with tumor from the paraglottic space.

There is no demonstrable correlation between invasion of the laryngeal framework and neck node status. Forty-nine percent of patients with framework invasion, however, had spread of tumor through the cartilage and into prelaryngeal strap muscles. Seventy-five percent of transglottic lesions had framework invasion, a number that exceeded the incidence of invasion from tumors at all other sites. There was no correlation in this series,

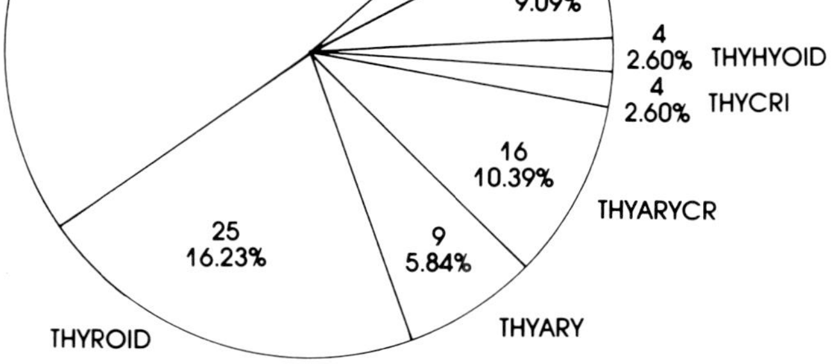

Figure 3–2. Frequency of cartilage invasion: ARY: arytenoid alone; ARYCRI: arytenoid and cricoid; THYARY: thyroid and arytenoid; THYARYCR: thyroid, arytenoid and cricoid; THYCRI: thyroid and cricoid; and THYHYOID: thyroid and hyoid.

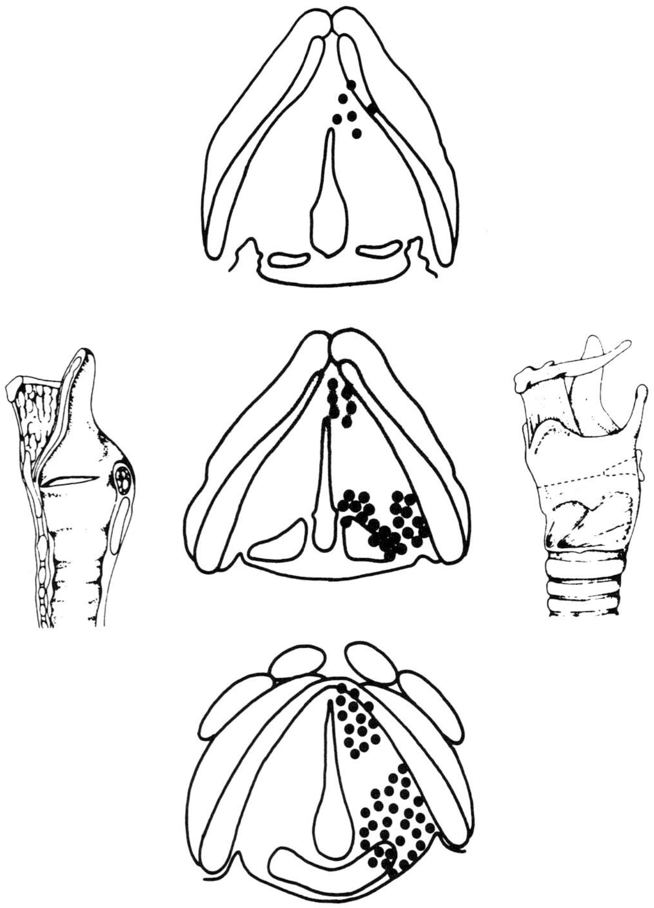

Figure 3–3. Tumors that produce framework invasion. Each dot represents the center of a tumor that produced framework invasion. In some cases, invasion was produced in more than one cartilage.

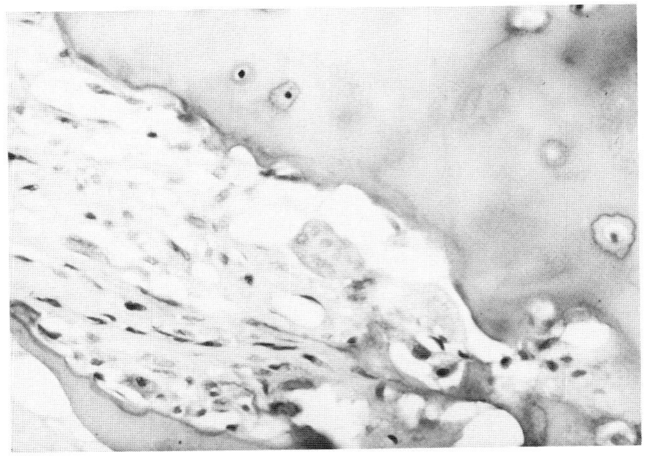

Figure 3–4. This photomicrograph shows a multinucleated osteoclast in the center of the field. Above this area, there is scalloping of the laryngeal framework, which is being eroded.

however, between framework invasion and survival or local control of disease.

HISTOLOGIC FEATURES

Framework invasion varied from massive through and through involvement to microinvasion. The mechanism of invasion was easier to appreciate in the cases with early invasion as opposed to those with massive destruction. The destructive process almost invariably involved the ossified portions of the laryngeal cartilage.

Focal ossification occurred extensively in the specimens studied. The areas involved generally conformed to the pattern described by Harrison and Denny[11] and Keen and Wainwright.[10] In these areas the normal bone structure was reproduced with striking accuracy; with bone trabeculae enclosing spaces containing fatty and hemopoietic marrow. These spaces usually did not show much activity, but in the presence of tumor nearby an intense stromal reaction was seen with numerous osteoblasts, osteoclasts, mixed inflammatory cells, and collagen bundles. This effect was often seen even before the tumor had penetrated the perichondrium. These findings have confirmed the findings of Carter and Tanner,[8] who reported osteoclastic activity eroding bone trabeculae well in advance of the edge of the tumor (Fig. 3–4).

In those larynges in which relatively little bony metaplasia had occurred, a process of microinvasion was seen that appeared to explain the mechanism of invasion. In Figure 3–5 the tumor is some distance away, separated by periosteum from the cartilage that is being eroded. A very reactive stroma has developed within the spaces in the cartilage and osteoblasts are actively laying down bony trabeculae. In other areas, osteoclasts are resorbing newly formed trabeculae. As the process continued, eventually only fragments of bone were left, surrounded by the reactive zone of tissue; later, the tumor penetrated the perichondrium. These appearances suggest that the mechanism of cartilage invasion involves an osteoblastic phase, followed by an

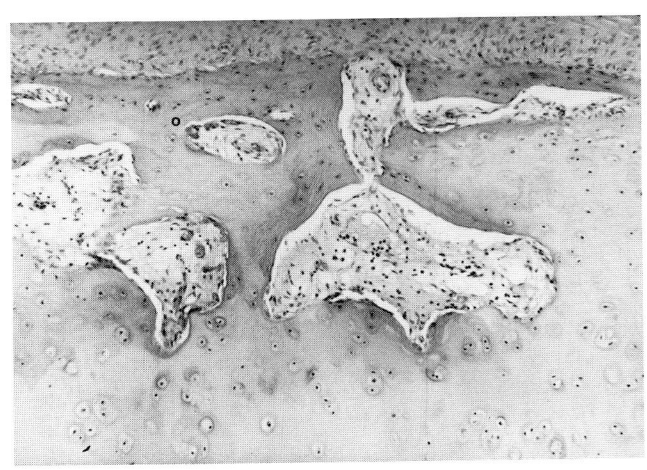

Figure 3–5. Microinvasion of the laryngeal framework. The carcinoma is outside the perichondrium and not shown in this field. In this area an ingrowth of stroma into the laryngeal framework is seen. Most of the framework is still cartilaginous, but in the area surrounding the stromal ingrowth trabeculae of bone are being formed. In other areas, marked O, multinucleate osteoclasts are eroding away the newly laid-down bony trabeculae.

osteoclastic phase. That is, cartilage is first changed to bone, which is then eroded by osteoclastic activity by the "host," presumably due to some tumor humoral factors, which eventually allows the invasion by tumor cells.

Another mechanism of cancer invasion that was more direct was also noted. Tumor cells were seen to find a route to the anterior thyroid cartilage via the collagen bundles in the conus elasticus (vocal ligament) and thus reach the area of the framework where there was no perichondrium (the anterior commissure tendon area). This confirmed the work of Yeager and Archer.[12]

BIOCHEMICAL INVESTIGATION

In all specimens examined the concentration of ALP was highest in the tumor tissue, intermediate in the control tissue, and lowest in the extrinsic muscle. Differences between the tumor and control tissue levels were statistically significant ($p = 0.005$). From these results, it would appear that some tumors may produce ALP that diffuses into the normal adjacent tissue. There appears to be a correlation between the ALP levels and the degree of framework invasion in these cases.

TETRACYCLINE LABELING

Tetracycline labeling was carried out in two patients to show activity of ossification in the framework of their larynges. Both larynges showed extensive tetracycline fluorescence, with double lines in keeping with the interval during which no tetracycline was given. The bone formation rate was estimated for one specimen and confirmed that the arytenoid on the tumor-invaded side had markedly increased osteoblastic activity. The tetracycline-labeled trabeculae showed "scalloping" due to the osteoclastic action (Fig. 3–6).

SUMMARY OF RESULTS

About half of the specimens demonstrated invasion of the laryngeal framework. The commonest area to be involved was the glottic level; the thyroid cartilage being the usual structure invaded, usually at the lower or upper midline portion at its angle. The arytenoid-cricoid complex was the next most common site, with involvement of the posterior inferior lamina of the thyroid related to this area. This pattern basically confirms the findings of previous authors.[6,7,12,13] Strap muscle was invaded in nearly half of the cases with framework invasion (48.7%). These findings differ from Harrison's,[7] which suggest that framework invasion in itself is not sufficient grounds for the T_4 grading. The exception to this is where only the arytenoid was involved.

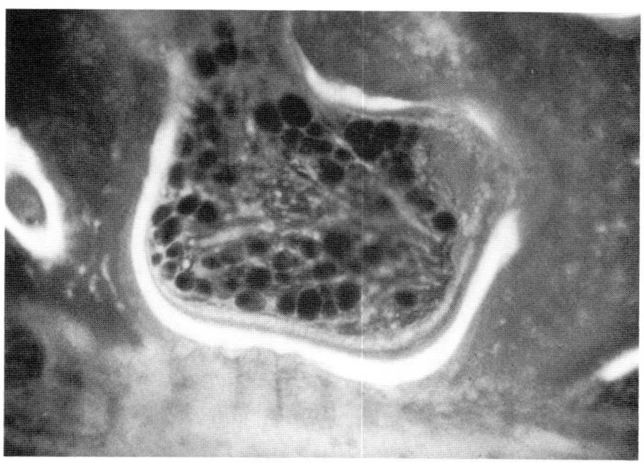

Figure 3–6. Bony trabeculae labeled with tetracycline under ultraviolet light. In the lower portion, scalloping of the newly deposited lamellae is seen.

Discussion

Our studies have confirmed the previously discussed observation that cartilage that has not undergone calcification or metaplastic bone formation is almost never invaded, and confirmed the conclusions of Carter et al[8,18] and McGavran et al[17] that early metaplastic bone invasion starts with the tumor separated from the framework by an intact perichondrium, and of Bennett et al[20] that tumors produce a prostaglandin-like material that stimulates osteoclastic activity. The presence of osteoblastic activity has been shown to be an early feature of framework invasion, particularly where metaplastic bone was not already present. Histologic evidence has been presented that shows early osteoblastic activity associated with osteoclastic activity in the framework invasion process. Biochemical assay has shown that the tumors appear to produce ALP. The activity of ALP was found to be higher in tumor tissue than in corresponding control tissues and was lowest outside the larynx, unless the outer tissues were invaded. Electrophoretic studies showed no apparent difference between ALP in normal and cancerous tissue; the mobility of the major band of activity appeared to correspond to that of the bone form of ALP. ALP activity seems to be associated with active deposition of bone and the enzyme may act by hydrolyzing pyrophosphate, which is an inhibitor of bone mineralization.[41] There is a possibility that two enzymes with pyrophosphatase activity may exist, one identical to ALP and one a separate protein. It has been suggested that ALP may play a central role in controlling DNA synthesis.[41] The enzyme is capable of dephosphorylating thymidylate, which may impair DNA synthesis.

Tumor forms of serum ALP have been found in bronchogenic carcinoma.[42] This isoenzyme is similar to the placental form of ALP, but quite different from the hepatic form; and has been found in breast, genitourinary, and gynecologic cancers.[41] Another isoenzyme has been found in hepatoma.[41] We found no previous report of an osseous type of ALP produced by squamous carcinomas of the larynx.

Further evidence of intense osteoblastic activity was shown by tetracycline labeling in two cases with framework invasion. The presence of active osteoblastic activity coupled with osteoclastic activity and scalloping of the recently laid down lamellae was shown. Estimations of the BFR showed increase in the arytenoid involved with tumor compared with the arytenoid on the opposite (uninvolved) side.

The evidence suggests that as part of the mechanism of framework invasion, tumors produce various substances that stimulate "host" cells to alter the framework in such a way that erosion of the bony lamellae by osteoclastic activity is a preliminary step to penetration of the framework. An important step of this process appears to be one of intense osteoblastic activity, in which ALP, presumably produced by the tumor, may play a part. This process may explain the often observed fact that unossified cartilage is not invaded: the cartilage appears to be first mineralized or ossified under stimulation by humoral factors, some of which may be produced by the tumor, and is then eroded mainly by means of osteoclastic activity mediated by a prostaglandin-like substance. This theory may explain the observation of increased ossification, seen on CT, in the framework closely related to laryngeal tumors. This may be a marker of early tumor invasion, or of aggressiveness of a laryngeal carcinoma.

CONCLUSIONS

Framework invasion occurs mainly at the glottic level and exclusively involves calcified or ossified cartilage. This type of spread is highest in transglottic tumors and is associated with a high degree of penetration through to strap muscles, justifying the T_4 classification. Framework invasion is associated with osteoblastic activity, seen histologically, and measured by tetracycline labeling in two cases. In ten patients studied, the tumor appeared to produce ALP of an osseous type; the levels of ALP were lower in control tissue from the larynx, and lowest outside the larynx, except where tumor had spread through to the extralaryngeal tissues. Osteoclastic activity with characteristic "scalloping" of the bone trabeculae occurred simultaneously with the above features, while tumor remained outside the perichondrium. Penetration of the perichondrium occurred as a late feature.

The results suggest the presence of a mechanism for invasion of the laryngeal framework, which involves an osteoblastic phase and which is probably under at least the partial control of tumor-produced ALP, followed by an osteoclastic phase. The presence of a localized increase in density of the framework, particularly the arytenoids, in close apposition to tumor is usually associated with early invasion of these structures by tumor. The mechanism appears to involve the production of ALP by the laryngeal tumor, resulting in active bone deposition. This feature may be a marker of tumor aggressiveness, and, since the osteoclastic phase is mediated by prostaglandin, this tendency could be delayed by the use of prostaglandin E_2 antagonists, such as indomethacin. This drug may therefore have a therapeutic indication in laryngeal cancer.

REFERENCES

1. Olofsson J, van Nostrand AWP. Growth and spread of laryngeal and hypopharyngeal carcinoma with reflections on the effect of preoperative irradiation. Acta Otolaryngol Suppl (Stockh) 1973;308:1.
2. Kirchner JA. One hundred laryngeal cancers studied by serial section. Ann Otol 1969;78:689–709.
3. Kirchner JA. Two hundred laryngeal cancers: Patterns of growth and spread as seen in serial section. Laryngoscope 1977;87:474–82.
4. Micheau C, Luboinski B, Sancho H, Cachin Y. Modes of invasion of cancer of the larynx. Cancer 1976;38:346–60.
5. Olszewski E. Vascularisation of ossified cartilage and the spread of cancer in the larynx. Arch Otolaryngol 1976;102:200–3.
6. Kirchner JA. Invasion of the framework by laryngeal cancer. Acta Otolaryngol (Stockh) 1984;97:392–7.
7. Harrison DFN. Significance and means by which laryngeal cancer invades thyroid cartilage. Ann Otol Rhinol Laryngol 1984;93:293–6.
8. Carter RL, Tanner SB. Local invasion by laryngeal carcinoma—the importance of focal (metaplastic) ossification within laryngeal cartilage. Clin Otolaryngol 1979;4:283–90.
9. Folkman J, Merler E, Abernathy C, et al. Isolation of a tumor factor responsible for angiogenesis. J Exp Med 1971;133:275–88.
10. Keen JA, Wainwright J. Ossification of the thyroid, cricoid and arytenoid cartilages. S Afr J Lab Clin Med 1958;4:83.
11. Harrison DFN, Denny S. Ossification within the primate larynx. Acta Otolaryngol (Stockh) 1983;95:440–6.
12. Yeager VL, Archer CR. Anatomical routes for cancer invasion of laryngeal cartilage. Laryngoscope 1982;92:449–52.
13. Archer CR, Yeager V, Herbold DR. Computed tomography vs. histology of laryngeal cancer: Their value in predicting laryngeal cartilage invasion. Laryngoscope 1983;93:140–7.
14. Broyles EN. The anterior commissure tendon. Ann Otol 1943;52: 342–5.
15. Pittam MR, Carter RL. Framework invasion by laryngeal carcinomas. Head Neck Surg 1982;4:200–8.
16. Ogura JH. Surgical pathology of cancer of the larynx. Laryngoscope 1955;65:867–926.
17. McGavran MH, Bauer WC, Ogura J. The incidence of cervical lymph node metastases from epidermoid carcinoma of the larynx and their relationship to certain characteristics of the primary tumor. Cancer 1961;14:55–66.
18. Carter RL, Tanner NSB, Clifford P, Shaw HJ. Direct bone invasion in squamous carcinomas of the head and neck: Pathological and clinical implications. Clin Otolaryngol 1980;5:107–16.
19. Tsao SW, Burman JF, Easty DM, et al. Some mechanisms of local bone destruction by squamous carcinomas of the head and neck. Br J Cancer 1981;43:392–401.
20. Bennett A, Carter RL, Stamford IF, Tanner NSSB. Prostaglandin-like material extracted from squamous carcinomas of the head and neck. Br J Cancer 1980;41:204–8.
21. Galasko CSB. Mechanism of bone destruction in the development of skeletal metastases. Nature 1976;263:507–8.
22. Galasko CSB, Bennett A. Relationship of bone destruction in skeletal metastases to osteoclast activation and prostaglandins. Nature 1976;263:508–10.
23. Galasko CSB. The pathological basis for skeletal scintigraphy. J Bone Joint Surg 1975;57B:353–9.
24. Orr W, Varani J, Gondek MD, Ward PA, Mundy GR. Chemotactic responses of tumor cells to products of resorbing bone. Science 1979;203:176–9.
25. Abramson M, Schiling RW, Huang CC, Salome RG. Collagenase activity in epidermoid carcinoma of the oral cavity and larynx. Ann Otol 1975;84:158–63.
26. Brem H, Folkman J. Inhibition of tumor angiogenesis mediated by cartilage. J Exp Med 1975;141:427–39.
27. Hately W, Evison G, Samual E. The pattern of ossification in the laryngeal cartilages: A radiological study. Br J Radiol 1965;38:585–91.
28. Archer CA, Yeager VL. Evaluation of laryngeal cartilages by computed tomography. J Comput Assist Tomogr 1979;3:604–11.
29. Nathan MD, El Gammal T, Hudson J. Computerized axial tomography in the assessment of thyroid cartilage invasion by laryngeal carcinoma: A prospective study. Otolaryngol Head Neck Surg 1980;88:726–33.
30. Mafee MF, Schild JA, Michael AS, et al. Cartilage involvement in laryngeal carcinoma correlation of CT and pathologic macrosection studies. J Comput Assist Tomogr 1984;8:969–73.
31. Lloyd GAS, Michaels L, Phelps PD. The demonstration of cartilaginous involvement in laryngeal carcinoma by computerized tomography. Clin Otolaryngol 1981;6:171–7.
32. Hoover LA, Calcaterra TC, Walter GA, Larson S. Preoperative CT scan evaluation for laryngeal carcinoma: Correlation with pathological findings. Laryngoscope 1984;94:310–5.
33. Gamsu G, Webb WR, Shallit JB, Moss AA. CT in carcinoma of the larynx and pyriform sinus: The value of phonation scans. AJR 1981;136:577–84.
34. Archer CR, Yeager VL, Herbold DR. Improved diagnostic accuracy in the TNM staging of laryngeal cancer using a new definition of regions based on computed tomography. J Comput Assist Tomogr 1983;7: 610–7.

35. Archer CR, Yeager VL. Computed tomography of laryngeal cancer with histopathological correlation. Laryngoscope 1982;92:1173–80.
36. Schild JA, Valvassori GE, Mafee MF, Bardawil W. Laryngeal malignancies and computerized tomography. A correlation of tomographic and histologic findings. Ann Otol 1982;91:571–5.
37. Gregor RT, Lloyd GAS, Michaels L. Computed tomography of the larynx: A clinical and pathologic study. Head Neck Surg 1981;3:284–96.
38. Michaels L, Gregor RT. Examination of the larynx in the histopathology laboratory. J Clin Pathol 1980;33:705–10.
39. Gregor RT, Hammond K. Framework invasion by laryngeal carcinoma. Am J Surg 1987;154:452–8.
40. Gregor RT. Unpublished data. Presented for PhD (Med) thesis at the University of the Witwatersrand, Johannesburg, 1986.
41. Crofton PM. Biochemistry of alkaline phosphatase isoenzymes. Crit Rev Lab Sci 1982;16:161–94.
42. Fishman WH, Inglis MI, Stolbach LL, Kraut MJ. A serum alkaline phosphatase isoenzyme of human neoplastic cell origin. Cancer Res 1968;28:150–2.

4

Cervical Lymph Node Disease in Laryngeal Cancer

Jonas T. Johnson, Eugene N. Myers

There is general agreement that the stage of laryngeal carcinoma that exists at the time of therapy is the most important identifiable factor in predicting prognosis. Therefore a staging system is commonly used to communicate treatment results with other investigators and as a basis for therapeutic decisions. In the TNM staging systems commonly employed, the clinically evident size and nature of the primary tumor (T), size, location, and number of metastatic nodes (M), and presence or absence of distant metastases are considered. The presence of cervical metastasis (N stage) has a greater impact on prognosis than the characteristics of the primary tumor (T stage). In this chapter we shall examine the risk of developing cervical metastasis as it relates to site and stage of the primary tumor. Management options for patients with cervical metastatic disease include surgery, radiation therapy, or a combination of the two.

Patients who undergo surgical therapy for cervical metastasis, either suspected or known, may benefit from subsequent histologic evaluation of the operative specimen. A growing body of knowledge currently suggests that histologic information generated from radical neck dissection may, in a far more subtle way, have implications for therapeutic decision-making than the TNM staging systems currently in use.

INCIDENCE OF CERVICAL METASTASIS

The risk of metastatic carcinoma to cervical lymphatics is of vital importance to the patient with squamous cell carcinoma of the larynx. There is universal agreement that the presence of cervical metastasis reduces survival. Extracapsular spread (ECS) of tumor in cervical metastasis may further reduce survival by 50%.

Our present ability to detect cervical metastasis is, unfortunately, limited. Clinical assessment of the neck is inexact. Bocca et al[1] report that 12% of patients treated for carcinoma of the neck initially judged N_0 on physical examination were subsequently found to have metastatic carcinoma following elective neck dissection, whereas 34% of 62 patients judged to have clinically suspicious palpable adenopathy had no histologic evidence of metastatic disease.

Cachin et al[2] found ECS of tumor in 20% of patients with no palpable metastasis. Synderman et al[3] observed that 20% of patients with supraglottic carcinoma initially staged N_0 had histologic evidence of metastasis when elective neck dissection specimens were evaluated. Half of these patients had ECS of tumor.

Attempts to improve diagnostic accuracy employing lymphangiography or radionuclide scanning have been imprecise and expensive. Computed tomography and magnetic resonance imaging may improve our ability to identify patients with disease that is not palpable, although small tumor metastasis continues to evade detection. To date, more sensitive methods to detect microscopic disease have been frustrated by lack of a suitable marker.

In view of these problems, the head and neck oncologist has been forced to approach cervical metastasis in patients with laryngeal carcinoma in three general groups. These include patients with palpable operable disease, patients with inoperable disease, and patients with no evidence of metastatic disease who must be managed according to the treating physician's assessment of the risk of potential metastatic disease.

The larynx should be considered according to its anatomic subunits, particularly when discussing the probability of cervical metastasis. Cancer of the larynx is described as supraglottic, glottic, or subglottic. This apparently simple scheme is complicated by the fact that some cancers are transglottic in location, involving more than a single anatomic site. Various investigators have reported that the risk of cervical metastasis varies according to the site of the primary tumor (Table 4–1).

Carcinoma of the Glottic Larynx

True glottic lesions rarely metastasize until cartilage invasion develops or there is extension into the supraglottic or subglottic

Table 4-1. Risk of Cervical Metastasis According to Site and Size of Primary Tumor

SITE	STAGE	RISK OF CERVICAL METASTASIS (%)
Glottis	T_1	<5
	T_2	<8
	T_3	15
	T_4	40
Subglottis	All stages	<10*
Supraglottis	T_1	25-40
	T_2	40-70
	T_3	65-80

*This figure does not account for the 65% incidence of paratracheal node involvement in subglottic carcinoma.

larynx. Leroux-Robert[4] observed metastasis in only 2.5% of 620 patients with carcinoma of the glottic larynx. This included one patient with a T_2 lesion, seven patients with T_3 lesions, and seven with T_4 lesions. Hawkins[5] reported cervical metastases in 7% of 800 patients with glottic carcinoma. The majority of metastases developed in patients with T_3 and T_4 lesions. Daly and Strong[6] noted metastases in fewer than 5% of patients with T_1, 8% of patients with T_2, and 15% of patients with T_3 glottic cancers.

It has been suggested that the relative paucity of metastasis in glottic carcinoma reflects the fact that the true vocal cords have little or no venous or lymphatic drainage. The region at the anterior commissure is an area of relatively increased risk in that the true vocal cords are attached anteriorly by a tendon (Broyle's ligament) that inserts into the internal perichondrium of the thyroid cartilage. Tumors may spread through Broyle's ligament into the anterior subglottic region with potential involvement of the delphian node overlying the cricothyroid membrane. The probability of cervical node metastases from glottic carcinoma increases with depth of invasion of the primary tumor. The incidence of lymph node metastases in carcinoma superficial to the conus elasticus is under 2%. Advanced glottic carcinoma with invasion of the thyroid cartilage is associated with an increased risk of cervical metastasis. Jesse[7] observed 19% incidence of metastases in patients with T_4 lesions with subsequent metastases in 20% more.

Elective therapy of the cervical lymphatics is not indicated in patients with superficial carcinoma limited to the true vocal cords. More invasive tumors with involvement of the anterior commissure and cricothyroid membrane may be associated with metastasis to the delphian node. Subsequent spread may include the thyroid gland, paratracheal nodes, and the mediastinum. Management options will be addressed later.

Subglottic Carcinoma

Metastatic disease from subglottic carcinoma is related to depth of invasion. Penetration of the conus elasticus and inner perichondrium of the thyroid cartilage results most commonly in involvement of the thyroid gland, paratracheal nodes, and upper mediastinum. Harrison[8] reports an incidence of paratracheal node involvement in as many as 65% of patients with subglottic carcinoma.

The jugular chain of lymphatics should be considered a secondary site of metastatic spread. Lederman[9] noted cervical metastasis in only six (4.3%) of 140 patients with subglottic tumors. Similarly, only five (9.2%) of 54 patients with subglottic carcinoma were reported by Pietrantoni et al[10] to have cervical metastasis.

Supraglottic Carcinoma

Lindberg[11] reported metastatic disease in 147 (55%) of 267 patients reviewed with carcinoma of the supraglottic larynx. The risk of metastatic disease in the neck varied according to the size of the primary tumor. Thirty-nine percent of patients with T_1 lesions had cervical metastases, whereas 65% of patients with T_3 and T_4 lesions had metastatic disease. Bocca et al[1] analyzed retrospectively the risk of cervical metastasis in 407 patients with carcinoma of the supraglottic larynx. Metastases were observed in 25% of patients with T_1 lesions and 69% of patients with T_2 lesions. Shah and Tollefsen[12] reported a respective incidence of metastatic disease of 40, 42, 55, and 65% in a series of 352 patients with T_1, T_2, T_3, and T_4 lesions, respectively. These authors noted that the risk of cervical metastasis varied according to the anatomic area involved with tumor. The supraglottic larynx confined within the free edge of the epiglottis, aryepiglottic fold, and arytenoid with no extension beyond these margins was termed "endolarynx." Only 34% of patients with carcinoma of the endolarynx developed cervical metastases. Carcinoma of the so-called "exolarynx" with tumor involving adjacent sites such as the tongue base, valleculae, pyriform sinus, or postcricoid region was associated with cervical metastases in 69% of patients.

Jorgensen et al[13] separated the supraglottic larynx into "suprahyoid" and "infrahyoid" portions. Ten of 25 patients with tumor involving the suprahyoid epiglottis, and 10 of 25 with carcinoma of the aryepiglottic fold had cervical metastasis. In contrast, only 25% of patients with infrahyoid epiglottic and 15% of patients with ventricular lesions had adenopathy. Similar findings were reported by Marks et al[14] in a retrospective study of 540 patients with squamous carcinoma of the supraglottic larynx. These authors noted that the presence of palpable metastasis varied according to the site of the primary tumor. The highest incidence of palpable adenopathy occurred in patients with carcinoma of the pyriform sinus (69%). Carcinoma of the suprahyoid epiglottis, valleculae, and tongue base had metastatic disease at the time of presentation in 57% of cases, and 48% of patients with carcinoma of the aryepiglottic fold, arytenoid, or free margin of epiglottis had palpable nodes. Only 32% of patients with infrahyoid epiglottic carcinoma presented with palpable nodes. Further study of this large series of patients revealed, however, that the location of the primary tumor did not correlate with the incidence of metastasis that developed subsequent to presentation. The risk of recurrence in the neck following therapy for pyriform sinus carcinoma was 15%; marginal epiglottis, 20%; suprahyoid epiglottis, 8%; transglottic carcinoma, 8%; and infrahyoid epiglottis, 11%.

Since assessment of risk is often complicated by the fact that patients frequently present with involvement of more than one anatomic site, these observations appear to simplify the situation by concluding that variations in risk reflect the variable incidence of metastatic disease at the time of presentation. The statistical risk of subsequent development of metastatic disease would appear to be similar without regard to the supraglottic site of the primary tumor.

Transglottic Carcinoma

Evaluation of transglottic carcinoma is difficult because of confusion surrounding its definition. Transglottic tumors represent a heterogenous group of lesions primarily involving the glottic larynx with supraglottic extension. A reasonable definition is tumor that involves both the true and false vocal cords. The term, however, is often employed to describe glottic carcinoma with subglottic extension.*

MANAGEMENT

The N_1 Neck

Therapy of involved cervical lymphatics cannot be undertaken without consideration of the primary lesion. This reality has been underscored by Mendenhall et al,[15] who noted in a study of 161 patients that neck metastases were not controlled by radical radiation therapy in 47% of 30 patients in whom radiation failed to control the primary lesion. In contrast, 86% of 91 patients whose primary tumors were successfully controlled by radiation also achieved control of cervical metastases. The effectiveness of radiation in controlling laryngeal lesions diminishes markedly in advanced disease stages. Olofsson[16] reported a 47% 3-year primary tumor control rate for patients with T_1 and T_2 lesions after initial irradiation. Lauerma[17] noted that 69% of T_1 and 48% of T_2 laryngeal tumors were controlled with irradiation. Henk[18] reported that tumor control was achieved in 73% of T_1 and T_2 patients and only in 51% of T_3 and T_4 patients. Hansen[19] retrospectively reviewed 511 patients with supraglottic carcinomas, treated primarily by irradiation. Five-year survival rate was 68% for stage I, 35% for stage III, and 10% for stage IV. Wang[20] reported cure rates for T_1 and T_2 lesions of 74%, whereas only 23% of patients with T_3 and T_4 lesions were controlled. Vermund[21] concluded, after an extensive literature review, that primary irradiation therapy is inadequate to treat stages III and IV laryngeal carcinomas.

Because of these reported results obtained with radiation alone, we advocate radical neck dissection for management of palpable cervical metastasis in patients with carcinoma of the larynx. When bilateral metastases are clinically evident, bilateral radical neck dissection should be undertaken. Since simultaneous bilateral radical neck dissection may be associated with increased intracranial pressure, prolonged facial edema, papilledema, and even blindness, we advocate preservation of one or both internal jugular veins, if possible, when bilateral neck dissections are to be performed in a single stage.

Surgical management of cervical metastasis offers the patient another advantage by permitting detailed pathologic evaluation of the specimen with consequent accurate assessment of the nature and extent of disease. Snow et al[22] in a retrospective review of 326 patients who underwent radical neck dissection found that ECS of tumor in cervical lymph nodes occurred in 23% of nodes under 3 cm in diameter. Subsequent studies reported by Johnson et al[23] indicate that ECS may be detected in as many as 65% of lymph nodes staged clinically N_1 (Figs. 4–1, 4–2). Both groups of authors concur that histologic demonstration of ECS of tumor is a predictor of poor prognosis. In a study of 105 patients with proven cervical node metastases treated by combined neck dissection and elective postoperative radiation therapy, our group[23] reported 3-year survival rate of 73% of 44 patients without ECS compared with 49% of 61 patients in whom ECS was demonstrated. These differences were statistically significant ($p < 0.03$).

Other authors have documented that extension of cervical metastasis out of the node into the soft tissue has a negative effect on survival. Noone et al[24] noted a 70% 5-year survival rate in patients with tumor limited to the node, with reduction to 48% with invasion of the nodal capsule, and further reduction in survival to 27% when ECS was identified. Shah et al[25] concur that cervical metastasis with involvement of the soft tissue of the neck correlates with poor prognosis. Sessions[26] retrospectively evaluated 791 patients. When cervical metastases were associated with soft tissue invasion by tumor, effectiveness of subsequent treatment decreased by a factor of 5.

Histopathologic assessment of the condition of the cervical lymphatics within the neck dissection specimen allows the surgeon to adjust management to the needs of the individual patient. Postoperative radiation therapy can be employed when circumstances dictate. We have reported preliminary results of a proposed program of postoperative radiation therapy with adju-

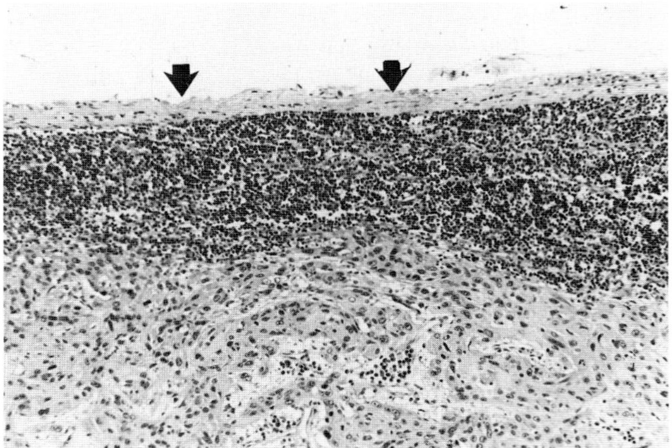

Figure 4–1. Cortical replacement of a cervical node by squamous cell carcinoma. Note that the capsule (arrows) is intact. This node demonstrates metastasis without extracapsular spread.

*Editors note: I would add to the confusion noted by the authors of this chapter by suggesting that the term "transglottic" coined by McGavran et al (Cancer 1961;14:55–66) is commonly employed to describe tumors that cross the ventricle, involving glottic and supraglottic sites. Many of these tumors are thought to arise within the ventricle and have a characteristic pattern of spread (see Chapter 2), but the term is applicable to any tumor that involves both glottic and supraglottic sites, regardless of origin. Confusion is heightened by the fact that a category of "transglottic" is not included in the standard TNM staging systems.

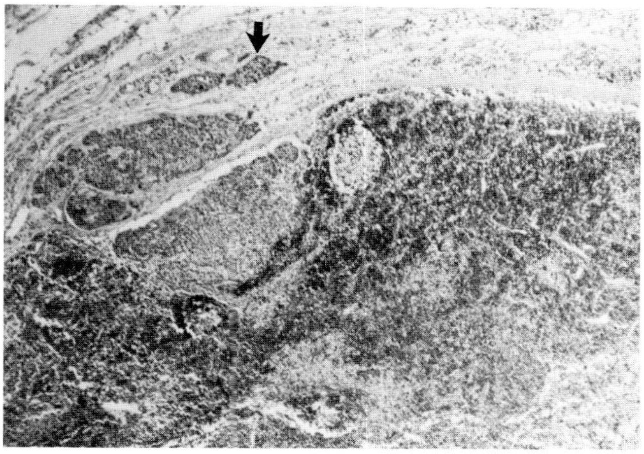

Figure 4–2. The capsule is disrupted and invaded by nests of tumor (arrow), which appear both within and outside the node.

vant chemotherapy for patients with ECS of tumor.[27] In a prospective clinical trial, patients with operable squamous cell carcinoma of the head and neck underwent resection of the primary tumor in continuity with radical neck dissection. Histologic confirmation of ECS of tumor in cervical lymph node metastasis was required for participation in the adjuvant chemotherapy protocol. Patients with ECS were referred for postoperative irradiation therapy delivered in 180 to 200 rad fractions to a total of 50 to 60 Gy in 5 to 6 weeks. Subsequent to the completion of radiation, adjuvant chemotherapy was instituted employing methotrexate (250 mg/m^2) followed 1 hour later by 5-fluorouracil (600 mg/m^2). Leucovorin rescue (10 mg/m^2) was administered at 24 hours and repeated every 6 hours for a total of six doses. Therapy was administered weekly with a 1 week rest following every two courses. A total of 18 courses of chemotherapy was administered over 6 months.

Fifty patients were eligible for this protocol, which was completed by 38 patients (76%). The 12 patients who failed to complete the protocol included three (6%) who developed recurrent carcinoma while on study, five (10%) who died of causes unrelated to cancer or the treatment before completion of chemotherapy, one (2%) in whom therapy was stopped due to toxicity, and three (6%) who refused to complete the adjuvant protocol. All patients were followed longer than 24 months after treatment. Sixty-seven percent (28 of 42) of assessable patients treated with adjuvant chemotherapy remained free of disease. This compares to an expected 2-year disease-free survival of approximately 38% previously observed in patients with ECS. This trial, although clearly needing further evaluation in a prospective randomized format, suggests that this program of adjuvant chemotherapy for patients with ECS of tumor may be effective. The results further stress the value of histologic assessment of cervical lymphatics in treatment planning.

The N_0 Neck

When no palpable or detectable cervical metastases are present, the head and neck oncologist has three reasonable therapeutic alternatives to offer; elective radiation therapy, elective neck dissection, or no immediate therapy but close follow-up with treatment of the neck to be withheld until metastatic disease is encountered.

Patients with squamous cell carcinoma confined to the true vocal cords do not require elective neck treatment. We advocate removal of the primary tumor with close follow-up of the neck. When glottic carcinoma involves supraglottic structures such as with so-called transglottic carcinoma, elective ipsilateral neck dissection is appropriate. For glottic carcinoma extending more than 2 cm subglottically, the risk of metastasis to the thyroid, paratracheal nodes, and upper mediastinum is increased. Under these circumstances, elective postoperative radiation therapy including an upper mediastinum portal is advocated.

Carcinoma of the supraglottic larynx has the propensity for early and bilateral cervical metastasis. In a recent review of 200 patients with squamous cell carcinoma of the supraglottic larynx treated at our institution with surgery alone or surgery plus postoperative radiation therapy, we observed recurrence in the larynx or pharynx in only 2% of cases. In contrast, nearly 20% of patients developed recurrent carcinoma in the contralateral neck when only an ipsilateral radical neck dissection had been perfomed. This observation held true without regard to the site of the primary supraglottic tumor. Laterally based tumors involving the aryepiglottic fold and arytenoid produced similar risk to the contralateral neck. Therefore we recommend elective bilateral neck dissection for all patients with squamous cell carcinoma of the supraglottic larynx. Spinal accessory nerves should be identified and preserved unless involved with metastatic carcinoma. The jugular vein should be skeletonized and preserved on the side with no clinical evidence of metastases. If bilateral elective neck dissection is undertaken, the internal jugular vein may be preserved bilaterally.

Squamous cell carcinoma arising in the subglottic larynx behaves similarly to glottic carcinoma with subglottic extension. These tumors metastasize to the thyroid bed, paratracheal lymphatics, and upper mediastinal nodes. Since block resection of these structures is difficult, the region is best treated with elective postoperative radiation therapy. Radiation should be delivered to portals designed to treat both the neck and the upper mediastinum.

The Inoperable Neck

When squamous cell carcinoma is considered inoperable because of fixation of cervical metastasis, we advocate neoadjuvant chemotherapy. If, following chemotherapy, the cervical metastases are judged to be operable, radical neck dissection may be performed followed by postoperative radiation therapy. Although it is unclear at this time whether multimodality therapy truly improves the outlook for patients with inoperable cervical disease, early results have been encouraging, particularly with patients who have achieved complete response of the tumor to chemotherapy. It would appear that prognosis may be improved in this group of patients.

Patients with inoperable cervical metastases remain a clinical dilemma of considerable significance. These patients should be offered treatment in accordance with investigative protocols as they become available.

CONCLUSIONS

Management of laryngeal carcinoma frequently requires concurrent treatment of the cervical lymphatics for apparent or potential metastatic disease. The laryngeal oncologist must be familiar with the patterns of spread associated with primary sites of tumor within the larynx. In our opinion elective treatment of the neck is indicated for most laryngeal cancers with the exception of tumors limited to the true vocal cord.

Surgical treatment of cervical lymphatics is advocated because it allows the head and neck oncologist the most complete assessment of disease stage, which, in turn, facilitates future treatment planning.

REFERENCES

1. Bocca E, Pignataro O, Oldini C. Supraglottic laryngectomy: 30 years of experience. Ann Otol Rhinol Laryngol 1983;92:14.
2. Cachin Y, Sancno-Garnier H, Micheau C, Marandas P. Nodal metastasis from carcinomas of the oropharynx. Otolaryngol Clin North Am 1979;12:145.
3. Synderman NL, Johnson JT, Schramm VL Jr, et al. Extracapsular spread of carcinoma in cervical lymph nodes: impact upon survival in patients with carcinoma of the supraglottic larynx. Cancer 1985;56:1597.
4. Leroux-Robert J. A statistical study of 620 laryngeal carcinomas of the glottic region personally operated upon more than five years ago. Laryngoscope 1975;85:1440.
5. Hawkins NV. The treatment of glottic carcinoma: an analysis of 800 cases. Laryngoscope 1975;85:1485.
6. Daly JF, Strong EW. Carcinoma of the glottic larynx. Am J Surg 1975;130:489.
7. Jesse RH. The evaluation of treatment of patients with extensive squamous cancer of the vocal cords. Laryngoscope 1975;85:1424.
8. Harrison DFN. The pathology and management of subglottic cancer. Ann Otol Rhinol Laryngol 1971;80:6.
9. Lederman M. Radiotherapy of cancer of the larynx. J Laryngol Otol 1970;84:867.
10. Pietrantoni L, Agazzi C, Fior R. Indications for surgical treatment of cervical lymph nodes in cancer of the larynx and hypopharynx. Laryngoscope 1962;72:1511.
11. Lindberg RD. Sites of first failure in head and neck cancer. Cancer Treat Symp 1983;2:21.
12. Shah JP, Tollefsen HR. Epidermoid carcinoma of the supraglottic larynx: role of neck dissection in initial surgical treatment. Am J Surg 1974;128:494.
13. Jorgensen K, Munk J, Andersen JE, Hjelm-Hansen M. Carcinoma of the larynx: series of 410 patients treated primarily with Co^{60} irradiation. Acta Radiol Oncol 1984;23:321.
14. Marks JE, Breaux S, Smith PG, et al. The need for elective irradiation of occult lymphatic metastases from cancers of the larynx and pyriform sinus. Head Neck Surg 1985;8:3.
15. Mendenhall WM, Million RR, Cassisi NJ. Squamous cell carcinoma of the head and neck treated with radiation therapy: the role of neck dissection for clinically positive neck nodes. Int J Radiat Oncol Biol Phys 1986;12:733.
16. Olofsson J. Specific features of laryngeal carcinoma involving the anterior commissure and the subglottic region. In: Alberti PW, Bryce DP, eds. *Workshops from the Centennial Conference on Laryngeal Cancer:* New York: Appleton-Century-Crofts, 1976.
17. Lauerma S. Treatment of laryngeal cancer: a study of 638 cases. Acta Otolaryngol Suppl (Stockh) 1967;225:1.
18. Henk JM. The influence of oxygen and hypoxia on laryngeal cancer management. Laryngoscope 1975;85:1134.
19. Hansen HS. Supraglottic carcinoma of the aryepiglottic fold. Laryngoscope 1975;85:1667.
20. Wang CC. Radiation therapy in the management of oral malignant disease. Otolaryngol Clin North Am 1979;12:73.
21. Vermund H. Role of radiotherapy in cancer of the larynx as related to the TNM system of staging: a review. Cancer 1970;25:485.
22. Snow GB, Annyas AA, VanSlooten EA, et al. Prognostic factors of neck node metastasis. Clin Otolaryngol 1982;7:185.
23. Johnson JT, Myers EN, Bedetti CD, et al. Cervical lymph node metastasis. Arch Otolaryngol 1985;111:534.
24. Noone RB, Bonner H Jr, Raymond S, et al. Lymph node metastases in oral carcinoma. Plast Reconstr Surg 1974;53:158.
25. Shah JP, Cendon RA, Farr HW, Strong EW. Carcinoma of the oral cavity—factors affecting treatment failure at the primary site and neck. Am J Surg 1976;132:504.
26. Sessions DG, Ogura JH, Fried MP. Laryngeal carcinoma involving the anterior commissure and subglottis. In: Alberti PW, Bryce DP, eds. *Workshops from the Centennial Conference on Laryngeal Cancer*. New York: Appleton-Century-Crofts, 1976:674.
27. Johnson JT, Myers EN, Schramm VL Jr, et al. Adjuvant chemotherapy for high-risk squamous-cell carcinoma of the head and neck. J Clin Oncol 1987;5:456.

5

Pathologic and Cytometric Indicators of Biologic Behavior in Laryngeal Cancer

Manning M. Goldsmith, Harold C. Pillsbury

Stage per stage, laryngeal squamous cell carcinoma is one of the more curable head and neck cancers. The tumor often presents at a relatively early stage because of hoarseness, and the cartilaginous framework that houses the tumor prevents local spread of the disease and facilitates en bloc resection.

Nevertheless, comparably staged patients with laryngeal malignancy frequently have a diverse clinical course and response to similar treatment. Although outcome is greatly influenced by stage of disease, the TNM system is an imperfect prognostic indicator. Descriptive pathologic morphology has been correlated with biologic behavior and prognosis for certain tumors of the aerodigestive tract.[1–3] Both TNM staging and pathologic morphology, however, are semiquantitative and fall short of defining determinants of tumor response expressed at a cellular level, which include both differentiable and proliferative properties within heterogeneous tumor cell populations.

This chapter will focus on pathologic morphology and DNA flow cytometry as they relate to biologic behavior of squamous cell carcinoma of the larynx.

DESCRIPTIVE PATHOLOGY

Several studies[1–5] have employed histologic grading systems based on various morphologic parameters of the tumor cell population and its relationship to adjacent tissues, correlating the total score of malignancy grade with prognosis for squamous cell carcinoma of the head and neck. Generally, these grading systems provide more objective and accurate criteria relating morphologic findings to biologic activity and growth patterns of head and neck tumors than histologic differentiation alone. However, morphologic criteria remain subjective, poorly standardized, and relatively crude approximations of tumor cell kinetics and biologic behavior of the cancer.

Since Broders'[6] original grading scale for squamous cell carcinoma, developed in the 1920s, pathologists have generally simplified the grading scale into three grades of poorly, moderately, and well-differentiated neoplasms on the basis of keratinization and nuclear atypia. The continued basis for grading squamous cell carcinoma has been its value in predicting biologic behavior. Generally, well-differentiated neoplasms grow in a slow predictable fashion with less propensity for regional spread than higher grade, poorly differentiated neoplasms.

An additional prognostic pathologic parameter relates to the tumor host interface and the pattern of tumor infiltration at the periphery. Tumors with large pushing borders and broad cords of cells with a well-defined tumor stromal interface appear to have a better prognosis than neoplastic cells that invade as single cells or small irregular cords.[7–9] Crissman[9] has found that pushing tumors tend to produce more basement membrane and that basement membrane is a good marker of tumor differentiation. Infiltrative squamous cell tumors appear to have a greater propensity for penetration and invasion of blood and lymph structures, and thus have a poor prognosis.[7–11]

Other pathologic parameters that have been found to affect prognosis include the identification of vascular and perineural invasion. Both of these features have been found to correlate with lymph node metastasis and poor prognosis.[7,8,10,12]

Our studies[7,8] demonstrated no significant correlation between histopathologic grading scales and prognosis for laryngeal cancer. Only three of the pathologic variables in our studies exhibited a meaningful relationship with clinical outcome. These were grade of tumor-associated tissue eosinophilia (TATE), the pattern of tumor infiltration at the periphery, and perineural invasion. Fifteen of 16 patients (94%) with perineural invasion fared poorly, whereas 62 of 105 (59%) without perineural invasion did so ($p < 0.005$). A pushing pattern of tumor spread at the periphery was associated with favorable clinical outcome ($p < 0.001$). There was no correlation between any of the remaining pathologic parameters and prognosis (Table 5–1).

Infiltration of the tumor periphery by lymphoreticular cells is a common feature of many human malignant neoplasms. Generally, dense lymphoplasmacytic invasion of the surrounding tumor stroma is considered to be a favorable prognostic sign, presumably indicative of good host immunologic response to the cancer.[13] Recently, attention has been directed to the degree of TATE in these inflammatory infiltrates. Several studies have suggested that TATE may be a favorable prognostic indicator for tumors of the bladder,[14] uterine cervix,[15] colon,[16] and stomach.[17,18]

The pattern of failure for 78 patients with poor clinical outcome in our study[7,8] was correlated with grade of TATE. Seventeen patients failed by distant metastasis and 61 failed local-regionally. All 17 patients who developed distant metastasis had very low-grade TATE (grades 0–1). None of 11 patients with higher-grade TATE (grades 2–4) failed by distant metastasis. Thus, high-grade TATE appeared to have a protective effect against distant metastasis ($p < 0.05$). High-grade TATE (grades 3–4) correlated with a favorable clinical outcome ($p < 0.001$). When a stepwise logistic regression analysis of the clinical pathologic variables in the study was applied, high-grade TATE proved to be the most influential variable affecting clinical outcome, followed by pattern of tumor infiltration at the periphery, stage, and perineural invasion.

To our knowledge, there is only one study in the English literature that relates TATE to prognosis in head and neck squamous cell carcinoma. Lowe and Fletcher[19] studied five oral cavity tumors with massive TATE (defined as greater than 100 eosinophils/high-powered field in ten fields). None of their patients had systemic eosinophilia or second primary tumors. The five patients survived an average of 5 years. One, with tongue cancer, lived 8 years despite distant metastases. The study was hampered by its small sample and no mention is made of the stage of disease and of mode of therapy for the tumors presented. Of interest may be the fact that all of the tumors in this study demonstrating massive TATE were large cell poorly keratinizing, moderately differentiated carcinomas. The authors postulated that TATE may be a tissue response to a particular pattern of squamous differentiation.

Lowe et al,[20] in an excellent review of TATE, state that only a small percentage of specific tumors have this response. The percentage of tumors exhibiting high grades of TATE in our study (12.5%) is in agreement with others.[14–20] The common feature of the types of tumor that show marked TATE is that they all derive from body surfaces. In the cervix and lung these tumors are usually of the large cell and nonkeratinizing type,[20] whereas in stomach the tumors are usually poorly differentiated adenocarcinomas.[17] In the present study we found no correlation between the presence or grade of TATE and the degree of differentiation or keratinization of the tumor.

Several studies[16,20] have suggested that TATE may have a protective effect on development of distant metastasis, although one[21] suggests that the opposite may be true. Interestingly, TATE and tumor-associated blood eosinophilia (TABE) may occur independently and appear to have opposite clinical significance. Most tumors with marked TABE have late disease, widespread metastasis, and poor outcome.[15,22] The pathogenesis of TABE is not known.

The reason that some tumors invoke a predominant eosinophilic response in their inflammatory infiltrates is also unknown. Wasserman et al[23] and Goetzl et al[24] isolated an eosinophilotactic factor from lung carcinomas, which suggests that the attraction of a marked eosinophilic infiltrate may be a function of the tumor cells. Similar eosinophilotactic factors have been isolated from Hodgkin's tumor cells[25] and from gastric tumors.[17] Alternatively, the eosinophilia may be part of a modulatory response to the immunologic interactions of the lymphoplasmocytic cells with tumor antigens. This is in keeping with the general role of the eosinophil to contain and terminate hypersensitivity reactions, especially those of the immediate type.[26] Several studies have suggested that T lymphocytes might be responsible for an antigen-induced local eosinotaxis that is blocked by antithymocyte globulin.[27,28]

In our study we found the eosinophilic response in corresponding lymph node metastases to be of the same grade as their respective primary sites. Bostrom and Hart[29] found the nodal eosinophilic response in five of their patients with cervical carconima. In four of the five, metastatic tumor cells were not found in the respective nodes with the eosinophilic response. These data suggest that the eosinophilic response is not site specific and may be indicative of the transport of eosinophilotactic factors to regional nodes.

The relationship of increased eosinophilic stromal reactions and host response to the tumor is unclear. Goswami[30] demonstrated that the growth of implanted murine tumors is inhibited if the implantation site has tissue eosinophilia. Eosinophils have recently been found to have cytotoxic properties for mammalian cell lines.[31–33] A major basic protein from the crystalloid core of the eosinophil normally acts to neutralize heparin released in immediate hypersensitivity reactions. Butterworth et al[32] recently demonstrated that this protein was the eosinophilic mediator of damage to schistosomula of *Schistosoma mansoni*. They also found that the major basic protein could cause nonspecific damage to murine ascites tumor cells as well as other mammalian cells. Another study demonstrated that eosinophils could be cytotoxic to mammalian tumor cells via the eosinophil-hydrogen peroxide-halide system.[33] This reaction could be inhibited by catalase, azide, and aminotriazole.

In conclusion, it appears that the presence of intense eosinophilia in the stroma of head and neck squamous cell carcinoma may be a useful and exciting new indicator of favorable prognosis and diminished tendency to develop distant metastasis. This may have significant implications for the future

Table 5-1. Histolopathologic Variables

Broder's scale
Bauer's scale
Grade of tumor-associated tissue eosinophilia (TATE)
Pattern of tumor spread at the periphery
Pleomorphism
Inflammation
Desmoplasia
Koilocytosis
Perineural invasion
Vascular invasion

evaluation and treatment of squamous cell carcinoma of the larynx, particularly with regard to the selection of patients for adjuvant chemotherapy. Further study is warranted to corroborate and further elucidate the mechanism of action of the eosinophil in the tumor-host interaction.

DNA FLOW CYTOMETRY

Recently, DNA flow cytometry has been used to elucidate objectively the phenotypic cellular parameters of tumors that may have both differentiable and prognostic significance. Flow cytometry can be broadly defined as the objective measurement of specific cellular features of a sample in an automated fashion as the sample moves past a stationary detector. Incident light is used to activate naturally occurring or added cellular fluorochromes, so that in theory any feature of a cell that can be caused to fluoresce may be detected and objectively measured. Intrinsic properties that can be measured by flow cytometry include cell size and granularity, among others, and these are generally used as "gate parameters" in the analysis of heterogeneous clinical specimens. Extrinsic properties include the analysis of cell surface antigens and nucleic acid quantitation, and these parameters have been extensively studied for many different tumors over the past decade.

Flow cytometric DNA analysis has been the most clinically applicable parameter to date. Figure 5–1 illustrates a pie graph of a replicating cell population and its corresponding DNA histogram. Gap 0 (G_0) represents a resting phase for the cell prior to its entry into gap 1 (G_1), or the presynthetic phase. The number of chromosomes for G_0 and G_1 is 2C (diploid). Once the cell enters the synthetic phase (S), the DNA of the cell increases until twice the normal complement of DNA (4C) is reached, at which point the cell exits gap 2 (G_2) to complete the cycle with mitosis (M). It then enters G_0 or G_1 at 2C. Corresponding sites of a replicating cell population are depicted on the DNA histogram in Figure 5–1.

Normal non-neoplastic cells contain a normal diploid quantity of DNA (euploid), whereas malignant cells frequently demonstrate abnormal DNA content (aneuploid). DNA index has been introduced as a measure of the degree of ploidy abnormality, denoting the ratio of DNA flourescence of abnormal to normal G_1G_0 cell populations (Fig. 5–2).

There is considerable variation in the reported incidence of

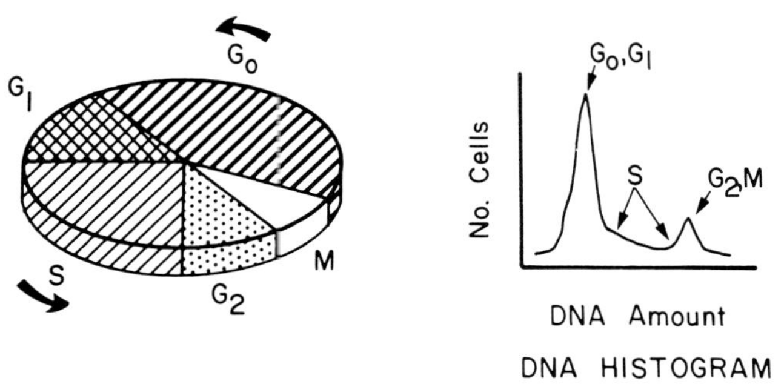

Figure 5–1. Diagram of cell cycle and corresponding DNA histogram.

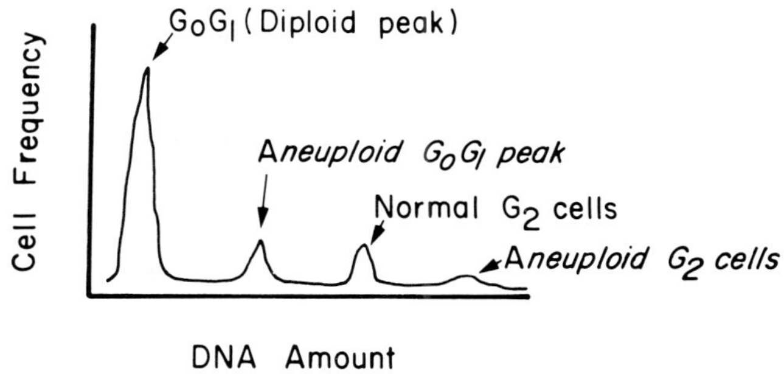

Figure 5–2. Aneuploid population demonstrated on DNA histogram.

DNA aneuploidy among malignancies studied in the current literature. It is generally agreed that Hodgkin's lymphoma, chronic lymphocytic leukemia, and the benign phase of chronic myelogenous leukemia are diploid tumors, where a 15 to 30% aneuploidy rate exists for the acute leukemias and indolent non-Hodgkin's lymphomas.[34] Aggressive lymphomas and multiple myelomas have a 50 to 80% rate of aneuploidy, and a 60 to 100% aneuploidy rate has been found in some solid tumors.[34]

Numerous investigators have reported results indicating a relationship between the DNA content of tumor cells and prognosis of the malignancy. Generally, the prognosis for solid tissue neoplasms is adversely affected by aneuploidy, as demonstrated by tumors of the bladder,[35] prostate,[36,37] colon,[38] and breast cancer.[39] On the other hand, neuroblastomas with aneuploid indices have a significantly improved prognosis compared with diploid tumors.[40] Prognostic implications of DNA index in acute leukemia and brain tumors are not yet settled.[34,41] Thus, it is possible that similar abnormalities in DNA content may have different prognostic implications for different malignancies.

Several issues become apparent on reviewing the literature on DNA flow cytometry of head and neck tumors. Terminology is poorly standardized; a "high" DNA amount or content may refer to the calculated DNA index or an integration of the modal peaks beyond the diploid peak. The definition of aneuploidy and the distinction between tetraploid G_1G_0 and diploid G_2 populations are also not standardized and are often subjective evaluations. The few studies in the literature relating ploidy to prognosis are poorly standardized and not well validated; coefficients of variation for histograms are often not reported. In addition, the few quantitative studies of DNA in squamous cell carcinomas of the aerodigestive tract have shown great diversity of DNA values and discrepant results with regard to the prognostic meaning of ploidy.[14,42–45] Some of these studies will be summarized.

In one of the early investigations of DNA analysis of oral cavity cancers, Holm[43] reported that cellular DNA amounts were of greater prognostic value than the type of ploidy. Holm found that oral cavity tumors with low DNA amounts (defined as less than 50% of the cells, with DNA values more than DNA G_1G_0 plus 2 SD) had a favorable prognosis. Patients with low DNA amounts had 96% 4-year survival rate compared with 36% survival rate for those with tumors with high DNA amounts ($p < 0.05$). Diploid carcinomas in Holm's study tended to have a better prognosis than aneuploid tumors, but the difference was not statistically significant. Interestingly, the few laryngeal tumors were aneuploid and had a favorable prognosis, but clearly the numbers were not large enough to reach statistical significance. Gussack et al,[46] using a formalin-fixed, paraffin-embedded (FFPE) technique for flow cytometric analysis, found that aneuploidy correlated with poor prognosis in 12 of 16 patients with laryngeal squamous cell carcinoma.

In contrast to the studies just mentioned, several investigators have reported entirely different conclusions with respect to the prognostic significance of ploidy in squamous cell carcinoma of the aerodigestive tract. Goldsmith et al,[7,8] employing the FFPE technique, found that aneuploid laryngeal squamous cell carcinoma had a better prognosis than diploid laryngeal tumors, but found an opposite trend for a smaller group of oral cavity tumors. A study by Roa et al[44] demonstrated that in vitro cell lines established from metastatic and recurrent squamous cell cancers usually had lower DNA content and chromosome number and exhibited more aggressive in vitro growth patterns than the primary tumor or earlier recurrence. Ensley et al,[47] using fresh tissue or formalin-fixed specimens for flow cytometric analysis in a larger number of patients with squamous cell carcinomas of the head and neck, determined that recurrent tumors and those refractory to cytotoxic therapy were predominantly diploid. Those tumors had a rather low S phase fraction, and perhaps the lower proliferative state accounts for their biologic behavior.

Nielsen et al[48] studied 50 patients with squamous cell carcinoma of the head and neck by DNA flow cytometric analysis using the FFPE technique. Patients with aneuploid tumors, who died with disease, had a statistically significant prolonged interval from time of diagnosis to death. It was concluded that aneuploid tumors demonstrated an overall favorable prognosis. Guo et al[49] studied 296 patients with squamous cell carcinoma of the head and neck using the FFPE technique. Sixty-one percent of patients with diploid tumors survived 5 years, compared with 28% of patients with aneuploid carcinomas. The authors concluded that patients with nondiploid tumors have a worse prognosis for survival and tumor recurrence than patients with diploid tumors, but that nondiploid may be more sensitive than diploid tumors to radiation therapy.

Careful analysis of the potential pitfalls involved in the DNA flow cytometric analysis of cellular parameters is instructive in analyzing the discrepancies in conclusions drawn in the studies mentioned relating DNA flow cytometry to head and neck cancer. These pitfalls have been reviewed by Ensley et al,[47] and the following discussion incorporates their outline with modifications and additions.

Instrumentation

The choice of instrumentation, experience of the operator and the individual analyzing the data, techniques for alignment and standardization, demonstration of accuracy and precision as well as interoperator variability are all sources of potential error independent of factors inherent in tissue preparation.

Tissue Preparative Technology

Solid tumor flow cytometry is hindered by the difficulty of obtaining high yield, unaltered, viable, single cell preparations. Because of desmosomes and dense intercellular stroma, connective tissue preparation of squamous cell carcinoma is particularly difficult.

As Ensley states: "It has been assumed that dissociation techniques that produce enough cells to obtain a DNA histogram are 'ipso facto' validated. One can take serious issue with this axiom and ask is 'enough cells to run, enough?' As with any quantitative analytical technique, the maximum recovery of the species of interest and representivity must be demonstrated. Every attempt should be made to determine the theoretical cellular (nuclear) yield of the tissue of interest and develop dissociation techniques that approach that figure. In addition, dissociation techniques must not be selective, particularly with respect to the cellular parameter that is to be determined. Artifacts may also be introduced by techniques of fixation and staining."

Since its introduction by Hedley et al,[50] the determination of ploidy on FFPE specimens has gained popularity for a variety of solid tumor systems. FFPE has the advantage of permitting assessment of ploidy for large archival data for which clinical outcome is already available. Histograms of comparable quality to those derived from fresh tissue have been demonstrated with the FFPE technique. Standardization of the FFPE histogram, however, has been the greatest drawback of this technique to date, since there is considerable intersample variability of the diploid peak with respect to the calculated locus using fresh internal standards. This phenomenon of intersample variability has been described by Schutte et al[51] and is attributed to varying conditions of formalin fixation with resultant variation in DNA staining intensity. Attempts to circumvent this problem by using standards that have been processed in the same fashion as the tumor specimen have been generally successful,[43,51] but problems may arise with pseudoaneuploidy, which has been identified in certain nonmalignant epithelia.[47]

When normal tissue is not available within the FFPE specimen for use as a standard, some authors assume that the first modal DNA peak of the tumor histogram corresponds to the G_1G_0 channel number, or diploid peak. Another common practice is to consider all monoclonal (single DNA histograms) DNA populations as diploid. These assumptions are predicated on studies with fresh solid tumors employing internal standards that have revealed the universal presence of diploid G_1 peaks and the rarity of true hypodiploidy. These assumptions can lead to erroneous determinations of ploidy, since such specimens may contain abnormal amounts of DNA, resulting in underestimation of true tumor aneuploidy. This type of error may account, in part, for the discrepancy of results in the head and neck flow cytometery literature to date.

As summarized by Ensley et al, appropriate flow cytometry technique must include the following:

1. Demonstration of adequate and representative nuclear yields.
2. Demonstration of uniform effects of formalin fixation and proteolytic enzyme treatment on DNA fluorochrome staining intensity.
3. Demonstration of appropriate diploid standards that are processed identically to FFPE samples.
4. Demonstration that the DNA and coefficient of variation of fresh and FFPE specimens are comparable from the same tissues.

Patient Population Chosen for Study

As has been pointed out, early or advanced disease may express differences with respect to cellular DNA content parameters, with more advanced and recurrent disease tending to be diploid. Therefore flow cytometric studies of squamous cell carcinomas of the head and neck restricted to patients with negative surgical margins or tumors with prior cytotoxic therapy may define a different population of tumors with respect to DNA parameters. This could consequently affect clinical conclusions made with regard to the prognostic significance of ploidy in these settings.

Thus, the current prognostic significance of ploidy in head and neck cancer remains unsettled. Our personal feeling is that aneuploidy probably indicates a more biologically aggressive tumor, yet one that is potentially more sensitive to cytotoxic therapy. Evidence exists in other tumor models that biologic factors that have a favorable impact on natural history may also adversely affect cytotoxic responses to therapy. The natural history of early stage, surgically removed diploid squamous cell carcinoma of the head and neck may be associated with superior survival when compared with aneuploid tumors. The lower S phase fraction of these diploid tumors, however, with consequent lower proliferative state may signify an unfavorable response to cytotoxic therapy.

CONCLUSIONS

It appears that the TNM staging system remains the best prognostic indicator for squamous cell carcinoma of the larynx. Although somewhat semiquantitative and subjective, several descriptive pathologic features seem to correlate with prognosis for this disease. Of these, tumor-associated tissue eosinophilia is a recently appreciated feature that has been described for other tumor systems and will require further corroboration before its full significance has been established.

Although aneuploidy is determined by considerably more objective methods, its prognostic significance in laryngeal squamous cell carcinoma is not yet clear. It appears, at present, that aneuploidy may indicate the more biologically aggressive tumors, yet those more likely to respond to cytotoxic therapy. Prospective studies utilizing fresh tissue, as opposed to paraffin-embedded specimens, with appropriate standards for determination of the diploid state, will be necessary to clarify the role of aneuploidy as an indicator of prognosis.

REFERENCES

1. Bauer WC. Varieties of squamous carcinoma—biologic behavior. Front Radiat Ther Oncol 1974;9:164–86.
2. Holm LE, Lundquist PG, Silfversward C, et al. Histological grading of malignancy in squamous cell carcinoma of the oral tongue. Acta Otolaryngol (Stockh) 1982;94:185–92.
3. Jakobson P, Killander D, Moberger G, et al. Histologic classification and grading of malignancy in carcinoma of the larynx. Acta Radiol 1973;12:1–8.
4. Broders AC. Carcinoma of the mouth; types and degrees of malignancy. Am J Roentgenol Radium Ther 1927;17:90–8.
5. Krause CJ, Carey TE, Ott RW, et al. Human squamous cell carcinoma. Arch Otolaryngol 1981;107:703–10.
6. Broders AC. Carcinoma. Grading and practical application. Arch Pathol 1926;2:376–81.
7. Goldsmith MM, Cresson DH, Arnold LA, et al. Part I. DNA flow cytometry as a prognostic indicator in head and neck cancer. Otolaryngol Head Neck Surg 1987;96:307–18.
8. Goldsmith MM, Cresson DH, Askin FB. Part II. The prognostic significance of stromal eosinophilia in head and neck cancer. Otolaryngol Head Neck Surg 1987;96:319–24.
9. Crissman JD, Liu WY, Gluckman JL, Cummings G. Prognostic value of histopathologic parameters in squamous cell carcinoma of the oropharynx. Cancer 1984;54:2995–3001.
10. McGavran MH, Bauer WC, Ogura JH. The incidence of cervical lymph node metastases from epidermoid carcinoma of the larynx and their relationship to certain characteristics of the primary tumor. A study based on the clinical and pathological findings from 96 patients treated by primary en bloc laryngectomy and radical neck dissection. Cancer 1961;14:55–66.
11. Kashima HK. The characteristics of laryngeal cancer correlating with cervical lymph node metastasis (analysis based on 40 total organ sections). In: Alberti PW, Bryce DP, eds. *Centennial Conference on Laryngeal Cancer*. New York: Appleton-Century-Crofts, 1976: 855–64.
12. Poleksic S, Kalwaic HJ. Prognostic value of vascular invasion in squamous cell carcinoma of the head and neck. Plast Reconstr Surg 1978;61:234–40.
13. Underwood JCE. Lymphoreticular infiltration in human tumors. Prognostic and biologic implications: a review. Br J Cancer 1974;30:538–48.
14. Lowe D, Fletcher CDM, Gower RL. Tumor-associated eosinophilia in the bladder. J Clin Pathol 1984;37:500–2.
15. Kapp DS, Livolsi VA. Intense eosinophilic stromal infiltrate in carcinoma of the uterine cervix: a clinicopathologic study of 14 cases. Gynecol Oncol 1983;16:19–30.
16. Pretlow TP, Keith EF, Cryar AK, et al. Eosinophil infiltration of human colonic carcinomas as a prognostic indicator. Cancer Res 1983;43:2997–3000.
17. Iwasaki K, Torisu M, Fujimura T. Malignant tumor and eosinophils. Cancer 1987;58:1321–7.
18. Yoon IL. The eosinophil and gastrointestinal carcinoma. Am J Surg 1959;97:195–200.
19. Lowe D, Fletcher CDM. Eosinophilia in squamous cell carcinoma of the oral cavity, external genitalia and anus—clinical correlations. Histopathology 1984;8:627–32.
20. Lowe D, Jorizzo J, Hutt MSR. Tumor-associated eosinophilia: a review. J Clin Pathol 1981;34:1343–8.
21. Lange P. Clinical and histological studies on cervical carcinoma: precancerosis, early metastasis, and tubular structures in lymph nodes. Acta Pathol Microbiol Scand 1960;50(Suppl 143):1–162.
22. Isaacson NH, Rapoport P. Eosinophilia in malignant tumors: its significance. Ann Intern Med 1946;25:893–902.
23. Wasserman SI, Goetzl EJ, Ellman L, Austen KF. Tumor associated eosinophilic factor. N Engl J Med 1974;290:420–4.
24. Goetzl EJ, Tashjian AH, Rubin RH, Austen KF. Production of a low molecular weight eosinophil polymorphonuclear leukocyte chemotactic factor by anaplastic squamous cell carcinoma of human lung. J Clin Invest 1978;61:770–80.
25. Kay AB, McVie JG, Stuart AE, et al. Eosinophil chemotaxis of supernatants from cultured Hodgkin's lymph node cells. J Clin Pathol 1975;28:502–5.
26. Weller PF, Goetzl EJ. The human eosinophil. Am J Pathol 1980;100:794–820.
27. Litt M. Eosinophils and antigen-antibody reactions. Ann NY Acad Sci 1964;116:964–85.
28. Parish WE. Substances that attract eosinophils in vitro and in vivo, and that elicit blood eosinophilia. Antibiot Chemother 1974;19:233–70.
29. Bostrom SG, Hart WR. Carcinomas of the cervix with intense eosinophilia. Cancer 1981;47:2887–93.
30. Goswami PK. Local leukocyte reaction to implants of carcinogen treated cells. Ind J Med Sci 1965;19:900–5.
31. Gleich GJ, Frigas E, Loegering DA, et al. Cytotoxic properties of the eosinophil major basic protein. J Immunol 1979;123:2925–7.
32. Butterworth AE, Wassom DL, Gleich GJ, et al. Damage to schistosomula of *Schistosoma mansoni* induced directly by eosinophil major basic protein. J Immunol 1979;122:222–9.
33. John EC, Klebanoff SJ. Eosinophil-mediated mammalian tumor cell

cytotoxicity: role of the peroxidase system. J Immunol 1980;124:1949–53.
34. Barlogie B, Raber MN, Schumann J, et al. Flow cytometry in clinical cancer research. Cancer Res 1983;43:3982–97.
35. Tribukait B, Gustafson H, Esposti P. Ploidy and proliferation in human bladder tumors as measured by flow cytofluorometric DNA-analysis and its reactions to histopathology and cytology. Cancer 1979;43:1742–51.
36. Tribukait B, Esposti P, Ronstrom L. Tumor ploidy for characterization of prostatic carcinoma: flow cytophotometric DNA studies using aspiration biopsy material. Scand J Urol Nephrol Suppl 1980;55:59–64.
37. Bichel P, Frederiksen P, Kjaer T, et al. Flow microfluorometry and transrectal fine needle biopsy in the classification of human prostatic carcinoma. Cancer 1977;40:1206–11.
38. Woiley RC, Schreiber K, Koss LG, et al. DNA distribution in human colon carcinoma and its relationship to clinical behavior. J Natl Cancer Inst 1982;69:15–22.
39. Atkin NB. Modal deoxyribonucleic acid value and survival in carcinoma of the breast. Br Med J 1972;1:271–2.
40. Look TA, Hayes FA, Nitschke R, et al. Cellular DNA content as a predictor of response to chemotherapy in infants with unresectable neuroblastoma. N Engl J Med 1984;311:231–5.
41. Laerum OD, Farsund T. Clinical application of flow cytometry: a review. Cytometry 1981;2:1–13.
42. Hellquist H, Olofsson J. Photometric evaluation of laryngeal epithelium exhibiting hyperplasia, keratosis, and moderate dysplasia. Acta Otolaryngol (Stockh) 1981;92:157–65.
43. Holm LE. Cellular DNA amounts of squamous cell carcinomas of the head and neck region in relation to prognosis. Laryngoscope 1982;92:1064–9.
44. Roa RA, Carey TE, Passamani PP, et al. DNA content of human squamous cell carcinoma cell lines. Arch Otolaryngol 1985;111:565–75.
45. Holm LE, Jackobsson P, Killander D, et al. DNA and its synthesis in individual tumor cells from human upper respiratory tract squamous cell carcinomas. Laryngoscope 1980;90:1209–24.
46. Gussack GS, Donnely K, Hester R, Donnell CA, Dowling EA. Flow cytometric DNA analysis of laryngeal carcinomas. Unpublished paper presented at the American Laryngological Association Meeting. April, 25, 1988, Palm Beach, FL.
47. Ensley JF, Maciorowski Z, Hassan M, et al. The potential and pitfalls of solid tumor flow cytometry with respect to squamous cell cancers of the head and neck. Unpublished data.
48. Nielsen MD, Caldarelli DD, Hutchinson JC Jr. Flow cytometric analysis of DNA contents in squamous cell carcinoma of the head and neck. Clinical correlates. Second International Conference on Head and Neck Cancer. Boston, MA 1988; abstract 216.
49. Guo, Y-C, DeSanto LW, Osetinsky GV. Prognostic implications of nuclear DNA content in squamous cell carcinoma of the head and neck. Second International Conference on Head and Neck Cancer. Boston MA, 1988: abstract 155.
50. Hedley DW, Freidlander ML, Taylor IW, et al. Methods for analysis of cellular DNA content of paraffin-embedded pathological material using flow cytometry. J Histochem Cytochem 1983;31:1333.
51. Schutte B, Reynders MMJ, Bosman FT, et al. Flow cytometric determination of DNA ploidy levels in nuclei isolated from paraffin-embedded tissue. Cytometry 1985;6:26–30.

6

Unusual Tumors of the Larynx

Idel I. Moisa, Panna Mahadevia, Carl E. Silver

Squamous cell carcinoma represents the most common type of laryngeal malignancy, accounting for approximately 90 to 95% of all cases. The remaining laryngeal cancers comprise a diverse group derived from various cell types within the larynx. The most frequently described entities within this latter group include verrucous carcinoma, salivary gland cancers, cartilaginous neoplasms, and neuroendocrine tumors. These will be discussed in this chapter. Other laryngeal malignancies are occasionally encountered and have been listed in Table 6–1.

VERRUCOUS CARCINOMA OF THE LARYNX

Verrucous carcinoma has been recognized as a distinct variant of squamous cell carcinoma with characteristic gross and microscopic findings since its original description by Ackerman in 1948.[1] The first description of this tumor occurring in the larynx was by Kraus and Perez-Mesa in 1966[2] and, since then, this tumor has been estimated to account for approximately 1 to 3.4% of laryngeal squamous cell carcinomas.[3,4] The lesion occurs most frequently in patients over the age of 50 years.[5,6] There is a male predominance, with 163 cases reported in males and only 19 in females.[7]

Although the etiology of this tumor is unclear, papilloma virus may be a possible factor. Using DNA hybridization, Abramson et al[7] demonstrated human papillomavirus (HPV-16-related) sequences in five consecutive patients with this laryngeal neoplasm. Similar findings have been reported in oral verrucous carcinomas. Most patients are cigarette smokers.

Verrucous carcinoma of the larynx is slow growing but relentlessly progressive and will cause death if untreated. The tumor is considered not to metastasize, although inflammatory cervical lymphadenopathy may often be present.[4,6,8] Fisher[5] reported five cases with proven cervical node metastases. The lymph node tumor maintained a verrucous pattern in three cases and grades I and II squamous cell carcinoma in two. It has been suggested, however, that Fisher's series may have included several cases of well-differentiated squamous cell carcinoma.[3]

Table 6–1. Primary Laryngeal Cancers

Squamous cell carcinoma	Carcinosarcoma
Verrucous carcinoma	Spindle cell (pleomorphic) carcinoma
Salivary gland tumors	Clear cell carcinoma
Adenoid cystic carcinoma	Osteosarcoma
Mucoepidermoid carcinoma	Fibrosarcoma
Acinic cell carcinoma	Fibrous histiocytoma
Cartilaginous tumors	Rhabdomyosarcoma
Chondroma	Liposarcoma
Chondrosarcoma	Plasmacytoma
Neuroendocrine tumors	Malignant lymphoma
Paraganglioma	Giant cell carcinoma
Large cell (carcinoid) neuroendocrine tumor	Melanoma
Small cell (oat cell) neuroendocrine tumor	Malignant ganglioneuroma
	Malignant mixed carcinoma

Diagnosis

Verrucous carcinoma of the larynx is usually an exophytic, grayish white tumor with filiform projections. The tumor is predominantly one of the upper larynx, occurring at or above the level of the vocal cords.[5,9] A warty appearance accounts for the name given to this tumor. Histologically, exophytic papillary fronds of extremely well-differentiated keratinizing squamous epithelial tumor cells grow inwardly with a "pushing border" into the surrounding tissue (Fig. 6–1).[4,5] As the tumor advances, keratin debris provokes an inflammatory reaction, which may produce micro- or macroabscesses. Eventually, pressure necrosis of cartilage may occur as the tumor extends into the thyroid lamina.[6]

Although pathologists have little difficulty diagnosing verrucous carcinoma when an entire surgical specimen is studied, it is often perplexing to diagnose this neoplasm accurately from a biopsy specimen. The tumors lack the usual histologic features of malignancy and are often misdiagnosed as benign epithelial lesions, such as squamous cell hyperplasia with or without keratosis, squamous cell papilloma, and pseudoepitheliomatous hyperplasia. On the other hand, the exophytic nature of the lesions can cause a fairly impressive clinical picture. Fisher's statement that "the grading of malignancy of verrucous carcinoma is often overestimated by the clinician examining the endolarynx and the biopsy section is often underdiagnosed by the surgical pathologist" accurately reflects the experience of most surgeons.[5] Nuclear DNA analysis[10] and image analysis of cells of verrucous carcinoma[11] may assist in the early histologic diagnosis of this tumor. The latter may be particularly helpful in distinguishing verrucous carcinoma from benign squamous papilloma.

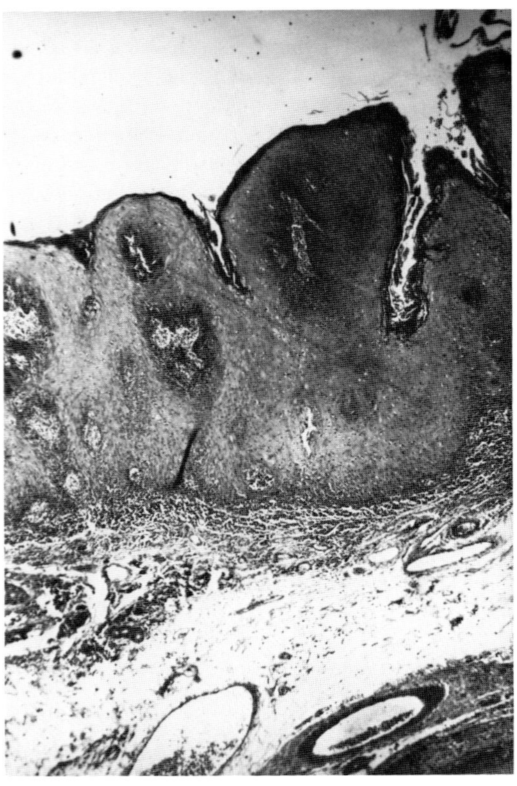

Figure 6–1. Verrucous carcinoma: Representative field of a large warty lesion showing papillary squamous epithelial proliferation characterized by excessive keratinization on the surface, extremely bland cytology, and noninfiltrating "pushing" type of lower border. (Hematoxylin & eosin; × 55.)

Treatment

Although radiation therapy continues to be recommended, this modality remains controversial because verrucous carcinoma has been reported to undergo anaplastic change after radiation and because this tumor is often radioresistant. The potential for radiation-induced anaplastic transformation, originally reported by Perez et al[12] in three of eight cases of oral verrucous carcinoma, has been subsequently noted in the larynx. Although the reason for this anaplastic transformation remains unclear, several possibilities exist. Smith et al[13] identified epithelial membrane antigen and cytokeratin, two established markers of epithelial differentiation, in the cytoplasm of their anaplastic carcinoma specimens and concluded that radiation directly transforms the well-differentiated squamous proliferation into an anaplastic carcinoma. Abramsom et al[7] have suggested that radiation may have the potential to activate or alter HPV-16-related sequences in verrucous carcinoma, resulting in anaplastic transformation.

On the other hand, examples of anaplastic transformation of verrucous carcinoma following radiation may represent cases in which foci of poorly differentiated carcinoma coexisted with verrucous carcinoma.[14] In a review of verrucous carcinoma of the oral cavity by McDonald et al,[15] approximately 30% of cases did not fulfill the diagnostic criteria for verrucous carcinoma and many of these cases had histologic foci of apparent well-differentiated squamous cell carcinoma. Of 53 verifiable lesions treated with radiation, anaplastic transformation occurred in only four. Eleven cases previously reported to be examples of radiation-induced anaplastic conversion appeared to have been initially inappropriately diagnosed as verrucous carcinoma. The coexistence of foci of less differentiated squamous cell carcinoma within verrucous lesions of the oral cavity has been reported to be as high as 20%.[16]

Notwithstanding these arguments, conversion of verrucous carcinoma of the larynx to a more aggessive lesion following radiation has been clearly documented by several authors. Biller et al[17] reported that radiation appeared to enhance local invasion in all three cases thus treated. Anaplastic transformation following radiotherapy was reported in one of four cases by Van Nostrand and Olofsson[18] and in one case by Smith et al.[13] Edstrom et al[19] reported the development of regional metastases of poorly differentiated carcinoma in two of six patients treated with radiation. In view of this, it may be safe to conclude that there is a small, but nevertheless definite, risk of conversion of verrucous carcinoma of the larynx to a significantly more aggressive tumor following radiation therapy.

An additional, perhaps less controversial, objection to radiotherapy in the treatment of verrucous carcinoma of the larynx is the high rate of failure following this therapeutic modality. Among 29 cases of verrucous carcinoma of the larynx reported in the literature with sufficient detail to assess treatment, Biller and Bergman[4] noted that four patients were treated with radiotherapy and 25 were treated surgically. Irradiation achieved two 3-year cures and there were two recurrences before 3 years. Twenty-three of the surgically treated patients remained tumor-free for periods of 1 to 10 years, and two developed recurrence within 1 year of treatment. The authors also noted that the majority of extralaryngeal lesions treated by irradiation had failed.

Lundgren et al[9] reported failure of response to radiotherapy in 13 (46%) of 28 patients and recurrence after radiotherapy in an additional three patients; there were no recurrences among the 16 patients treated surgically. These authors believe that surgery is more effective for primary control of verrucous carcinoma, since this tumor, although not radioresistant, seems less radiosensitive than ordinary squamous cell carcinoma. They concluded that the mainstay of treatment for this tumor should be conservation laryngeal surgery, saving radiotherapy for more extensive lesions that would otherwise require total laryngectomy. Total laryngectomy would be indicated for large lesions that fail to respond to radiation or when other considerations preclude partial laryngectomy.

Perhaps the highest incidence of radiation failure has been demonstrated by Ferlito and Rechner.[3] In their review of 90 reported cases of verrucous carcinoma initially treated with irradiation, the neoplasm persisted or recurred in 64 (77.1%).

Although a few authors believe this laryngeal tumor should be treated by repeated endoscopic resections in the form of vocal cord stripping, endolaryngeal laser surgery, cryosurgery, or suction diathermy, such procedures result in a high rate of recurrence.[20–22] One reported patient required 16 procedures within a 5-year period.[20] Although endoscopic laser surgery may be acceptable in managing certain small lesions, most authorities are of the opinion that conservation surgery remains the therapeutic modality of choice for verrucous carcinoma of the larynx. The excellent cure rates achieved with these procedures have already been discussed. The surgery should preserve as much laryngeal structure and function as possible. Since cervical lymph node metastases are rare, if not nonexistent, elective neck dissection is not indicated. Because inflammation secondary to the tumor often causes impressive reactive lymphadenopathy, however, a neck dissection may occasionally be performed. For large lesions, total laryngectomy may be preferable to radiation in view of the small but definite risk of anaplastic transformation following the latter. Kanee[10] has reported response of verrucous carcinoma to methotrexate and Biller and Bergman[4] have suggested this may be the treatment of choice for inoperable lesions.

SALIVARY GLAND CANCERS OF THE LARYNX

The larynx possesses a rich supply of mucous glands that are of the mixed seromucous type and are exocrine in function. These glands are most concentrated in the ventricular folds, the subglottic surface of the anterior commissure, and the saccules, and are more sparsely distributed on the free portion of the epiglottis, aryepiglottic folds, arytenoids, and ventricles. They are usually absent on the true cords.[23]

Although the histologic pattern of salivary gland cancers of the larynx is diverse, the most commonly reported malignancies include adenocarcinoma, adenoid cystic carcinoma (cylindroma) and mucoepidermoid carcinoma. Each has been reported with approximate equal frequency (Table 6–2). Because of their rarity, much of the early information regarding these tumors was derived from grouping these malignancies under the general category of adenocarcinoma or salivary gland tumors of the larynx.[24,25] Treatment suggestions have thus ranged from the most conservative surgery feasible regardless of histopathologic type[25] to total laryngectomy with ipsilateral radical neck dissection, without regard to the stage of disease.[24] At the present time, it appears that laryngeal adenocarcinoma, adenoid cystic carcinoma, and mucoepidermoid carcinoma represent distinct clinical entities. Although surgery is the generally preferred modality of treatment, the type of operation should depend on the histologic type and extent of the tumor.

Adenocarcinoma

A review of the literature has revealed 75 cases of adenocarcinoma of the larynx.[24–33] This malignancy usually occurs in patients in the sixth decade[28,29,34] and shows a significant male predominance (Table 6–2). A supraglottic, submucosal mass often described as large, bulky, smooth, and nonulcerated is characteristic. Histologically, these tumors form glandular structures lacking specific features to categorize them further. The extent of glandular differentiation varies. The poorly differentiated tumors show solid aggregates of epithelial tumor cells with little or no obvious glandular lumina (Fig. 6–2). Such a diagnosis requires exclusion of large cell neuroendocrine carcinoma and metastatic carcinoma. Most patients present with advanced disease. Cervical metastasis is present at initial presentation in the majority of cases; in the remainder, adenopathy usually develops subsequently. The average duration of symptoms may range from 15 months[7] to 33 months.[24]

Table 6-2. Salivary Gland Cancers of the Larynx

CANCER	NO. CASES	MALE (%)	SUPRAGLOTTIC (%)	GLOTTIC (%)	TRANSGLOTTIC (%)	SUBGLOTTIC (%)
Adenocarcinoma	75	86	81	4.2	8.5	6.3
Adenoid-cystic carcinoma	74	59	39	5.3	1.7	54
Mucoepidermoid carcinoma	77	84	59	28	7	6

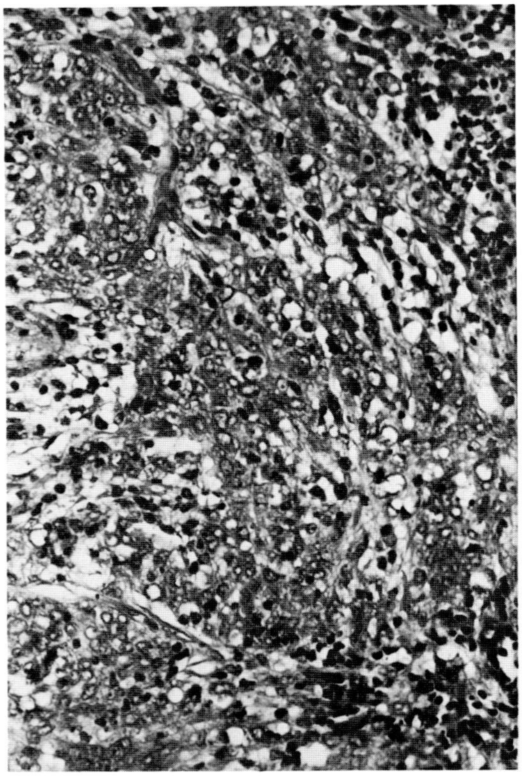

Figure 6–2. Poorly differentiated adenocarcinoma: ill-defined groups of cohesive polygonal cells with vesicular nuclei, nucleoli, and moderate amount of pale vaculolated cytoplasm. Lymphoplasmacytic cells are seen in and around the groups of carcinoma cells. (Hematoxylin & eosin; × 352.)

As a result of advanced disease at initial presentation, most patients require total laryngectomy and radical neck dissection. Radiation is suggested as palliative therapy for patients who are considered inoperable or as postoperative therapy in an attempt to improve survival. Despite such aggressive treatment, most patients die from distant metastases (primarily to the lungs and liver) within 2 years.[24,26,30,34] Whicker et al[28] have suggested that this tumor may have a greater tendency for noncontiguous spread so that block excision with clear margins may not constitute adequate treatment of this disease; thus explaining, in part, the dismal prognosis. Five-year survival rate is approximately 12.5%.[26]

Adenoid Cystic Carcinoma

A review of the literature has revealed 74 cases of adenoid cystic carcinoma of the larynx.[29,32,35,36] This tumor usually occurs in patients in the fifth decade,[29,35] mostly male. The observation that patients with adenoid cystic carcinoma of the larynx tend to be younger than those with adenocarcinoma has been noted in several studies. The majority of tumors are either subglottic or supraglottic. Of 60 cases, in which the site of origin was indicated, 31 were subglottic and 22 were supraglottic (Table 6–2).

These tumors tend to be large and advanced, presenting as a firm, smooth mass at direct laryngoscopy. Airway obstruction is commonly produced by subglottic tumors.[26,35] Pain is a prominent symptom and may be attributed to the propensity of adenoid cystic carcinoma for perineural invasion.[28,35,36] The average duration of symptoms is estimated to be 16 to 20 months.[26,35]

Adenoid cystic carcinomas of the larynx arise submucosally. Microscopically, they are composed of small uniform cells arranged in one or more of three patterns; tubular, cribriform (including cylindromatous), and solid (Fig. 6–3). Perineural and intraneural invasion by tumor is frequently seen with extension of tumor well beyond the clinically visible tumor mass. This makes clinical diagnosis and complete resectability difficult and places the patient at a high risk for local recurrence.[25,35] In one study three of four patients with this pathologic feature experienced local recurrence and ultimately died from disease, whereas three of four patients without this feature survived.[29]

The treatment of choice, according to most authorities, is surgical; total or partial laryngectomy for control of the primary tumor. Since the frequency of clinical adenopathy associated with this tumor is low (10 to 15%), prophylactic neck dissection is not generally advocated.[29,36] In the presence of palpable cervical lymphadenopathy, radical neck dissection and postoperative radiation therapy is recommended.[37] Postoperative irradiation should also be considered when there is evidence of perinueral invasion, when margins of resection are inadequate, or as palliation for inoperable lesions.[36]

Although Toomey et al,[26] in 1967, reported a 5-year survival

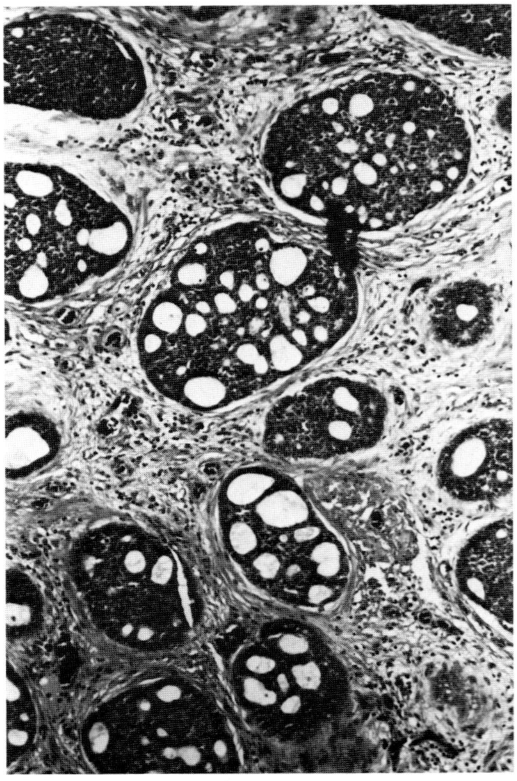

Figure 6–3. Adenoid cystic carcinoma: Rounded groups of small uniform tumor cells arranged in the classic cribriform pattern. (Hematoxylin & eosin; × 140.)

rate of only 28.6%, recent results have been more encouraging. Cohen et al,[29] in 1985, reported 2- and 5-year survival rates of 87.5 and 44.4%, respectively. The latter figure did not seem to decrease at 8 years. Patients with adenoid cystic carcinoma of the larynx tend to live for relatively long periods despite frequent local recurrences or distant metastases to the lungs. In Cohen's series, patients survived an average of 38.4 months after the first recurrence and 36 months from the time of the appearance of pulmonary metastases.[29] Recurrent disease must therefore be treated aggressively. Local recurrences should be treated with cure as the goal, whereas the presence of pulmonary metastases should not deter adequate local treatment.[29,37] Resection of a solitary pulmonary lesion in patients with adenoid cystic carcinoma of the larynx may be justified.

Mucoepidermoid Carcinoma

A literature review has revealed 77 cases of mucoepidermoid carcinoma of the larynx.[38–42] This tumor demonstrates a significant male predominance and occurs most often in the seventh decade in males and the sixth decade in females (Table 6–2).[42] One instance occurred in a 13-year-old boy.[41] The majority of cases have been supraglottic, with most of the remainder glottic. Forty-two of 71 cases, where such information was available, were supraglottic; 20 were glottic.

The histopathologic picture of better-differentiated low-grade mucoepidermoid carcinoma is distinctive (Fig. 6–4). In the larynx, however, this tumor, particularly when of high grade, has often been mistaken for squamous cell carcinoma (Fig. 6–5).[39,42] This was most striking in the report by Ferlito et al[43] in which 10 of 11 cases were initially diagnosed as squamous cell carcinoma. For this reason, Ho et al[39] recommend more frequent employment of mucicarmine stains in histologic study of laryngeal carcinomas, emphasizing the importance of this distinction since mucoepidermoid carcinoma is thought to respond poorly to radiation therapy.

The clinical course and prognosis of patients with mucoepidermoid carcinoma of the larynx are determined by the histologic grade of the tumor.[38] Overall, this tumor carries a better prognosis than does adenocarcinoma of the larynx.[44] Damiani et al[38] reported 3-, 5-, and 10-year survival rates of 100% regardless of clinical stage in eight patients classified as having low-grade mucoepidermoid carcinoma of the larynx; a literature review revealed 91% 5-year survival rate in patients with similar lesions. In contrast, only five of ten patients with adenosquamous high-grade mucoepidermoid carcinoma and 50% of patients with comparable histologic picture reported in the literature survived 3 years.

The treatment of mucoepidermoid carcinoma of the larynx is mainly surgical because this tumor is at best only partly radiosensitive.[42] The exact nature of the operation should

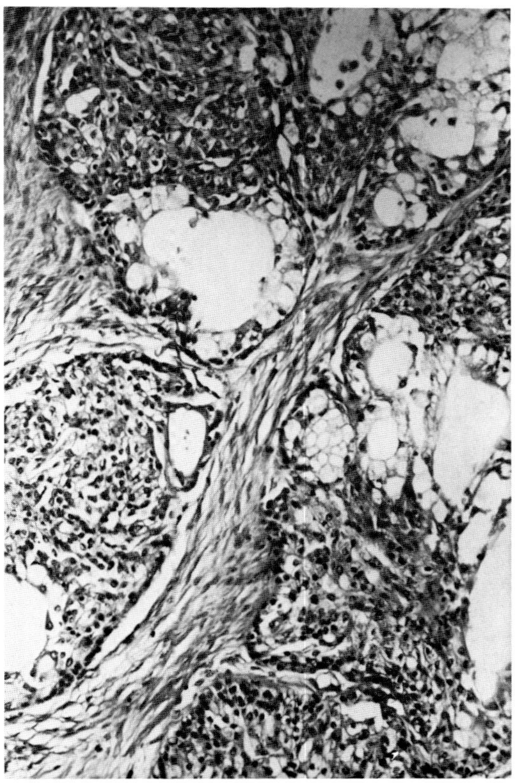

Figure 6–4. Low-grade mucoepidermoid carcinoma: Glandular structures formed by mucous cells with vaculolated-to-clear cytoplasm are seen to merge imperceptibly with intermediate type polygonal cells. (Hematoxylin & eosin; × 140.)

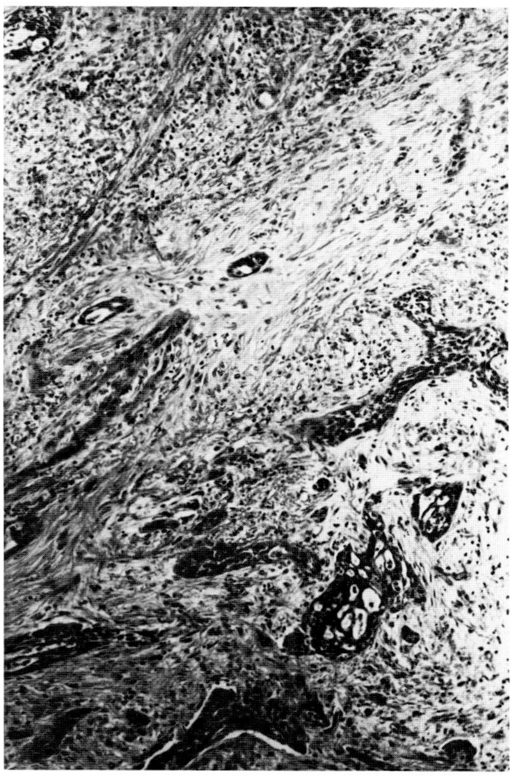

Figure 6–5. High-grade mucoepidermoid carcinoma: Irregular nests of infiltrating epidermoid cells without evident keratinization are seen with a prominent fibrous and inflammatory stromal reaction. A few nests exhibit glandular lumina, which were shown to contain mucin by special staining; intracellular mucin was also demonstrable in these areas. (Hematoxylin & eosin; × 140.)

depend on histologic grade, extent of tumor involvement, and status of the neck.[44] Low-grade tumors confined to the supraglottis may be adequately treated by partial laryngectomy, whereas larger tumors or those involving the subglottis may require total laryngectomy.[38,44] On the other hand, high-grade mucoepidermoid carcinoma of the larynx should be treated by total laryngectomy and postoperative radiation therapy.[22,30,45] Although radical neck dissection is reserved for situations in which there is palpable lymphadenopathy, Ferlito et al[43] and Barnes[46] have advocated elective neck dissection in high-grade tumors. Spiro et al[30] found that treatment failure was often due to uncontrolled cervical node metastases or distant spread, rather than local recurrence, and suggested that results might have been improved if regional nodes had been treated more aggressively, either by more liberal use of elective radical neck dissection or by combinations of radiation therapy and surgery.

CARTILAGINOUS TUMORS OF THE LARYNX

Most cartilaginous tumors of the larynx occur in males over the age of 50 years.[47] Lesions may arise in elastic cartilage (epiglottis and vocal process of arytenoid) or in hyaline cartilage (cricoid, thyroid, and arytenoid body cartilages). The former are small, do not recur after simple excision, and may represent foci of metaplastic elastic cartilage rather than tumor.[48–50] The true cartilaginous neoplasms of the larynx, on the other hand, originate from the hyaline cartilage of the cricoid cartilage (70%), thyroid cartilage (20%), and body of arytenoid cartilage (10%).[51–55] Of 157 cases reported in the literature, 37 were classified as chondrosarcomas, whereas the others appeared histologically benign.[47,51] For clinical purposes, the majority of chondromatous tumors are considered to be low-grade malignancies, because their benign-looking histologic appearance often does not reflect their actual biologic behavior. Actually, the histopathologic distinction between chondroma and low-grade chondrosarcoma is often difficult and may even differ among pathologists. Although Goethals et al[51] believed that 18 of 22 cartilaginous laryngeal tumors showed histologic features of malignancy, none of these lesions metastasized and only six recurred locally. A significant proportion of "well-differentiated" lesions may recur locally, metastasize, and eventually cause death.[48,55,56]

Diagnosis

Cartilaginous tumors of the cricoid usually arise from the posterior plate, extending into the airway, with resultant airway obstruction, dysphagia, or hoarseness.[47,51] The most common physical finding is a subglottic, smoothly rounded submucosal mass. In contrast, cartilaginous tumors of the thyroid ala commonly protrude laterally, presenting as a cervical mass.[56] Radiographs are helpful in establishing the diagnosis and usually show an opaque rounded mass, often with mottled calcification.[11] Biopsy may be difficult and often unsuccessful because of the hardness and submucosal depth of the mass. Histologically, the tumors resemble hyaline cartilage, but exhibit excessive cellularity and atypical nuclear features that increase in degree with increasing grade of malignancy (Fig. 6–6).

Treatment

Benign chondromas and chondrosarcomas should be treated similarly. Surgery is the only available treatment and must be used because even benign cartilaginous tumors are uniformly lethal without treatment.[56] In general, complete excision of the lesion with its perichondrial capsule and a reasonably generous margin of normal tissue is the treatment of choice.[51,52] Most cases can be successfully managed by conservative resection (laryngofissure or thyrotomy with local resection). Despite the high recurrence rate, it appears that this conservative approach is justified in most cases, since the overwhelming majority of lesions (85%) are clinically low-grade malignancies that do not metastasize. Recurrences usually appear after reasonably long intervals and are usually treatable by further conservative surgery.[53] This point of view has been disputed by Chambers and Friedel,[47] who believe that a more aggressive surgical approach should be adopted because of the high recurrence rate reported in the literature. For poorly differentiated (high-grade) chondrosarcomas, however, or for extensive tumors involving more than half the cricoid cartilage, total laryngectomy is recommended.[52,53,55]

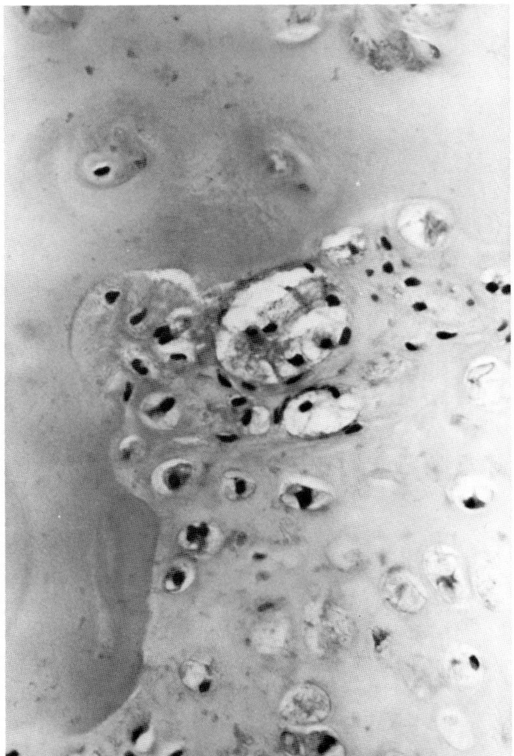

Figure 6–6. Low-grade chondrosarcoma: The tumor cartilage in the lower right two thirds appears cellular with frequent binucleated chondrocytes and a mild degree of nuclear pleomorphism. (Hematoxylin & eosin; × 140.)

NEUROENDOCRINE TUMORS OF THE LARYNX

Neuroendocrine neoplasms are derived from cells belonging to the dispersed neuroendocrine system, a diverse group of cells widely distributed throughout the body and sharing the ability to synthesize, store, and in some instances secrete a variety of biogenic amines and peptides[57,58] (Table 6–3). In the larynx, two such cells, the paraganglion chief cell and the Kulchitsky cell, have been identified and three types of neuroendocrine tumors have been described. Paragangliomas of the larynx arise from the paraganglion chief cell while large and small cell neuroendocrine tumors are thought to arise from the Kulchitsky cell. Although demonstrating similar neuroendocrine features according to ultrastructural and histochemical studies, the neoplasms represent distinct clinical entities.

Paragangliomas of the Larynx

The paraganglion chief cell is the characteristic cell in paraganglia, vascular structures located throughout the body. This cell appears to be derived from neural crest cells that migrate along the route of the vagus and then the superior and recurrent laryngeal nerves, aggregating to form superior and inferior pairs of paraganglia in the larynx.[59–62] The former are subepithelial structures on either side of the midline just above the anterior ends of the false vocal cords, whereas the latter are more variable in location, occurring bilaterally anywhere from the inferior horn of the thyroid cartilage to the cricotracheal area. Unusual locations of laryngeal paraganglia include the midline of the cricothyroid membrane, the pyriform sinus, within branches of the superior and recurrent laryngeal nerves, and the capsule of the thyroid gland.[63–65]

The nomenclature regarding tumors arising from laryngeal paraganglia is confusing. Terms such as "chemodectoma," "glomus tumor of the larynx," "chromaffinoma," or "nonchromaffin paraganglioma of the larynx" are misleading because they imply properties that do not apply to laryngeal paraganglia or to tumors derived from these structures. In the larynx, a more logical nomenclature emphasizing the anatomic site seems appropriate. Tumors arising from laryngeal paraganglia are therefore best termed "paragangliomas of the larynx" (PGL).

A recent review of the literature revealed 68 reported cases of PGL.[64,66,67] Although occasionally found in children, PGL occur most commonly in adults and have an approximately equal sex distribution. This tumor develops most often in the supraglottic region, with the aryepiglottic fold representing the single most common site of involvement. Hoarseness, dysphagia, throat or ear pain, and respiratory complaints were often present for long periods prior to tumor recognition (average, 42.4 months). Our review supports the opinion that the symptoms of throat pain and referred otalgia indicate a poor prognosis.[68,69] In this study, nine of 15 (60%) patients reporting these symptoms succumbed to the disease. In most, the endoscopic appearance was that of a reddish or bluish, submucosal, smooth swelling of the supraglottic larynx. Profuse bleeding was frequently reported at biopsy. Microscopically, laryngeal paragangliomas appear similar to paragangliomas elsewhere in the body (Fig. 6–7). Cervical metastasis at initial presentation was reported in 15 of the 68 patients; 11 had metastasis to lymph nodes and four of the cervical masses were due to extralaryngeal extension of tumor to the cervical region or thyroid gland. The determinate survival for the entire group at 1, 5, and 10 years was 90, 60, and 50%, respectively.

The classification of PGL as benign or malignant remains controversial. Some authors believe that the behavior of PGL is similar to the majority of paragangliomas, which are benign and rarely metastasize, and the PGL reported to have a malignant course probably represent misdiagnosed lesions.[70,71] Others have reported a significantly higher metastatic rate for PGL.[69,72,73] In this review, PGL were characterized by cervical lymph node metastasis at initial presentation in 22% of cases, subsequent distant metastasis in 22%, and overall mortality of 24%. This suggests that PGL have considerable malignant potential and that biologic behavior must be considered "indeterminate" in cases that present without initial metastatic disease.

NEUROENDOCRINE STUDIES

Of the 68 PGL reported in the literature, 17 were studied ultrastructurally. All demonstrated neurosecretory vesicles characterized by a centrally located electron-dense core surrounded by a limiting membrane with an intervening lucent halo. Ten PGL were studied cytochemically (histochemically or immunohistochemically). Seven demonstrated evidence of a variety of biogenic amines or peptides; most cases demonstrated more than one such substance.[67]

Clinical hormonal activity resulting from noradrenaline[74] and calcitonin[72] secretion was demonstrated in two patients with PGL; in three others hypertension and tachycardia disappeared after tumor removal. Elevated urinary levels of catecholamines were noted, suggesting catecholamine secretion.[75,76]

TREATMENT

PGL appear to be radioresistant and are best managed surgically.[63,64,74,77,78] Because of their vascularity, PGL may

Table 6–3. Neuroendocrine Tumors of the Larynx

CANCER*	NO. CASES	MALE (%)	SUPRAGLOTTIC (%)	GLOTTIC (%)	TRANSGLOTTIC (%)	SUBGLOTTIC (%)	NSV*	PCF*
PGL	68	49	90	1	1	8	17/17	7/10
LCT	42	68	85	0	10	5	30/30	14/14
SCT	74	72	52	15	15	18	23/23	6/6

*PGL: paraganglioma of the larynx; LCT: large cell neuroendocrine tumor of the larynx; SCT: small cell neuroendocrine tumor of the larynx; NSV: neurosecretory vesicles; PCF: positive cytochemical findings.

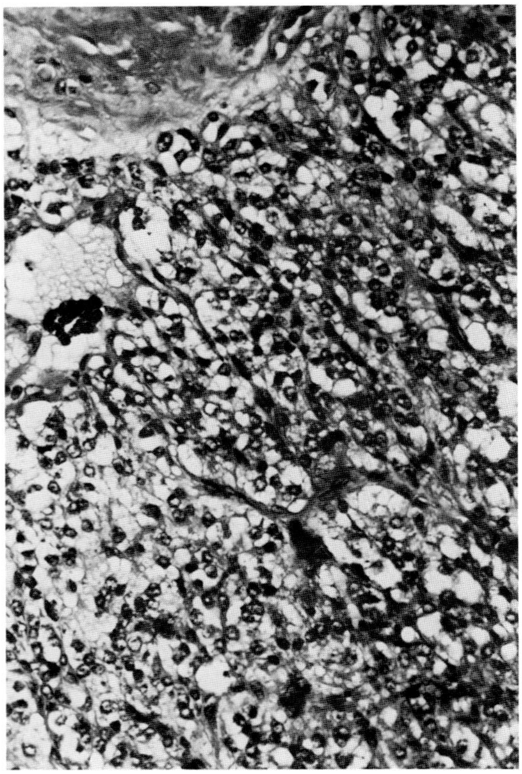

Figure 6–7. Paraganglioma: Trabecular and occasional rounded nests of tumor cells with very delicate and vascular supporting stroma. Immunoperoxidase stain for chromagranin was positive in a large number of tumor cells and for S_{100} protein positive in a few scattered sustentacular cells. (Hematoxylin & eosin; × 352.)

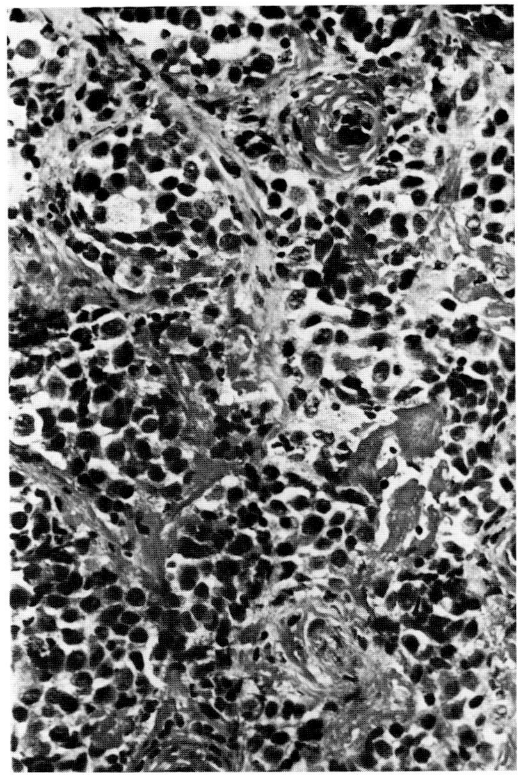

Figure 6–8. Large cell neuroendocrine carcinoma: Tumor exhibits an organoid growth pattern; nests of polygonal to round tumor cells are seen. Grimelius stain demonstrated abundant argyrophilic granules. Using immunoperoxidase method, diffuse positive cytoplasmic staining was observed for neuron-specific enolase, chromagranin, calcitonin, and cytokeratin. (Hematoxylin & eosin; × 352.)

cause profuse bleeding at biopsy. These tumors may be delineated by angiography and may be dissected more easily following embolization.[79–81] Chemotherapy has not been shown to be effective in the management of PGL.[24]

Large Cell Neuroendocrine Tumors of the Larynx

The Kulchitsky cell, which is thought to give rise to carcinoid tumors and oat cell carcinomas in the gastrointestinal and respiratory tracts, has been identified in the respiratory epithelium of the larynx.[82–84] Carcinoid tumors and oat cell carcinomas are considered to be the well-differentiated and the poorly differentiated ends of a spectrum of tumors derived from the Kulchitsky cell.[85–88] Histologically, these neuroendocrine laryngeal tumors have been more appropriately classified as large cell and small cell neuroendocrine tumors of the larynx (Figs. 6–8, 6–9).[71]

A comprehensive review of the literature revealed 42 large cell neuroendrocrine tumors of the larynx (LCT).[67,71] These neoplasms occurred exclusively in adults, demonstrated a male predominance, and occurred more frequently in the supraglottis. A prolonged period (average, 22.6 months) of hoarseness, dysphagia, and throat and ear pain was characteristic prior to tumor recognition. LCT often presented as a polypoid or sessile mass. Cervical metastasis at initial presentation in 39% of cases and a mortality rate of 45% was reported. The determinate survival rate for these patients at 1, 5, and 10 years was 82, 34, and 28%. Recurrences, usually in regional lymph nodes, and distant metastases, frequently to skin, were often noted.

NEUROENDOCRINE STUDIES

Thirty of the 42 LCT reported in the literature were studied ultrastructurally.[67] All demonstrated neurosecretory vesicles similar to those described for PGL. Fourteen LCT were studied cytochemically (histochemically or immunohistochemically); all demonstrated evidence of biogenic amines or peptides, or both.

LCT did not exhibit clinical hormonal activity, although elevated urine levels of 5-hydroxyindoleacetic acid, a serotonin metabolite, was reported in two cases.[89,90]

TREATMENT

LCT are radioresistant and should be managed surgically.[69,91–94] Because they may have prominent perineural extension peripheral to the main tumor mass, these tumors should be resected beyond the clinically detectable tumor margins.[94] Since this tumor shows a high likelihood of early

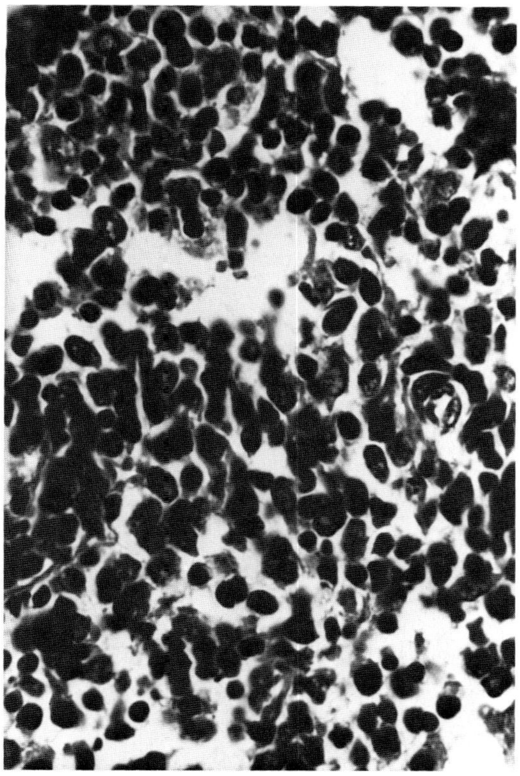

Figure 6–9. Lymph node metastasis of small cell neuroendocrine carcinoma of epiglottis. Tumor cells exhibit anaplastic nuclei and very scanty cytoplasm, resembling oat cell carcinoma. (Hematoxylin & eosin; × 880.)

cervical metastasis, some authors advocate elective neck dissection.[86,95] Chemotherapy has not proven effective in the management of LCT.[74]

Small Cell Neuroendocrine Tumors of the Larynx

A literature review revealed 74 small cell neuroendocrine tumors (SCT) of the larynx.[67,96,97] These neoplasms occurred most commonly in adult males. The tumor occurred more often in the supraglottic regions, but other regions of the larynx were commonly affected. In our review, a brief period (average, 3.8 months) of hoarseness and dysphagia was characteristic prior to tumor recognition. SCT are the most aggressive neuroendocrine cancers of the larynx. They are characterized by cervical metastasis at initial presentation in 59% of cases, subsequent distant metastasis in 55% of cases, and a mortality rate of 73%. The determinate survival rates for these patients at 1 and 5 years were 54 and 14%, respectively. The majority of patients were dead of disease within 13 months. Although there were local and regional recurrences, most patients developed diffuse metastasis to liver and bone.

NEUROENDOCRINE STUDIES

Twenty-three of the 74 SCT reported in the literature were studied ultrastructurally.[67] All demonstrated neurosecretory vesicles similar to those described for PGL and LCT. All six cases studied cytochemically (histochemically or immunohistochemically) demonstrated evidence of a variety of biogenic amines and peptides.

Clinical hormonal activity was reported in four cases of SCT; two patients demonstrated clinical and chemical evidence of the syndrome of inappropriate secretion of antidiuretic hormone,[98,99] one developed the myasthenic Eaton-Lambert syndrome,[100] and one demonstrated clinical and chemical evidence of elevated levels of corticotropin.[101]

TREATMENT

SCT, because of its very aggressive nature, should be considered to have metastasized at initial presentation. A thorough metastatic workup therefore is indicated. The use of radiation and chemotherapy has resulted in improved survival. Based on this review, it would appear that therapeutic irradiation to the larynx and neck and adjuvant chemotherapy offer the least disabling and most effective form of therapy.[95,97,102] The role of surgery for this tumor is limited and may include cases of early localized disease in which conservative resection can potentially remove all tumor before dissemination has occurred or cases of recurrent or persistent local or regional disease after radiation or chemotherapy.

FUTURE STUDIES

Neuroendocrine tumors are demonstrably capable of producing a broad spectrum of immunoreactive substances, the monitoring of which may be useful in diagnosis, prognostication, and therapy evaluation.[97,103–105] At present, however, several difficulties exist. First, to be useful as a tumor marker, the substance in question should vary with disease activity and response to treatment and should be produced in amounts that can be measured in the serum. Although several potential neuroendocrine tumor "markers" have been proposed, a characteristic one having all these properties has not yet been found. Second, as most neuroendocrine tumors and the overwhelming majority of neuroendocrine tumors of the larynx are not hormonally active, monitoring a secretory product would be difficult.

Ultrastructural and cytochemical data, however, may be clinically useful. The demonstration of neuroendocrine features by these techniques on a biopsy specimen may be a useful method of following patients with these laryngeal neoplasms. Also, although no characteristic "marker" for these neuroendocrine tumors was clearly evident in this review, neurospecific enolase (NSE) was demonstrated in all 11 LCT and all five SCT in which it was studied. Although not investigated in the cases of PGL reviewed here, this enzyme has been consistently demonstrated in each of 18 paragangliomas of other head and neck sites.[67,103,104] Thus, at present, NSE appears to be the most characteristic chemical indicator for neuroendocrine tumors of the larynx. It is hoped that the future discovery of neuroendocrine markers may aid in detection as well as monitoring of patients with these laryngeal neoplasms.

REFERENCES

1. Ackerman LV. Verrucous carcinoma of the oral cavity. Surgery 1948;23:670–8.

2. Kraus FT, Perez-Mesa C. Verrucous carcinoma. Clinical and pathologic study of 105 cases involving the oral cavity, larynx and genitalia. Cancer 1966;19:26–38.
3. Ferlito A, Rechner G. Ackerman's tumor (verrucous carcinoma) of the larynx. Cancer 1980;46:1617–30.
4. Biller HF, Bergman JA. Verrucous carcinoma of the larynx. Laryngoscope 1975;85:1698–700.
5. Fisher HR. Verrucous carcinoma of the larynx—a study of its pathologic anatomy. Can J Otolaryngol 1975;4:270–7.
6. Batsakis JG, Hybels R, Crissman JD, et al. The pathology of head and neck tumors: XV. Verrucous carcinoma. Head Neck Surg 1982;5:29–38.
7. Abramson AL, Brandsma J, Steinberg B, Winkler B. Verrucous carcinoma of the larynx. Possible human papillomavirus etiology. Arch Otolaryngol 1985;111:709–15.
8. Ryan RE, DeSanto LW, Devine KD, Weiland LH. Verrucous carcinoma of the larynx. Laryngoscope 1977;87:1989–94.
9. Lundgren JAV, Van Nostrand P, Harwood AR, et al. Verrucous carcinoma (Ackerman's tumor) of the larynx: diagnostic and therapeutic considerations. Head Neck Surg 1986;9:19–26.
10. Kanee B. Oral florid papillomatosis complicated by verrucous squamous carcinoma. Treatment with methotrexate. Arch Dermatol 1969;99:196.
11. Michaels L, Cooper J, Brewer CJ, et al. Image analysis in histological diagnosis of verrucous squamous carcinoma of the larynx. J Pathol 1984;143:329.
12. Perez CA, Kraus FT, Evans JC, et al. Anaplastic transformation in verrucous carcinoma of the oral cavity after radiation therapy. Radiology 1966;86:108–15.
13. Smith RRL, Kuhajda F, Harris A. Anaplastic transformation of verrucous carcinoma following radiotherapy. Am J Otolaryngol 1985;6:448–52.
14. Rider WD. Toronto experience of verrucous carcinoma of the larynx. In: Alberti PW, Bryce DP, eds. *Workshops from the Centennial Conference on Laryngeal Cancer*. New York: Appleton-Century-Crofts, 1976:460.
15. McDonald J, Crissman J, Gluckman J. Verrucous carcinoma of the oral cavity. Head Neck Surg 1982;5:22–7.
16. Medina JE, Dichtel W, Luna MA. Verrucous squamous carcinomas of the oral cavity. Arch Otolaryngol 1984;110:437–40.
17. Biller HF, Ogura JH, Bauer WC. Verrucous cancer of the larynx. Laryngoscope 1971;81:1323–9.
18. Van Nostrand AWP, Olofsson J. Verrucous carcinoma of the larynx. Cancer 1972;30:691–702.
19. Edstrom S, Johansson SL, Lindstrom J, Sandin I. Verrucous squamous cell carcinoma of the larynx: evidence for increased metastatic potential after irradiation. Otolaryngol Head Neck Surg 1987;97:381–4.
20. Lee RJ. Verrucous carcinoma of the larynx. Otolaryngol Head Neck Surg 1988;98:593–5.
21. Glanz H, Kleinsasser O. Verrucous carcinoma of the larynx—a misnomer. Arch Otorhinolaryngol 1987;244:108–11.
22. Maw RA, Cullen RJ, Bradfield JWB. Verrucous carcinoma of the larynx. Clin Otolaryngol 1982;7:305–11.
23. Nassar VH, Bridger P. Topography of the laryngeal mucous glands. Arch Otolaryngol 1971;94:490–8.
24. Cady B, Rippey JH, Frazell EL. Non-epidermoid cancer of the larynx. Ann Surg 1968;167:116–20.
25. Sessions DG, Murray JP, Bauer WC, Ogura JH. Adenocarcinoma of the larynx. Can J Otolaryngol 1975;4:293–6.
26. Toomey JM. Adenocarcinoma of the larynx. Laryngoscope 1967;77:931–61.
27. Bloom J, Behar AJ, Zikk D, Shanon E. Adenocarcinoma of the epiglottis. Report of a case and review of the literature. Arch Otolaryngol Head Neck Surg 1987;113:1330–3.
28. Whicker JH, Neel HB, Weiland LH, Devine KD. Adenocarcinoma of the larynx. Ann Otol 1974;83:487–90.
29. Cohen J, Guillamondegui OM, Batsakis JG, Medina JE. Cancer of the minor salivary glands of the larynx. Am J Surg 1985;150:513–8.
30. Spiro RH, Lewis JS, Hajdu SI, Strong EW. Mucous gland tumors of the larynx and laryngopharynx. Ann Otol 1976;85:498–503.
31. Dogra TS. Adenocarcinoma of the larynx. J Laryngol Otol 1973;87:685–9.
32. Houle JA, Batsakis JG. Primary adenocarcinoma of the larynx. J Laryngol Otol 1976;90:1159–63.
33. Ferlito A. Histological classification of larynx and hypopharynx cancers and their clinical implications. Acta Otolaryngol (Suppl) 1976;342:1–88.
34. Fechner RE. Adenocarcinoma of the larynx. Can J Otolaryngol 1975;4:284–9.
35. Olofsson J, Van Nostrand AWP. Adenoid cystic carcinoma of the larynx. A report of four cases and a review of the literature. Cancer 1977;40:1307–13.
36. Tewfik TL, Novick WH, Schipper HM. Adenoid cystic carcinoma of the larynx. J Otolaryngol 1983;12:151–4.
37. Eschwege F, Cachin Y, Micheau CH. Treatment of adenocarcinomas of the larynx. Can J Otolaryngol 1975;4:290–2.
38. Damiani JM, Damiani KK, Hauck K, Hyams VJ. Mucoepidermoid-adenosquamous carcinoma of the larynx and hypopharynx: a report of 21 cases and a review of the literature. Otolaryngol Head Neck Surg 1981;89:235–43.
39. Ho KJ, Jones JM, Herrera GA. Mucoepidermoid carcinoma of the larynx: a light and electron microscopic study with emphasis on histogenesis. South Med J 1984;77:190–5.
40. Supiyaphun P, Vaewuichit K, Pongsupat T, et al. Mucoepidermoid carcinoma of the larynx: report of 2 cases. J Med Assoc Thai 1986;69:500–4.
41. Mitchell DB, Humphreys S, Kearns DB. Mucoepidermoid carcinoma of the larynx in a child. Int J Pediatr Otorhinolaryngol 1988;15:211–5.
42. Cumberworth VL, Narula A, MacLennan KA, Bradley PJ. Mucoepidermoid carcinoma of the larynx. J Laryngol Otol 1989;103:420–3.
43. Ferlito A, Rechner G, Bottin R. Mucoepidermoid carcinoma of the larynx. A clinicopathological study of 11 cases with review of the literature. ORL 1981;43:280–99.
44. Binder WJ, Som P, Kaneko M, Biller HF. Mucoepidermoid carcinoma of the larynx. A case report and review of the literature. Ann Otol 1980;89:103–7.
45. Thomas K. Mucoepidermoid carcinoma of the larynx. J Laryngol Otol 1971;85:261–7.
46. Barnes L. Mucoepidermoid carcinoma. In: *Surgical Pathology of the Head and Neck*, Vol. 1. New York: Marcel Dekker, 1985:187.
47. Chambers RG, Friedel W. Chondrosarcoma of the larynx. Laryngoscope 1976;86:713–7.
48. Hyams VJ, Rabuzzi DD. Cartilaginous tumors of the larynx. Laryngoscope 1970;80:755–67.
49. Fechner RE. Chondrometaplasia of the larynx. Arch Otolaryngol 1984;110:554.
50. Hill MJ, Taylor GL, Scott GBD. Chondromatous metaplasia in the human larynx. Histopathology 1980;4:205.
51. Goethals PL, Dahlin DC, Devine KD. Cartilaginous tumors of the larynx. Surg Gynecol Obstet 1963;117:77–82.
52. Batsakis JG. *Tumors of the head and neck*. 2nd ed. Baltimore: Williams & Wilkins, 1979:52.
53. Cantrell RW, Reibel JF, Jahrsdoerfer RA, Johns ME. Conservative surgical treatment of chondrosarcoma of the larynx. Ann Otol Rhinol Laryngol 1980;89:567–71.
54. Gorenstein A, Neel HB, Weiland LH, Devine KD. Sarcomas of the larynx. Arch Otolaryngol 1980;106:8–12.
55. Huizenga C, Balogh K. Cartilaginous tumors of the larynx: a clinicopathologic study of 10 new cases and a review of the literature. Cancer 1970;26:201.
56. Cocke EW. Benign cartilaginous tumors of the larynx. Ann Otol Rhinol Laryngol 1962;72:1678–730.
57. Pearse AGE. The APUD cell concept and its implications in pathology. Pathol Annu 1974;9:27–41.
58. Pearse AGE, Takor TT. Embryology of the diffuse neuroendocrine system and its relationship to the common peptides. Fed Proc 1979;38:2288–94.
59. Glenner GG, Grimely PM. Tumors of the extra-adrenal paraganglionic system (including chemoreceptors). In: *Atlas of tumor pathology*, 2nd series, fascicle 9. Washington, DC: AFIP, 1974.
60. Lawson W. The neuroendocrine nature of the glomus cell: an experimental, ultrastructural and histochemical tissue culture study. Laryngoscope 1980;90:120–44.
61. Pearse AGE, Polak JM, Rost FWD, et al. Demonstration of the neural

crest origin of type I (APUD) cells in the avian carotid body, using a cytochemical marker system. Histochemie 1973;34:191–203.
62. Lawson W, Zak F. The glomus bodies (paraganglia) of the human larynx. Laryngoscope 1974;84:98–111.
63. Zak FG, Lawson W. Glomic (paraganglionic) tissue in the larynx and capsule of the thyroid gland. Mt Sinai J Med 1972;39:82–90.
64. Zak FG, Lawson W. *The paraganglionic chemoreceptor system: physiology, pathology, and clinical medicine*. Heidelberg: Springer-Verlag, 1982.
65. Dahlquist A, Carlson B, Hellstrom S. Paraganglia of the human recurrent laryngeal nerve. Am J Otolaryngol 1985;7:366–9.
66. Hanna GS, Ali H. Chemodectoma of the larynx. J Laryngol Otol 1986;100:1081–7.
67. Moisa I. Neuroendocrine tumors of the larynx. Head and Neck (to be published).
68. Ali S, Aird DW, Bihari J. Pain-inducing laryngeal paragangliomas (non-chromaffin). J Laryngol Otol 1983;97:181–8.
69. Stanley JS, Weiland LH, Neel HB. Pain-inducing laryngeal paraganglioma: report of the 9th case and review of the literature. Otolaryngol Head Neck Surg 1985;95:107–12.
70. Batsakis JG. *Tumors of the head and neck, clinical and pathological correlations*, 2nd ed. Baltimore: Williams & Wilkins, 1979:377.
71. Woodruff JM, Shah JP, Huvos AG, et al. Neuroendocrine carcinomas of the larynx. Am J Surg Pathol 1985;9:771–90.
72. Justrabo E, Michaels R, Calmettes C, et al. An uncommon apudoma: a functional chemodectoma of the larynx, report of a case and review of the literature. Acta Otolaryngol (Stockh) 1980;89:135–43.
73. Lawson W. Glomus bodies and tumors. NY State J Med 1980;80:1567–75.
74. Vetters JM, Toner PG. Chemodectoma of larynx. J Pathol 1970;101:259–65.
75. Ishida M, Hasegawa S, Sato T, Tateishi R. Glomus tumor (nonchromaffin-paraganglioma) of the larynx. Laryngoscope 1971;81:957–61.
76. Harrison DFN. Unusual tumors. In: Suen JY, Myers EN, eds. *Cancer of the head and neck*. New York: Churchill Livingstone, 1981: 663–4.
77. Hooper R. Chemodectoma of the glomus laryngicum superior. Laryngoscope 1972;82:686–92.
78. Uvarov AA, Ogoltsova ES. Malignant paraganglioma of the larynx. Vestn Otorinolaringol 1983;1:76–7.
79. Sneige N, Mackay B, Ordonez NG, Batsakis JG. Laryngeal paraganglioma. Arch Otolaryngol 1983;109:113–7.
80. Basset JM, Paraire F, Francois M, Fleury P. Deux novelles tumeurs rares du larynx; un lipome, un chemodectome. Ann Otolaryngol 1982;99:151–8.
81. Klap P, Reizine D, Monteil JP, et al. Tumors and vascular malformations of the larynx. Angiographic aspects and therapeutic implications. Ann Otolaryngol 1984;101:579–83.
82. Ewen SWB, Bussolotti G, Pearse AGE. Uptake of 1-DOPA and 1-5-hydroxytryptophan by endocrine-like cell in the rat larynx. Histochem J 1971;4:103–10.
83. Kirkeby S, Romert P. Argyrophilic cells in the larynx of the guinea-pig demonstrated by the method of grimelius. J Anat 1977;123:87–92.
84. Lewis DJ, Prentice DE. The ultrastructure of rat laryngeal epithelia. J Anat 1980;130:617–32.
85. Bensch KG, Corrin B, Pariente R, Spencer H. Oat-cell carcinoma of the lung—its origin and relationship to bronchial carcinoid. Cancer 1968;22:1163–78.
86. Goldman NC, Katibah GM, Medina J. Carcinoid tumors of the larynx. Ear Nose Throat J 1985;64:52–8.
87. Gould VE, Linnoila I, Memoli VA, Warre WA. Neuroendocrine components of the bronchopulmonary tract: hyperplasias, dysplasias, and neoplasms. Lab Invest 1983;49:519–37.
88. Gould VE, Memoli V, Chejfic G, Johannessen JV. The APUD cell system and its neoplasms, observations on the significance and limitations of the concept. Surg Clin North Am 1979;59:93–107.
89. Carles D, Devars F, Traissac L, et al. Carcinoide primitif du larynx. Ann Pathol 1983;3:65–8.
90. Blok PHHM, Manni JJ, Borek PVD, et al. Carcinoid of the larynx: a report of three cases and a review of the literature. Laryngoscope 1985;95:715–9.
91. Goldman NC, Hood CI, Singleton GT. Carcinoid of the larynx. Arch Otolaryngol 1969;90:90–3.
92. Gapany-Gapanavicius B, Kenan S. Carcinoid tumor of the larynx. Ann Otol 1981;90:42–7.
93. Tamai S, Iri H, Maruyama T, et al. Laryngeal carcinoid tumor: light and electron microscopie studies. Cancer 1981;48:2256–9.
94. Mills SE, Johns ME. Atypical carcinoid tumor of the larynx, a light microscopic and ultrastructural study. Arch Otolaryngol 1984;110:58–62.
95. Snyderman C, Johnson JJ, Barnes L. Carcinoid tumor of the larynx: case report and review of the world literature. Otolaryngol Head Neck Surg 1986;95:158–64.
96. Ferlito A. Diagnosis and treatment of small cell carcinoma of the larynx: a critical review. Ann Otol Rhinol Laryngol 1986;95:590–600.
97. Baugh RF, Wolf GT, Beals TF, et al. Small cell cancer of the larynx: results of therapy. Laryngoscope 1986;96:1283–90.
98. Trotoux J, Glicmananas M, Sterkers O, et al. Syndrome der schwartz-bartter: revelateur d'un cancer larynge sons-glottique a petites cellulles. Ann Otolaryngol 1979;96:349–58.
99. Pazdur R, Bonami P, Gould VE, et al. Neuroendocrine small cell carcinoma in miscellaneous primary sites: implications for staging and therapy. Anticancer Res 1981;1:335–40.
100. Medina JE, Moran M, Goepfert H. Oat cell carcinoma of the larynx and Eaton-Lambert syndrome. Arch Otolaryngol 1984;110:123–6.
101. Bishop J, Osamura RY, Tsutsumi Y. Multiple hormone production in an oat cell carcinoma of the larynx. Acta Pathol Jpn 1985;35:915–23.
102. Vrabec DP, Bartels LJ. Small cell anaplastic carcinoma of the larynx: review of the literature and report of a case. Laryngoscope 1980;90:1720–6.
103. Warren WH, Caldarelli DD, Javid H, et al. Neuroendocrine markers in paragangliomas of the head and neck. Ann Otol Rhinol Laryngol 1981;94:555–9.
104. Warren WH, Lee I, Gould VE, et al. Paragangliomas of the head and neck: ultrastructural and immunohistochemical analysis. Ultrastructural Pathol 1985;8:333–43.
105. Baugh RF, Wolf GT, McClatchey KD. Small cell carcinoma of the head and neck. Head Neck Surg 1986;8:343–54.

PART TWO

Imaging

7

Evaluation and Staging of Laryngeal and Hypopharyngeal Cancer by Computed Tomography and Magnetic Resonance Imaging

Anthony A. Mancuso

This chapter has several goals: to show state-of-the-art images and describe how they may be obtained on virtually all but the oldest computed tomography (CT) and magnetic resonance imaging (MRI) equipment; to demonstrate the natural history and typical spread patterns of laryngeal and hypopharyngeal cancer; to identify areas where imaging can critically influence treatment decisions; and to set in perspective the role of CT relative to other imaging techniques, in particular MR.

Because of the technical demands required to obtain accurate information, detailed protocols have been developed to exploit the full potential of current CT and MRI units[1–3] (Table 7–1). Results are best when such protocols are supervised and interpreted by a physician who fully understands the implications of the data being gathered, the natural history of the disease, and the limitations of the imaging techniques.

ANATOMY

This section emphasizes those aspects of laryngeal and hypopharyngeal anatomy that are essential to understanding the predominantly cross-sectional imaging techniques used. The axial plane shows the deep spread patterns of tumors in the larynx to the best advantage with few exceptions. With MR multiplanar images with good contrast resolution are possible. The indications and real need for coronal and sagittal images are limited and may be most useful for reviewing pathoanatomic studies, such as those shown in Chapter 2, and for gaining a three-dimensional concept of the spread patterns of the disease. Because of CT and MRI, the third dimension (deep spread) of tumor can now be seen routinely in exquisite detail.

The larynx and hypopharynx are intimately related and may be thought of as one unit. The anterior wall of the hypopharynx forms the posterior wall of the larynx. The lateral portions of the hypopharynx, and the pyriform sinuses, extend anteriorly, coming to lie between the deep spaces of the larynx and its framework to some extent. The mucosal surfaces and landmarks in the larynx are well known to those diagnosing and treating cancer and will not be reviewed here. The emphasis in modern cross-sectional imaging is on evaluation of tumor spread to and beyond the deep tissue planes that lie between the mucosa and laryngeal framework, as well as to and beyond the framework itself.[4–17] These are areas of spread that cannot be adequately evaluated by physical examination or older diagnostic imaging techniques. Mucosal spread is evaluated by modern endoscopic techniques. With this combination, the team treating laryngeal cancer can now know the full anatomic extent as well as the depth of penetration and volume of tumor. Imaging of the deep extent of laryngeal and hypopharyngeal cancer has limitations and pitfalls. These will be discussed as the pertinent anatomy and spread patterns are presented.

Mucosa

Modern contrast-enhanced CT normally shows the mucosal surfaces of the larynx as smooth and nonenhancing (Figs. 7–1 to 7–4). The hypopharyngeal mucosa, however, frequently "enhances" (concentrates intravenous medium). This is usually most obvious along the posterior pharyngeal wall and in the postcricoid region (Fig. 7–5). It is more obvious in the pyriform sinuses when they are collapsed rather than distended. This tendency for enhancement is normal and varies among individuals and with the rate and timing of contrast injection. The

Table 7-1. CT Protocols

EXTENT OF STUDY	GANTRY ANGLE	SLICE THICKNESS	FOV	REFORMATIONS	BONE ALGORITHM USED	COMMENT
Larynx and hypopharynx (a) 1 cm above hyoid to 1 cm above FVC	(a) Parallel to TVC or C4-C5/C5-C6 disc (obtain scout during suspended inspiration). See text This is a must	(a) 3 mm contigious	(a) 14-16 cm for larger patients 12-14 cm for smaller patients	(a) Reformations for transglottic tumor may be done (evaluate ventricle) Sagittal reformation may be done for PES or anterior commissure spread	(a) Rarely for cartilage detail	In supraglottic lesions look for tongue base/preepiglottic spread. In glottic lesions evaluate ventricle, subglottic extent carefully. In hypopharynx note extent in postcricoid-apex region and exolaryngeal spread 1.5-2.0 mm sections are sometimes necessary in these areas
(b) FVC to bottom of cricoid	(b) As in a.	(b) 3 mm contiguous	(b) 14-16 cm; 12-14			In all lesions carefully evaluate cartilages
(c) Optional: Repeat FVC to mid-cricoid during quiet breathing	(c) As in a (may want to retake scout in quiet breathing to reangle gantry and localize FVC-TVC levels)	(c) 3 mm contiguous	(c) 14-16 cm; 12-14	(c) No		Quiet breathing and suspended inspiration help in evaluation of laryngeal ventricle, anterior and posterior commissure, upper subglottic regions
Node survey C1-C2 posterior belly digastric to sternal notch. See comments	Parallel to TVC or C4-C5	3 mm thick by 5 mm increments	14-16 cm; 12-14	No		Most nodes will be covered by laryngeal sections complete by adding additional cuts—above higher sections to look for retropharyngeal nodes if advanced neck disease is present; below lowest sections to finish staging of lower neck. Good contrast enhancement is mandatory

FOV: field of view; TVC: true vocal cords; PES: preepiglottic space; FVC: false vocal cords.

enhancing mucosal surface is usually slightly irregular and less than 1 to 2 mm thick.

Deep Spaces

The paraglottic (paralaryngeal) and preepiglottic spaces lie between the mucosa and the laryngeal framework (cartilages and connecting membranes and ligaments). Over the years, there has been some debate over whether these should be subcompartmentalized or named differently but, at this time, these terms are generally well accepted.[4,18–22]

The paraglottic (paralaryngeal) space is paired and roughly symmetrical (Fig. 7–6). It is the largest connecting space in the larynx. In the supraglottic larynx it surrounds the laryngeal ventricle and continues cephalad adjacent to the preepiglottic space. There is no substantive boundary between the preepiglot-

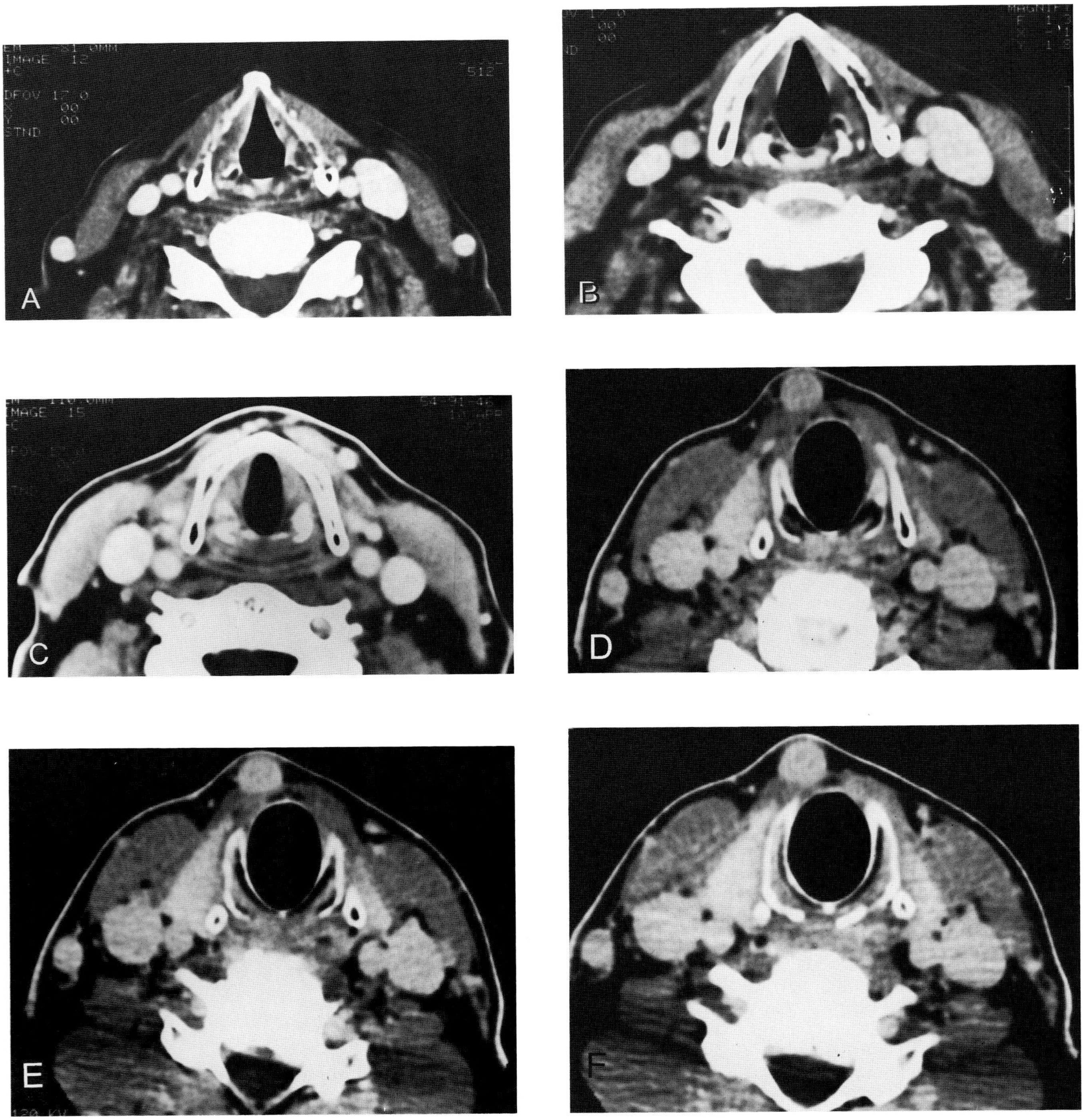

Figure 7–1. Axial computed tomography images from the false cord level through the subglottic region. Levels correlate with labeled anatomic diagram in Figure 7–2. (From Mancuso.[1] Reprinted with permission.)

tic and paraglottic spaces (Figs. 7–3, 7–4). This also means that the paraglottic spaces freely communicate across the midline via the preepiglottic space. Some authors suggest that the quadrangular membrane be considered the medial border of the paraglottic space and the space between the mucosa and quadrangular membrane be called the supraglottic space.[4] This probably is a needless exercise because the quadrangular membrane is neither visible on imaging studies nor does it seem to serve as a significant boundary to tumor spread.[18–22]

The paraglottic space may be thought of as extending "into" the aryepiglottic folds to surround the laryngeal vestibule posteriorly (Fig. 7–5). In this manner it lies deep to the endolaryngeal surface of the aryepiglottic folds medially and to the mucosa of the medial wall of the pyriform sinus laterally. It also lies

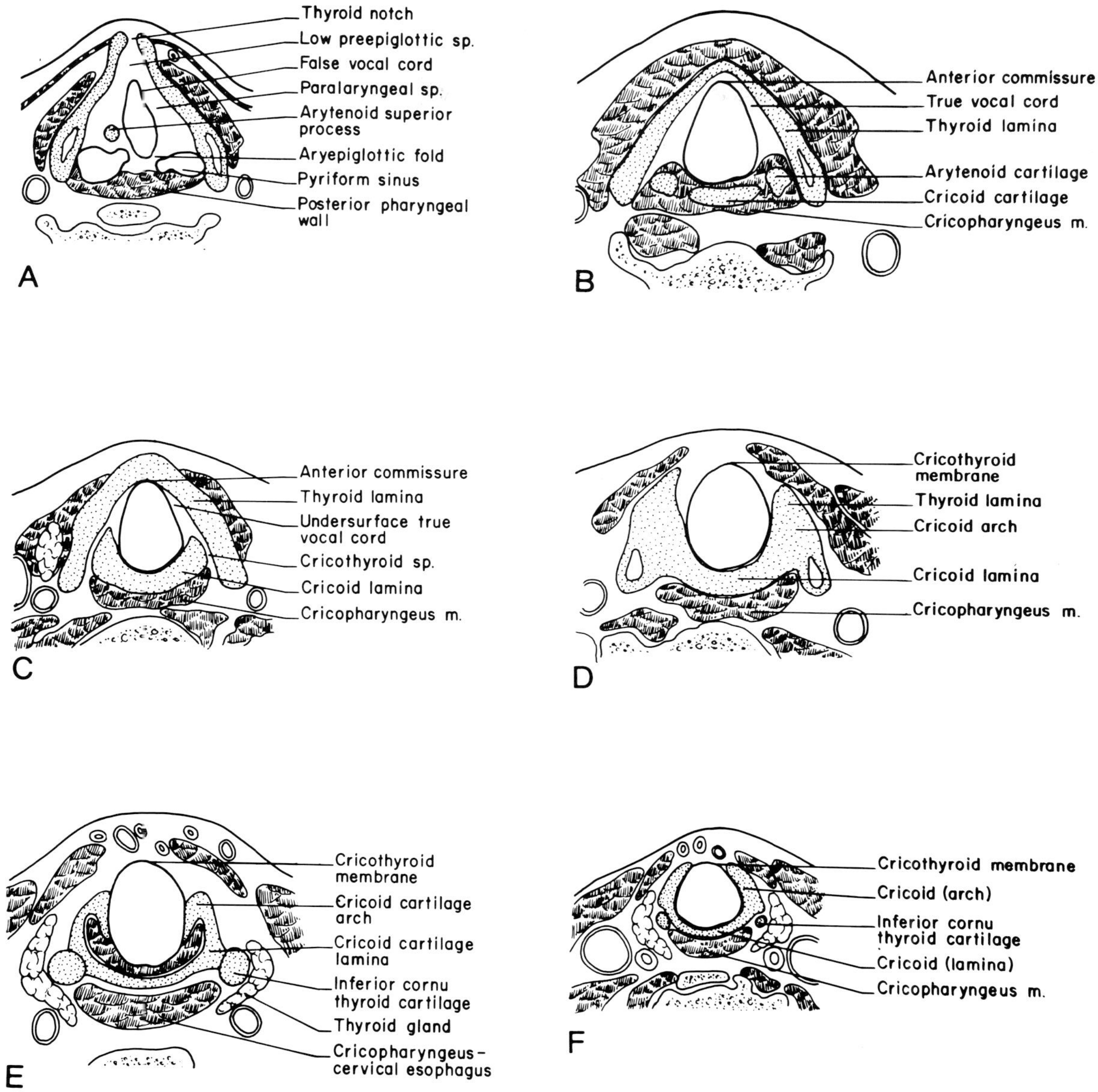

Figure 7–2. Labeled anatomic diagram to correlate with sections shown in Figure 7–1. sp: space; m: muscle. (From Mancuso.[1] Reprinted with permission.)

anterior to the pyriform sinus. The paraglottic spaces are in continuity anteriorly via the preepiglottic space but are discontinuous posteriorly where they are separated by the arytenoid, corinculate, and cuneiform cartilages and their associated ligaments (Fig. 7–5). In the supraglottic larynx the paraglottic space mainly contains fat (Fig. 7–3). There is an extensive interface between the fat-containing space and the perichondrium of the thyroid cartilages as well as the thyrohyoid membrane. At and above the level of the false cords, one may see thin bands of muscle within the fat (Figs. 7–1, 7–3, 7–5). The appendix of the laryngeal ventricle (saccule) may appear as a round or oval air space in the anterior third of the paraglottic space, a common normal variant (Fig. 7–5).

At the glottic level, the medial boundary of the paraglottic space is the conus elasticus (Fig. 7–6). This elastic cone extends from the vocal ligament, which runs the full length of the true vocal cord, to the upper edge of the cricoid cartilage. The elastic cone is an important barrier to tumor spread, which can be seen on high-resolution MRI of laryngeal specimens but to date is not consistently visualized in vivo on CT or MRI. The elastic cone blends with the cricothyroid membrane anterolaterally; their condensation anteriorly is named the cricothyroid ligament. More posterolaterally, the thinner cricothyroid membrane forms the lateral boundary of the paraglottic space. At the true cord level, the medial thyroarytenoid muscle occupies most of the volume of the paraglottic space (Fig. 7–5). A thin band of fat may be visible between the muscle and the thyroid cartilage.

The subglottic space lies medial to the elastic cone (Fig. 7–6). In contrast to the supraglottic space already discussed in the subglottic region the elastic cone presents a significant boundary

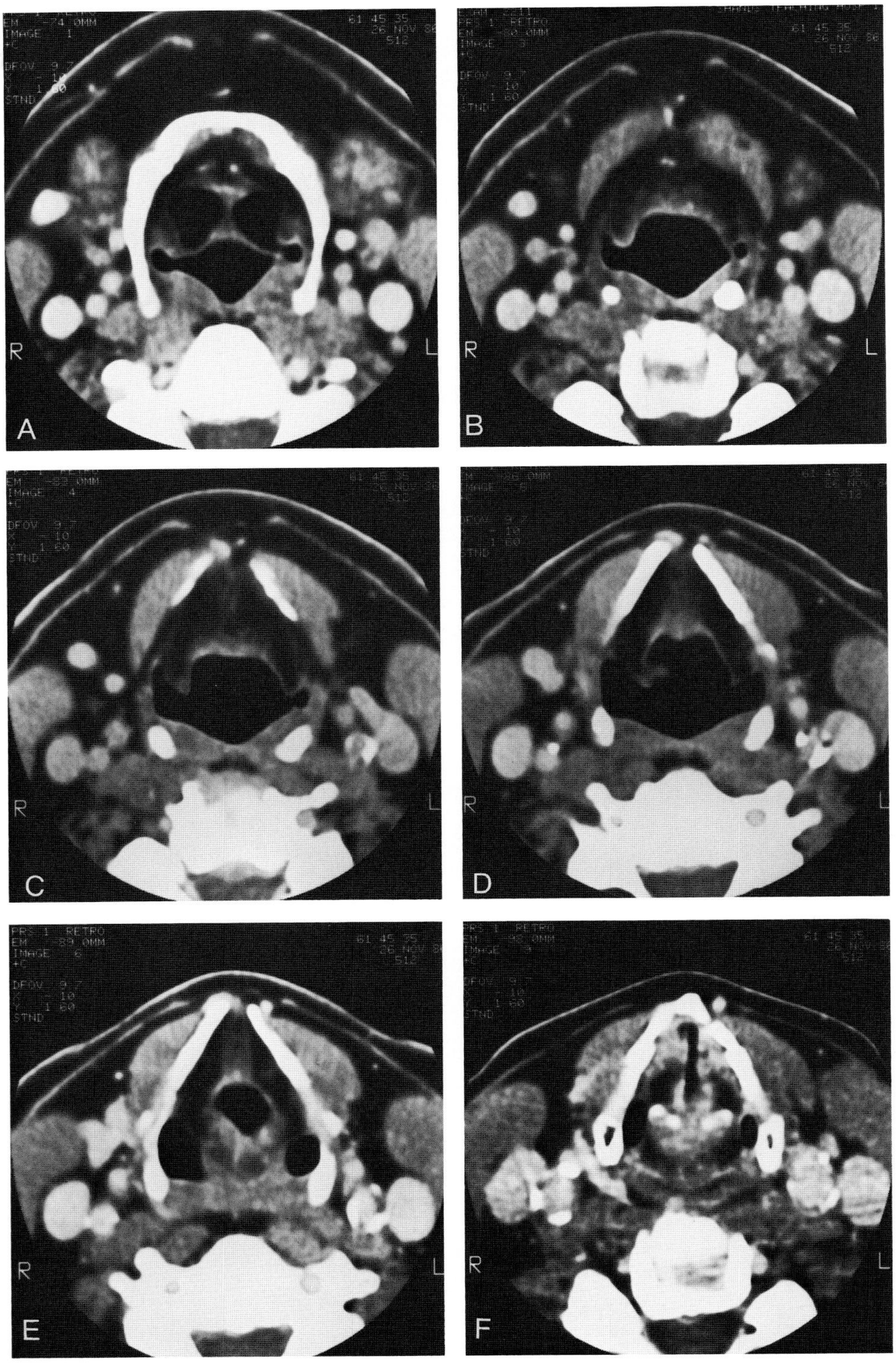

Figure 7–3. Axial computed tomography images through the supraglottic larynx. Correlate anatomy with labeled line diagrams in Figure 7–4. (From Mancuso.[1] Reprinted with permission.)

to tumor spread. In the subglottic space the mucosa is closely applied to the elastic cone, cricothyroid membrane, or perichondrium of the cricoid cartilage. As a result, there is normally no radiographically visible tissue thickness between the cricoid cartilage and the airway (Figs. 7–1, 7–2), and there is no barrier to contralateral spread of tumor in the subglottic region.

The preepiglottic space is the other important deep space of the larynx (Fig. 7–7). This fat-filled space lies between the infrahyoid epiglottis and the thyroid laminae inferiorly, and the infrahyoid epiglottis and thyrohyoid membrane superiorly (Figs. 7–3, 7–4). The preepiglottic space is bounded cranially by the thin hyoepiglottic ligament, which presents no significant

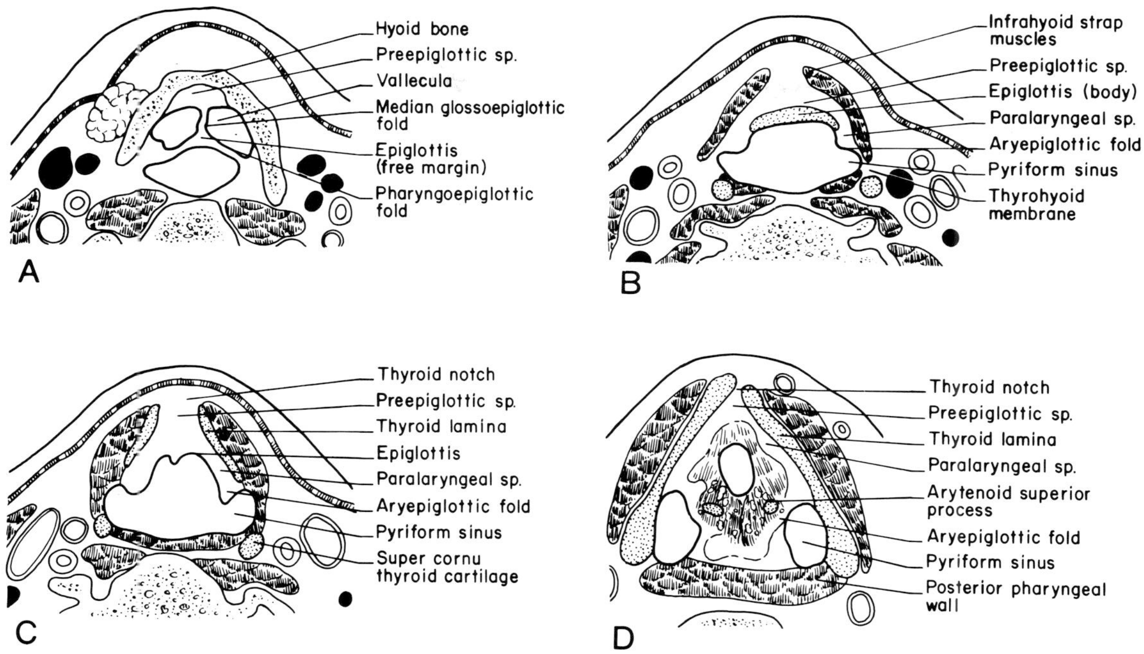

Figure 7–4. Labeled anatomic diagram of the supraglottic larynx to correlate with sections shown in Figure 7–3. sp: space. (From Mancuso.[1] Reprinted with permission.)

barrier to tumor spread[18–22] and is essentially in continuity with the core of intrinsic muscles which make up the tongue base. Caudally, the preepiglottic space ends at the petiole of the epiglottis. The infrahyoid epiglottis tapers considerably from its cranial to caudal aspects; it may be considered as an inverted pyramid with its base at the tongue base and apex immediatedly superior to the anterior commissure. The thyroepiglottic ligament attaches the epiglottis to the thyroid cartilage.

Laryngeal Framework

The cricoid cartilage surrounds the airway and is the base of the laryngeal framework. The cricoid has two ossification centers on each side, one above and one below the cricothyroid joint. Ossification is not complete in men until the fifth and women until the eighth decades of life.[4] The cricothyroid membrane runs from the inferior margin of the thyroid cartilage to the superior margin of the cricoid, and is pierced by neurovascular bundles (Figs. 7–1, 7–2). The thyroid cartilage overlies and protects the airway anterolaterally. Its appearance and that of the cricoid cartilage change dramatically on serial axial sections, and thus serve as useful landmarks for identifying the level of the section. The superior and inferior cornua, as well as the cricoid lamina, mark the most posterior extent of the laryngeal skeleton. The thyroid cornua articulate with the cricoid (cricothyroid joint) inferiorly and are attached to the greater horns of the hyoid bone superiorly via the thyrohyoid ligaments. Ossification of thyroid cartilage, like cricoid, is age- and sex-dependent. In males, ossification begins posteriorly and inferiorly with a second ossification center arising more anteriorly.[4] By 30 to 40 years of age, all but the upper anterior edges are usually ossified. In women, the second (more anterior) ossification center seldom forms. The arytenoid cartilage is usually heavily calcified and may, if large enough, have a visible marrow cavity. The epiglottic cartilage calcifies enough to be seen on CT in about 1 to 2% of patients.

The degree of variation in mineralization of the laryngeal cartilages should be obvious from this discussion. This variation is reflected and magnified by CT cross-sections. In any patient the calcification/ossification of the thyroid and cricoid cartilages will be roughly symmetrical, but often the larynx is tilted slightly relative to the axial scan plane. Moreover, the constantly curving contours of the cartilages in any plane sectioned often results in an asymmetrical or incompletely mineralized appearance. All these factors produce difficulty in diagnosing subtle cartilage invasion on CT. Some of these may be overcome with MRI. An ossified area may contain a visible fat-filled marrow space. Consideration of all possible variations must be left to the reader.

The connecting membranes of the larynx are not visualized on CT or MR images. Their location can be estimated by the position of the infrahyoid strap muscles. These muscles are visible on all sections through the larynx and hypopharynx, but are most obvious on the sections where there are gaps between the hyoid bone and thyroid cartilage and the cricoid and thyroid cartilages (Fig. 7–3). They are seen as oblong, tissue-density structures usually outlined by fat on either side. The connecting membranes are situated on the deep surface of the muscle.

TECHNIQUES OF EXAMINATION

Computed Tomography

From 1973 to 1985, CT equipment was in a rapid state of evolution. Expensive equipment often became obsolete by the

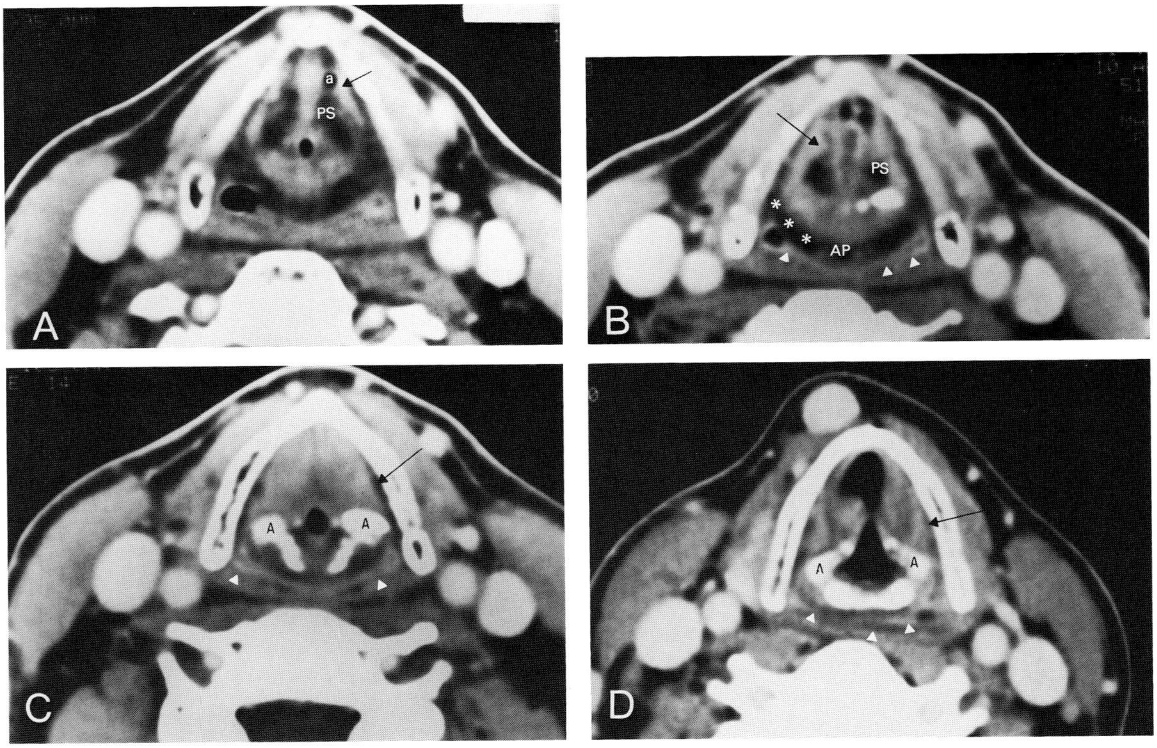

Figure 7–5. Additional axial computed tomography sections to supplement basic normal anatomy shown in Figures 7–1 to 7–4. These scans were done during breathholding to reduce motion artifacts. Breathholding may cause the false cord, ventricular, and true cord sections to appear as if the airway is nearly obliterated, as seen above. One must become familiar with these appearances for reasons outlined in the text. **A**: The false cords are apposed in the midline. Deeper structures, including the appendix of the laryngeal ventricle (a), paraglottic space (PS) fat, and lateral thyroarytenoid muscle (arrow) are clearly visible. **B**: At the level of the ventricle-undersurface of the false cord, the lateral thyroarytenoid muscle occupies a larger proportion of the paraglottic space (PS). Fat within the arytenoid pad or posterior laryngeal wall (AP) is in continuity with that in the paraglottic space (***). The mucosa of the posterior pharyngeal wall (arrowheads) can be seen as separate from the mucosa of the posterior laryngeal wall (that mucosa covering the arytenoid pad). The muscle of the posterior pharyngeal wall (inferior constrictor) is the band of tissue density just posterior to the enhancing hypopharyngeal mucosa (arrowheads). **C,D**: The true cords are apposed in the midline so that the anterior commissure cannot be evaluated. The arytenoids (A) are rotated medially. The paraglottic space (arrow) is now only a thin band of fat lying between the true cord musculature and the thyroid lamina. The muscle and enhancing mucosa of the upper postcricoid region (arrowheads) are now visible. (From Mancuso.[1] Reprinted with permission.)

time it was delivered. CT technology has now "matured." Although refinements are being constantly made, they do not alter basic system capabilities. Equipment sold by major manufacturers since 1985 is capable of producing excellent images of the larynx and hypopharynx. Units placed before this time lacked sufficient speed to eliminate motion artifacts. Thin sections with high resolution are also required for satisfactory imaging of the head and neck region. Recent generation units create such thin-section, small field of view (FOV) images in 1 to 3 seconds at totally acceptable doses of radiation. Moreover, variation of the scanning parameters that affect imaging quality has been simplified. Excellent quality images are the routine when operator-dependent variables are optimized for each patient with the help of baseline protocols (Table 7–1). This requires physician supervision and well-trained, motivated technologists. Lack of attention to these details often produces a useless study. Important machine-dependent variables such as the tube-detector efficiency, scan speed, and reconstruction time must be considered at the time of purchase. Although clinicians rarely have control over these details, they may demand from the radiologist images and interpretation of high quality.

With that background, let us consider the specifics of making good quality images. The basic requirements for head and neck imaging are:

1. Slice thickness: 1.5 to 2 mm for high detail work; 3 to 4 mm for routine studies.
2. Field of view: 9 to 18 cm.
3. Matrix: 512 × 512.
4. Scan time: 1- to 3-second routine; 4 to 6 seconds for high detail work (eg, temporal bone).
5. Capacity for doing dynamic vascular studies.

Certain steps should be followed in the planning and execution of any CT study (Table 7–2). These are more critical in the head and neck region than elsewhere in the body because a key

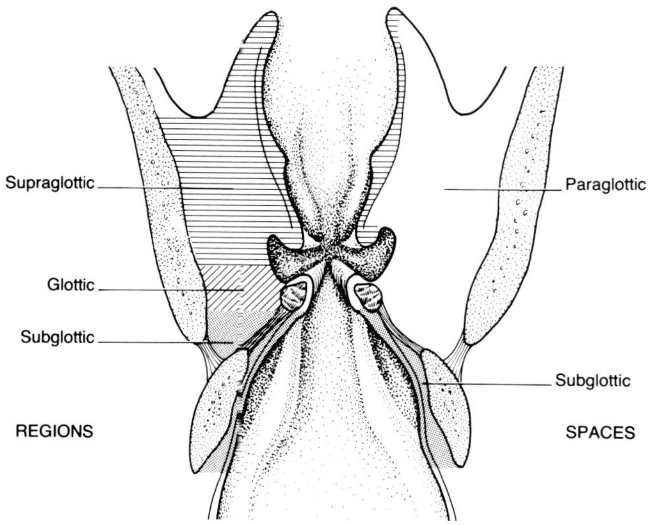

Figure 7–6. Coronal midplane diagram of the larynx. One needs to understand fully the relationship of the paraglottic and subglottic spaces to the surrounding laryngeal framework and regions in order to interpret images of the larynx.

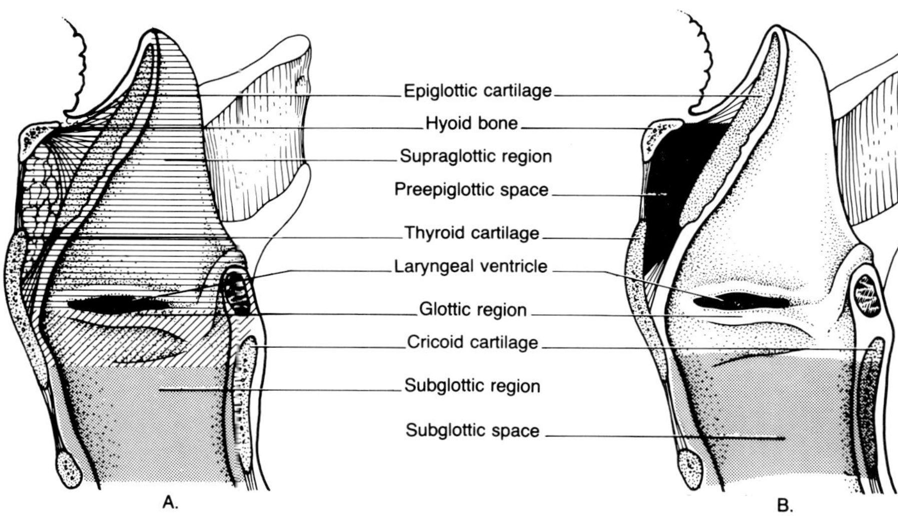

Figure 7–7. Sagittal midplane diagrams of the larynx showing its regions (A) and spaces (B). A three-dimensional concept of the relationship of the deep spaces to the laryngeal framework and regions is essential for accurate interpretation of sectional images.

Table 7–2. Steps for Planning CT Examination*

1. Adequate definition of clinical questions to be answered by the study
   a. From referring physician
   b. From talking with and examining the patient
2. Planning the study
   a. Proper positioning
   b. Preliminary view—select gantry angles, slice thickness
   c. Set technique factors according to demands of study and dose considerations
   e. Choose appropriate primary reconstruction algorithm
3. Execute study
   a. Reduction of motion artifacts—patient restraint, shoulders down, breathholding
   b. Proper use of intravenous contrast
   c. Constant physician supervision; repeat or add views as needed
4. Recording the data
   a. Proper photography
   b. Magnify areas of interest
   c. Save and reconstruct raw data whenever necessary

*Adapted with permission from Mancuso[1].

management decision may rest on the status of structures or spaces a millimeter or two in size. Moreover, seemingly simple things like how the gantry is angled relative to the structure of interest may vastly alter the appearance of normal and deranged anatomy. Precise surgery and radiotherapy are often required in treating head and neck cancer; they should be matched by equally precise diagnostic imaging. Each step in Table 7–2 should be followed in conjunction with the more specific protocols in Table 7–1.

In the larynx and hypopharynx, positioning and gantry angle are critical (Fig. 7–8). The neck should be slightly hyperextended. This will draw the larynx up higher in the neck, helping to avoid streak artifacts produced when sections are made through the shoulders. Slight hyperextension will also place the plane of the true cords roughly parallel to the C4-C5 or C5-C6 disc space. The chin and head should be immobilized and the shoulders relaxed and displaced as far inferiorly as possible. Optimal and suboptimal positioning are shown in the digital radiographs in Figure 7–8. The plane of section for laryngeal and hypopharyngeal studies must be absolutely parallel to the true vocal cords or ventricle. The angle is chosen from the lateral, digital radiograph (Fig. 7–8) either based on laryngeal

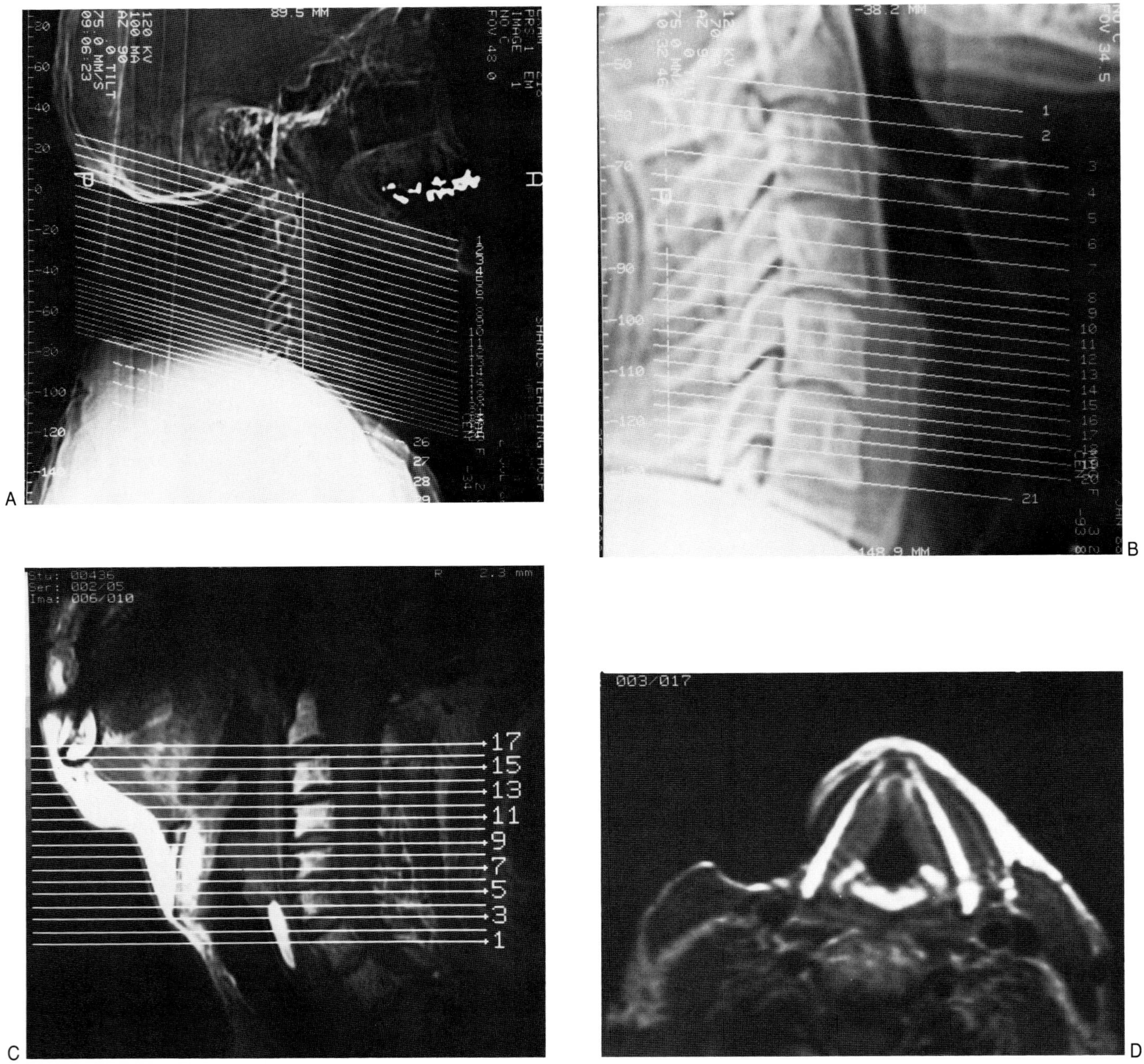

Figure 7–8. **A:** Lateral digital radiograph used to plan the computed tomography examination. Note that: (1) the neck is comfortably extended; (2) the sections are made *precisely* parallel to the true to false vocal cord (TVC-FVC) horizontal plane; (3) the extent of the study has been planned in advance with some economy of sections above and below the main area of interest. An average laryngeal study has 30 to 40 sections; and (4) it would have been better if this patient's shoulders were lower, but this was the best she could do. **B:** A close-up view of the larynx, demonstrating usual extent of the laryngeal portion of the examination. (Higher and lower sections might be used if detailed neck survey is necessary.) Neck scans are parallel to the TVC-FVC horizontal plane and this approximates the plane of the C4-C5 and C5-C6 disc spaces. **C,D:** Preliminary sagittal MRI showing suboptimal angle of axial sections. Note, in particular, sections 4 to 6, which are through the low supraglottis anteriorly and the true cords posteriorly. This is reflected on the confusing axial image in D, showing the cricoarytenoid joint level posteriorly and fat *above* the anterior commissure anteriorly (arrow). This is poor technique.

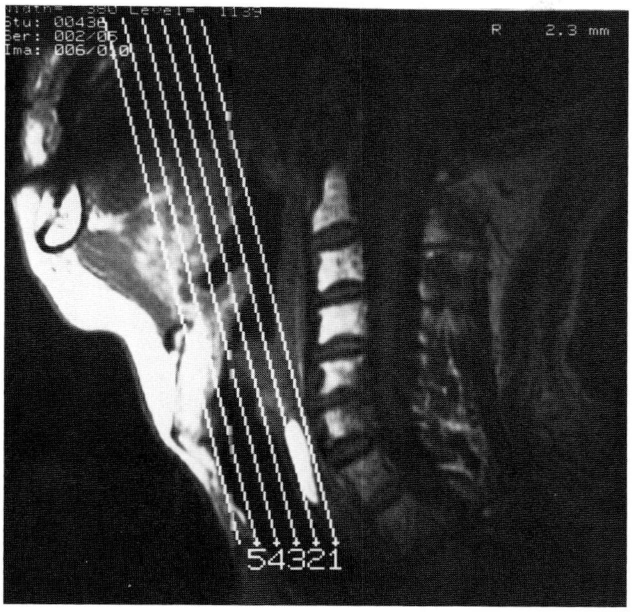

E

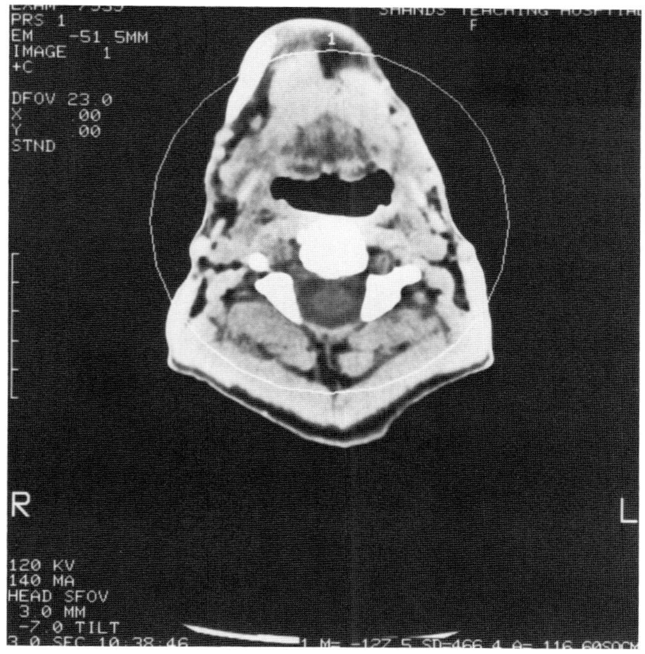

F

Figure 7–8 (*continued*). E: The same patient as seen in C and D with optimal selection of the plane for coronal sections. F: The circular cursor indicates a proper selection of field of view (FOV). When the selected FOV is programmed, the entire frame will be filled with the area inside the circle. This markedly improves spatial resolution. A small picture with a lot of black space (air) surrounding it represents substandard, suboptimal selection of FOV and can lead to serious interpretive errors because subtle findings may go unrecognized on these small pictures with relatively low spatial resolution. The results of *optimal* selection of FOV are illustrated throughout the chapter (see Figure 7–5).

landmarks or by making the scans parallel to the C4-C5 or C5-C6 disc space. Sections made off axis relative to the transglottic region can cause major interpretive errors. These skewed images can, for example, make the false cords appear to be at the same level as the undersurface of the true cords.

After the gantry angle is selected, one must program the extent of the study. A typical study planned for laryngeal cancer is shown in Figure 7–8. If first-order nodal sites are to be included, sections usually begin at, or slightly above, the angle of the mandible and end at the clavicles. Sections through the larynx should be contiguous (no gaps) and no more than 3 to 4 mm apart. Thinner (1.5 or 2 mm) sections may be employed if required, although, in my experience, 3 mm sections suffice for the vast majority of cases.

FOV between 14 and 16 cm, if centered properly, will usually cover the lymph node-bearing areas of the neck as well as the larynx. This may be done prospectively or retrospectively. Retrospective magnification should not be substituted for proper selection of FOV. A reduction in FOV improves spatial resolution if the matrix size is held constant. Pixel magnification averages and blurs data; this may be desirable to enhance presentation of images, but it is a needless sacrifice if substituted for a true reduction in the FOV. Laryngeal studies should be reconstructed with standard soft tissue algorithms. Bone algorithms may be used, as indicated, to improve cartilage detail but rarely make a difference in accuracy of diagnosis. However, when cartilage invasion is suspected, the images should be filmed at both "bone" and "soft tissue" window settings.

Intravenous contrast is used for most studies. It is mandatory when the neck is being studied for possible nodal metastases. Many primary tumors will enhance, especially at their margins, and this will improve tumor conspicuity, especially at tumor-muscle interfaces. The effect is most noticeable in supraglottic and hypopharyngeal primates or any other tumor that is ulcerative. Either rapid drip infusion or a power injector may be used.

Magnetic Resonance Imaging

MRI studies should be done with localized receiver coils capable of being closely coupled to the neck. Optimal designs are just now becoming available from manufacturers. FOV and slice thickness should be about the same as for CT, although 1.5 to 2 mm thick sections are not practical. Sections should never be thicker than 5 mm. Standard T_1 and T_2 weighted images are usually sufficient. The choice of imaging plane should be based on the information necessary for treatment planning. This is discussed later in the chapter. MRI is an "immature" technology at present, and technical advances are likely to lead to future improvement.

GLOTTIC CANCER

Patterns of Tumor Spread

There is generally good correlation between the extent of intralaryngeal tumor demonstrated by CT or MRI with that determined by whole organ serial section (Chapter 2). Thus, these modalities may serve as valuable clinical tools. Small, obvious T_1 lesions of the true vocal cord often do not require such expensive studies unless the endoscopist is not sure of the subglottic extent, or if submucosal spread or the status of the laryngeal ventricle is in question (Fig. 7–9). The anterior commissure can be easily evaluated clinically so that imaging also seems unnecessary for this alone. Cartilage invasion at the anterior commissure is highly unlikely if the cord is mobile and the tumor is confined to the glottis. One should be highly skeptical about the interpretation of a minor area of lack of mineralization as representing cartilage invasion in such limited lesions (Figs. 7–10, 7–11). This is more likely a normal variant. These limited lesions must be distinguished, however, from the very aggressive cancers at the anterior commissure which spread cephalad in the low preepiglottic space to attack the petiole of the epiglottis (see "Transglottic Lesions").

Spread of endolaryngeal carcinoma may be horizontal (anterior and posterior) or vertical (cephalocaudal). Spread to the anterior commissure is the primary ventral, horizontal path of tumors limited to the true cord.[4,18–24] This horizontal spread pattern tends to predominate in the earlier stages, whereas vertical spread will tend to prevail at later stages of growth. The concept of the aggressive anterior commissure tumor just discussed is a prime example of a lesion that can exhibit an advanced growth pattern at an early stage (small volume) (Figs. 7–12, 7–13). In glottic cancer this tendency for early vertical spread also occurs in tumors arising at the posterior wall of the

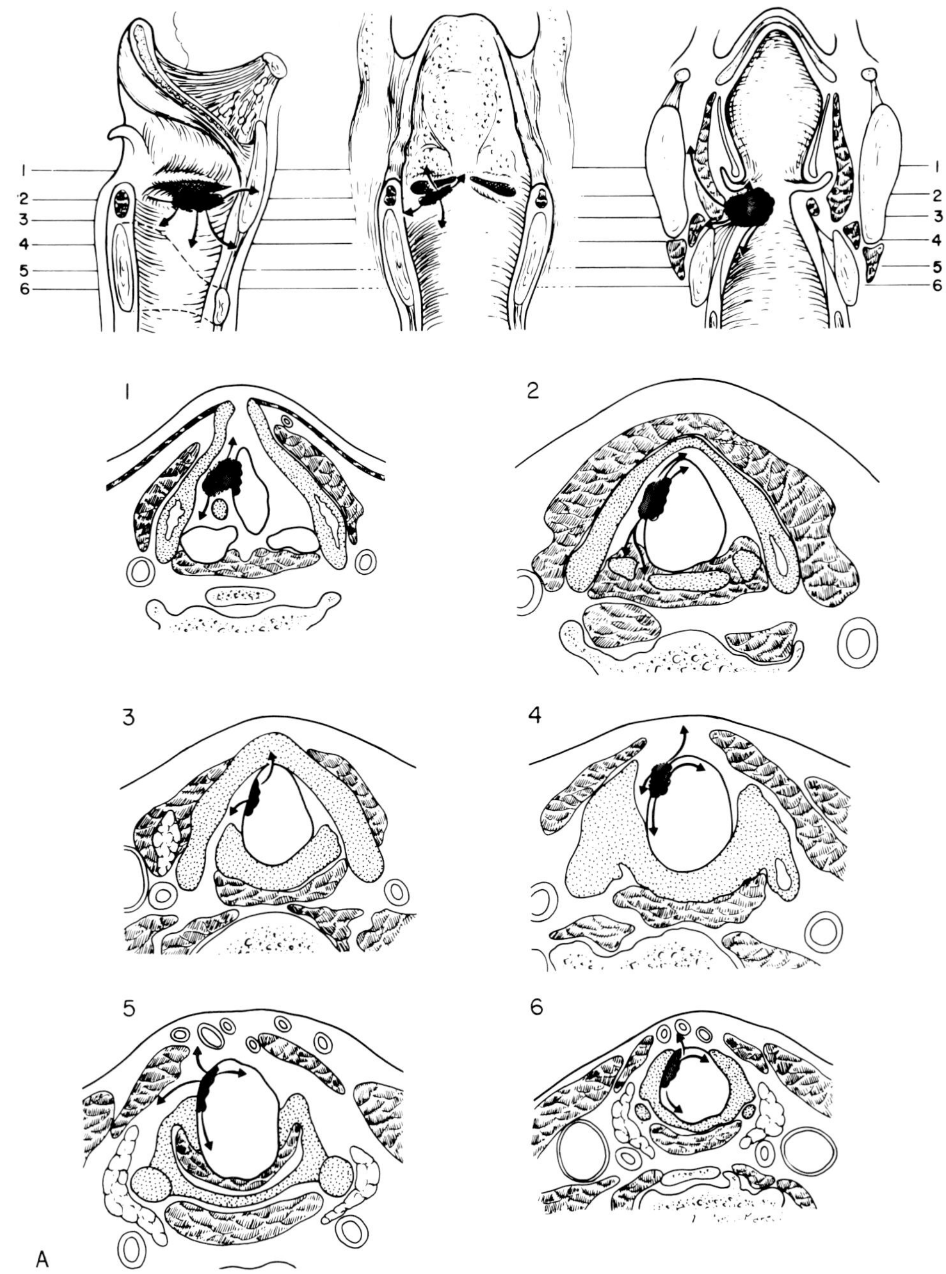

Figure 7–9. A: These axial images (1–6) are made at levels indicated on the three diagrams at the top. They illustrate the basic spread patterns of glottic primary tumors. (From Mancuso and Hanafee.[2] Reprinted with permission.)

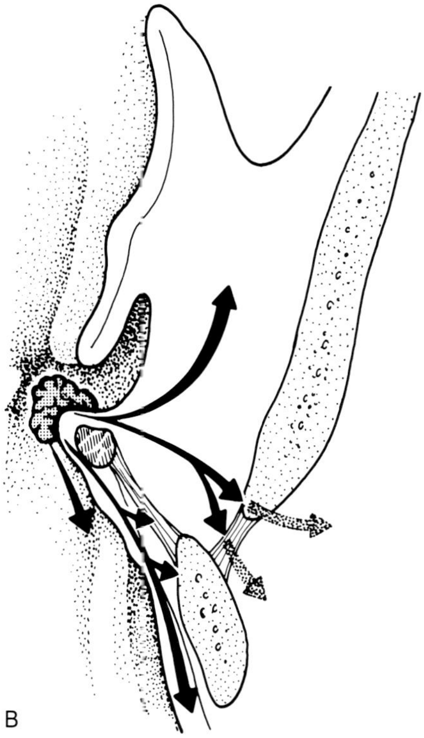

B

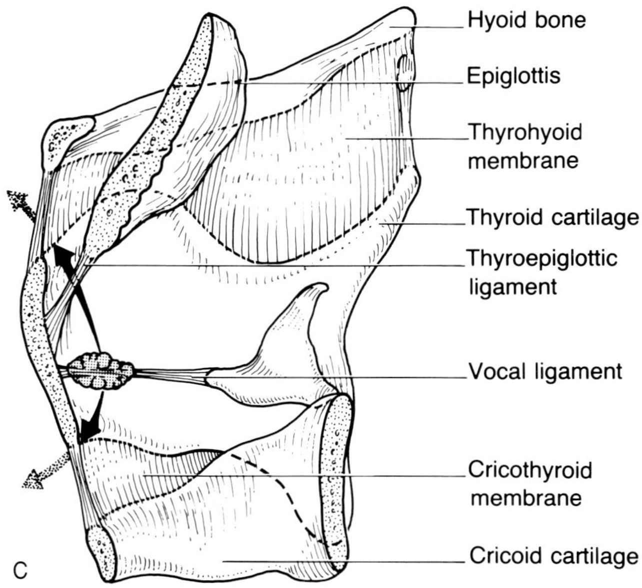

C

Figure 7-9 (*continued*). B: Illustrates deep spread patterns of glottic cancer. Submucosal subglottic disease and that in the paraglottic space cannot be directly detected by the endoscopist, although a "submucosal bulge" or reduced cord mobility may imply the presence of such disease. Spread in the paraglottic space is a primary pathway for lesions to become transglottic. C: Anterior glottic lesions may spread vertically to become transglottic (arrows). More advanced tumors can spread through the cricothyroid membrane or attack the thyrohyoid membrane-thyroid cartilage junction in the thyroid notch region. These spread patterns were largely undetectable prior to CT (unless very advanced).

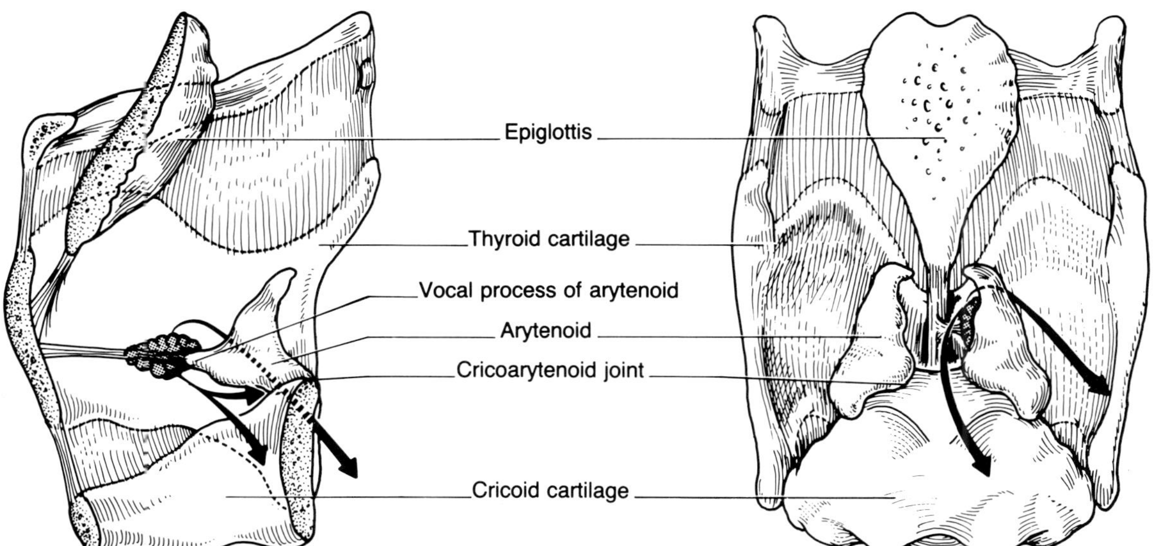

D. E.

Figure 7-9 (*continued*). D,E: Glottic cancers infrequently arise posteriorly. When significant tumor burden is noted on the posterior true cord, one or more of the indicated spread patterns may be present. Notice how even early lesions do not have far to go to reach the cricoid. (From Mancuso and Hanafee.[2] Reprinted with permission.)

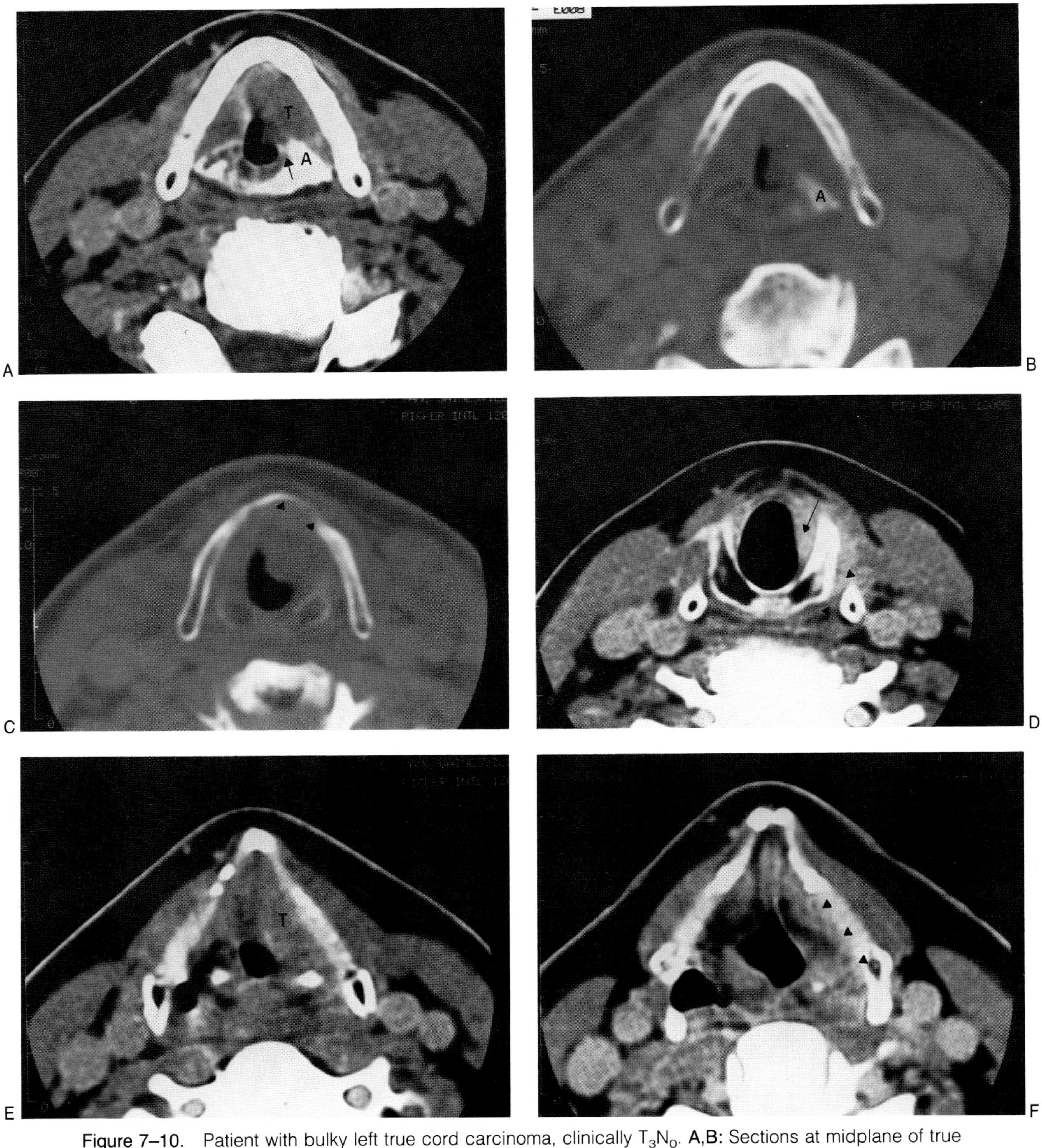

Figure 7–10. Patient with bulky left true cord carcinoma, clinically T_3N_0. **A,B:** Sections at midplane of true vocal cords photographed at narrow (A) and wide (B) windows show tumor (T) involving the entire true vocal cord with tissue thickening over the medial aspect of the cricoarytenoid joint (arrow). The arytenoid (A) is sclerotic. The thyroid cartilages are symmetrical. **C:** At the undersurface of the true cords, the thyroid cartilage appears "saucerized" (arrowheads). There was proven cartilage invasion at this point, although CT findings are equivocal. **D:** Mid to low subglottic section shows submucosal (no mucosal lesion present at gross pathologic examination) subglottic spread (arrow) and sclerosis of the cricoid with a subtle suggestion of obliteration of the fat plane near the cricothyroid joint (arrowheads) compared with the normal side. Cricoid cartilage invasion and extralaryngeal spread were confirmed pathologically. **E,F:** At the ventricular level (E) and false cord level (F), extensive tumor (T) spreads within the paraglottic space. A broad zone of tumor lies adjacent to the thyroid cartilage perichondrium (arrowheads) and the cartilage appears indistinct but really differs little in appearance from the normal side. Tumor was confirmed but there was no cartilage invasion at this level.

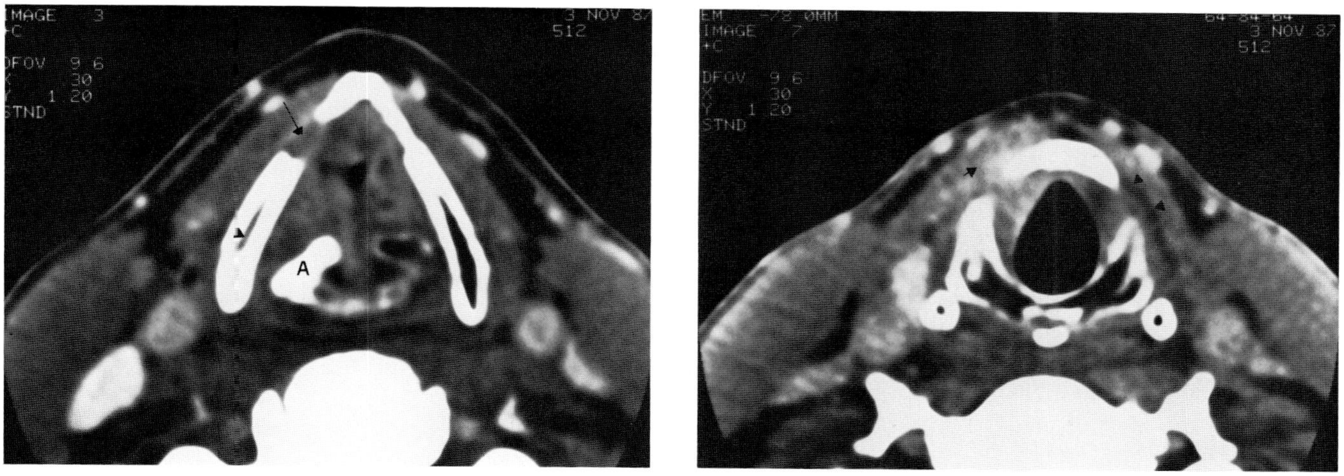

A B

Figure 7–11. Patient with right-sided T_3 glottic carcinoma. Thyroid cartilage was *not* tender and no prelaryngeal abnormalities were palpable. **A**: At glottic level, there is a focal defect (arrow) in an otherwise well-ossified thryoid cartilage. This should be considered highly suspicious for cartilage invasion but occasionally such focal defects are seen as a normal variation. Further inspection shows the marrow space obliterated (arrowhead) and the arytenoid (A) sclerotic and displaced. **B**: Tumor penetrates the cricothyroid membrane and obliterates the fat deep to the infrahyoid strap muscles (arrow). Compare with the normal side (arrowheads). Point of cartilage attack was probably the insertion of cricothyroid membrane on inferior margin of the thyroid cartilage. Cricoid showed reactive sclerosis but no tumor invasion. All findings were pathologically confirmed following total laryngectomy. Patient also received postoperative radiotherapy.

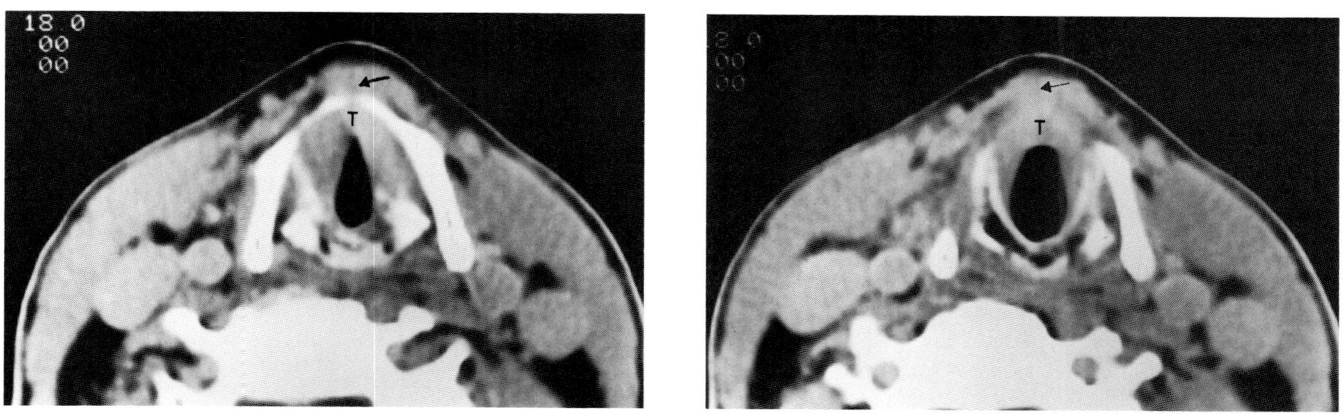

A B

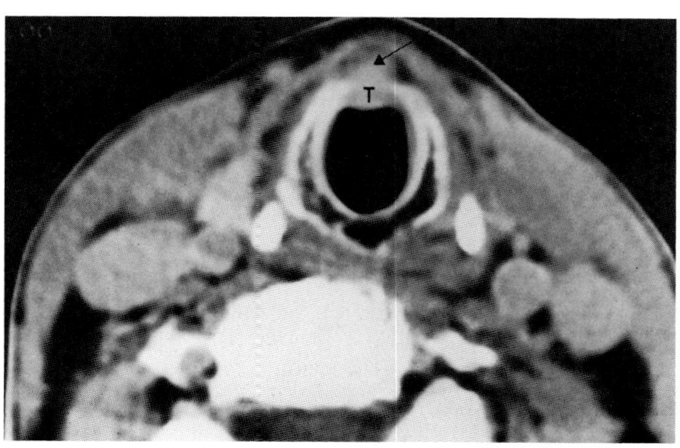

C

Figure 7–12. A 55-year-old man with a carcinoma of the right true cord (TVC) with anterior commissure involvement. The lesion, at laryngoscopy, was considered an early T_2 on the basis of minimal subglottic spread anteriorly. There was *no* palpable fullness or tenderness in the prelaryngeal soft tissues. **A,B,C**: Pretreatment scans through the TVC, mid and low subglottis show tumor (T) infiltrating the prelaryngeal soft tissues (arrow) after spreading through the cricothyroid membrane.

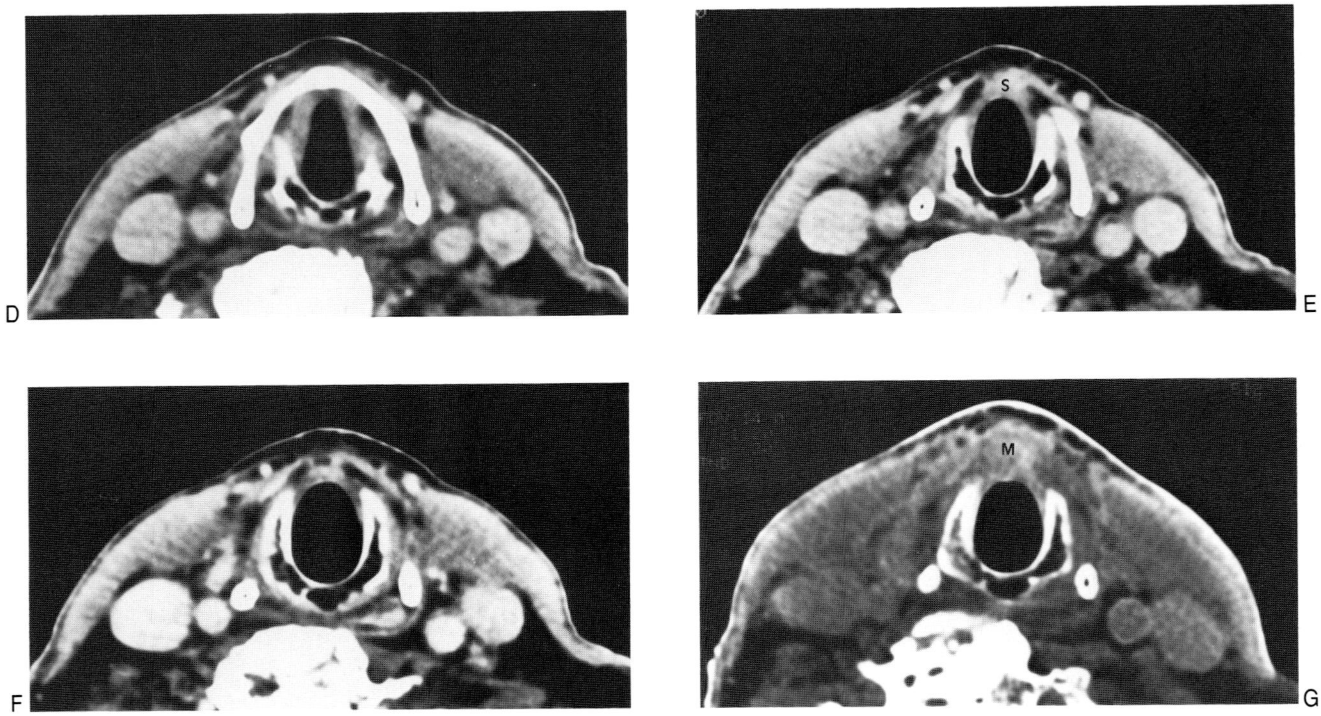

Figure 7-12 (*continued*). D,E,F: Scans corresponding to levels in A through C done 3 years postradiotherapy (RT). In E there is minimal residual scarring (S). Patient is tumor-free 4 years after treatment. G: Scan at same level as in B and E done 6 weeks post-RT. Residual mass (M) was still present but involuted after 3- to 6-month period.

larynx and in the region of the vocal process of the arytenoid (Fig. 7–14); fortunately, primary tumors *arising* at this site are relatively uncommon.

Vertical spread beyond the horizontal plane of the true vocal cords results in a primary lesion being staged at least T_2. The most common form of this is subglottic spread. If the tumor spreads subglottically from the anterior commissure, it will frequently be seen as irregular thickening of the cricothyroid membrane (Figs. 7–12, 7–13). CT or MRI may show early extension of such lesions into the prelaryngeal soft tissues (Fig. 7–12). The cricothyroid membrane is a strong boundary against tumor growth, and such spread probably occurs through natural defects for neurovascular bundles or at the attachment of the membrane to the undersurface of the thyroid cartilage.[25] Cartilage invasion at the anterior commissure is likely only if there is subglottic spread or if the tumor is over 2.0 cm in its greatest dimension.[26] Once significant (10 mm) anterior subglottic spread is noted, areas of demineralization in and about the anterior commissure are more likely to herald early cartilage invasion. Supplemental MR examination may help detect such early cartilage invasion in properly imaged patients if well-localized, highly detailed studies are done.[27]

Both horizontal and vertical spread patterns are less common posteriorly. The key anatomic areas of interest here are the body, vocal process, and lateral process of the arytenoid as well as the posterior wall of the larynx and the posterior commissure.[28,29] The posterior commissure comprises the mucosa overlying the medial face of the arytenoid while the posterior wall of the larynx consists of the mucosa overlying the posterior surface of the arytenoid. Tumors usually do not originate at this site, but secondary involvement is common in advanced lesions (Fig. 7–14). Scans performed during quiet respiration (glottis open) are essential for evaluating this region, because during adduction, the mucosa of the posterior commissure (intra-arytenoid area) bunches up, simulating tumor pathologic thickening. When obvious tumor is noted in this location, subtle arytenoid and cricoid invasion is present in about 20% of cases.[4] Cartilage invasion in the region of the cricoarytenoid joint is difficult to detect with CT (Fig. 7–14). Posterior tumors may also spread laterally to invade the paraglottic space. From here, they can grow vertically downward toward the cricothyroid joint (Fig. 7–15). Laterally, these tumors can infiltrate the submucosa surrounding the pyriform sinus apex, thereby gaining access to its lymphatic drainage. Continued growth at either of these sites can lead to thyroid and cricoid cartilage invasion and/or exolaryngeal spread.

Laterally situated vocal cord cancer tends to grow vertically either in a cephalad or caudad direction (Fig. 7–9). In general, the deep spread pattern will be reflected by the mucosal disease, although spread in the paraglottic space may "hide" a considerable volume of tumor from view. At times, entirely occult spread deep to the laryngeal ventricle and/or subglottically (deep to the elastic cone) will only be detectable on CT (or MRI). This is one situation in which coronal MRI might be of benefit over CT (Fig. 7–16). A focused MRI study can be of value if the vertical extent of the lesion is not clear on axial CT. Some authors[4] suggest that this vertical pattern be called a paraglottic, rather than transglottic, growth pattern. There is a

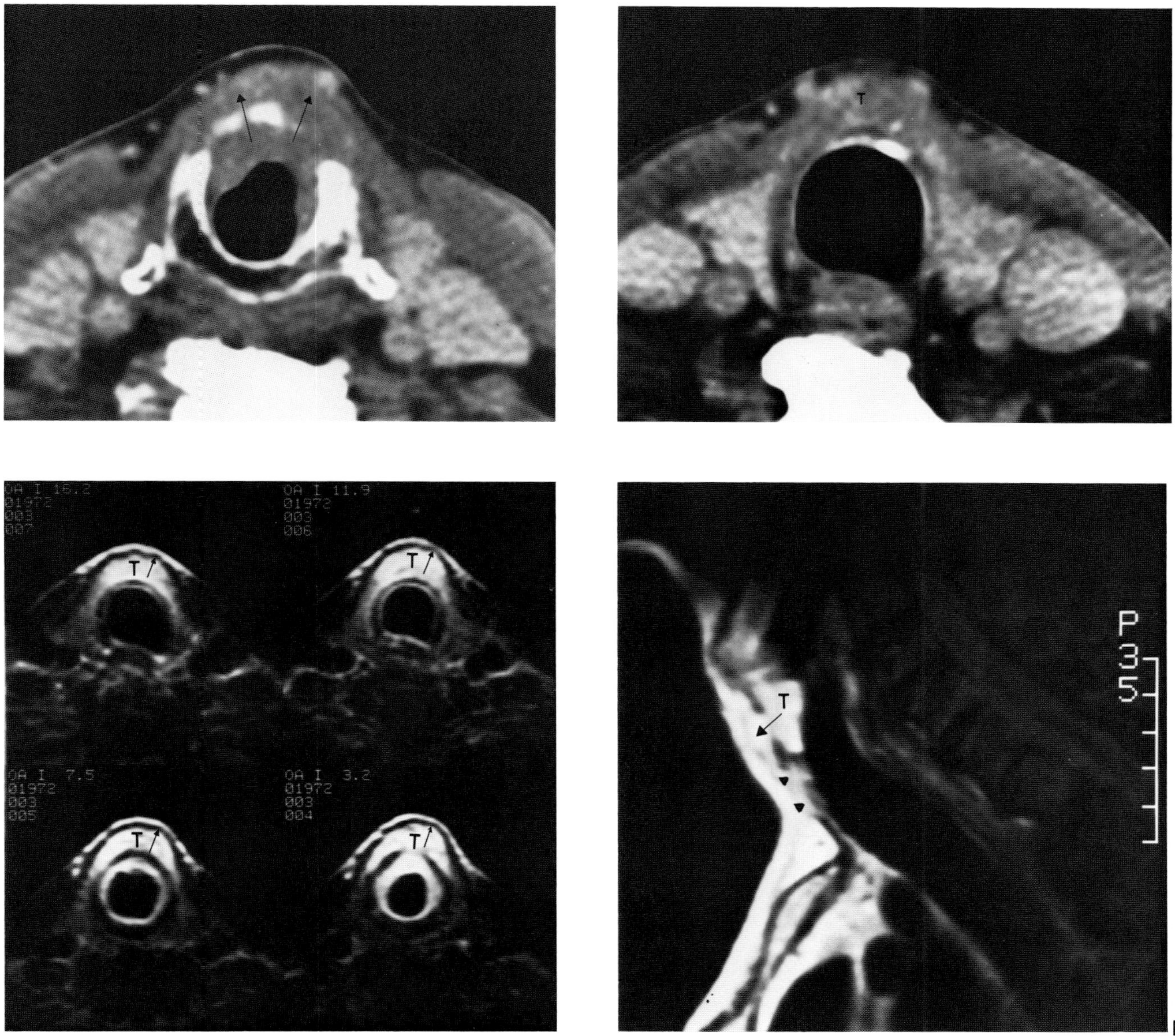

Figure 7–13. Patient with glottic cancer and a "vague fullness" in the prelaryngeal soft tissues noted on physical examination. Direct laryngoscopy showed an advanced glottic cancer with 10 to 15 mm of subglottic spread and a fixed right true vocal cord. Lesion was a T_3 (suspicious T_4) clinically. **A**: Computed tomography (CT) section in low subglottis shows nearly circumferential subglottic spread and extensive tumor in the prelaryngeal soft tissues (arrows). **B**: Extralaryngeal pretracheal tumor (T) at the first-second ring junction is present. **C**: Four-on-one composite view of axial T_2 weighted images. Section in upper left matches Figure 7–13B; that in lower right matches Figure 7–13A. Extralaryngeal tumor (T) displaces and lies deep to infrahyoid strap muscles (arrows). **D**: Sagittal T_2 weighted image shows intraluminal subglottic cancer (T), extralaryngeal tumor at cricothyroid membrane level (arrow) and pretracheal tumor (arrowheads). Comment: Without CT and magnetic resonance imaging study, this patient may have had tracheotomy performed too close to the tumor. Such error is particularly likely when patients require urgent tracheostomy and imaging cannot be performed.

high frequency of both cephalad and caudal spread in more advanced, laterally placed, glottic lesions. One group[4] has shown that paraglottic spread is present in one third of T_3 and T_4 glottic cancers and that caudal paraglottic spread occurs in 50% of cases with a "transglottic" mucosal pattern. Moreover, there may be unsuspected paraglottic spread in T_2 lesions (Fig. 7–17). The highly refined depiction of this on high-quality CT and MR images may help to improve selection criteria for surgery or radiation therapy in these patients.[30–33]

Subglottic spread occurs frequently in glottic cancer. It tends to be anterolateral but may be predominantly lateral. Subglottic spread may be deep or superficial to the mucosa or elastic

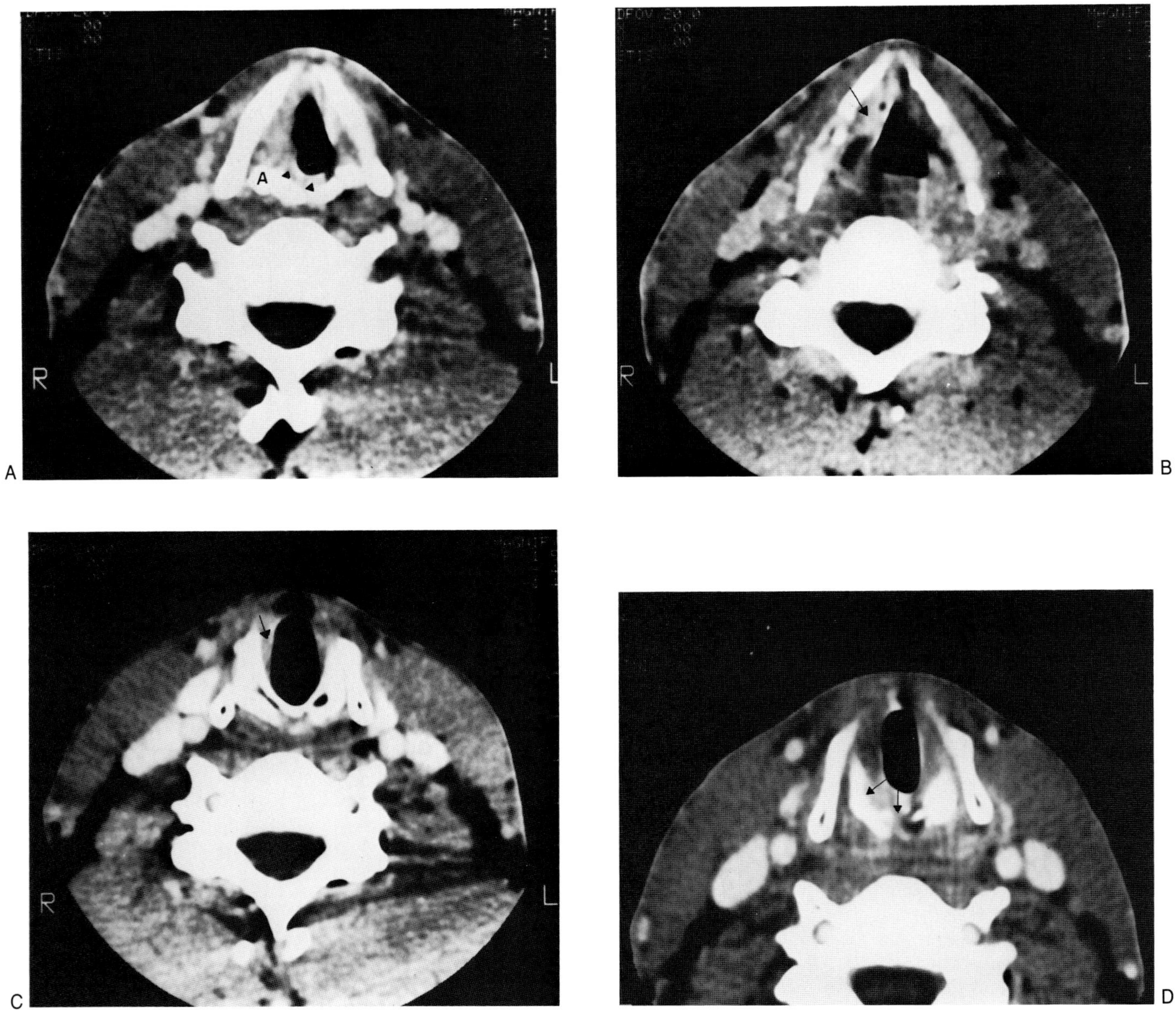

Figure 7–14. A 60-year-old man with T_3 glottic cancer with minimal extension to the ventricle and no subglottic disease at direct laryngoscopy. Limited mucosal disease was noted over the medial aspect of the arytenoid. **A**: At true vocal cord level, the right arytenoid (A) is displaced compared with the left. There is extensive abnormal thickening of the soft tissues in the interarytenoid region (arrowheads). **B**: At the false vocal cord level, tumor has infiltrated the paraglottic space (arrow). **C**: Subtle, but definite, evidence of 7 to 9 mm of lateral subglottic spread (arrow). **D**: Scan 12 weeks postradiotherapy (RT). Persistent tumor invades the cricoid cartilage (arrows). Comment: In reality, this is a low-volume transglottic lesion. Patient was treated with RT and followed closely with computed tomography (CT). The CT done 12 weeks post-therapy showed obvious cricoid cartilage destruction. This was probably due to unrecognized cricoarytenoid joint invasion. Prompt salvage laryngectomy following biopsy confirmation revealed extensive tumor invading the cricoid. The patient is free of tumor 5 years after treatment.

cone.[18–22] When deep, it may not be seen clinically and a serious underestimation of subglottic involvement can occur (Fig. 7–18). Imaging is essential to avoid such understaging. At the University of Florida, subglottic spread is described in millimeters from the undersurface of the true cord. In addition to the linear extent of subglottic spread, the relationship of tumor to the cricoid is of critical importance. This relationship is beautifully displayed on axial images (Fig. 7–10 to 7–18). Coronal sections are not very helpful in assessment of subglottic spread, since they can only be easily assessed in the midcoronal plane; this precludes evaluation of the more anterior or posterior components of subglottic spread. Sagittal views are similarly only really useful in the midsagittal plane. Sagittal views are occasionally valuable for assessing anterior prelaryngeal spread

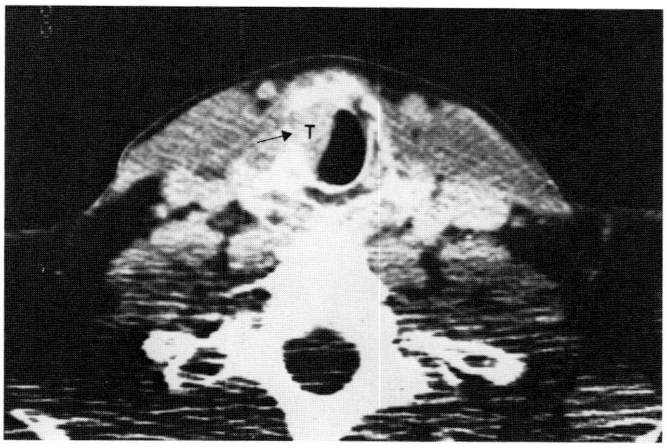

A

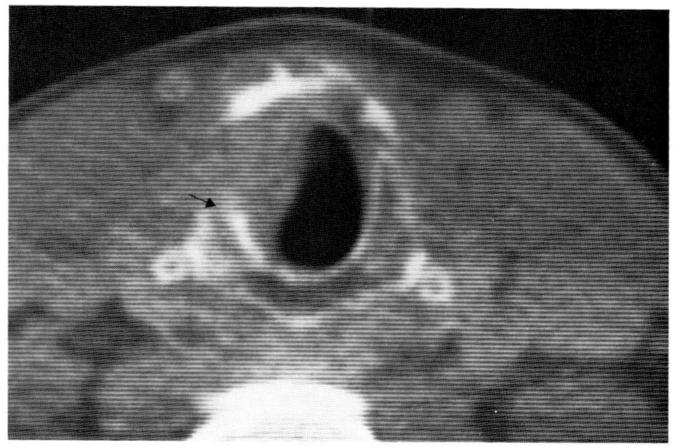

B

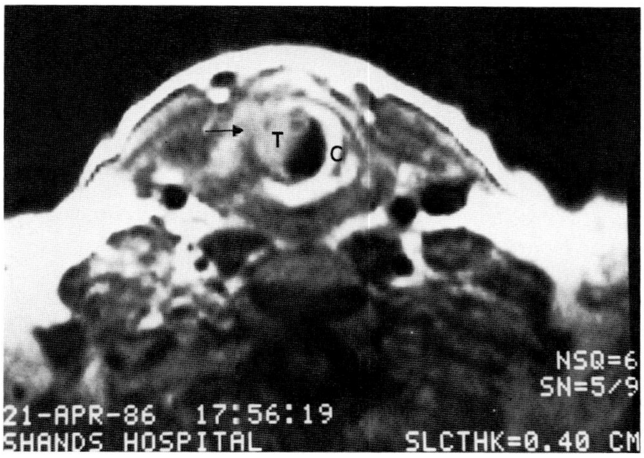

C

Figure 7–15. Patient with clinically T_3 glottic cancer. **A,B:** Soft tissue and "bone window" views from a marginal-quality computed tomography (done outside our institution). Intraluminal subglottic tumor (T) is obvious and destruction of the cricoid is likely (arrow). **C:** Low-field magnetic resonance (MR) imaging study shows intraluminal tumor (T), extralaryngeal tumor (arrow), and complete replacement of the right side of the cricoid by abnormal signal (compare with normal cricoid (C) on the left).

of tumor (Fig. 7–13). Large-volume subglottic disease is a predictor of increased risk for cartilage invasion or exolaryngeal spread.[18–22] When present on CT, large-volume or inferior subglottic disease might suggest that a focused, supplemental MRI be done to look for cartilage invasion or exolaryngeal spread that is not apparent on CT (Fig. 7–15). Extensive subglottic disease also places nodes at higher risk. Spread to the trachea is unusual but, again, is easily assessed on axial images. MRI is superior to CT for demonstrating invasion of tracheal rings, a rare phenomenon.

The diagnosis of vocal cord fixation is made by endoscopic or physical examination. Scans attempted during phonation are often degraded by motion and are time consuming. They are impractical on MRI at the present time. There are several possible reasons for fixation and any one or all may be operative in a given patient. A careful imaging assessment of the possible reasons for fixation is absolutely essential in the choice of radiation therapy or conservation surgery for selected patients with fixed cords. Fixation is caused by some form of deep infiltration. Most common is spread to the paraglottic space with infiltration of the thyroarytenoid muscle. This can be implied on CT, but contrast between tumor and muscle is not sufficient to demonstrate muscle invasion; it can be predicted if the paraglottic space is obliterated at the true vocal cord level (Fig. 7–10). Good quality MRI can show muscle invasion.[27] Fixation may also be due to spread to the cricoarytenoid joint, which is difficult to demonstrate on CT (see before). Spread lateral, medial, or posterior to the arytenoid may be a predictor of this mechanism of fixation. Vocal cord fixation is not usually associated with anterior commissure spread even if cartilage invasion is present, although in advanced lesions at this site the cords may show "reduced mobility." High-volume paraglottic spread usually indicates thyroarytenoid muscle involvement and possibly other reasons for vocal cord fixation in advanced lesions (Fig. 7–10). Tumor can infiltrate the course of the recurrent laryngeal nerve, but these lesions are usually so advanced that multiple possible causes of cord fixation will be visible.

Integration of Imaging and Treatment in Glottic Carcinoma

Treatment options for limited (CT) glottic lesions are discussed elsewhere in the text. Cure rates are high for any method. There is little role for diagnostic imaging in these patients. If, for some reason, the clinician believes that the lesion may be more extensive than the endoscopic examination suggests, then CT (or MRI) might be of value. This usually occurs due to a lack of confidence in the evaluation of the subglottic region or reduced

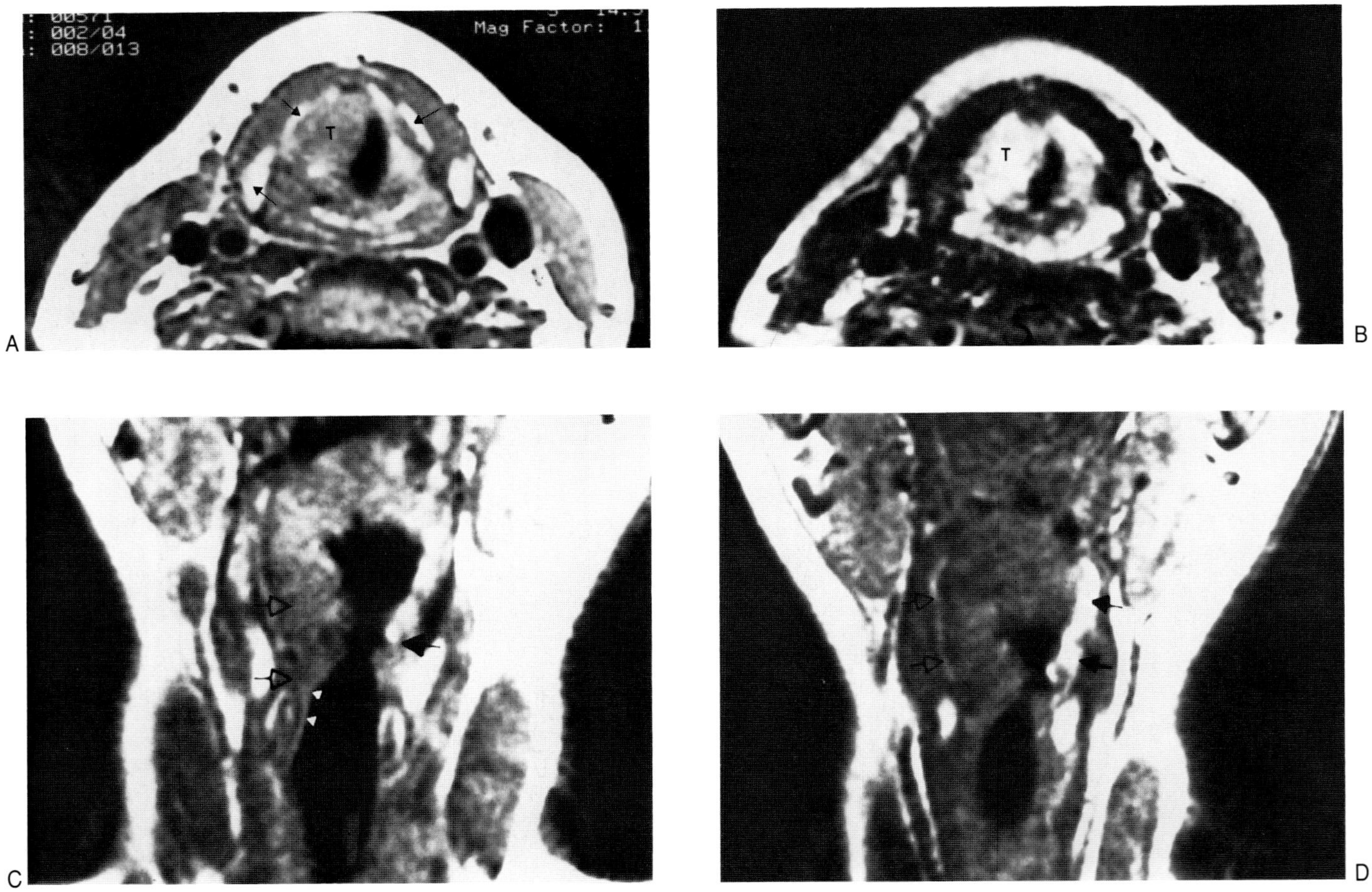

Figure 7–16. Magnetic resonance imaging study done on a 1.5 T unit on a patient with transglottic cancer. **A,B:** T_1 and T_2 weighted images at the ventricular level show bulky tumor (T). Thyroid cartilages contain fat (arrows); it is difficult to be sure if right thyroid lamina is invaded. **C,D:** Adjacent T_1 weighted images near the midcoronal plane of the larynx. **C:** Tumor infiltrates the paraglottic space (open arrows), crosses the true vocal cord level (closed arrow), and spreads subglottically (arrowhead). **D:** There is marked asymmetry of the marrow space of the right (open arrows) and fat on the left is in the paraglottic space. It is difficult to be certain whether this asymmetry is due to obliquity of the plane of section relative to the thyroid cartilage or tumor invasion. Comment: These are average-to-good MR images obtained on a high-field instrument. Comparison to routinely good computed tomography (CT) images throughout the chapter should show that, currently, CT images, properly done, are consistently of better quality than MR.

mobility of the true vocal cord. Cervical metastases rarely occur in these patients so that the detection of subclinical cervical metastases is not a justification for imaging.

Standard vertical hemilaryngectomy or radiotherapy may be used to treat limited T_2 and highly selected T_3 as well as T_1 cancers of the true vocal cord.[34–37] Tumor limits may be easily defined by CT in most cases. Standard vertical hemilaryngectomy requires an inferior margin at least 1 cm below the free margin of the true cord and 3 to 4 mm posterior margin. The posterior cut may transect the vocal process of the arytenoid. The superior margin is above the free edge of the false vocal cord. Occult spread to the ventricle or false cord can be seen easily on high-quality CT (Fig. 7–17). A bulky tumor may bulge upward, mimicking spread to the ventricle or false cord. In such cases coronal reformations or supplemental MRI may be done if this circumstance is likely to alter the therapeutic approach (Fig. 7–16). Axial CT will easily show subglottic spread and if this is adjacent or close to the cricoid, standard vertical hemolaryngectomy is not feasible (Fig. 7–18). Further anterior or posterior spread requires an extended variation of vertical hemilaryngectomy.[38–40] It is in the more advanced lesions that CT and MR imaging can be particularly useful in choosing a primary mode of therapy that will more likely cure the lesions as well as preserve function. Of course, the imaging findings must be integrated with myriad other factors, including patient desires, reliability, and physical condition, as well as relative local surgical and radiotherapy expertise.

For T_2 lesions, the therapeutic decision usually is between radiotherapy and a standard or extended vertical hemilaryngectomy. It is possible that CT evidence of an advanced T_2 lesion may help select patients for elective treatment of the neck. On occasion CT will detect nonpalpable metastatic nodes in patients with T_2 glottic cancer (Fig. 7–17).

It should be clear from the prior discussion on spread patterns

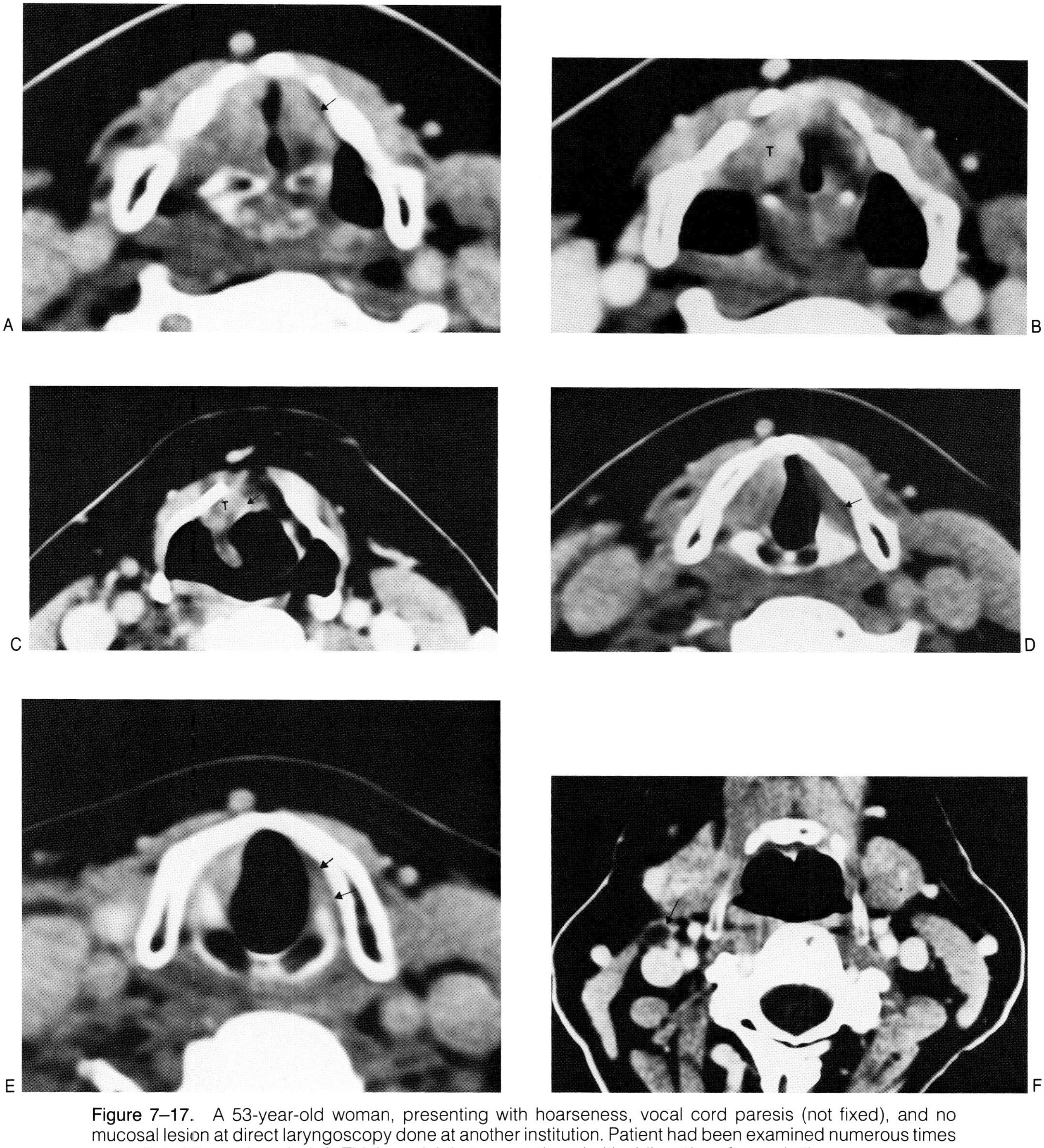

Figure 7–17. A 53-year-old woman, presenting with hoarseness, vocal cord paresis (not fixed), and no mucosal lesion at direct laryngoscopy done at another institution. Patient had been examined numerous times over a 6- to 12-month period. **A:** Thickened right true vocal cord with obliteration of paraglottic space; compare with paraglottic space on left (arrow). **B:** Tumor (T) infiltrates the right paraglottic space at false vocal cord level. **C:** Tumor (T) continues cephalad spread in low supraglottis and shows early spread into preepiglottic space (arrow). **D,E:** Spread also extends downward, obliterating paraglottic space at level of undersurface of true cords and upper subglottis. Note normal left paraglottic space (arrow) at both levels. **F:** Clinically occult 8 mm node (arrow) completely replaced by metastatic disease was also found by computed tomography (CT). Comment: Direct laryngoscopy at University of Florida also showed no mucosal lesion but a subtle submucosal bulge was noted. Because of CT findings, multiple *deep* biopsies were done. Invasive squamous cell carcinoma was diagnosed.

A 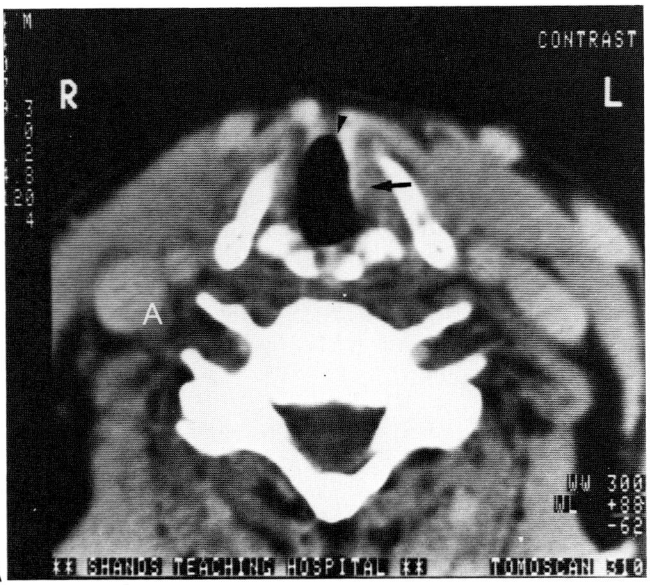

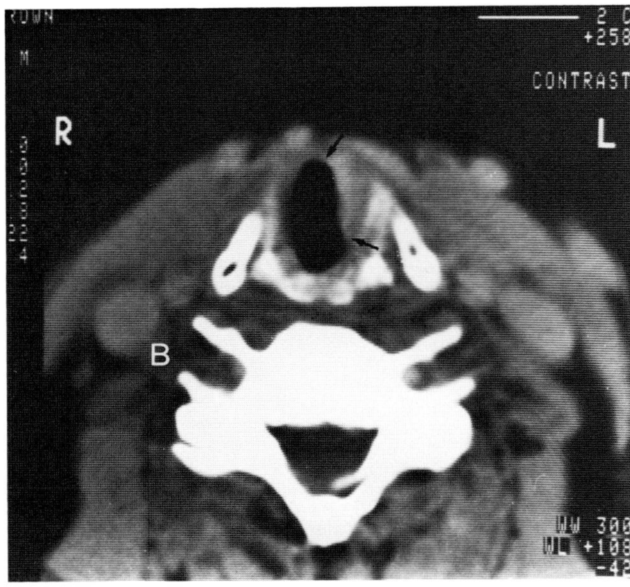 B

C 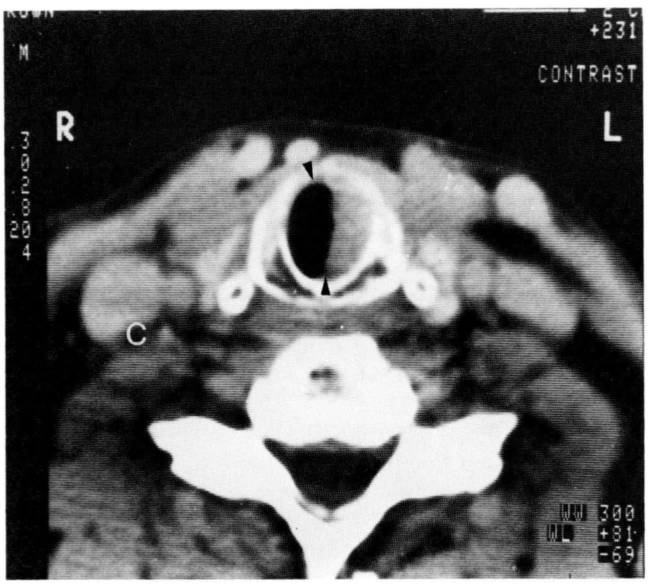

Figure 7–18. A 55-year-old man with left true vocal cord (TVC) carcinoma who was told, following laryngoscopy at another institution, that his lesion was suitable for vertical hemilaryngectomy. **A**: Thickened TVC (arrow) with gross thickening, ending at anterior commissure (arrowhead). **B**: Bulky subglottic tumor; arrows indicate its anterior and posterior limits. **C**: High-volume tumor in the low subglottis with spread across the midline anteriorly and posteriorly (arrowheads). Comment: Direct laryngoscopy at the University of Florida showed submucosal subglottic bulge. Total laryngectomy confirmed all findings. (From Mancuso and Hanafee.[2] Reprinted with permission.)

that, clinically, T_2 glottic cancer can have extensive submucosal spread that cannot be evaluated fully by physical examination or endoscopy. In a failure analysis of several series one group's findings suggest that unrecognized spread to the anterior subglottic wall probably accounts for failed conservation surgery in a significant number of patients.[4] With modern imaging, spread in this area is easy to evaluate except for subtle erosion of the anteroinferior margin of the thyroid cartilage (Figs. 7–12, 7–13). If radiotherapy is chosen as primary therapy, CT may be useful in follow-up and may help to detect or confirm recurrence faster than in previous times. Although controversial, at the University of Florida, radiotherapy has proven capable of controlling low-volume tumors with early prelaryngeal spread through the anterior subglottic wall (Fig. 7–12).

It should be apparent from this discussion that current staging schemes are quite limited as an aid to choice of therapy. Early prelaryngeal spread of tumor was almost never appreciated in the past. It is probably not correct to call these T_4 lesions on the basis of the CT because, in the past such a primary would have been staged T_2, and may stand a good chance for cure with radiotherapy alone, that is, the lesion behaves more like a T_2 than T_4 in its response to treatment. We are now in an era where uniformity of end-result reporting is in jeopardy unless the staging schemes are altered to account for information available on modern imaging techniques or a system of independent clinical and imaging staging is implemented.[41–44]

Spread to the arytenoid region requires extended vertical hemilaryngectomy or radiation therapy to control the primary tumor. Recall that this spread pattern is a particularly ominous one because of the tendency for occult submucosal spread and ready access to the cricoarytenoid joint. Obliteration of the fat pad around the arytenoid indicates significant tumor burden posteriorly (Fig. 7–10). Sometimes 01.5 to 2 mm sections will be necessary to determine the extent of tumor in this area. CT scan can show either unsuspected medial (posterior commissure or subglottic) or lateral (paraglottic) extensions that will obviate a safe margin even for extended vertical hemilaryngectomy.

Although most patients with T_3 glottic carcinoma are treated by total laryngectomy, at the University of Florida selected T_3 lesions are treated with radiotherapy producing roughly 67% cure by irradiation alone and overall cure rate of about 80%, with salvage laryngectomy for recurrences.[43] CT is most useful for selection of T_3 lesions likely to be amenable to radiation therapy. Those with low-volume lesions, no evidence of cartilage invasion, and limited vertical paraglottic spread are most favorable. Similar selection criteria can be used to identify a subgroup of patients with T_3 lesions that might be amenable to extended vertical partial laryngectomy.[45]

Advanced T_3 and T_4 glottic cancers are managed with total or near-total laryngectomy with or without postoperative radiotherapy. If near-total laryngectomy is planned, CT can show circumferential subglottic involvement, contralateral anterior subglottic wall extension, or extensive exolaryngeal spread that might contraindicate such an approach[35] (Fig. 7–18). Fortunately, these patterns are much less common than a unilaterally spreading tumor confined to the larynx with minimal, if any, exolaryngeal spread.

In advanced cancers, CT can also show inferior subglottic, tracheal, or exolaryngeal spread that requires lower than usual tracheal transection and possibly postoperative irradiation.[34] For patients with advanced lesions who present with airway obstruction, demonstration of the inferior extent of tumor by CT may help avoid placing the emergency tracheostomy too close to, or through, gross tumor.[46] On occasion, advanced glottic cancer will spread directly into the tracheoesophageal groove. Preoperative knowledge of this can help in planning the lower limit of resection and method of pharyngeal closure.

SUPRAGLOTTIC CARCINOMA

Patterns of Tumor Spread

Supraglottic tumors may arise from the epiglottis, aryepiglottic fold, false vocal cord, or posterior wall (interarytenoid area or "arytenoid pad"). There are distinctive spread patterns based on these sites of origin (Figs. 7–19, 7–20). I have concluded, on the basis of study of over 500 CT examinations of the larynx, that supraglottic spread patterns are best classified according to the method suggested by Meyer-Breiting and von Ilberg:[4]

1. Ventral (epiglottic) carcinoma
2. Lateral (false cord, laryngeal ventricle, aryepiglottic fold) carcinoma
3. Ventrolateral carcinoma (at the junction of the epiglottis and aryepiglottic fold)
4. Posterior wall carcinoma (arytenoid or interarytenoid region)

Ventral carcinomas arise on the laryngeal surface of the suprahyoid (free margin) or infrahyoid (fixed portion) of the epiglottis (Figs. 7–19, 7–20). Those of the fixed portion of the epiglottis frequently invade the preepiglottic space. They may either grow through the naturally occurring perforations in the epiglottic cartilage, erode through the cartilage, or skirt around its edges to get to the preepiglottic space (Figs. 7–21, 7–22). Ability to obtain axial CT images has simplified the previously difficult assessment of spread to the preepiglottic space. The normal fatty density is replaced by the tissue density of tumor. Examination of whole-organ sections corroborates accurate portrayal by CT of the extent of disease in the preepiglottic space. Occasional growth of an exophytic tumor into the laryngeal vestibule may be confused with preepiglottic space infiltration but may be distinguished by the normal volume of fat still present in the preepiglottic space (Fig. 7–23). MRI may prove to be superior to CT for this assessment. Although uncommon, tumor can spread to the tongue base via the preepiglottic space beneath intact mucosa (Fig. 7–24).[18,21] Such spread is usually obvious on axial sections but sagittal reformations or limited, supplemental MRI in the midsagittal plane can prove to be useful for confirmation in suspicious borderline cases.

Some authors have reported a high frequency of glottic involvement by epiglottic cancers.[4] These are usually tumors that originate in the region of the petiole. Thin (1.5 to 2 mm) sections will sometimes be required to show the relationship of tumor to the anterior commissure. Obliteration of the fat in the low preepiglottic space is the sign of involvement at the site (Fig. 7–25). The subtle symmetrical and relatively minimal findings may make it difficult for an inexperienced observer to diagnose such spread. With anterior commissure involvement, these lesions become transglottic (Fig. 7–21; see transglottic section). A relatively high rate of spread to the thyroid cartilage is seen in tumors that spread across and below the anterior commissure (Fig. 7–21). These low, ventral supraglottic lesions may also spread horizontally to involve the anterior false cords and laryngeal ventricles bilaterally and often symmetrically. Tumors with high-volume, preepiglottic space spread may penetrate the laryngeal framework. The favored site of invasion is at the transition from thyroid cartilage to thyrohyoid membrane, particularly in the region within 1 cm (Figs. 7–21, 7–26) from the thyroid notch. This may be difficult to demonstrate with CT. In suspicious cases, limited supplemental MRI may show early invasion of the infrahyoid strap muscles as a sign of framework penetration.[27] Direct invasion of the thyroid lamina below this junction without invasion of the anterior commissure or spread across the laryngeal ventricle (that is, transglottic cancer) is unusual in cancer of the infrahyoid epiglottis but probably not as rare as some authors suggest (Fig. 7–26). Ventral epiglottic lesions may rarely extend directly through the thyrohyoid membrane or involve the hyoid bone; this occurs only with massive lesions of the preepiglottic space. The subtle variations in density of the thyroid cartilage seen on sections through the supraglottis are almost always related to volume-averaging artifacts (sections skimming across a curving contour of the cartilage) or normal variation in mineralization. Clear findings indicting invasion of the laryngeal framework should be interpreted as strong evidence that the lesion is, in reality, transglottic, and some other evidence of this has gone undetected. If the lesion is not obviously transglottic, it is probably biologically aggressive (Fig. 7–26).

Lateral supraglottic cancers start at the false cord, laryngeal

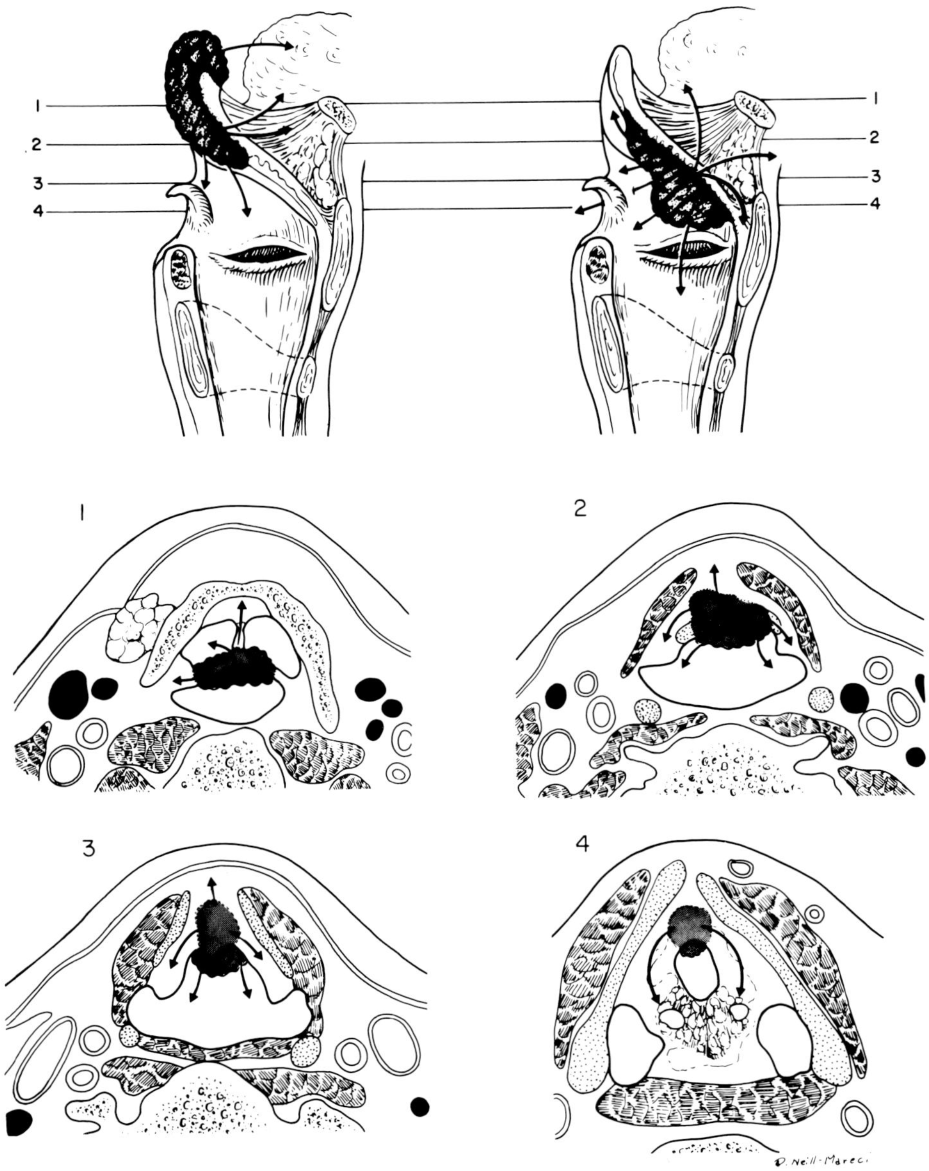

Figure 7–19. Spread patterns of anterior supraglottic cancers. Whole-organ figures at top show approximate levels of axial computed tomography sections. (From Mancuso and Hanafee.[2] Reprinted with permission.)

ventricle, or aryepiglottic fold and may grow superficially for some time (Figs. 7–17, 7–20, 7–27). Half of all lateral carcinomas, however, will show substantial growth in the paraglottic space, including spread to the glottic and subglottic regions, by the time they come to treatment (Figs. 7–17, 7–22). The submucosal spread of these lesions may be remote from the obvious mucosal disease, and it is in these cases that highly resolved, carefully interpreted images have much to offer. The primary sign of spread to the paraglottic space is obliteration of the fat within the space and loss of visualization of the superior extension of the lateral cricoarytenoid muscle when compared with the opposite side (Figs. 7–10, 7–17, 7–22). Anterolateral lesions tend to spread to the preepiglottic space while posterolateral tumors extend to the arytenoid and cricoarytenoid joint. The CT signs of spread to these regions and limitations of imaging within regions are identical to those discussed in the section of spread patterns of glottic cancer. The tendency to involve the cricoarytenoid region is most evident in aryepiglottic fold lesions, which may also spread submucosally to extralaryngeal sites as do pyriform sinus cancers. Bulky tumors can sometimes hang down into the laryngeal ventricle, mimicking invasion. Coronal MRI or CT reformations may, at times, help separate the bulky "hanging" lesions from truly infiltrative ones; however, this remains a limitation of any modern imaging technique.

Some authors have recognized a subtype of supraglottic carcinoma called the "Winkel carcinoma."[4] This is a useful classification because these tumors have a relatively distinctive growth pattern and may show a higher tendency for invading the laryngeal framework. On axial images, these legions appear to begin at the junction of the aryepiglottic fold and infrahyoid epiglottis. They spread to the preepiglottic space 70% of the time and usually extend around, rather than through, the epiglottic cartilage (Fig. 7–22). When high-volume, deep

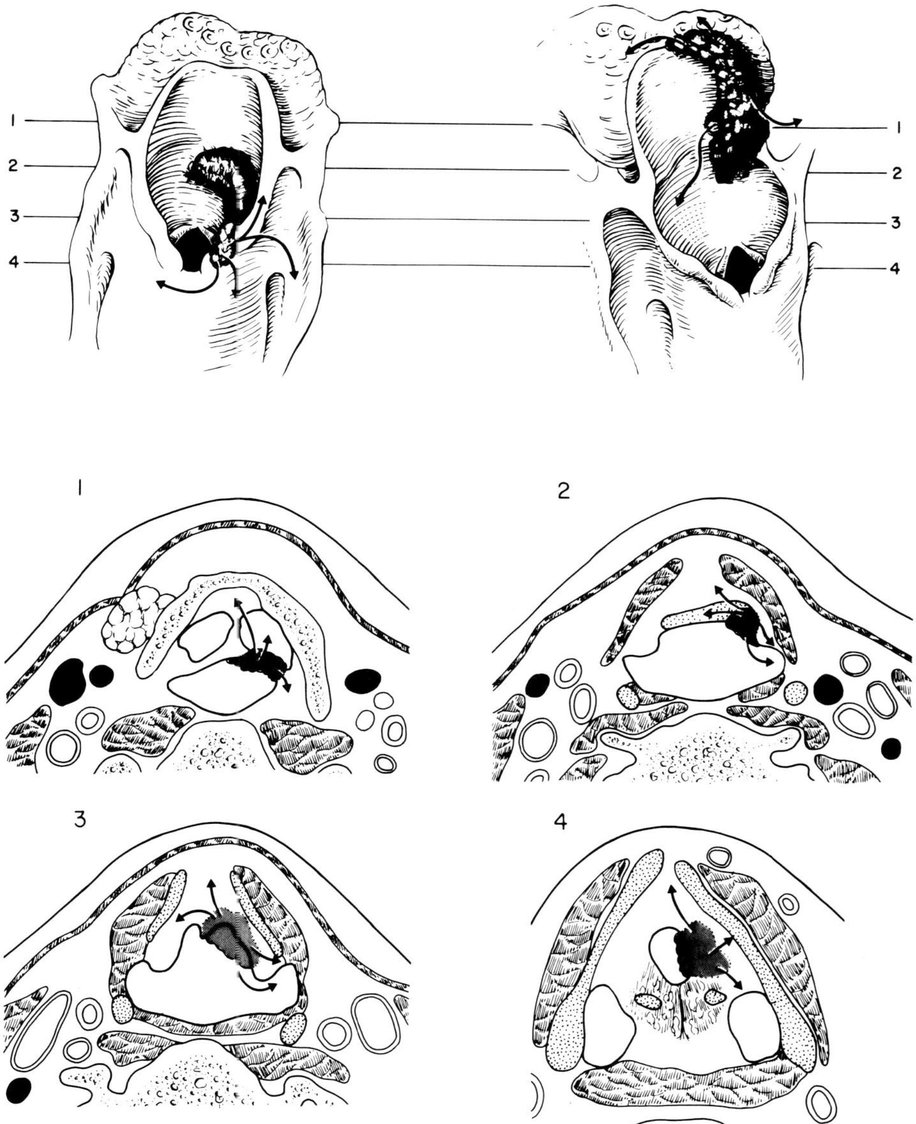

A

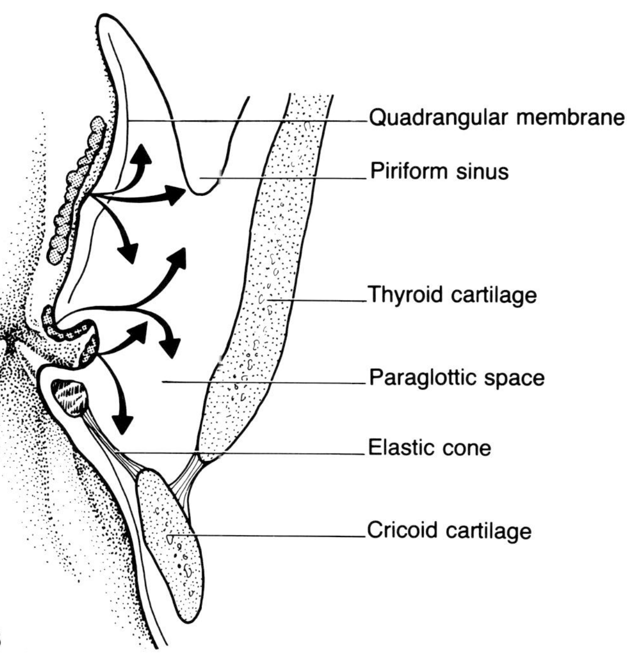

B

Figure 7–20. **A:** Spread patterns of lateral and anterolateral supraglottic cancers. Whole-organ pictures at top show approximate levels of axial computed tomography (CT) sections. **B:** Routes of deep spread of laterally situated supraglottic cancers. Note in particular that tumors arising on the mucosa lining the ventricle, especially those deep in its "fundus," can grow primarily into the paraglottic space and largely be hidden from the endoscopist's view. (From Mancuso and Hanafee.[2] Reprinted with permission.)

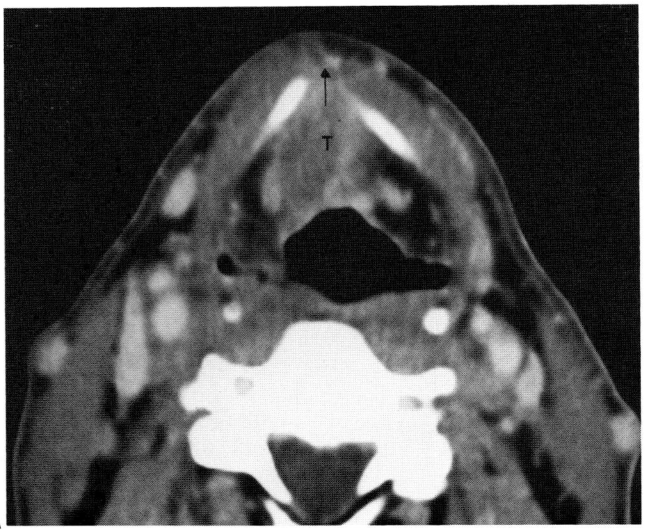

A

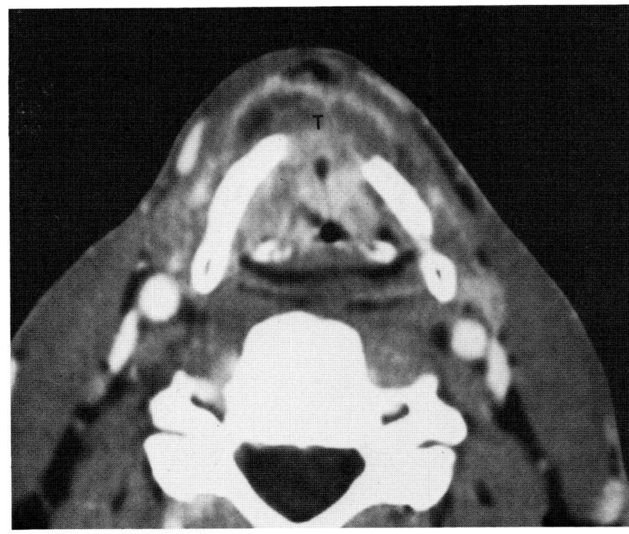

B

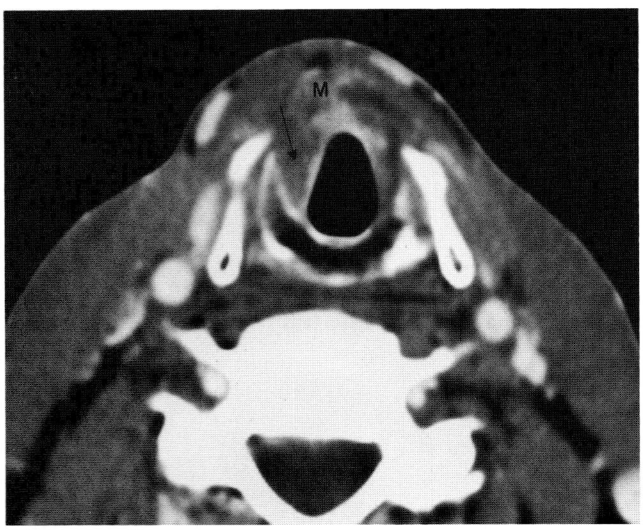

C

Figure 7–21. A 63-year-old man with bulky, ulcerative carcinoma of the infrahyoid epiglottis. Inferior limit uncertain at indirect laryngoscopy. Dorsolateral view showed anterior commissure spread. There was no mass or tenderness in the prelaryngeal soft tissues according to highly experienced examiners. **A**: Tumor (T) fills the preepiglottic space and spreads through the upper thyroid notch (arrow). There is asymmetry of the infrahyoid strap muscles and subcutaneous fat. **B**: At false vocal cord-ventricle level, the thyroid cartilage is destroyed and an obvious tumor mass (T) infiltrates the prelaryngeal soft tissues. **C**: In the upper subglottis, tumor or edema, or both, thicken the endolaryngeal soft tissues (arrow) and a prelaryngeal mass (M) is still present. Comment: All findings were confirmed following total laryngectomy.

spread is present, one should look carefully for evidence of invasion of the laryngeal framework at the attachment of the thyrohyoid membrane along the upper edge of the thyroid cartilage (Figs. 7–22, 7–26). When these cancers become transglottic, thyroid cartilage invasion at other points is possible. As with ventral carcinomas, limited MRI focused on the area of potential invasion may show infiltration of the infrahyoid strap muscles as a sign of penetration of the laryngeal framework (Fig. 7–26). These lesions also tend to involve the pharyngoepiglottic fold and vallecula; this is best evaluated by the endoscopist but is almost always visible on good quality CT (Fig. 7–23).

Posterior supraglottic cancer arising in the arytenoid and interarytenoid region is unusual. These lesions tend to spread subepithelially, and their full extent is usually best appreciated on MRI or CT (Fig. 7–28). These lesions can invade the anterior wall of the postcricoid portion of the hypopharynx; if this spread is submucosal, it may only be appreciated by MRI or CT (Figs. 7–18 to 7–21). If such findings are suspected but not clearly evident on CT, a focused MRI study done with 3 to 4 mm sections and moderately T_2 weighted images can be used for confirmation.

Integration of Imaging and Treatment in Supraglottic Carcinoma

CT remains the most useful imaging study for supraglottic cancer and is far better than MRI in evaluation of cervical adenopathy (see Chapter 8). CT is more likely to produce a study free of significant motion artifact and is at least 20 to 30% less expensive than MRI. With future improvements, particularly in speed, MRI will assume a more important role.

Supraglottic cancer treated with the intent to preserve laryngeal function may be managed with radiotherapy or a variety of subtotal supraglottic laryngectomies. The basic conservation surgical procedure is the horizontal subtotal supraglottic laryngectomy, which may be extended to include the ipsilateral

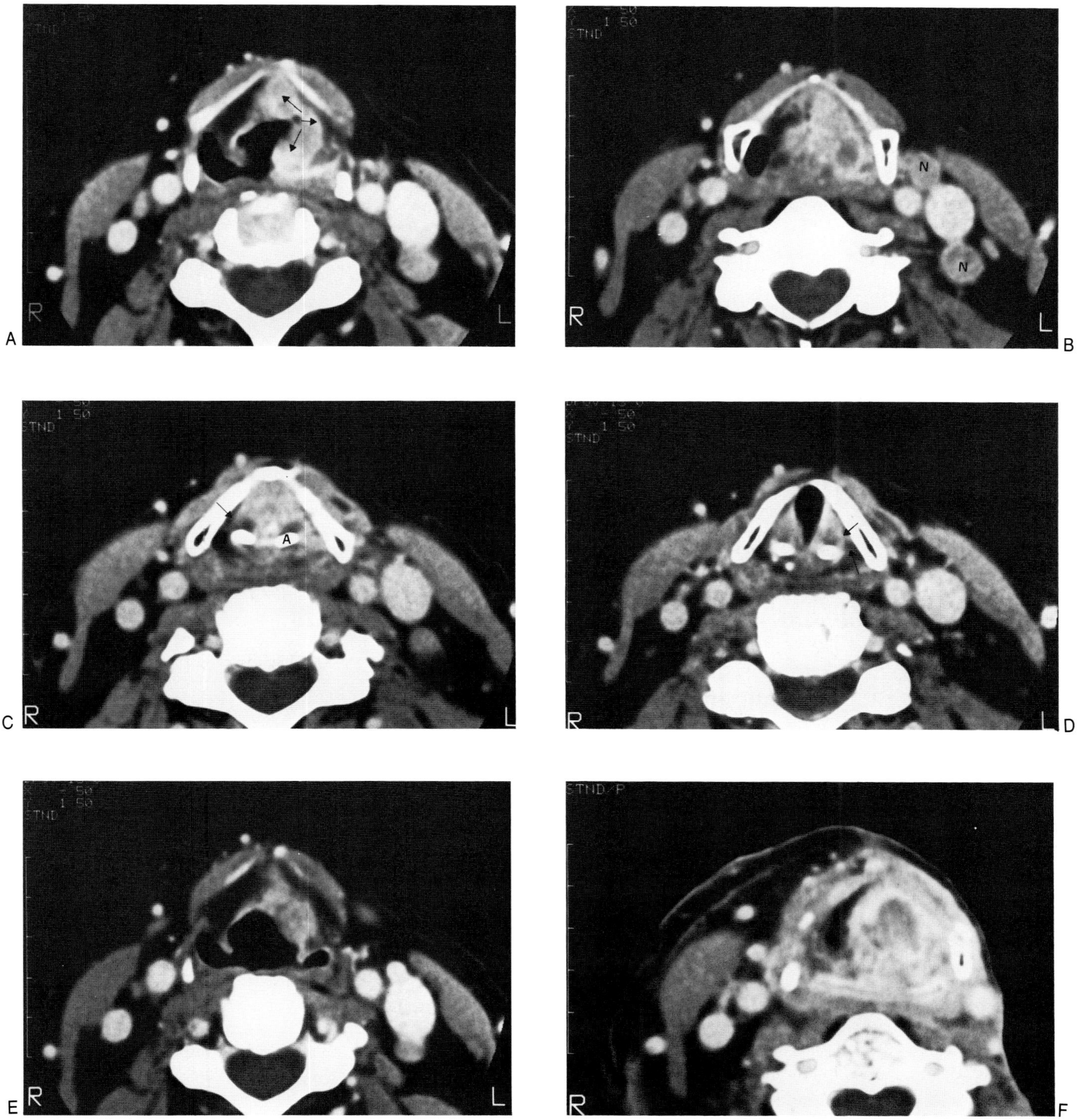

Figure 7–22. A 58-year-old woman with supraglottic carcinoma arising at the junction of the aryepiglottic fold and infrahyoid epiglottis. **A:** Typical spread pattern of the lesion (arrows): anteriorly, to the preepiglottic space; laterally, directly into the paraglottic space; posteriorly, to the aryepiglottic fold. **B:** At upper false vocal cord (FVC) level, the paraglottic space is full. Note the tumor deep to the anterior wall of the pyriform sinus within the paraglottic space. Neck was N_1 clinically. Computed tomography showed two positive nodes (N). **C:** At low FVC-ventricular level, there is still tumor obliterating the paraglottic space (compared with normal right side; see arrow) and lateral to the arytenoid (A). **D:** At the ventricular level, there is perhaps minimal edema (arrow) lateral to the arytenoid. No definite, deeply infiltrating tumor is visible. **E:** Level above that in A shows continual cephalad growth in paraglottic and preepiglottic spaces. **F:** Persistent submucosal cancer following treatment for cure with radiotherapy (RT), followed by radical neck dissection. Comment: This was a high-volume cancer, probably better suited to surgery than RT for definitive management. Clinically, response of primary to RT was considered good. At the time of the CT in Figure 7–22F (done 12 weeks post-RT) there was only minimal friability of mucosa, suggesting persistence of tumor in a generally "edematous" larynx.

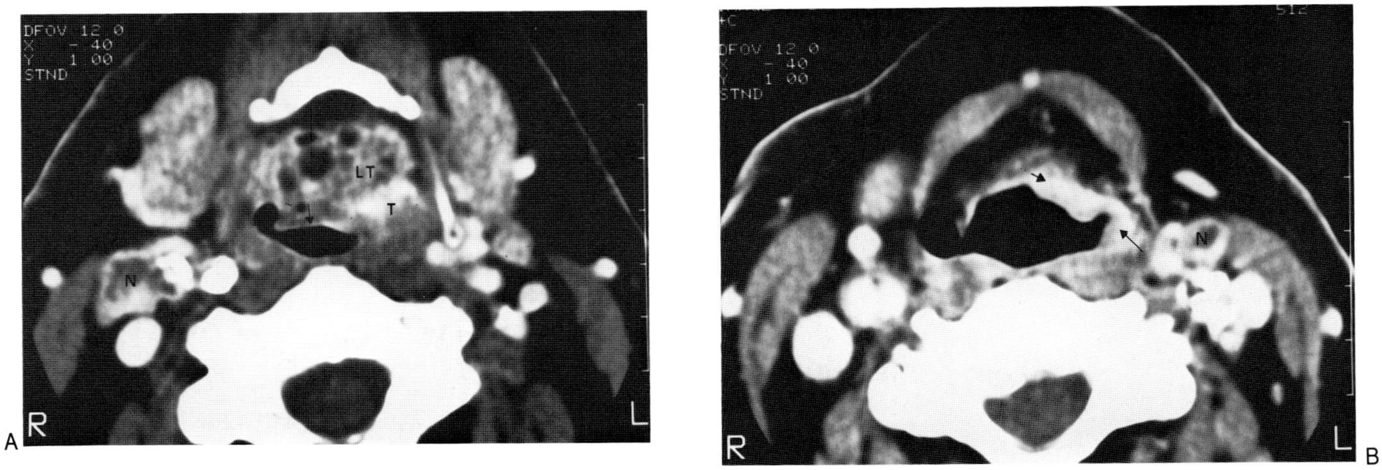

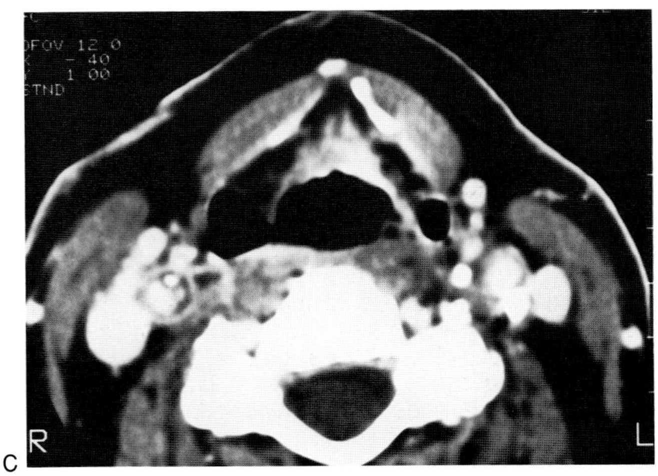

Figure 7–23. Example of a relatively superficially spreading carcinoma of the free margin of the epiglottis with spread to the upper aryepiglottic fold. **A**: Tumor (T) spilling into left vallecula is difficult to distinguish from lingual tonsillar (LT) tissue. Note slightly thickened (presumably edematous), but otherwise normal, free margin of epiglottis on right (arrow). Metastatic node (N) on right is difficult to tell from adjacent "soft" carotid plaque. **B**: Tumor is about 5 mm thick (note scale on left) and involves the infrahyoid epiglottis and aryepiglottic fold (from arrow to arrow). Note positive left neck node (N). **C**: There is *minimal*, if any, preepiglottic space spread. Note that nearly the full volume of fat normally present, in the preepiglottic space, at this level is uninvolved.

arytenoid or true cord and can also be modified to include the vallecula and tongue base.[46,47] All extended procedures carry an increased risk of failure, since the oncologically sound basic operation is being extended to deal with more advanced lesions that have a higher tendency for occult spread beyond the planned surgical margins. The sites of these possible "leaks" can be demonstrated on CT or MRI.

Radiation therapy offers an excellent chance for control of primary disease in many patients. This is especially true for superficial and low-volume tumors.[30–32,34] Laser excision may be as effective for very limited lesions, although treatment of the neck would require some additional procedure in many cases. Although spread to the preepiglottic space has often been considered a relative contraindication for radiotherapy, recent studies suggest that tumor volume may be a more important factor for predicting likelihood of radiotherapy control than whether preepiglottic or paraglottic space invasion is present.[30–32] This experience includes patients with 75 to 100% invasion of the preepiglottic space who achieved primary control with irradiation alone (Fig. 7–29). Since CT and MRI are sensitive and accurate tools for evaluating the preepiglottic space, previously employed methods of assessment such as palpation or gross findings on lateral plain films of the larynx or laryngograms, which could detect only the most high-volume preepiglottic spread, are obsolete. These larger-volume lesions, detectable by such methods, probably still are best treated by surgery (Figs. 7–21, 7–22, 7–26). Of course, further study of the significance of preepiglottic space involvement and tumor volume is required. Tumor volume is easy to determine with simple interactive computer programs available on most modern CT and MRI units. Preliminary data indicate that supraglottic cancers 8 cc or more in volume stand a 50 to 60% chance of failing therapy (Tables 7–3, and 7–4).[31–32] Other factors such as tumor differentiation, aggressiveness, and other parameters need to be considered in management decisions.

High-volume, deep spread of tumor beneath intact mucosa occurs frequently in supraglottic cancer, and this submucosal disease is easily and accurately evaluated with CT and MRI (Figs. 7–16 to 7–21). When present, high-volume, submucosal spread suggests that the tumor may have grown transglottically and/or penetrated the laryngeal framework (Figs. 7–17, 7–21 to 7–29). These two circumstances usually dictate a primarily surgical approach. Comprehensive evaluation by endoscopy and CT, with very thin sections and limited MRI study of

A
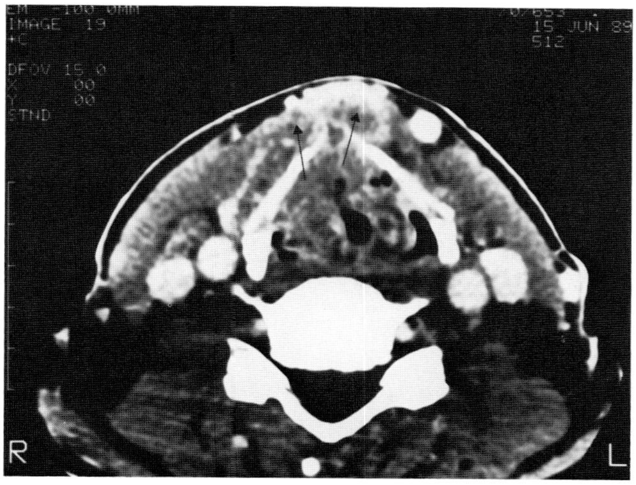

B
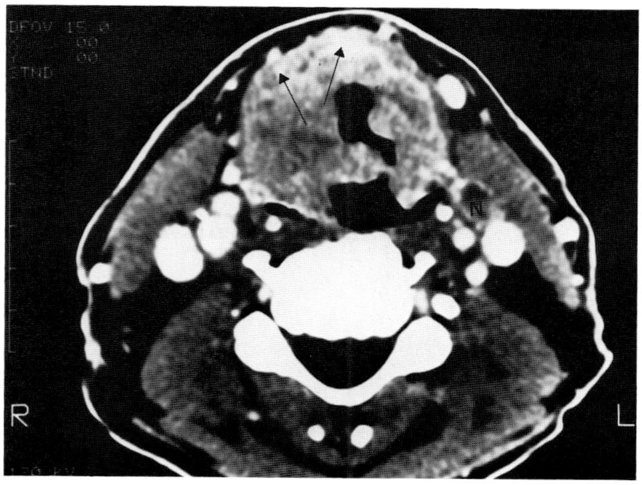

C
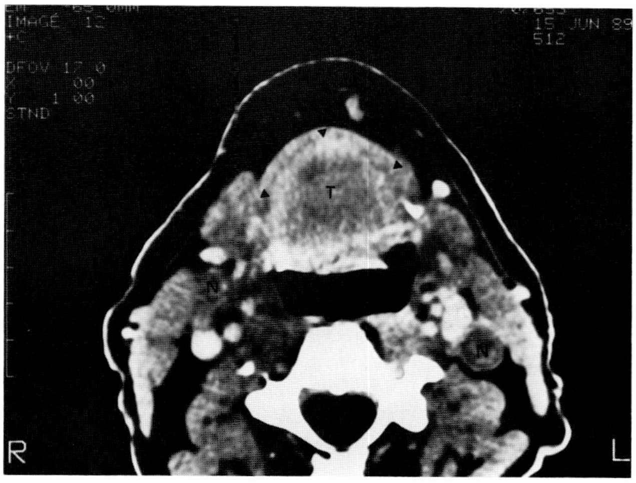

Figure 7–24. Patient with dysphagia and otalgia and obvious epiglottic carcinoma. No mucosal abnormality of the tongue base was seen at dorsolateral view. The vallecula was firm on palpation. **A,B:** Extensive epiglottic tumor fills the preepiglottic space, paraglottic spaces, and spreads to the prelaryngeal soft tissues (arrows). Computed tomography (CT)-positive node (N). **C:** Massive tumor (T) invades and replaces the deep tongue base (arrowheads show tumor limits). CT-positive node (N). Comment: Because clinical findings at tongue base were minimal, surgery was done. Massive, surgically incurable, tongue base invasion was confirmed. Margins were positive. Patient was sent for postoperative radiotherapy.

questionable areas, will help in many complex surgical decisions, particularly in choosing between extended conservation procedures and total extirpation of the larynx.

TRANSGLOTTIC CARCINOMA

Patterns of Tumor Spread

Transglottic carcinoma can be a somewhat ambiguous classification, depending on the experience and philosophic inclinations of the person using the term.[18–22,33] There is general agreement that the term "transglottic" indicates involvement of glottis and supraglottis. Some suggest this implies the tumor has crossed the laryngeal ventricle, but this is not necessarily true, since transglottic growth can occur anterior and posterior to the laryngeal ventricle. Although vocal cord fixation is present in the overwhelming majority of lateral and posterior transglottic lesions, fixation need not be present in lesions crossing the anterior commissure and in lower volume lateral lesions (Figs. 7–12, 7–17).

The notion that the term "transglottic" should be used for tumors beginning in the laryngeal ventricle is interesting and can further complicate communication. In fact, it is very useful to realize that tumors may begin in the ventricle and grow primarily submucosally in the paraglottic space (Fig. 7–17). This growth pattern may be obvious on CT and MRI studies because of obliteration of deep fat planes, and less obvious clinically, perhaps being recognized only as a submucosal bulge or suspected because the vocal cord is "sluggish" or fixed. By the time these ventricular primaries present clinically, they have usually grown transglottically. Practically speaking, some of these probably arise on the undersurface of the false cord and some represent lateral cephalad spread of a glottic primary in the paraglottic space. It is likely that a number of these actually begin in the fundus or floor of the ventricle but it is difficult to prove how many. In our experience, when a tumor is almost entirely submucosal, we assume it began in the ventricle; otherwise, the primary site is determined on the basis of the predominant mucosal component (Figs. 7–10, 7–17). For example, transglottic carcinoma with obviously mucosal disease at the glottic level and paraglottic extension to the supraglottis is

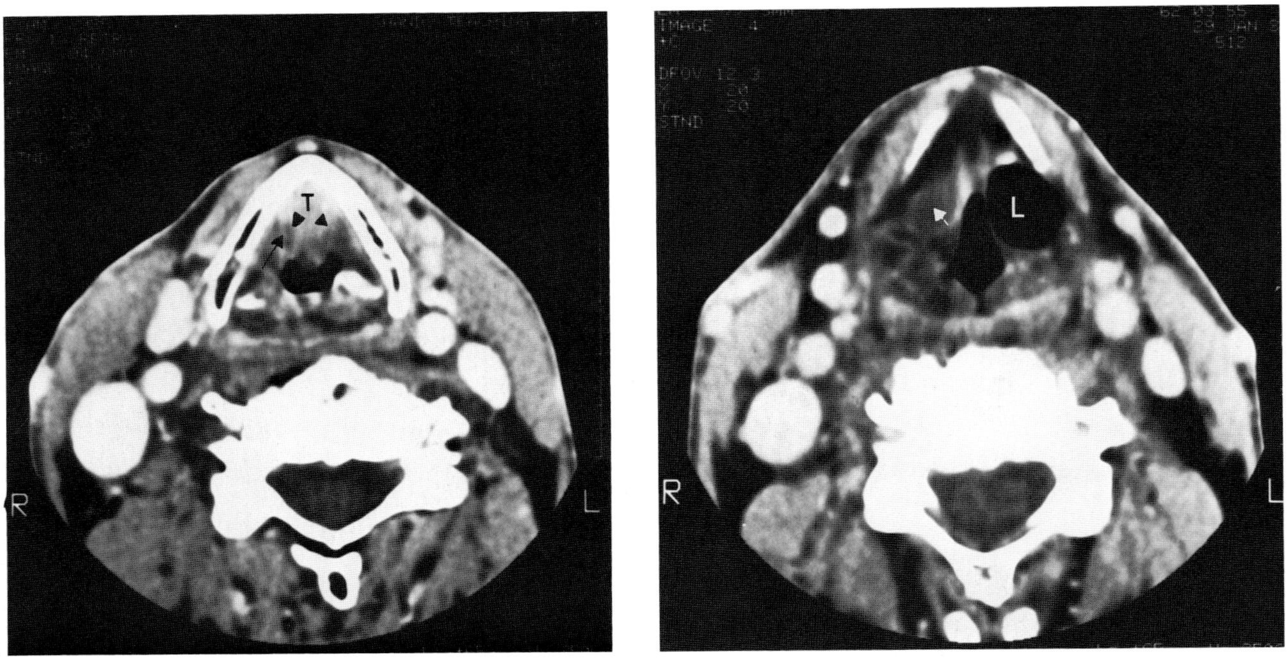

A B

Figure 7–25. A 46-year-old woman with carcinoma just above the anterior commissure. **A**: At the false vocal cord (FVC) level, there is a small tumor mass (T) that spreads to the anterior FVC bilaterally (arrowheads). Much of the soft tissue swelling is lower density than tumor, suggesting it is, at least in part, edema (arrow). **B**: A submucosal mass on the left turned out to be an air-filled laryngocele (L). A fluid-filled laryngocele is seen on the right (arrow). The preepiglottic space deep to the petiole is normal.

considered to be of true cord origin, whereas a transglottic lesion with a false cord mucosal component and predominantly paraglottic space spread to the glottic or subglottic level is considered a false cord primary. This group of lesions comprises the lateral transglottic cancers. CT and MRI show a lesion traversing the paraglottic space (Figs. 7–10, 17–17).

Although vocal cord fixation is usually present, roughly 10 to 15% of low-volume transglottic tumors have mobile cords.[31] The more posterior the lesion, the higher the likelihood of fixation. Sixty-five percent of transglottic lesions over 2 cm will have invaded the laryngeal framework.[20] This may not be visible on CT or MRI in many cases for reasons already discussed.

Anterior transglottic spread may occur due to vertical extension of glottic-subglottic or supraglottic carcinoma (Fig. 7–21). When anterior transglottic growth occurs, penetration of the laryngeal framework is likely. This is frequently obvious on imaging studies and can be manifested by defects in the thyroid cartilage, prelaryngeal spread through the cricothyroid membrane (Figs. 7–12, 7–13, 7–21), or exolaryngeal spread at the transition between the top of the thyroid cartilage and the thyrohyoid membrane (Figs. 7–21, 7–26). Supplementary MRI may be required to confirm early extralaryngeal spread as manifested by invasion of the infrahyoid strap muscles (Figs. 7–13, 7–15). On moderately T_2 weighted axial sections, the higher signal intensity tumor will be seen invading or displacing the muscle bundles. Anterior commissure cancer may be very aggressive. Kirchner and Fischer[23] described a tendency for some of these lesions to spread between intact layers of perichondrium, replacing the thyroid cartilage (Fig. 7–11). We have observed this in vivo and in each case the spread to the cartilage and extralaryngeal soft tissues was not anticipated from clinical examination alone (Figs. 7–11, 7–21). This finding has resulted in some of the most dramatic changes in treatment plans over the years of our experience with CT and MRI (Fig. 7–21).

Posterior spreading carcinomas, whether glottic or supraglottic in origin, may become transglottic at a low-volume stage (Fig. 7–14). Early transglottic spread in the region of the cricoarytenoid joint, interarytenoid area, or posterior laryngeal wall (arytenoid pad) may be difficult to identify on routine laryngeal images. Focused MRI or thin-section (1.5 to 2 mm) CT may be necessary in cases in which spread to this region might alter choice of therapy.

Integration of Imaging and Treatment in Transglottic Carcinoma

In general, transglottic cancers are advanced and will be treated with total, or near-total, laryngectomy and possibly postoperative radiotherapy.[4,34,35] The neck will be treated as well. Clinically occult transglottic spread demonstrated on CT is one reason a patient might be selected for total laryngectomy rather than definitive radiotherapy (Figs. 7–30 to 7–33).[44,48,49] If cartilage invasion and extralaryngeal spread have occurred, any type of conservation surgery is usually contraindicated. Unsuspected extralaryngeal or bilateral spread may obviate even near-total laryngectomy. In advanced lesions, preoperative

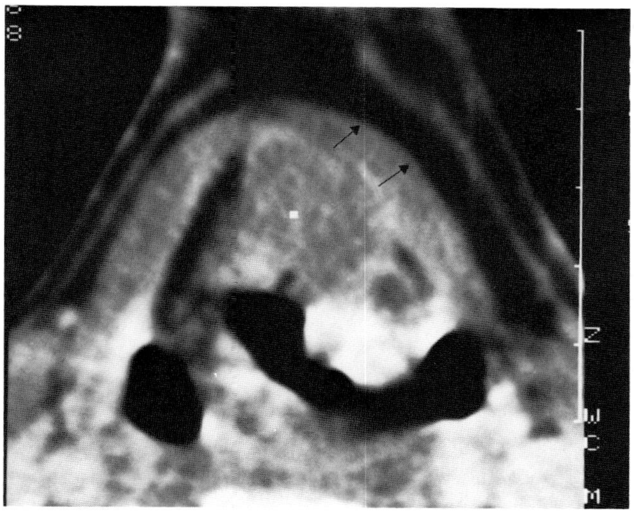

A

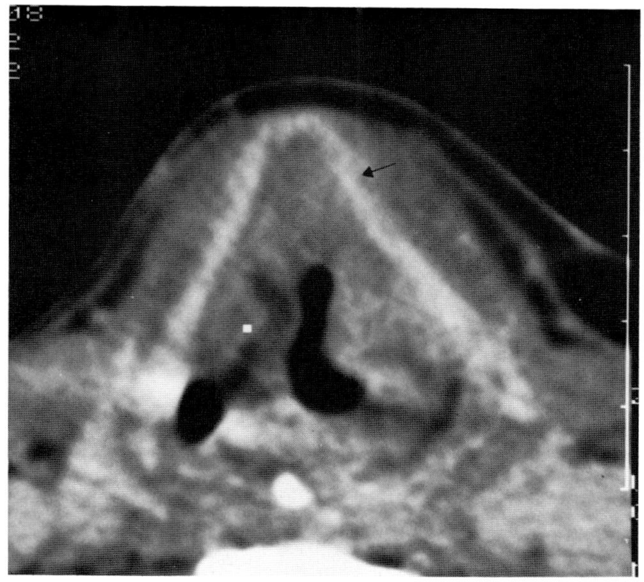

B

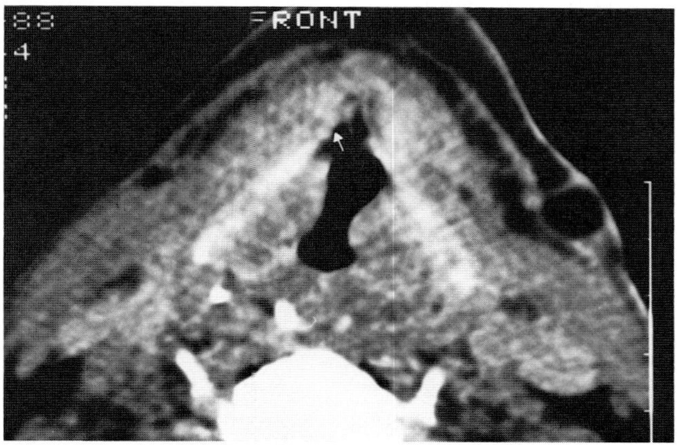

C

Figure 7–26. A 68-year-old man with carcinoma of the infrahyoid epiglottis. A: Midsupraglottic section shows high-volume, deeply infiltrating cancer filling the preepiglottic space and paraglottic space. Note the bulging of the infrahyoid strap muscles on the left (arrows). B: At the false vocal cord level, high-volume paraglottic spread is stil present, the infrahyoid strap muscles still appear thicker on the left, and there is subtle evidence of infracture of the thyroid cartilage (arrow). C: Following radiotherapy, the laryngeal cartilages are collapsing inward (compare position to that in Figure 7–26B, and air is present down to denuded surface of laryngeal framework (arrow). These are signs of gross condronecrosis. Comment: Because of findings suspicious for framework invasion on pretreatment computed tomography (CT), magnetic resonance imaging was requested. The patient was unable to tolerate the study. Definitive radiotherapy was attempted with resulting necrosis probably related to preexisting framework invasion. (This cannot be proven in this case.) The patient's larynx was functionally useless. Laryngectomy showed chondronecrosis and persistent tumor.

imaging may indicate the need for an inferiorly placed tracheostomy, or laryngopharyngectomy if submucosal disease approaches or involves the hypopharynx. At times, imaging may be the only means of anticipating that laryngopharyngectomy and myocutaneous flap, gastric pull-up, or other extensive pharyngeal reconstruction will be required in a transglottic laryngeal primary tumor (see "Hypopharyngeal Cancer").

There is a subgroup of transglottic lesions that may be managed with the intent of preserving the larynx.[33–36,44,48] Low-volume lesions with lateral spread in the paraglottic space with or without cord fixation may be cured with radiotherapy alone[33–36,44,48] (Fig. 7–17). These patients are highly selected on the basis of tumor extent, reliability for follow-up, and motivation for preserving the larynx, among other factors. Patients with high-volume, lateral or posterior transglottic patterns may not be good candidates for such an approach (Fig. 7–14); those with strictly lateral or anterolateral, low-volume disease may be (Fig. 7–12). To date, only preliminary data are available directly relating imaging findings to such patient selection.[30–33]

Transglottic cancer at any site has a relatively high rate of penetration of the laryngeal framework.[4,18–22,49] In some cases this will escape detection by CT. MRI may prove superior but has its limitations as well.[27] It is possible that subtle cartilage invasion is radiocurable,[42] although many studies have shown that penetration of the laryngeal framework is a reliable predictor of failure to control the primary site with radiotherapy alone. It will be necessary to develop profiles that will allow for conservation of the larynx with acceptable cure rates. Limited transglottic lesions with limited cartilage invasion may be one area where imaging will play a pivotal role in treatment planning.

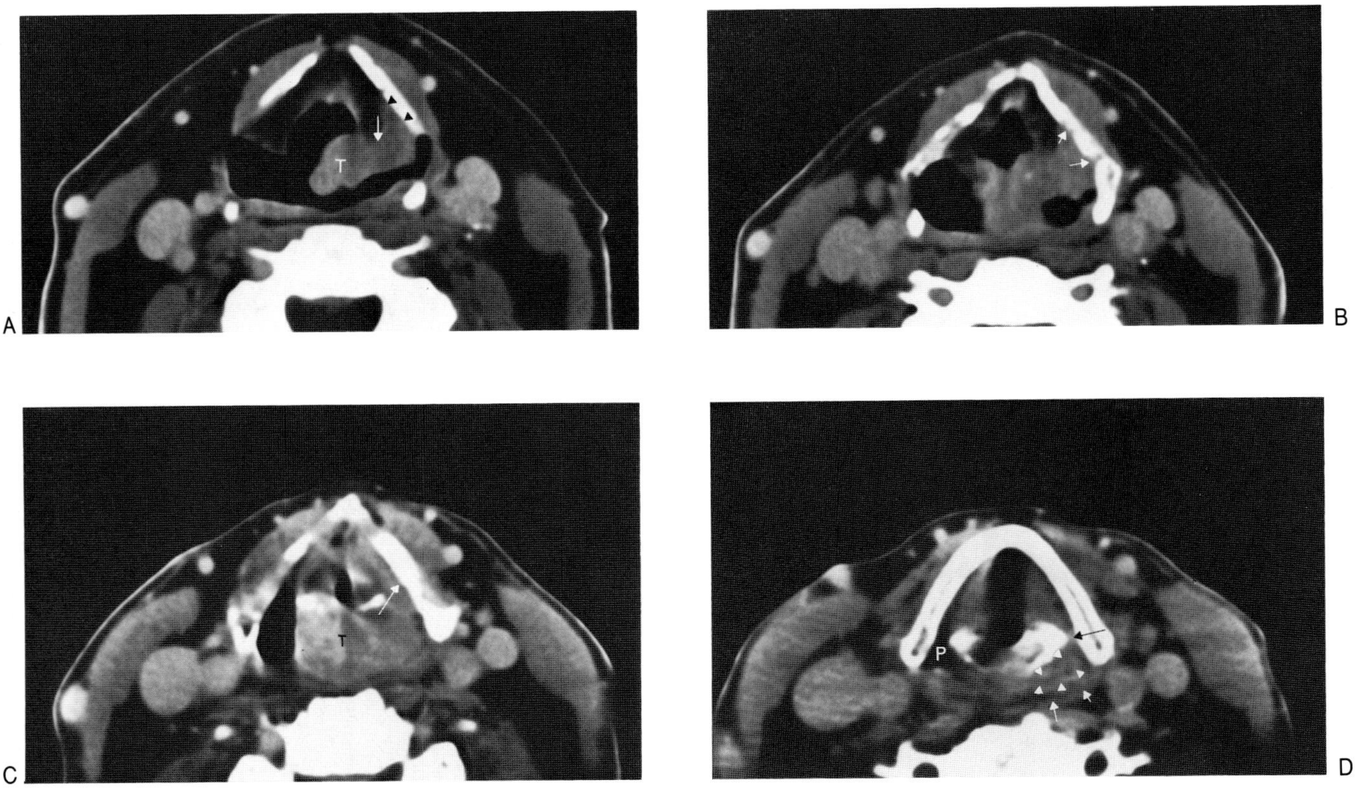

Figure 7–27. A 64-year-old man with carcinoma of the aryepiglottic fold (marginal supraglottic). A: Aryepiglottic fold is obviously thickened by tumor (T). Note the broad zone of tumor in the paraglottic space deep to the anterior wall of the pyriform sinus (arrow) and along the thyroid cartilage inner wall (arrowheads). B: At false vocal cord (FVC) level, there is a very broad interface between the tumor and thyroid cartilage as in Figure 7–27A. Focal areas of demineralization (arrows) are no different from the normal side and should *not* be interpreted as foci of cartilage invasion. These tumors almost never invade the cartilage at this location. C: At the ventricular level, there is a bulky tumor mass (T) on the posterior laryngeal wall. The paraglottic space is still obliterated (arrow), although the findings are fairly subtle. D: At the undersurface of the true vocal cord level, there is subtle obliteration of the paraglottic space between the cricoid and thyroid cartilages (black arrow) and equally subtle thickening of the soft tissues in the upper postcricoid region (arrowheads). Note normal posterior pharyngeal wall (white arrows) and normal position of pyriform sinus apex on right (P).

HYPOPHARYNGEAL CANCER

Patterns of Tumor Spread

Hypopharyngeal cancer arises in one of three sites: the pyriform sinus, posterior pharyngeal wall, or postcricoid region. The pattern of growth is influenced by the site of origin, aggressiveness of the particular tumor, and adjacent laryngeal anatomy (Fig. 7–34A,B). Hypopharyngeal cancers commonly spread to adjacent portions of the larynx and hypopharynx, penetrate the laryngeal framework, and grow in the extralaryngeal soft tissue.

Pyriform sinus cancers are the most common hypopharyngeal lesions encountered in the United States. Direct growth of tumor from the pyriform sinus to the larynx is possible via the paraglottic space (Fig. 7–34). A pyriform sinus cancer will typically appear (on axial sections) as a thick, infiltrating mass surrounding the pyriform sinus (Fig. 7–35). Involvement of the anterior, posterior, lateral, and medial walls is usually present, although two walls tend to dominate. Clinically inapparent spread to the endolarynx occurs when the tumor penetrates the anterior wall and grows ventrally into the paraglottic space (Fig. 7–35). This growth may extend to the preepiglottic space and onto the contralateral hemilarynx beneath intact mucosa. Ventral growth in the paraglottic space is usually restricted to that space and perhaps a small portion of the ipsilateral preepiglottic space (Fig. 7–34). Pyriform sinus cancer may also spill over or penetrate the aryepiglottic fold to involve the endolarynx. This is usually obvious at endoscopy. When the aryepiglottic fold is thickened on axial images, it is difficult to know whether mucosal spread is on one side or both. Once the tumor has grown to the apex of the pyriform sinus, it can continue this dorsal-caudal spread on the mucosa to the posterior wall of the larynx and postcricoid region (Figs. 7–28, 7–34 to 7–36).

Tumor may also grow caudally from the apex of the pyriform sinus to the cricothyroid joint, extralaryngeal soft tissues, and into the upper tracheoesophageal groove. This will be manifested by obliteration of fat planes, cartilage destruction, and

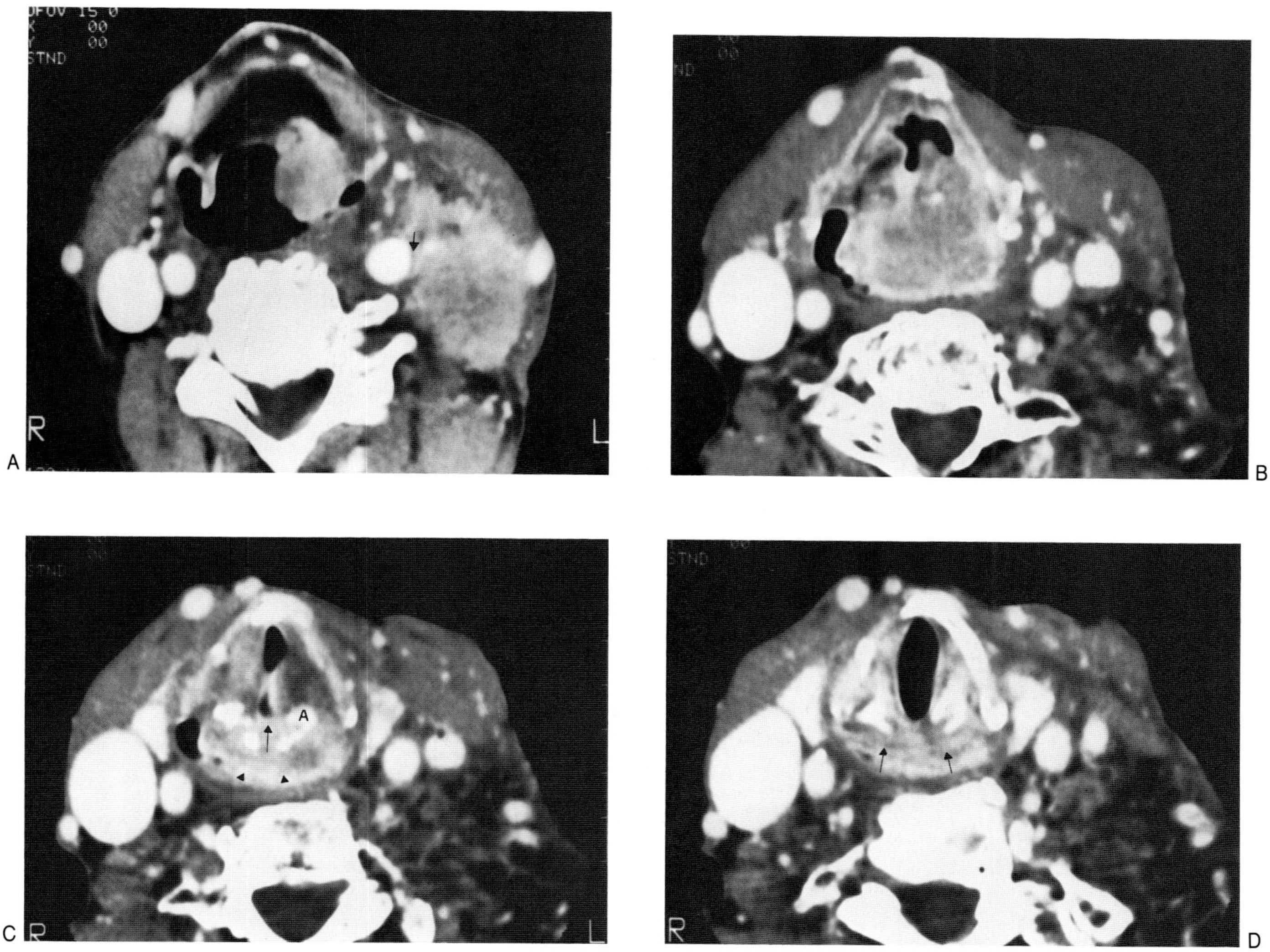

Figure 7–28. Patient with carcinoma of the posterior laryngeal wall. **A:** The aryepiglottic fold spread seen here frequently occurs in these lesions. The nodal metastatic disease is very aggressive; the surrounding edema and indistinct margins indicate obvious capsular penetration. The carotid is not encased; *focal* fixation is possible but unlikely from the appearance of the interface between the nodal mass or carotid (arrow). **B:** These masses are typically bulky and sometimes visually inseparable from the posterior pharyngeal wall. Of course, this is not a problem for the endoscopist. **C:** Extensive interarytenoid spread (arrow) is present at the true vocal cord (TVC) level as well as spread to upper postcricoid region (arrowheads). Musculature of the left TVC is atrophic (note decreased density compared with the right cord) and arytenoid (A) is fixed or displaced medially. All these findings strongly suggest cricoarytenoid joint invasion. **D:** Tumor spread to the midpostcricoid region (arrows).

displacement and swelling of adjacent structures, including the infrahyoid strap muscles, thyroid gland, and esophageal wall. T_2 weighted MRI can be especially helpful in showing early extralaryngeal spread and invasion of the muscular wall of the esophagus.

Spread from the lower postcricoid region to the esophageal verge and beyond may be undetectable by endoscopy, and CT findings may appear subtle to the untrained observer (Fig. 7–31). Obliteration of fat in the upper tracheoesophageal groove or asymmetrical thickening of the postcricoid soft tissue and upper cervical esophagus might be the only clues to such extension. T_2 weighted MR images, with their superior tumor muscle contrast, can confirm invasion of the postcricoid portion of the inferior constrictor (cricopharyngeus muscle) or muscular wall of the esophagus. This MRI study need only be limited to one or two acquisitions focused on the postcricoid region. Medial deep spread from the apex of the pyriform sinus will ultimately reach the arytenoid, cricoarytenoid joint, and subglottis (deep to the elastic cone). The cord may be fixed due to invasion of deep musculature, the cricoarytenoid region, or growth along the recurrent nerve. The last factor is uncommon and only occasionally can be anticipated by imaging.

Pyriform sinus carcinoma frequently penetrates the laryngeal framework. Favored sites laterally are at the cornua of the

A B C D E F

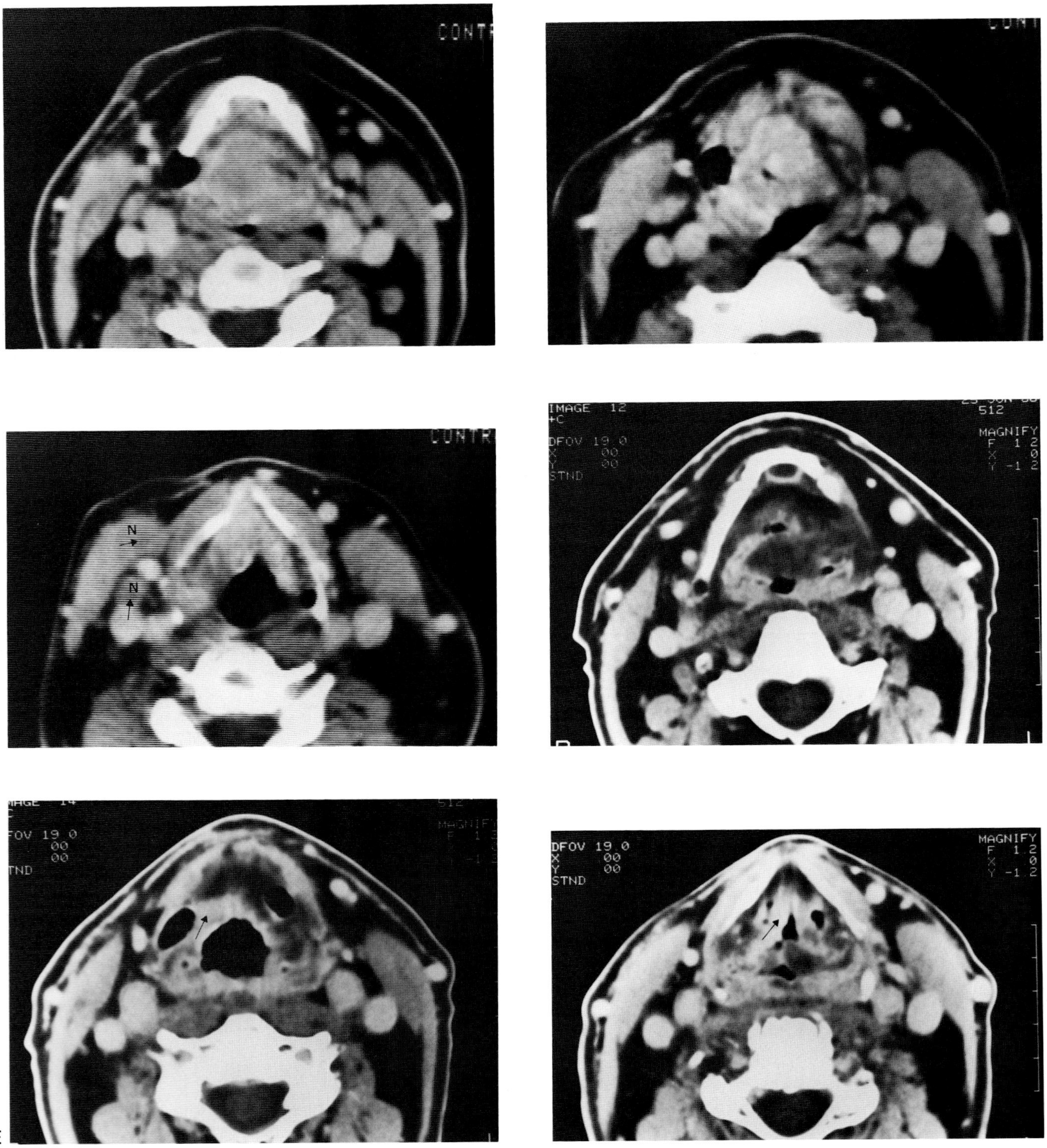

Figure 7–29. Patient with carcinoma of epiglottis who preferred radiation over supraglottic laryngectomy for primary attempt at control of his disease. **A, B, C:** Preradiotherapy study shows a high-volume cancer filling the entire preepiglottic space and extending to the paraglottic spaces bilaterally. The two computed tomography (CT)-positive nodes (N) in C were not palpable in this short, thick-necked patient; they measure 12 and 6 mm and contain metastatic foci (arrows). **D, E, F:** Postradiotherapy study 2 years after therapy shows diffuse edema or fibrosis, or both, and minor areas of focal increased density (arrows) but no evidence of recurrence. Note in E that the CT-positive nodes were controlled with radiotherapy. Patient has no evidence of disease at 5 years.

Table 7-3. Local Control in 31 Patients as a Function of T Stage for Low-Volume and High-Volume Lesions

STAGE	LOCAL CONTROL BY TUMOR VOLUME	
	<6 cc	≥6 cc
T_1	3/3	—
T_2	3/4	0/1
T_3	9/11	6/11
T_4	—	0/1
Total*	15/18 (83%)	6/13 (46%)

*p = 0.038.

Table 7-4. Local Control According to Degree of Preepiglottic Space Involvement and Tumor Volume for T_3 Lesions

PREEPIGLOTTIC SPACE INVOLVEMENT (%)	TUMOR VOLUME	
	<6 cc	≥6 cc
0-25	7/8	2/4
25-75	1/2	1/2
>75	1/1	3/5
Total*	9/11 (82%)	6/11 (55%)

*p = 0.181.

thyroid cartilage (Fig. 7–30). This thyroid cartilage invasion is usually easily recognized on CT. Frequently, tumor surrounds the superior horn of the thyroid cartilage. When large portions of the thyroid cartilage are destroyed, extralaryngeal spread is usually present. If the tumor has started in, or involves, the mid to upper pyriform sinus, it may invade the thyroid cartilage at its transition with the thyrohyoid membrane. Tumor must transgress the paraglottic space to invade the cartilage at that point. Extralaryngeal spread may also occur at the posterior aspect of the thyrohyoid membrane. Rarely, tumor may spread through the membrane along the point of penetration of the superior laryngeal neurovascular bundle (Fig. 7–31). Supplemental MRI may be used to confirm subtle extralaryngeal spread as described previously.

Posterior pharyngeal wall cancers commonly involve both the oropharynx and hypopharynx. These tend to be flat, thick cancers as seen on axial images and usually cause asymmetrical thickening of the entire posterior wall, although one side often is thicker than the other (Fig. 7–32). More lateral spread will involve the posterior wall of the pyriform sinus and circumferential submucosal involvement of a pyriform sinus is common. In the latter circumstance it may be difficult to decide whether

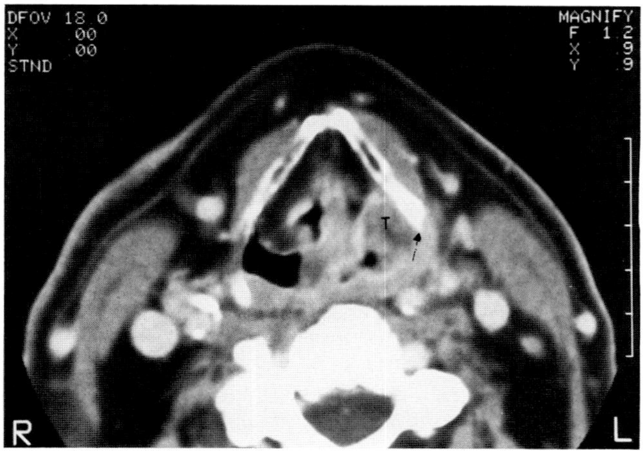

Figure 7–30. Clinically, T_2 pyriform sinus carcinoma. Tumor (T) obviously invades the thyroid cartilage (arrow). Gross cartilage invasion at this site was confirmed pathologically.

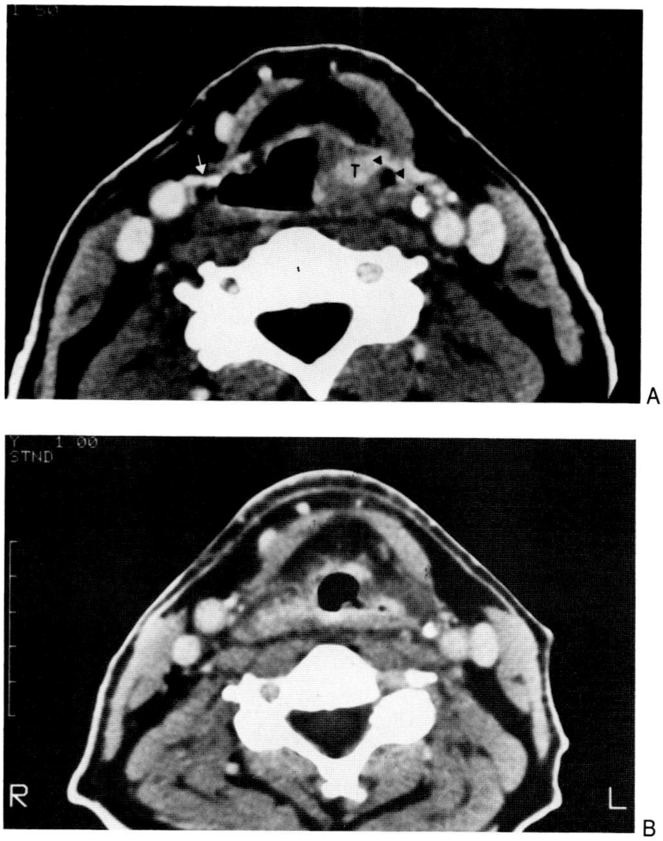

Figure 7–31. Clinically, T_2 pyriform sinus carcinoma. **A:** The main bulk of the tumor (T) involves the anterior and medial walls of the pyriform sinus. There is extralaryngeal spread through the thyrohyoid membrane along the superior laryngeal neurovascular bundle (arrowheads). Compare the pathologically involved left neurovascular bundle with the normal one (arrow) on the right. **B:** At 1 year postradiotherapy. Both the extralaryngeal spread and pharyngeal components of the tumor appear to have been controlled. Comment: This patient is free of disease at 2 years following radiation therapy. He was followed with computed tomography (CT) for 1 year at 3 month intervals and will have been followed with CT at 6-month intervals 2 more years (total of 3 years of imaging follow-up).

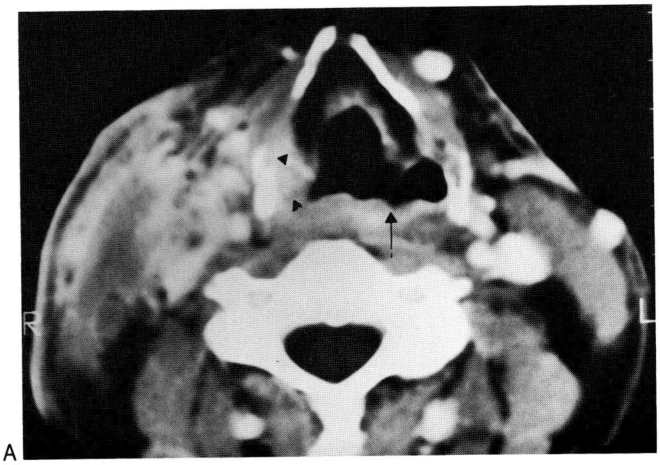

A

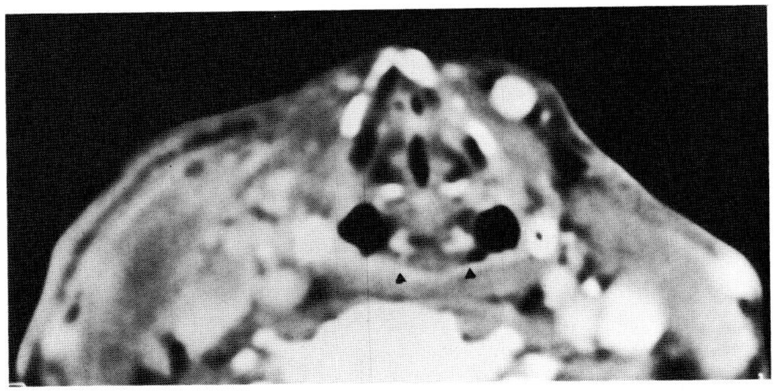

B

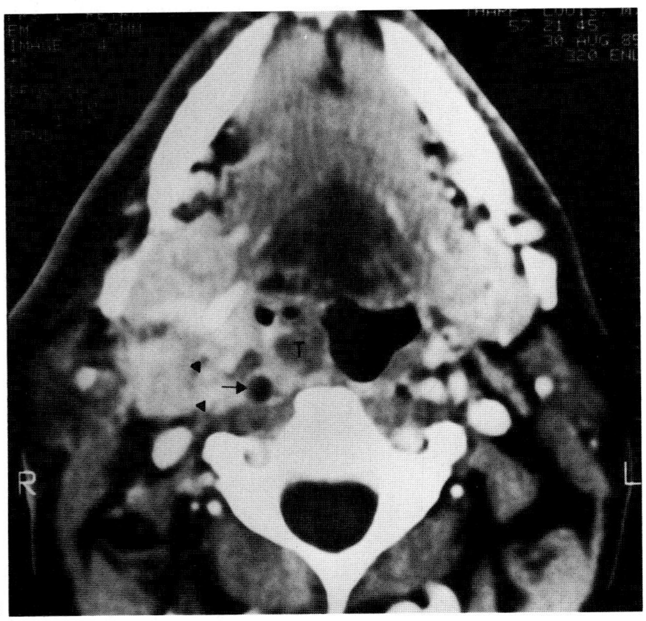

C

Figure 7–32. Posterior pharyngeal wall carcinoma with advanced neck disease. **A:** Typical plaque-like variety of posterior pharyngeal wall cancer; the lesion is predominantly on the right side but spreads across the midline (arrow) and involves the right pyriform sinus (arrowheads). Nodal mass (seen better in Figure 7–35C) is aggressive and has an extensive inflammatory component. **B:** These lesions typically end at the arytenoid level. No thickening of the pharyngeal wall is visible; its enhancement (arrowheads) is nonspecific. **C:** These lesions will often involve multiple levels of the pharynx. Here a more exophytic portion of the tumor (T) involves the low oropharyngeal wall. Note the necrotic, 7 mm retropharyngeal node (arrow). The neck node appears highly aggressive; inflammation and extracapsular tumor surround the internal and external carotid artery (arrowheads).

the lesion may be primary in the pyriform sinus with spread to the posterior pharyngeal wall (Fig. 7–36). Posterior pharyngeal wall lesions have a distinct tendency to end at about the arytenoid level (Fig. 7–32). Cephalad spread to involve the pharyngoepiglottic fold and beyond this to the posterior or oropharyngeal wall of glossotonsillar sulcus is common in advanced lesions (Fig. 7–32). Spread as far superiorly as the midnasopharynx may be present. Much of this growth may be submucosal and easier to detect on T_2 weighted MRI. Cartilage invasion is unusual and limited to the superior cornu of the thyroid cartilage in the rare instances when it is present. Invasion of the prevertebral muscles is unusual at initial presentation and probably occurs most frequently in post-treatment recurrences. Spread to the postcricoid region is uncommon. CT or MRI may detect involved retropharyngeal nodes in patients with posterior pharyngeal wall cancer (Fig. 7–32).

Primary postcricoid carcinoma is uncommon in the United States. It is a circumferentially spreading lesion. Much of this growth may be submucosal and visible only with imaging. It usually appears as diffuse thickening of the postcricoid soft tissues with this thickening frequently extending to involve the cervical esophagus. Cricoid cartilage invasion and local extralaryngeal spread may occur. Invasion of tracheoesophageal nodes may be detected with CT or MRI.

Bulky tumors of the posterior wall of the larynx may abut the posterior wall of the hypopharynx, making it difficult to determine the site of origin of the lesion (Figs. 7–28, 7–33). This should be clear to the endoscopist. If not, a modified valsalva maneuver may be done during scanning to distend the hypopharynx and aid in the differentiation.

Integration of Imaging and Treatment in Hypopharyngeal Cancer

CT is the preferred method of examination for hypopharyngeal cancer at the University of Florida. It almost always suffices for

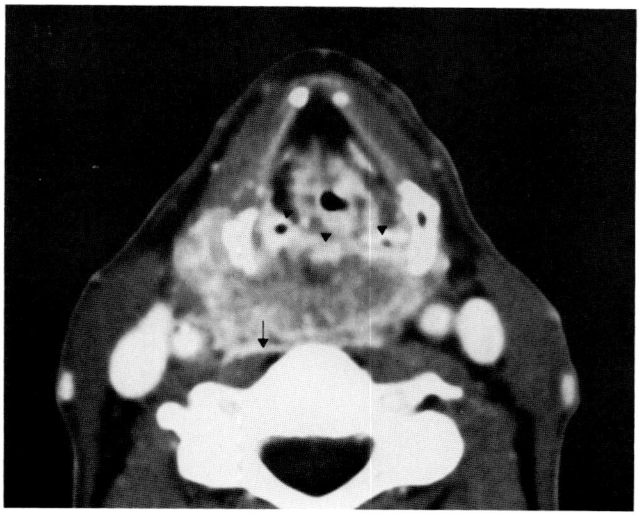
A

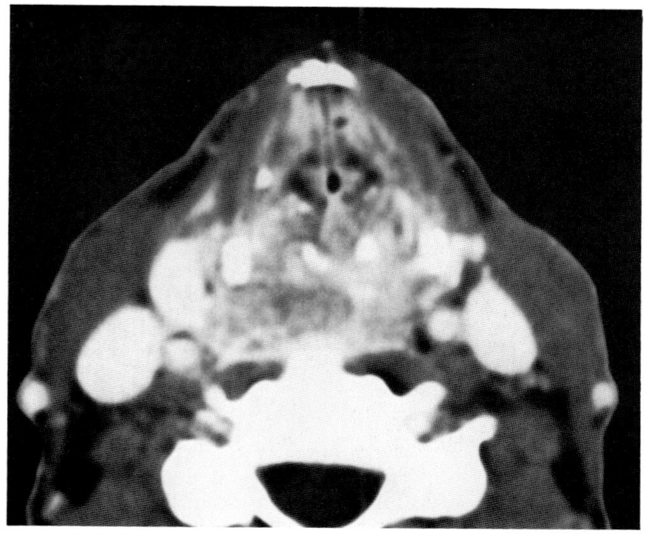
B

Figure 7–33. Low posterior pharyngeal wall cancer to compare with those arising more cephalad (see Fig. 7–32) and those originating on the posterior laryngeal wall (Fig. 7–28). A: False vocal cord level bulky tumor fills the hypopharynx. The enhancing posterior *laryngeal* wall (arrowheads) is seen as separate from the enhancing anterior margin of the tumor. The prevertebral fascia also enhances (arrow); this is unusual in an untreated patient and is probably reflective of a biologically aggressive tumor or associated inflammation. B: At the ventricular level, it would be difficult to know whether this was a posterior pharyngeal or laryngeal wall primary. C: There is extensive postcricoid tumor (T).

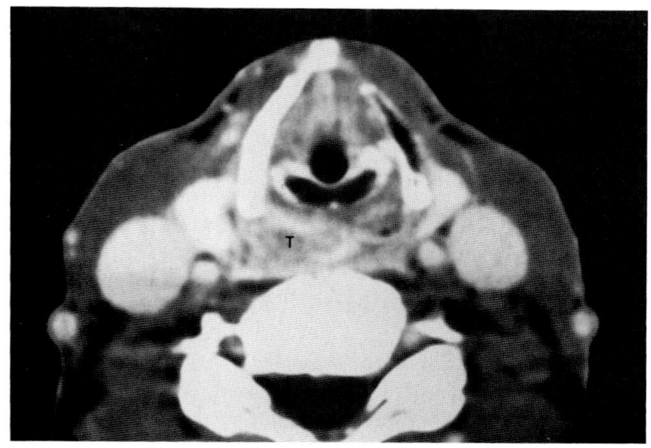

C

evaluation of the primary lesion, although we have an occasional (less than 10% of cases) need for focused supplemental MRI.

Pyriform sinus cancer is usually advanced at presentation and treated with surgery and postoperative radiotherapy. However, CT can help immeasurably in evaluating smaller lesions that may appear suitable for definitive radiotherapy or partial laryngopharyngectomy (Figs 7–30, 7–31). Cartilage invasion renders such lesions unsuitable for either partial laryngopharyngectomy or definitive irradiation. Although in laryngeal cancer, thyroid cartilage invasion is often difficult to detect with CT or MRI, this does not seem to be the case in pyriform sinus cancer. It is common for an apparent T_2 or T_3 lesion to be upstaged to T_4 on the basis of CT evidence of cartilage invasion (Figs. 7–30, 7–35, 7–35). In T_3 (fixed cord) pyriform sinus carcinoma the likelihood of cartilage invasion or extensive multidirectional spread at the level of the apex is increased. Spread to thyroid cartilage, postcricoid region, extralaryngeal soft tissues, or across the midline usually obviates even extended varieties of conservation surgical procedures.[34–36,50,51] The combination of CT and MRI can provide highly accurate appraisals of all these areas.

Most pyriform sinus cancer is treated with total laryngopharyngectomy or, in some institutions, with a near-total procedure.[50–52] Imaging can help select between these two by showing extensive extralaryngeal, caudal, or contralateral extensions and can also help in planning the margins of total resection and anticipating the method of pharyngeal reconstruction (Fig. 7–35). Unanticipated spread in the tracheoesophageal groove or thyroid gland invasion may be detected.

As for the supraglottic larynx, modern imaging has created some problems in relating the American Joint Commission (AJC) staging system to management decisions. Early exolaryngeal spread of tumor (eg, via the thyrohyoid membrane) may be detected with CT or MRI (Fig. 7–31). It is unclear whether subtle evidence of exolaryngeal spread justifies staging a lesion T_4, since the means of detecting extralaryngeal spread were far more limited when the staging system was adopted. Subtle extralaryngeal spread through the thyrohyoid membrane in an otherwise limited lesion may still be controllable with definitive radiotherapy (Fig. 7–31) or conservation surgery and postoperative radiotherapy. More experience is necessary to determine how these findings need to be weighted in management decisions. At some time, there will likely need to be formal

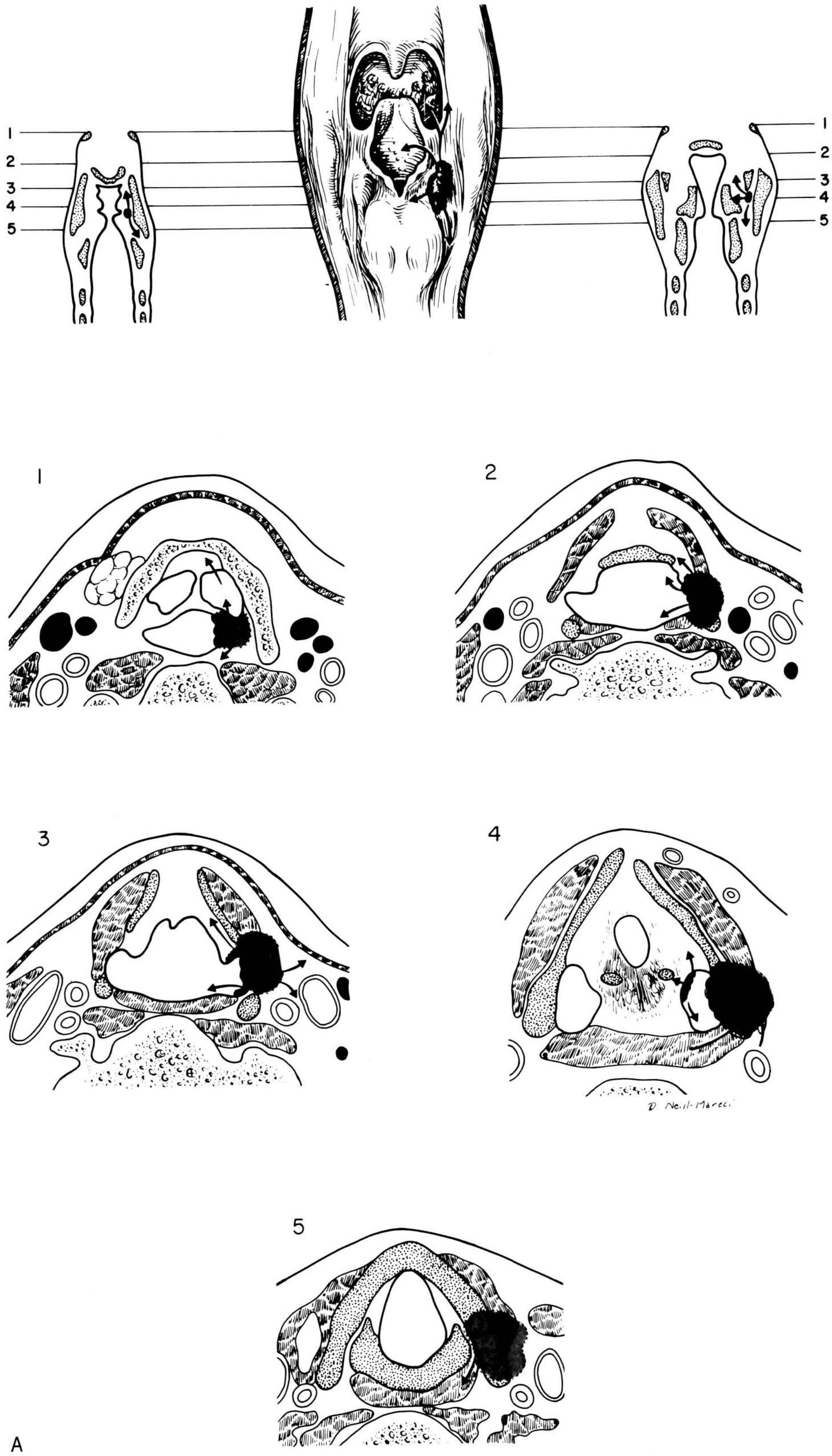

Figure 7–34. Spread patterns of hypopharyngeal cancer. **A**: Basic spread patterns. Figures at the top indicate approximate levels of the following axial sections (1–4).

A

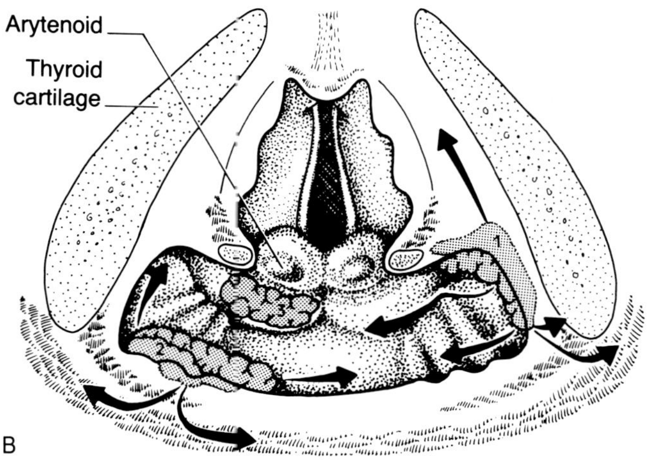

B

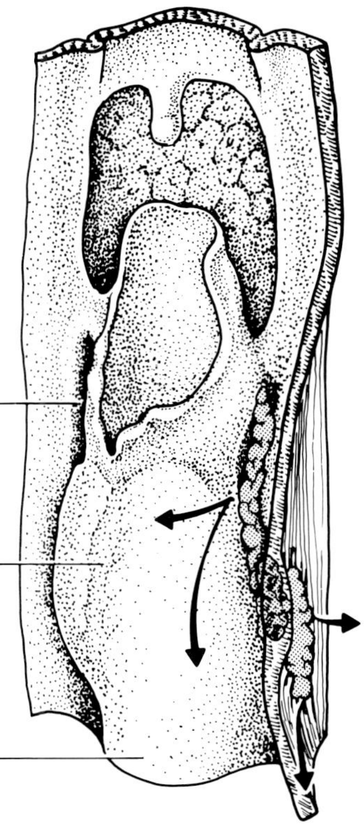

C

Figure 7-34 (*continued*). B: General trends of spread of pyriform sinus (1), posterior laryngeal wall (2), and posterior pharyngeal wall-postcricoid (3) tumors. C: Important spread patterns at and beyond the postcricoid and pyriform sinus apex. Mucosal spread is visible to the endoscopist; however, submucosal or extramural spread may not be appreciated, leading to underestimates of the lower extent of tumors. (From Mancuso and Hanafee.[2] Reprinted with permission.)

accommodations made in staging schemes for imaging findings in hypopharyngeal as well as laryngeal cancer and cervical metastatic disease.

Posterior pharyngeal wall cancer may be managed with surgery or radiotherapy; combined treatment is frequent.[34,35,53] Suprahyoid pharyngotomy with resection and preservation of the larynx is possible as a conservation method in early lesions. Imaging may show postcricoid, bilateral, laryngeal, or extralaryngeal spread that obviates this conservation procedure. Patients with these tumors are at high risk for "skip areas" or multifocal disease so that they are usually treated with definitive radiotherapy. At the University of Florida, it is thought that adjustments made in response to CT data showing retropharyngeal node involvement in these cancers have, in part, led to improved cure rates with radical radiotherapy.[54]

POST-TREATMENT EVALUATION

Evaluation After Radiation Therapy

At doses below 60 to 65 Gy, it is difficult to see any change in the larynx, hypopharynx, or neck on imaging studies done 8 to 12 weeks after completion of therapy. Higher dosage does lead to obvious and persistent alteration in the appearance of these structures. There is an evolution of the abnormalities caused by irradiation. The time course and specific appearance varies with individuals and their body habitus, but some general trends can be recognized.

From the end of therapy up to several months, there is usually swelling and intense enhancement (with intravenous contrast) of the submandibular glands due to radiation sialadenitis (Fig. 7–37). Over the next several months, the glands may return to a near-normal appearance, show increased fat content, or become completely atrophic, leaving behind only fat and some stromal elements. The parotid gland may show no change or evidence of mild sialadenitis, depending on the extent of the radiation ports. In patients with a large amount of fat, there is obvious edema or developing fibrosis or both, visible in the fat between the platysma and skin from the end of therapy onward (Fig. 7–37). This may diminish with time but may never resolve. Slim strands of presumed perilymphatic or other fibrosis run, in general, perpendicular to the platysma. This change is seen to a lesser extent in the fat deep to the investing layer of deep cervical fascia.

Following high-dose irradiation (greater than 65 Gy), the endolaryngeal soft tissues assume an almost characteristically "boggy" appearance (Figs. 7–29, 7–31, 7–37). This swelling is usually maximal from the end of therapy to 3 months posttherapy. The edema or fibrosis, or both, then involutes, but obvious changes persist indefinitely. At the University of Florida, we have followed patients up to 5 to 6 years postirradiation and have observed persistent, stable thickening of the free margin of the epiglottis, aryepiglottic folds, false cords, posterior wall of the larynx, and pharyngeal walls (Figs. 7–29, 7–31, 7–37, 7–38). During the 3 to 6 months following therapy, this increased thickness is accompanied by vague, increased density in the fat of the preepiglottic and paraglottic spaces, as well as the fat within the aryepiglottic folds (Figs. 7–29, 7–31, 7–37, 7–38). The presumed edematous changes tend to be most pronounced paraglottically and within the aryepiglottic folds. After 3 to 6 months, the fat planes become more distinct but a

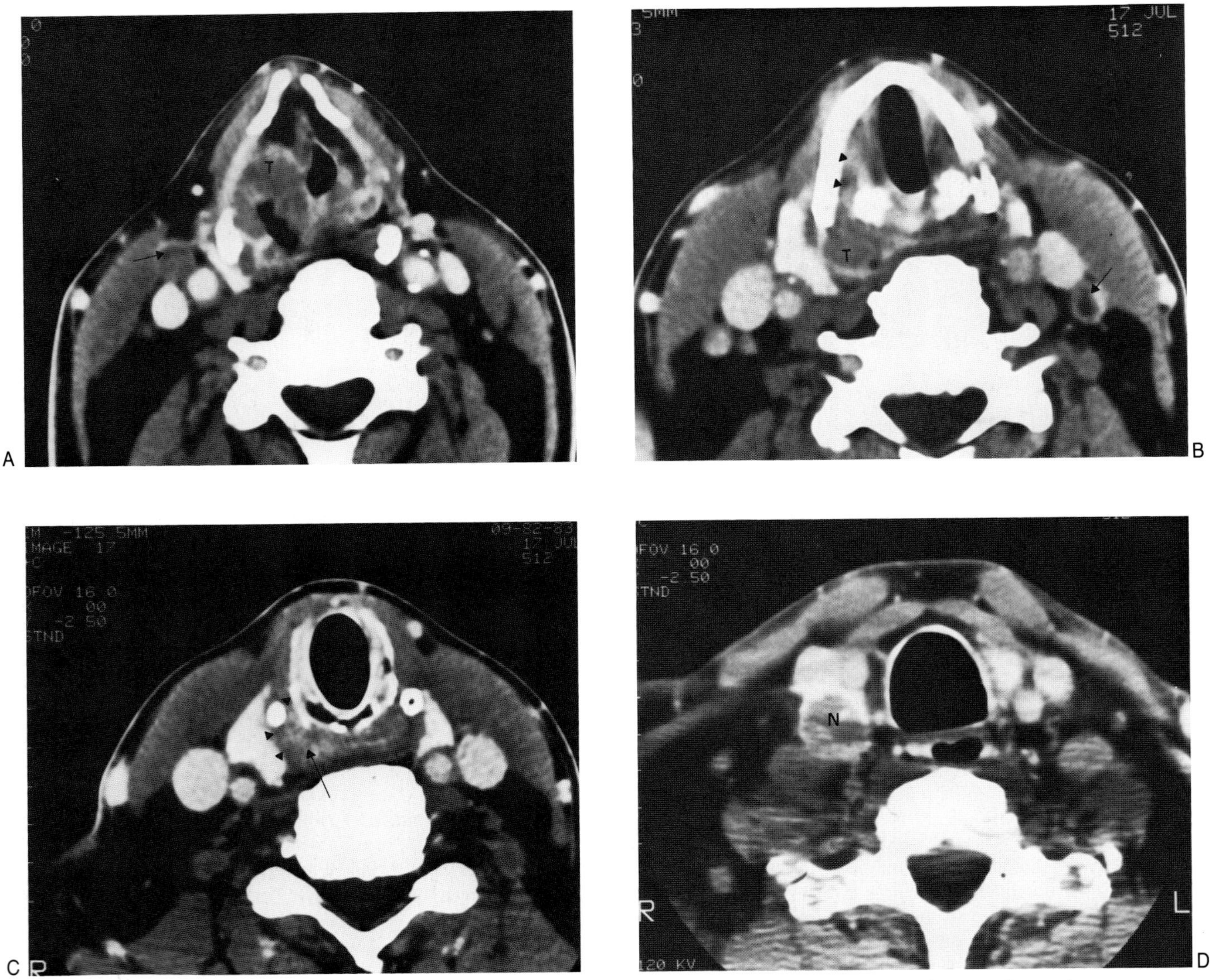

Figure 7–35. A patient with pyriform sinus carcinoma clinically staged T_3N_0. The apex of the pyriform sinus was difficult to evaluate but appeared to be involved at DL. **A:** Deep spread of tumor (T) is predominantly in the paraglottic space. Note first of three computed tomography (CT)-positive nodes. The peripheral lucency in the 10 mm node (arrow) is the pathologically proven metastasis. **B:** Obvious tumor is present in the pyriform sinus apex (T) and infiltrates the paraglottic space (arrowheads). A second *contralateral* CT-positive node is present (arrow); it is completely replaced by metastasis. **C:** Obliteration of the internal architecture of the low postcricoid-esophageal verge region (arrow) indicates a likely presence of tumor at this location. This is even more suspicious based on widening of right cricothyroid joint and indistinct tissue planes between the esophageal verge and thyroid gland (arrowheads). No mucosal lesion was seen at this level. Tumor was confirmed intraoperatively; CT allowed for anticipation of gastric pull-up for pharyngeal reconstruction. **D:** A 2.0 cm nodal metastasis (N) to the scalene node was not felt on physical examination, even retrospectively. Comment: The clinical T_3N_0 lesion was upstaged to T_4N_{2C} (right neck, N_{2B}; left N_1) and the patient was informed that gastric pull-up would be likely. All CT findings were confirmed pathologically.

vague, increased density is still visible within the deep fat spaces, probably representing perilymphatic or more diffuse fibrosis.

The intrinsic laryngeal musculature may become atrophic and replaced by fat, especially on the side of a fixed true cord, which does not become mobile following treatment (Fig. 7–37I). This atrophy is one possible reason for lack of return of normal function in a successfully treated patient. The subglottic larynx will often show persistent thickening of the mucosa adjacent to the cricoid perichondrium (Fig. 7–37); this is never "normal" in the untreated larynx. MRI is no more specific than CT in its rendering of these changes, except that T_2 weighted images will reveal edematous mucosa and fat by virtue of their increased water content and high signal (Fig. 7–38). Mucositis will be

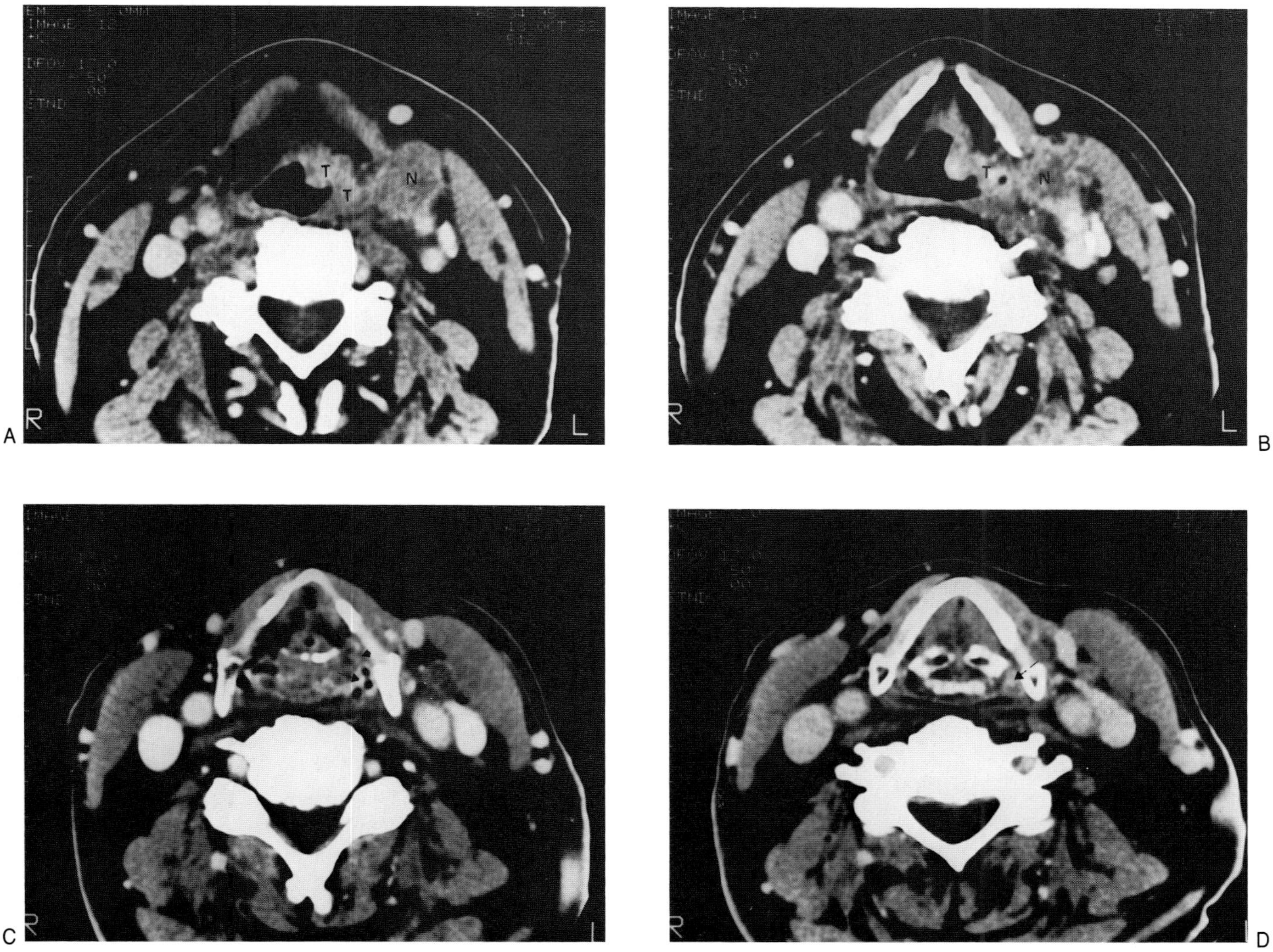

Figure 7–36. Two patients with relatively superficially spreading pyriform sinus carcinoma to contrast with deeper spread patterns seen in other patients. **A,B:** Primary tumor (T) involves the pyriform sinus and aryepiglottic fold. On physical examination, it was unclear whether the palpable neck mass was produced by extralaryngeal spread of tumor or by nodal metastatic disease. On computed tomography (CT), it is obvious that this is a node (N) with extracapsular spread of tumor to and probably through the thyrohyoid membrane. **C:** At the ventricular level, approaching the pyriform sinus apex, the fungating, superficially spreading cancer thickens the mucosa and enhances (arrow). There is still a plaque of abnormal tissue obliterating the paraglottic space adjacent to the left thyroid ala (arrowhead). **D:** At the pyriform sinus apex, note the submucosal cancer (arrow) in comparison to the normal side. This was confirmed at surgery.

seen as superficial, increased signal on T_2 weighted MRI and excessive contrast enhancement on CT. This is most marked during therapy and for 5 weeks post-therapy. Increased mucosal signal on MRI may persist for many months or years.

From the foregoing discussion, it should be clear that diffuse changes in the larynx and hypopharynx are common following high-dose radiotherapy. This means that diffuse changes cannot be interpreted as evidence of recurrent tumor. It also means that detection of recurrence is more difficult than the original evaluation of the untreated larynx and hypopharynx. The primary tumor mass gradually involutes during successful radiotherapy but an obvious focal mass can persist up to 3 months following successful therapy. Focal abnormalities can be relatively subtle after 3 months (Figs. 7–12, 7–29, 7–37).

A subtle, or even relatively obvious, focal abnormality should not be considered evidence of persistent tumor up to 3 months post-therapy (Figs. 7–12, 7–29, 7–37E–I). Obvious large (2 to 3 cm) masses or progressively enlarging masses are another matter (Fig. 7–22). It is probably best to avoid imaging at all until 3 months post-therapy so that one is not tempted to biopsy the more limited areas of CT or MRI abnormality (Figs. 7–12, 7–37E–I). Such a biopsy could lead to an otherwise avoidable case of perichondritis or chondronecrosis.[55] After 3 months, subtle focal abnormalities should be followed carefully

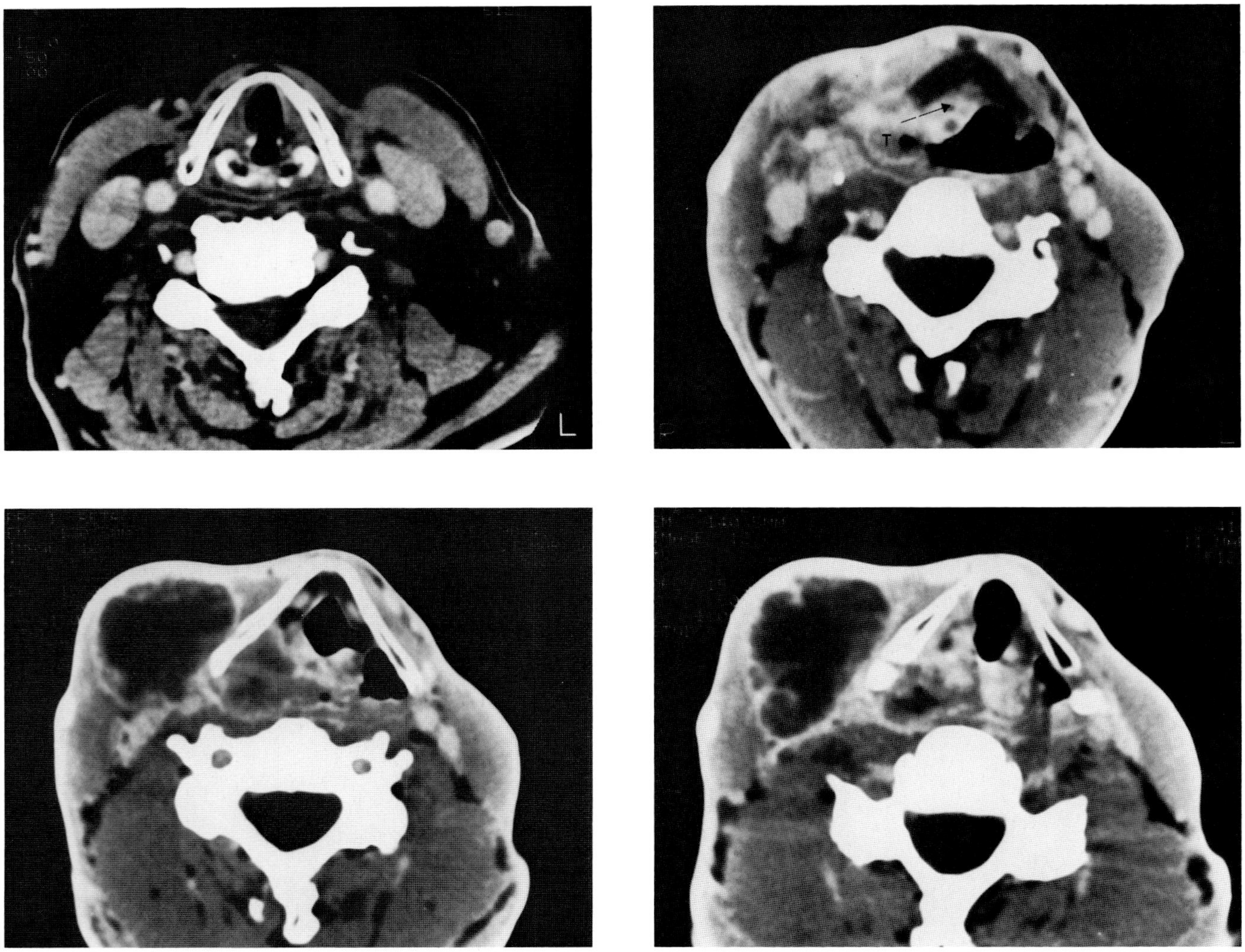

E F G H

Figure 7-36 (*continued*). **E:** At the level of the undersurface of the true cord (3 mm caudal to Figure 7–36D), tissue planes are near normal. **F:** Patient 2 has a bulky exophytic primary (T) with submucosal spread heading toward the preepiglottic space via the paraglottic space (arrow). **G, H:** As in patient 1, it was uncertain whether the neck mass was a node or extralaryngeal extension of the primary tumor; it is clearly a node on CT. Note the tendency of this type of pyriform sinus cancer to spread circumferentially, involving all walls. These lesions frequently have significant involvement of the posterior pharyngeal wall as well as the posterior wall of the larynx (that is, arytenoid pad).

clinically, perhaps with supplemental imaging. At the University of Florida, we have followed patients with routine CT at 3- to 6- month intervals for 2 years post-therapy. Based on this unpublished experience, we have concluded that it is unusual for CT to detect recurrence before it is clinically evident, although this occasionally may occur (Fig. 7–39). Serial CT is probably only cost-justifiable in highly selected patients who are treated with radiotherapy but are considered to be at high risk for failure.

After successful treatment, positive nodes under 2 cm in size usually involute to a size well under 1 cm. Normal nodes virtually disappear completely following radiotherapy (Fig. 7–29). Two to 3 cm or larger nodal masses often shrink below 1 cm, although occasionally they may persist without shrinkage. It is impossible to determine by imaging whether such masses have been sterilized by radiotherapy. Successfully treated, larger masses typically will become grossly necrotic. The inner wall often remains thick and irregular, whereas the outer wall will usually become smooth and better demarcated from surrounding soft tissues. Persistence of indistinct outer margins of a nodal mass several months after irradiation suggests active tumor. Postirradiation changes make physical examination of the neck difficult. Gross adenopathy may be visible on CT and not palpable. Spread to nodal sites outside the usually primary drainage areas (e.g., retropharyngeal nodes and contralateral neck) is more likely because tumor and therapy will alter drainage pathways.[34] Imaging can help avoid unnecessarily radical management of obviously incurable disease.

Radiation-induced perichondritis and chondronecrosis are uncommon complications of radiotherapy if patients are prop-

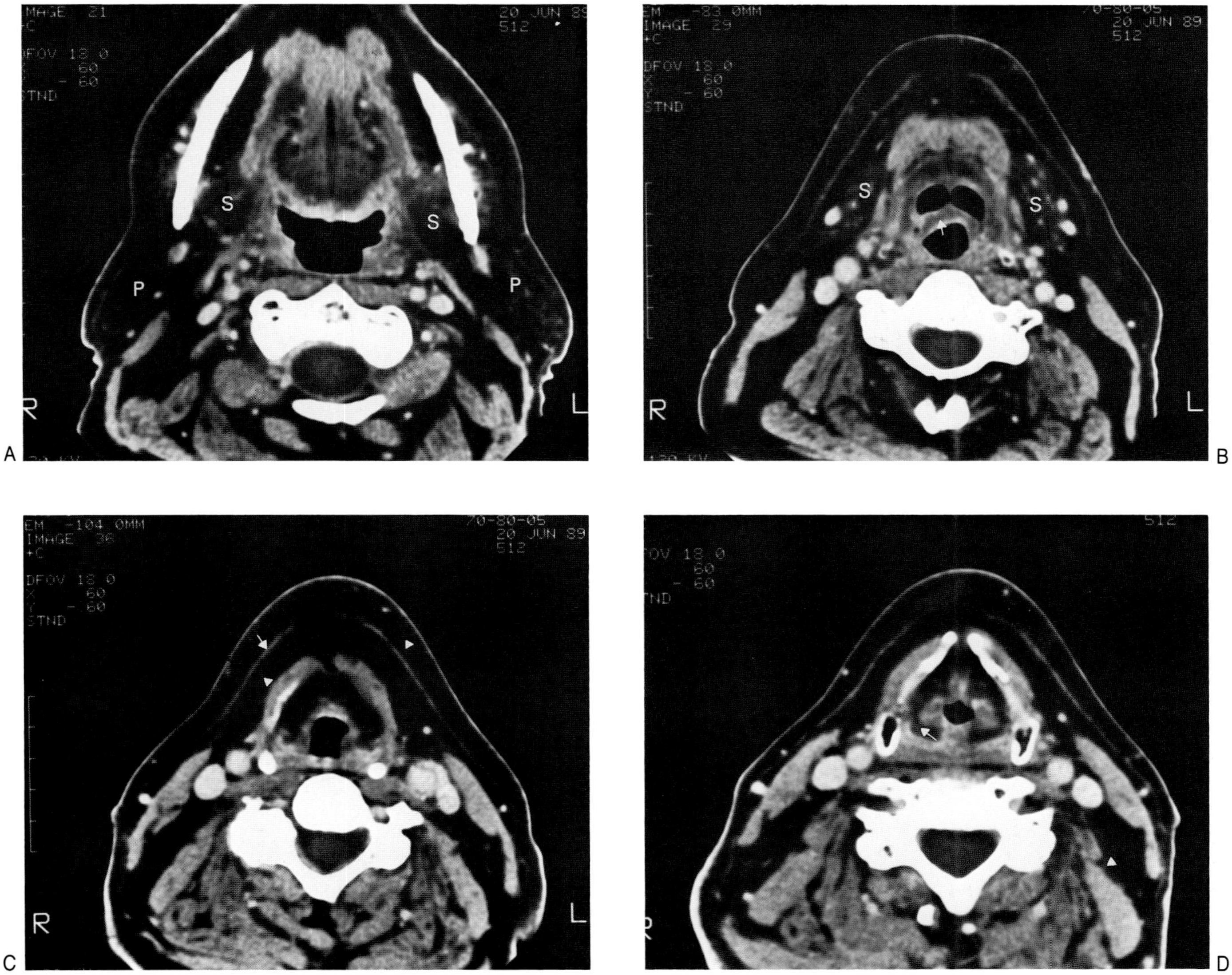

Figure 7–37. Two patients treated with high-dose, twice-a-day radiation therapy for laryngeal cancer. **A–D:** Patient 2 years after radiotherapy (RT), showing typical residual changes. **A:** Fatty replacement of parotid gland (P) and deep process of the submandibular glands (S). **B:** Thickened free margin of epiglottis (arrow) and fatty replacement of submandibular glands (S). **C:** Platysma (arrow) is about twice as thick as normal. Subtle strands of tissue in the subcutaneous and deeper fat (arrowheads) typically occur in fatter patients and probably represent perilymphatic fibrosis. Thicker than usual aryepiglottic folds and posterior pharyngeal wall musculature are also common findings. **D:** Aryepiglottic folds are two to three times thicker than usual. The fat with the folds (arrow) is increased in density, reflecting edema and/or fibrosis. Compare to normal fat in the paraglottic space.

erly selected for therapy.[34,55–58] It is often impossible to tell if one is dealing with a severe chondronecrosis alone or in combination with recurrence (Figs. 7–26, 7–40). The only sure sign of recurrence in such cases may be an obviously positive neck node (Fig. 7–39). CT can be used for careful monitoring of patients with chondronecrosis. If the laryngeal skeleton is obviously disrupted, with numerous areas of sequestration, the surgeon can confidently assume that the larynx will never be useful again and will remove it (Fig. 7–40). Alternatively, careful follow-up with imaging might show obvious growth of a laryngeal mass or subclinical adenopathy, indicating that the necrosis is coexistent with tumor.

Evaluation after Surgery or Combined Therapy

Postoperative evaluation of the larynx, hypopharynx, and neck is even more difficult than after irradiation. Laryngeal deformity produced by conservation surgery complicates interpretation of CT findings. Loss of symmetry after vertical hemilaryngec-

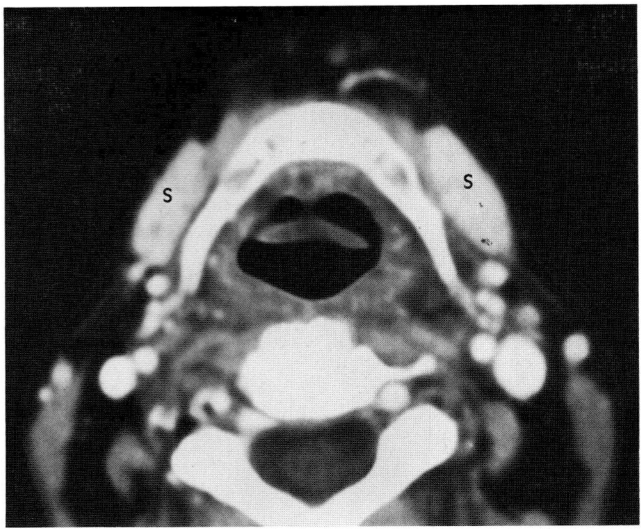

E

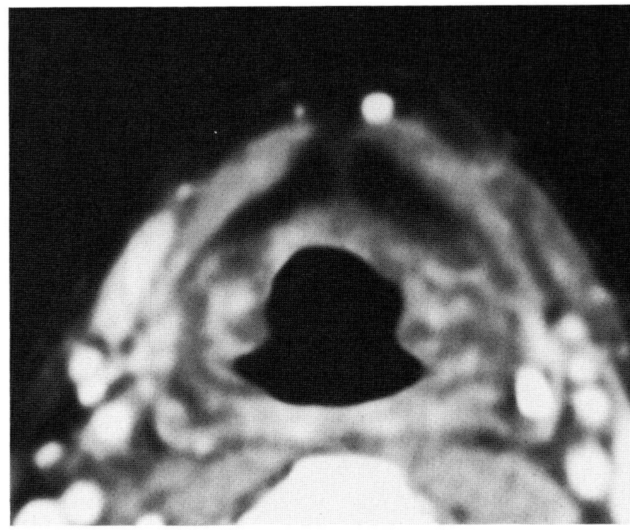

F

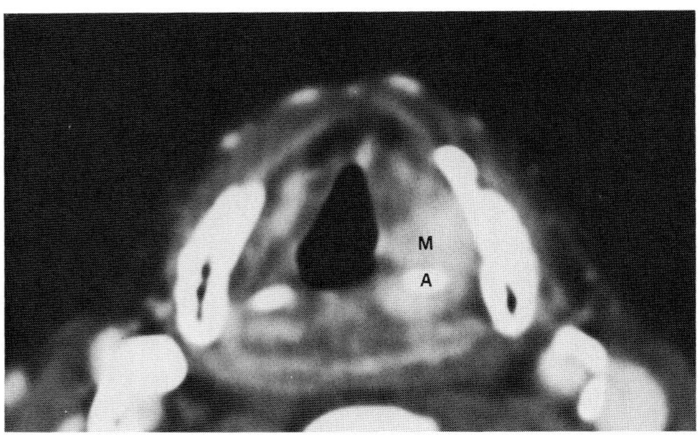

G

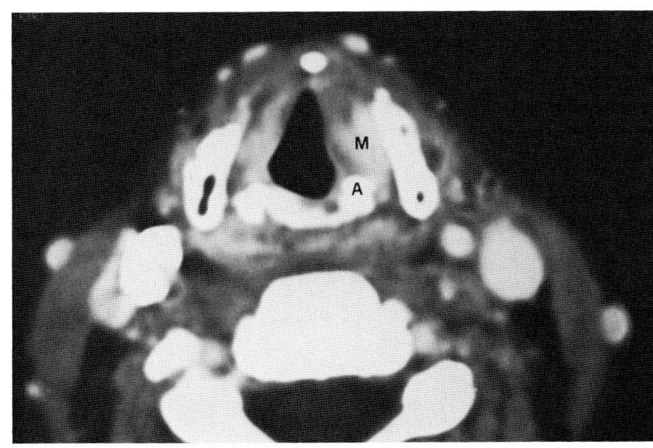

H

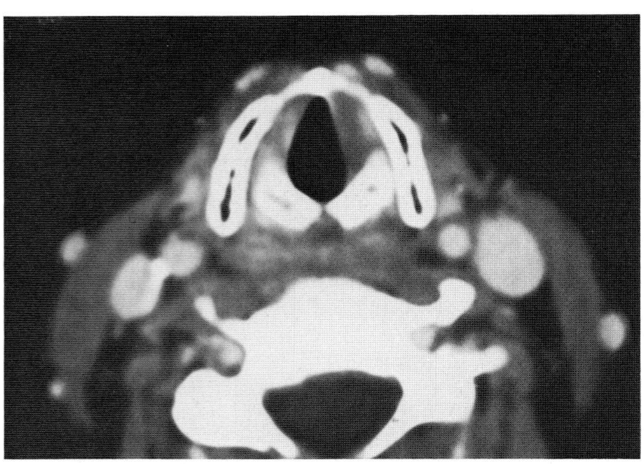

I

Figure 7-37 (*continued*). **E–I**: Patient 12 weeks post-RT for T_3 vocal cord cancer. **E**: Intense enhancement of submandibular glands (S) is due to radiation sialadenitis. Free margin of the epiglottis is thick. **F**: Marked, diffuse thickening of the aryepiglottic folds and increased density in the fat within the folds and paraglottic space is most likely related to edema. **G**: Focal mass (M) at false vocal cord (FVC)-ventricular level surrounds the arytenoid (A). This area was highly suspicious for persistent tumor clinically as well as by computed tomography. Note edema of the right FVC and posterior laryngeal wall. **H**: Focal mass (M) and displacement of arytenoid (A) persist at true vocal cord (TVC) level. **I**: Diminished density at undersurface of TVC level suggests atrophy of intrinsic musculature. Comment: Biopsy of focal mass was negative. Cord remains fixed. Follow-up scans showed resolution of "mass" and patient is free of disease at 3½ years.

tomy, obliteration, or alteration of deep tissue planes are important obstacles. Baseline studies are essential because of the loss of these normal interpretive aids.[59] These should be done in high-risk patients about 2 to 3 months postoperatively. In the absence of baseline examination, only an obvious infiltrating mass can be interpreted as recurrent tumor (Fig. 7–41). Clinically evident neck disease may lead the surgeon or radiation oncologist to suspect primary site failure. Similarly, subclinical neck disease seen on CT may lead to clinical or CT confirmation of otherwise subtle primary site failure.

CT and MRI are ideal for evaluating the patient suspected of failure following total laryngectomy or laryngopharyn-

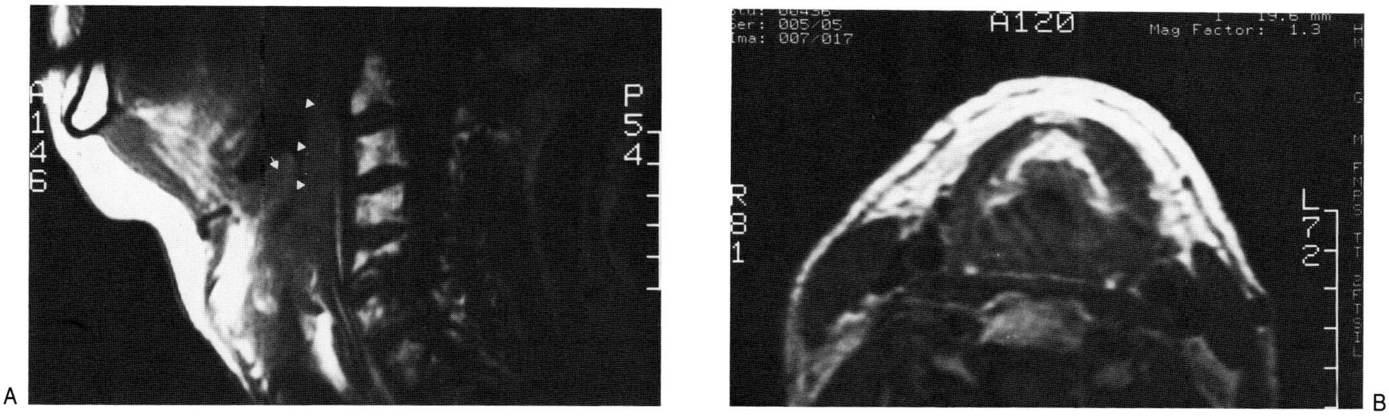

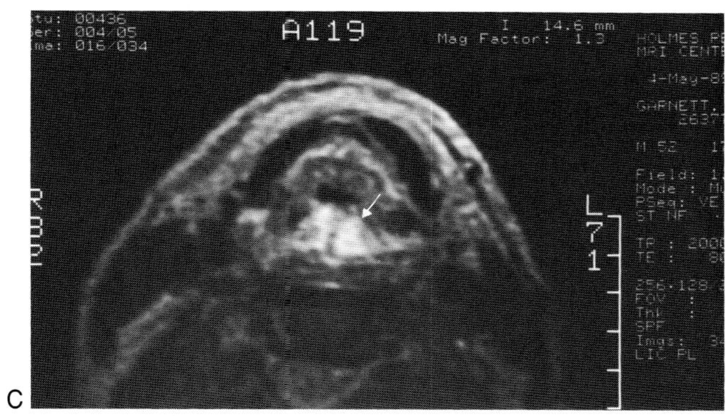

Figure 7–38. Magnetic resonance imaging (MRI) of patient following high-dose radiotherapy for supraglottic cancer. Scan findings described below were erroneously interpreted as recurrence at another insitution. **A:** Lateral view shows thick epiglottis (arrow) and posterior pharyngeal wall (arrowhead). **B, C:** T_1 and T_2 weighted images showing typical aryepiglottic fold thickening with edema more obvious on the T_2 weighted image (arrow). Comment: This study was done on a high-field unit with surface coils. Note the overall suboptimal quality relative to the CT images shown in Figure 7–37. This would be considered an average-to-good quality MRI examination.

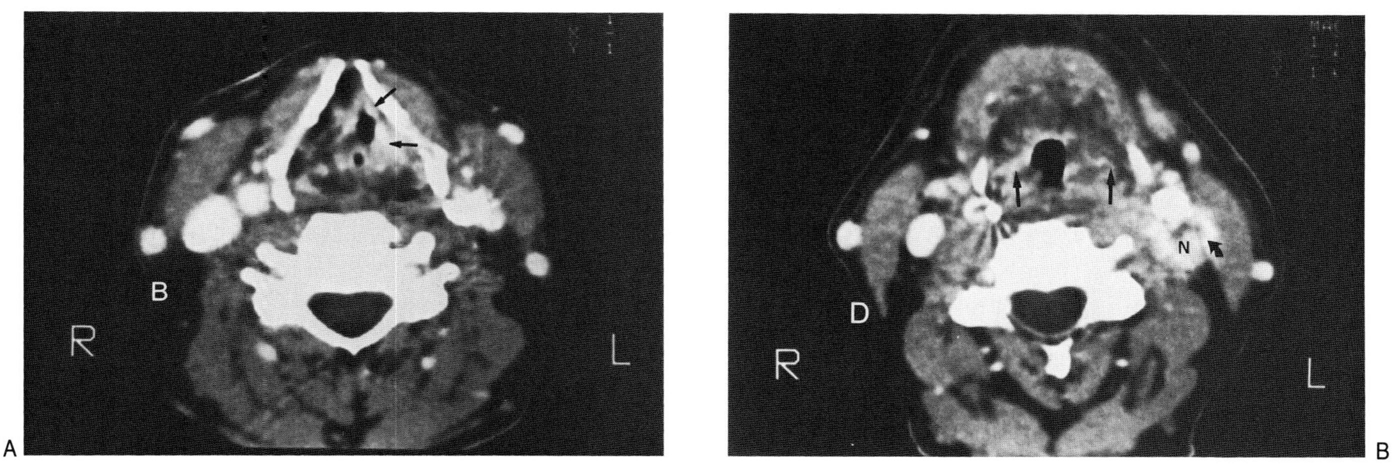

Figure 7–39. Patient treated with radiotherapy (RT) alone for supraglottic cancer. There was persistent edema 4 to 5 months post-RT but no focal laryngeal lesions were seen and the neck examination was negative except for post-RT changes. **A:** Focal mass infiltrates the paraglottic space (arrows). The remaining endolaryngeal soft tissues appear edematous. **B:** Typical, diffuse post-RT edema (arrow) but no focal masses are seen at this level. Computed tomography (CT)-positive node (N) with capsular penetration and sternocleidomastoid (curved arrow). Comment: Deep biopsy confirmed recurrence. All CT findings were confirmed pathologically. (From Mancuso and Hanafee.[2] Reprinted with permission.)

A

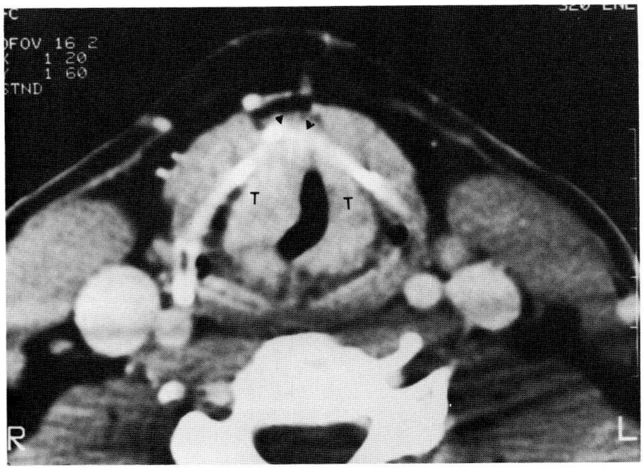

B

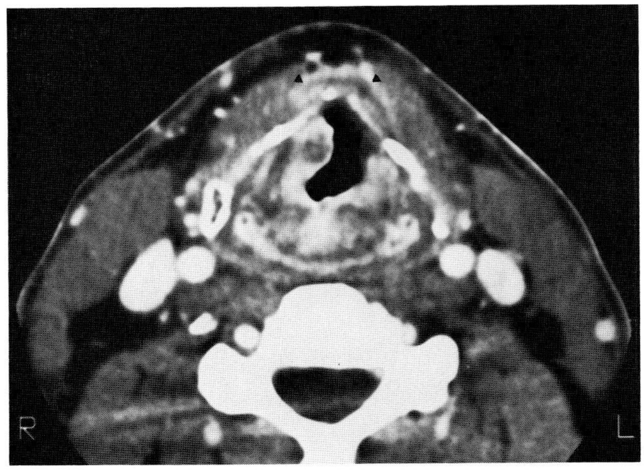

C

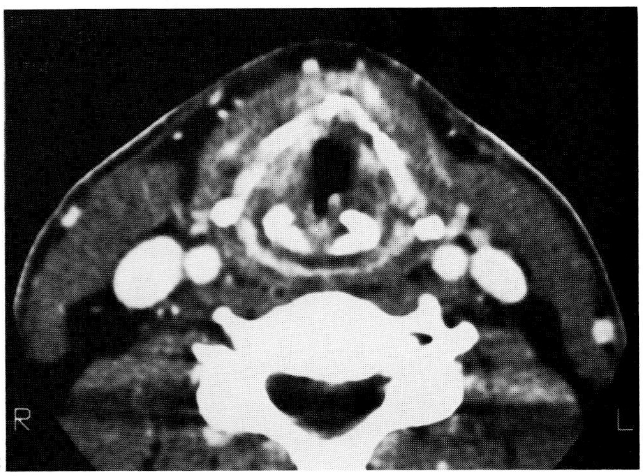

Figure 7–40. Patient with a high-volume carcinoma of the infrahyoid epiglottis. **A**: Preradiotherapy study at false vocal cord level shows extensive bilateral paraglottic tumor (T). Spread pattern suggests early invasion of thyrohyoid attachment near thyroid notch (arrowheads). **B**: Five months post radiotherapy there is extensive edema and soft tissue necrosis; abnormal tissue extends to perichondrial surface. There is also enhancement of the prelaryngeal soft tissues (arrowheads). **C**: Extensive glottic edema and prelaryngeal abnormality. Comment: Clinically, this was a useless larynx. Computed tomography is consistent with moderately advanced perichondritis and early chondronecrosis. Coexistent tumor could not be excluded. The patient was followed for several more months and because of increased pain and poor laryngeal function, a total laryngectomy was done. Pathologic examination revealed advanced perichondritis and chondronecrosis but no definite tumor.

gectomy.[60] Baseline studies are not necessary unless margins are unusually close or other risk factors are present. The reconstructed neopharynx and peristomal area are easy to evaluate (Fig. 7–42). If a peristomal biopsy shows recurrent cancer, CT—possibly with supplemental MRI—is necessary to determine its extent. Negative studies usually indicate minimal local disease. Unfortunately, however, the stomal focus is often the "tip of the iceberg" (Fig. 7–42). Cure is unlikely in advanced stomal or neopharyngeal recurrence, and the imaging can help select the least morbid means of palliation.[61] If aggressive palliative or attempted curative procedures are planned, imaging studies should include the entire neck and chest. The neck study should include the skull base to reveal all retropharyngeal nodes.[62,63] The entire neopharynx must be studied, since there are frequently "skip areas" between the more obvious masses (Fig. 7–42). This apparent multifocality might be the result of unrecognized perivascular or lymphatic spread. The stomal site and mediastinum must be studied in detail to determine the level of tracheal involvement, possible spread to the muscular wall of the esophagus, and encasement of the aorta or brachiocephalic vessels. One must also look for mediastinal adenopathy and pulmonary metastatic disease. The impact of any or all of these findings will vary with institutional biases relative to the management of recurrences. MRI is particularly useful for showing tracheal invasion, spread to the muscular wall of the esophagus, paravertebral or prevertebral muscle invasion, vascular encasement, and mediastinal or hilar adenopathy. CT is best for detecting nodal disease and pulmonary metastases.

Surgery, with or without radiation therapy, profoundly alters the neck. Extensive scarring may be present and this should not be overinterpreted as neck recurrence. MRI can help differentiate end-stage (dehydrated) scar from tumor; although it cannot distinguish active granulation tissue and tumor. Baseline studies with follow-up or imaging-directed needle biopsy may be necessary in suspicious cases. Functional neck dissection removes the fatty envelope around the node-bearing area of the neck, making detection of recurrent adenopathy more difficult with CT. Ultrasound or MRI might prove useful if neck recurrence is suspected on CT or clinically and if such confirmation is necessary.

In conclusion, evaluation of the postsurgical or postcombined-therapy larynx, hypopharynx, and neck for tumor recurrence is difficult. Baseline studies, experience and cooperation between the imagers and treatment team are necessary. Not all

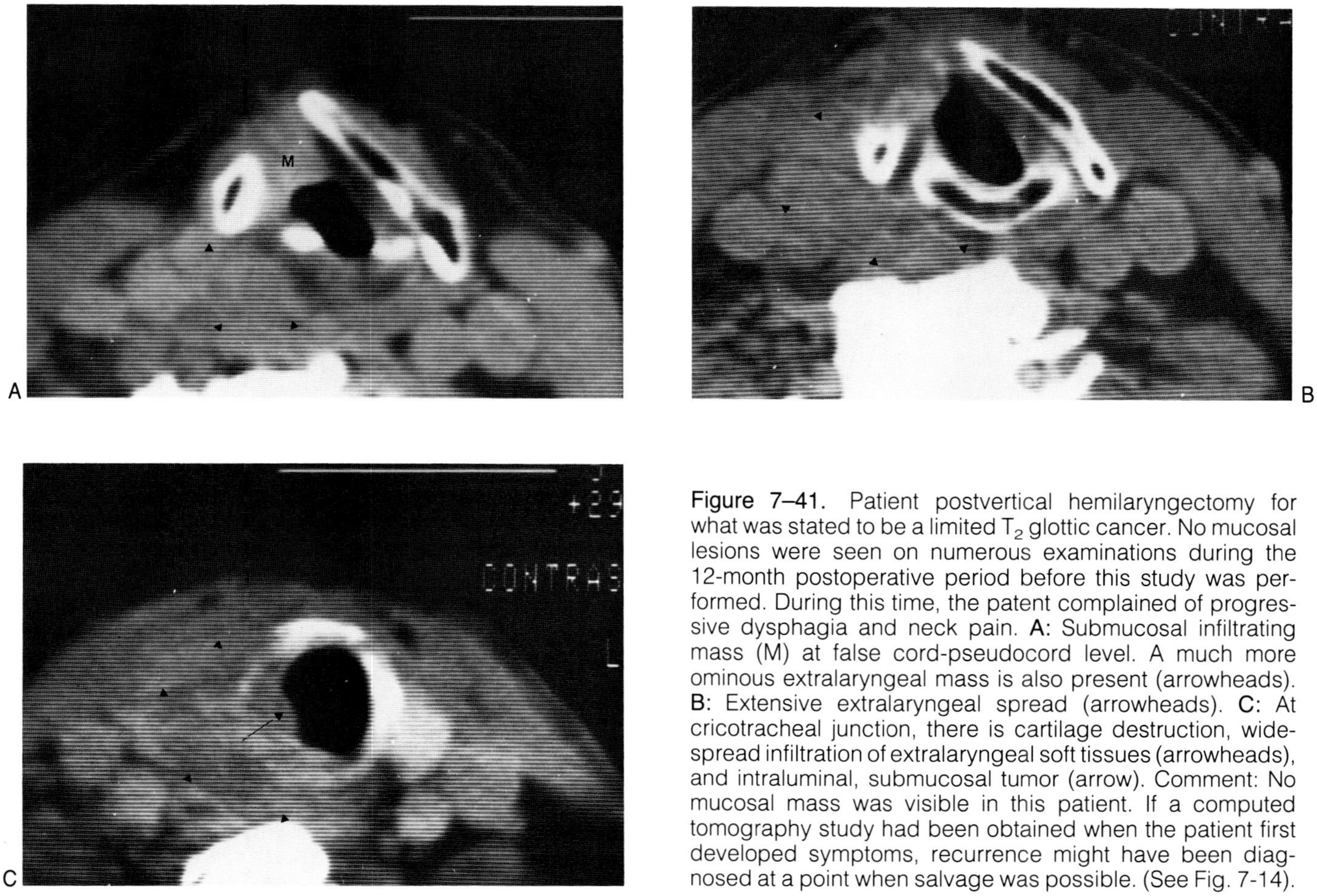

Figure 7–41. Patient postvertical hemilaryngectomy for what was stated to be a limited T_2 glottic cancer. No mucosal lesions were seen on numerous examinations during the 12-month postoperative period before this study was performed. During this time, the patent complained of progressive dysphagia and neck pain. **A**: Submucosal infiltrating mass (M) at false cord-pseudocord level. A much more ominous extralaryngeal mass is also present (arrowheads). **B**: Extensive extralaryngeal spread (arrowheads). **C**: At cricotracheal junction, there is cartilage destruction, widespread infiltration of extralaryngeal soft tissues (arrowheads), and intraluminal, submucosal tumor (arrow). Comment: No mucosal mass was visible in this patient. If a computed tomography study had been obtained when the patient first developed symptoms, recurrence might have been diagnosed at a point when salvage was possible. (See Fig. 7-14).

patients require intense follow-up with expensive imaging procedures, but it is indicated for individuals on the basis of clinical situation, pathologic evaluation, and whether careful physical examination is possible.[64,65] At the University of Florida, we usually begin this evaluation with CT and use a focused MRI study to resolve any residual issues that might critically affect management. Imaging-directed needle biopsy can be used for confirmation when tissue is not available by other, simpler, or less expensive approaches.

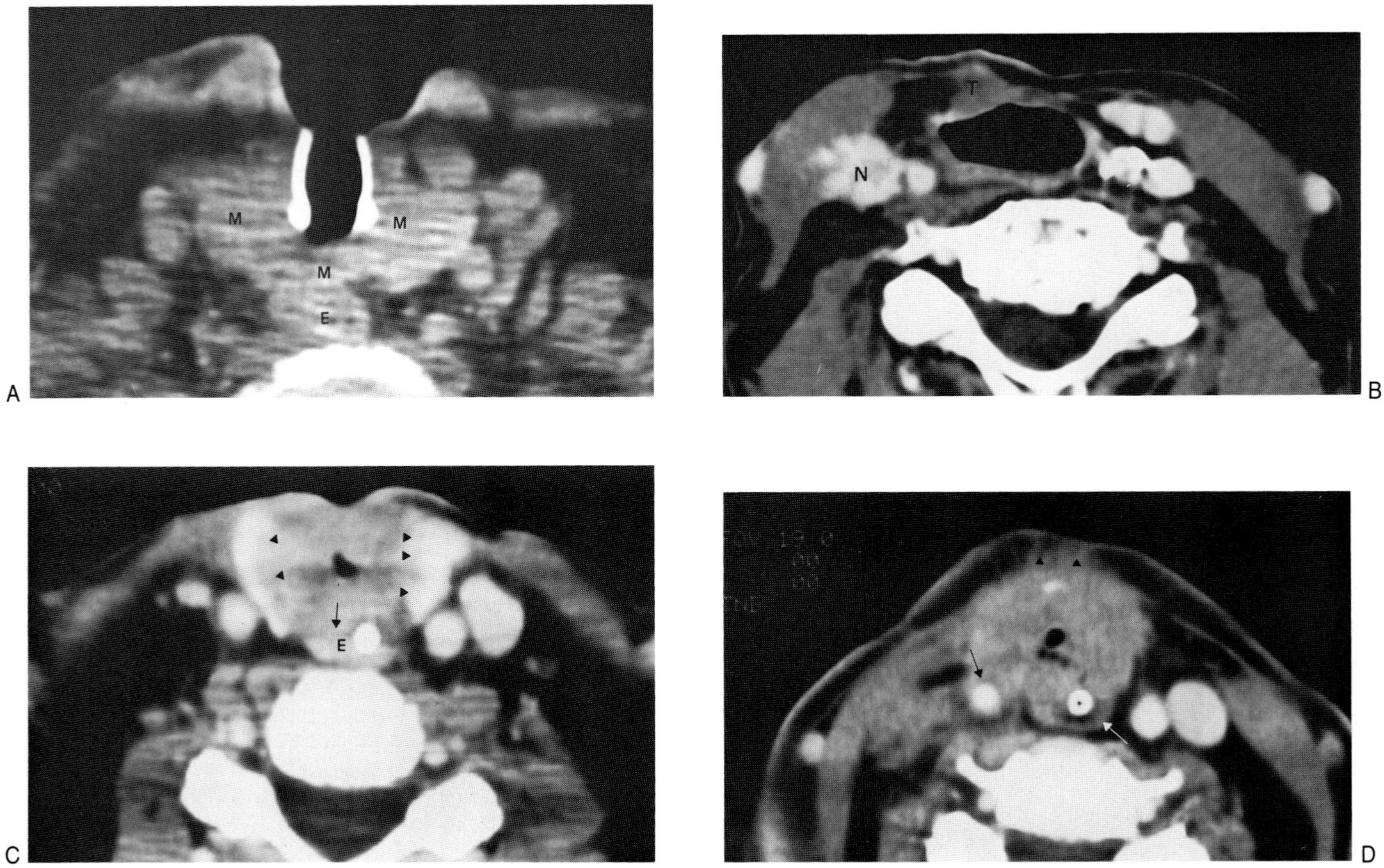

Figure 7–42. Four patients postlaryngectomy for carcinoma of the larynx. **A, B**: Clinically, there was only a "small right-sided area of friability" at the stomal site. Biopsy revealed invasive squamous cell carcinoma. **A**: There is a large, deep peristomal mass (M). **B**: On physical examination, the neck was negative and neopharynx appeared normal. A cord of tumor, however, had grown along the right anterior wall of the neopharynx (T). Nodal metastasis with strong evidence of capsular penetration was present on the right as well (N). **C, D**: A second patient who was believed to have a limited peristomal recurrence clinically. The neopharynx and neck were normal on physical examination. The patent had dysphagia. **C**: Extensive peristomal and perineopharyngeal disease invades the thyroid gland (arrowheads) and probably the anterior esophageal wall (arrow). **D**: On a more cephalad section, there is encasement of the right common carotid artery (black arrow) and spread to subcutaneous fat (arrowheads). Some of the normal neopharyngeal wall is visible posteriorly (white arrow). **E**: esophagus.

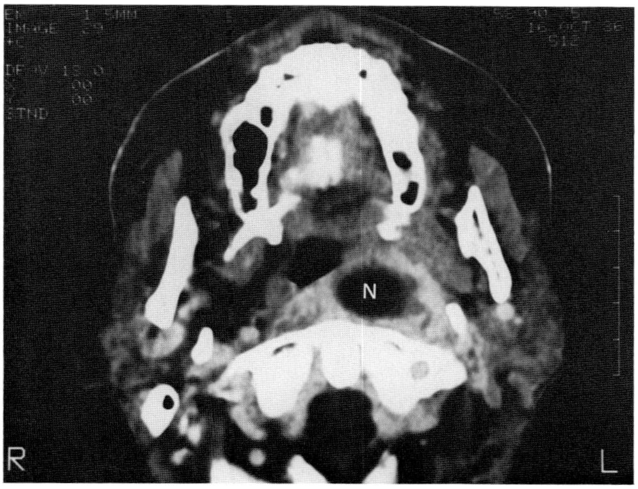

E

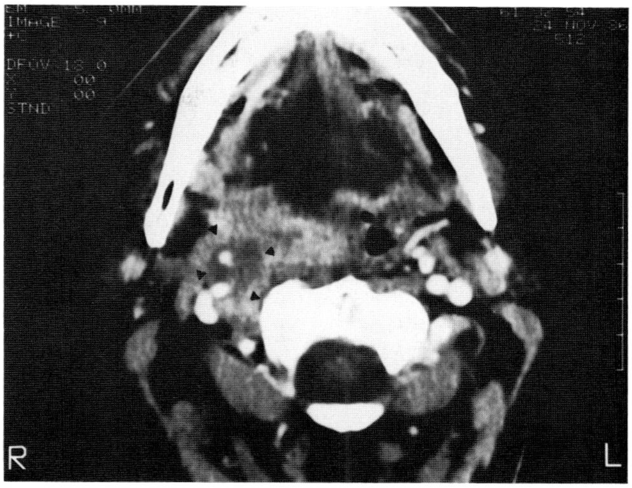

F

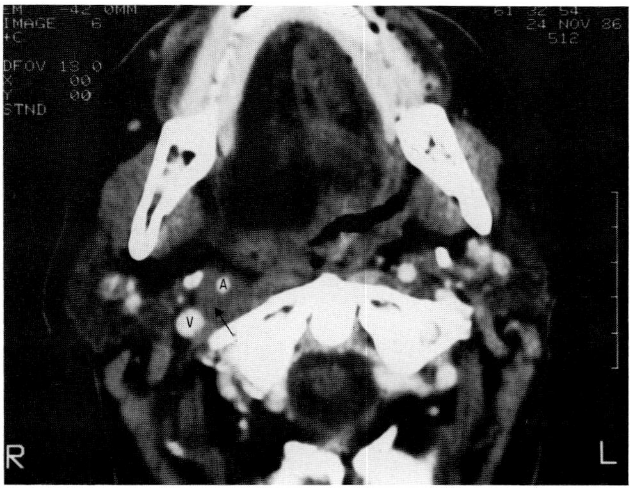

G

Figure 7-42 (*continued*). E: Third patient 1 year postlaryngectomy complaining of occipital headaches. Physical examination was normal except for postoperative changes. Metastasis to retropharyngeal lymph node with skull base invasion is present. F, G: Fourth patient with neopharyngeal recurrence. Sections show that tumor has spread around the structures of the carotid sheath, digastric muscle and those muscles arising on styloid process (arrowheads). Tumor (arrow) in between the carotid artery (A) and jugular vein (V) is most likely perineural extension along one of the lower cranial nerves.

REFERENCES

1. Mancuso AA. *Workbook for MRI and CT of the head and neck,* ed. 2. Baltimore: Williams & Wilkins, 1989.
2. Mancuso AA, Hanafee WN. *Computed tomography and magnetic resonance imaging of the head and neck,* ed. 2. Baltimore: Williams & Wilkins, 1985;1–503.
3. Dillon W, Mancuso AA. The nasopharynx and oropharynx. In: Newton TH, Hasso AN, Dillon WP, eds. *Modern neuroradiology—computed tomography of the head and neck,* vol. 3. New York: Raven Press, 1988:10.1–10.67.
4. Myer-Breiting E, Burkhardt A. Tumours of the larynx. *Histopathology and clinical inferences.* Berlin: Springer-Verlag, 1988.
5. Mancuso AA, Hanafee WN, Julliard GJF, et al. The role of computed tomography in the management of cancer of the larynx. Radiology 1977;124:243–4.
6. Mancuso AA, Calcaterra TC, Hanafee WN. Computed tomography of the larynx. Radiol Clin North Am 1978;16:195–208.
7. Sagel SS, AufderHeide JF, Aronberg DJ, et al. High resolution computed tomography in the staging of carcinoma of the larynx. Laryngoscope 1981;91:292–300.
8. Archer CR, Yeager VL. Computed tomography of the larynx with histopathological correlation. Laryngoscope 1982;92:1173–80.
9. Gregor RT, Lloyd GAS, Michaels L. Computed tomography of the larynx: a clinical pathologic study. Head Neck Surg 1981;3:284–96.
10. Mafee MF, Schild JA, Valvassari GE, Capek V. Computed tomography of the larynx: correlation with anatomic and pathologic studies in cases of laryngeal carcinoma. Radiology 1983;147:123–8.
11. Mafee MR, Schild JA, Michael AS, et al. Cartilage involvement in laryngeal carcinoma: correlation of CT and pathologic macrosection studies. J Comput Assist Tomogr 1984;8:969–73.
12. Schild JA, Mafee MF, Valvassari GE, et al. Laryngeal malignancies and computerized tomography: a correlation of tomographic and histopathologic findings. Ann Otol Rhinol Laryngol 1982;91:571–5.
13. Silverman PM, Bossen EH, Fisher SR. Carcinoma of the larynx and hypopharynx: computer tomographic-histopathologic correlations. Radiology 1984;151:697–702.
14. Reid MJ. Laryngeal carcinoma: high resolution computed tomography and thick anatomic sections. Radiology 1984;151:689–96.
15. Gerritsen GJ, Valk J, van Velzen DJ, et al. Computed tomography: a mandatory investigational procedure for the T-staging of advanced laryngeal cancer. Clin Otolaryngol 1986;11:307–16.
16. Hirano M, Kurita S, Cho JS, Tanaka H. Computed tomography in determining laryngeal involvement of hypopharyngeal carcinoma. Ann Otol Rhinol Laryngol 1988;97:476–82.
17. Sulfaro S, Barzan L, Querin F, et al. T staging of the laryngohypo-

pharyngeal carcinoma. Arch Otolaryngol Head Neck Surg 1989;115: 613–20.
18. Tucker GR Jr. The anatomy of laryngeal cancer. Can J Otolaryngol 1974;3:417–31.
19. Olofsson J, van Nostrand AWP. Growth and spread of laryngeal and hypopharyngeal carcinoma with reflections on the effect of preoperative irradiation. Acta Otolaryngol Suppl (Stockh) 1973;308:1–84.
20. Kirchner JA. Two hundred laryngeal cancers: patterns of growth and spread as seen in serial section. Laryngoscope 1977;87:1–9.
21. Lam KH, Wong J. The preepiglottic and paraglottic spaces in relation to spread of carcinoma of the larynx. Am J Otolaryngol 1983;4:81–91.
22. Welsh LW, Welsh JJ, Rizzo TA. Internal anatomy of the larynx and the spread of cancer. Ann Otol Rhinol Laryngol 1989;98:228–34.
23. Kirchner JA, Fischer JJ. Anterior commissure cancer—a clinical and laboratory study of 39 cases. Can J Otolaryngol 1975;4:637–43.
24. Bryce PD. The laryngeal subglottis. J Laryngol Otol 1979;89:667–85.
25. Yeager VL, Archer CR. Anatomical routes for cancer invasion of laryngeal cartilages. Laryngoscope 1982;92:449–52.
26. Archer CR, Yeager VL, Herbold DR. Improved diagnostic accuracy in laryngeal cancer using a new classification based on computed tomography. Cancer 1984;53:44–57.
27. Castelijns JA, Gerritsen GJ, Kaiser MC, et al. MRI of normal or cancerous laryngeal cartilages: histopathologic correlation. Laryngoscope 1987;97:1085–93.
28. Hirano M, Kurita S, Kiyokawa K, et al. Posterior glottis. Morphological study in excised human larynges. Ann Otol Rhinol Laryngol 1986;95:576–81.
29. Cerat J, Charlin B, Brazeau-Lamontagne L, Mongeau CJ. Assessment of the cricoarytenoid joint: high-resolution CT scan study with histoanatomical correlation. J Otolaryngol 1988;17:65–7.
30. Gilbert RW, Birt D, Shulman H, et al. Correlation of tumor volume with local control in laryngeal carcinoma treated by radiotherapy. Ann Otol Rhinol Laryngol 1987;96:514–8.
31. Isaacs J, Mancuso AA, Mendenhall WM, et al. Deep spread patterns in CT staging of T_{2-4} squamous cell laryngeal carcinoma. Otolaryngol Head Neck Surg 1988;99:455–64.
32. Freeman DE, Mancuso AA, Parsons JT, et al. Irradiation alone for supraglottic larynx carcinoma: can CT findings predict treatment results? Presented at the 31st Annual Meeting of American Society of Therapeutic Radiation Oncologists, San Francisco, October 1–6, 1989.
33. Mittal B, Marks JE, Ogura JH. Transglottic carcinoma. Cancer 1984;53:151–61.
34. Millon RR, Cassisi NJ. Larynx. In Million RR, Cassisi NJ, eds. *Management of head and neck cancer—a multidisciplinary approach*. Philadelphia: JB Lippincott, 1984:315–64.
35. Cummings CW, Sessions DG, Weymuller FA, Wood P. *Atlas of laryngeal surgery*. St. Louis: CV Mosby, 1984:209–62.
36. Ogura JH, Heeneman H. Conservation surgery of the larynx and hypopharynx—selection of patients and results. Can J Otolaryngol 1973;2:1–16.
37. Biller HF, Ogura JH, Pratt LL. Hemilaryngectomy for T_2 glottic cancers. Arch Otolaryngol 1971;93:238–43.
38. Biller HF, Lawson W. Partial laryngectomy for vocal cord cancer with marked limitation or fixation of the vocal cord. Laryngoscope 1986;96:61–4.
39. Som ML. Cordal cancer with extension to vocal process. Laryngoscope 1975;85:1298–1307.
40. Kirchner JA, Som ML. The anterior commissure technique of partial laryngectomy: clinical and laboratory observations. Laryngoscope 1975;85:1308–17.
41. Harrison DFN. Classification: the great deception. J Otolaryngol 1988;17:12–5.
42. Million RR. The myth regarding bone or cartilage involvement by cancer and the likelihood of cure by radiotheraapy. Head Neck 1989;11:30–40.
43. Parsons JT, Mendenhall WM, Mancuso AA, et al. Twice-a-day radiotherapy for T_3 squamous cell carcinoma of the glottic larynx. Head Neck 1989;11:123–8.
44. Karim ABMF, Kralendonk JH, Yap LY, et al. Heterogeneity of stage II glottic carcinoma and its therapeutic implications. Int J Radiat Oncol Biol Phys 1987;13:313–7.
45. Kessler DJ, Trapp TK, Calcaterra TC. The treatment of T_3 glottic carcinoma with vertical partial laryngectomy. Arch Otolaryngol Head Neck Surg 1987;97:1020–4.
46. Silver CE. Surgery for Cancer of the Larynx. New York: Churchill Livingstone, 1981.
47. Bocca E, Pignataro O, Oldini C, et al. Extended supraglottic laryngectomy—review of 84 cases. Ann Otol Rhinol Laryngol 1987;96:384–6.
48. Biller HF, Lawson W. Partial laryngectomy for transglottic cancers. Ann Otol Rhinol Laryngol 1984;93:297–300.
49. Kirchner JA. Pathways and pitfalls in partial laryngectomy. Ann Otol Rhinol Laryngol 1984;93:301–5.
50. Dumich PS, Pearson BW, Weiland LH. Suitability of near-total laryngopharyngectomy in pyriform carcinoma. Arch Otolaryngol 1984;110:664–9.
51. Laccourreye H, St Guily JL, Brasnu D, et al. Supracricoid hemilaryngopharyngectomy—analysis of 240 cases. Ann Otol Rhinol Laryngol 1987;96:217–21.
52. Million RR, Cassisi NJ. Radical irradiation for carcinoma of the pyriform sinus. Laryngoscope 1981;91:439–50.
53. Marks JE, Smith PG, Sessions DG. Pharyngeal wall cancer—a reappraisal after comparison of treatment methods. Arch Otolaryngol 1985;111:79–85.
54. Mendenhall WM, Parsons JT, Mancuso AA, et al. Squamous cell carcinoma of the pharyngeal wall treated with irradiation. Radiother Oncol 1988;11:205–12.
55. Ward PH, Calcaterra TC, Kagan AR. The enigma of postradiation edema and recurrent or residual carcinoma of the larynx. Laryngoscope 1982;92:449–52.
56. Chandler JR. Radiation fibrosis and necrosis of the larynx. Ann Otol Rhinol Laryngol 1979;88:509–14.
57. Goodrich WA, Lenz M. Laryngeal chondronecrosis following roentgen therapy. Am J Roentgenol Rad Ther 1948;60:22–8.
58. Keene M, Harwood AR, Bryce DP, et al. Histopathological study of radionecrosis in laryngeal carcinoma. Laryngoscope 1982;92:173–80.
59. DiSantis DJ, Balfe DM, Hayden R, et al. The neck after vertical hemilaryngectomy: computed tomographic study. Radiology 1984; 151:683–7.
60. DiSantis DJ, Balfe DM, Hayden R, et al. The neck after total laryngectomy: CT study. Radiology 1984;153:713–7.
61. Gluckman JL, Hamaker RC, Schuller DE, et al. Surgical salvage for stomal recurrence: a multi-institutional experience. Laryngoscope 1987;97:1025–9.
62. Mancuso AA, Harnsberger HR, Muraki AS, et al. Computed tomography of cervical and retropharyngeal lymph nodes. Part II - pathology. Radiology 1983;148:715–23.
63. Harnsberger HR, Mancuso AA, Muraki AS. The upper aerodigestive tract and neck: CT evaluation of recurrent tumors. Radiology 1983;149:503–9.
64. Foote RL, Buskirk SJ, Stanley RJ, et al. Patterns of failure after total laryngectomy for glottic carcinoma. Cancer 1989;64:143–9.
65. Lam KH, Lau WF, Wei WI. Tumor clearance at resection margins in total laryngectomy—a clinicopathologic study. Cancer 1988;61: 2260–72.

8

Evaluation of Cervical Nodes by Computed Tomography and Magnetic Resonance Imaging

Peter M. Som

The radiologist can provide the clinician with important information about the pathologic status of cervical lymph nodes in patients with primary head and neck cancer. This radiographic information can be used to stage a patient's disease more accurately, improve treatment planning, and to determine response to therapy more sensitively.

In the early days of computed tomography (CT), clinicians often doubted the usefulness of this modality. Crudity of images on early CT scanners, lack of experience in interpretation, and failure to appreciate the adjunctive rather than competitive roles of imaging and clinical examination all contributed to this attitude. More recently, marked refinement of CT images, development of magnetic resonance imaging (MRI), greater experience of diagnostic radiologists, and acceptance by clinicians of the reliability of imaging information have made imaging an essential part of the assessment of a patient with head and neck cancer.

There are situations in which imaging may be uniquely informative. Nodes with central necrosis that appear normal on physical examination can be identified. Imaging permits reliable evaluation of nodes in locations that are difficult to evaluate clinically, such as the retropharyngeal area, the tracheoesophageal groove, and the nodes immediately deep to the sternocleidomastoid muscle. Encasement of, or extension to, the internal carotid artery (ICA) or skull base by extranodal tumor spread can be accurately detected by imaging long before these features are clinically apparent. Imaging is of particular value in patients who have a mycocutaneous flap or scarring from prior surgery or irradiation; evaluation of subtle changes deep to these bulky or "woody" tissues may be otherwise impossible.[1,2]

CT has been available for clinical use for about a decade. The earliest reported application of this modality to evaluate cervical lymph nodes was as recent as 1981.[3] Prior to this time, the only available radiologic technique for evaluation of cervical lymph nodes was lymphangiography. This time-consuming study often failed because of the technical difficulty of identification and injection of the extremely small lymphatics in the neck. Reactive nodal disease could not be reliably distinguished from malignant nodal disease and many lymph nodes could simply not be visualized because of proximal obstruction to the flow of contrast material. These lymphatic pathways could not only be altered or blocked by tumor, but by prior surgery, irradiation, and infection.[4,5] Thus, it is easily understandable that lymphangiography has become obsolete. In comparison, imaging offers a quick, reliable, noninvasive, and easily reproducible method for examining cervical lymph nodes.

Angiography was previously employed to evaluate the carotid arteries. Gross arterial encasement or vessel deviation by tumor could be seen. However, subtle tumor encasement or tumor extension to the vessel's adventitia went undetected. Contrast-enhanced CT scans and MRI scans will accurately demonstrate the proximity of tumor mass to vessel and may suggest even subtle extension to the arterial wall. Recently, ultrasound has been employed to help distinguish tumor that is just positioned against the artery from actual tumor invasion.[6] At the present time, the use of arteriography is confined primarily to assessment of intracranial cross-circulation in patients who may require carotid artery sacrifice or grafting because of tumor invasion.

The radiologist faced with the task of specifically evaluating metastatic cervical lymph nodes must address several problems: the location of normal lymph nodes must be established so that nodes in unusual locations can be recognized; a nomenclature must be developed to facilitate precise communication between radiologist and clinician; and criteria for evaluating metastatic lymph nodes must be established so that uniformity and consistency can be realized not only between imaging examinations, but between different radiologists.

The fatty tissue of the neck provides an effective medium for smooth and easy motion of the muscles, vessels, and nerves. The same fat also serves as an excellent background medium for imaging the cervical lymph nodes. This occurs because of several factors: (1) the cervical lymph nodes are all situated within the fat of the head and neck; (2) the CT attenuation of fat is significantly lower than that of lymph nodes; and (3) the MR signal intensities of fat are different enough from those of lymph nodes to allow the nodes to be detected.

In patients with normal amounts of cervical fat, lymph nodes as small as 3 to 5 mm diameter can usually be demonstrated by imaging procedures. If the amount of fat is diminished, however, (as in normal children, very muscular or cachectic patients, or postoperative patients) or if the texture of the fat has been altered so that it has an abnormal CT attenuation or different MR signal intensities (as after operation, irradiation, or infection,) imaging sensitivity may be decreased, permitting small lymph nodes to remain undetected. However, CT and MRI still complement the clinical examination in these patients, because the same circumstances that alter the appearance and character of fat also increase the difficulty of physical examination. Thus, the status of cervical lymph nodes can be most accurately studied in all patients by a combination of both clinical and imaging findings. Such combined information provides a more detailed and accurate assessment than may be achieved by either method alone.

NOMENCLATURE

Standard nomenclature has been based on the work of Rouviere.[7] The most frequently used names of the nodal chains and the approximate number of lymph nodes in each chain are summarized in Figure 8–1.[8–12] More recently, a simplified nomenclature (Fig. 8–2, Table 8–1) has gained popularity.[1,13] As long as both radiologist and clinician employ the same system, information concerning nodal abnormalities can be exchanged with accuracy. Clear communication is essential, not only for relating information about suspicious lymph nodes, but for evaluating response to therapy.

EVALUATION OF CERVICAL NODES BY COMPUTED TOMOGRAPHY

Size and Shape

It has long been clinically observed that lymph nodes in the submandibular and jugulodigastric areas are larger and more consistently palpable than are other cervical nodes. These upper neck nodes tend to enlarge because of benign reactive hyperplasia in response to numerous common inflammatory episodes of the teeth, gums, tonsils, and pharynx. Clinical studies suggest that any upper cervical lymph node larger than 1.5 cm in diameter should be considered pathologic. Imaging studies have demonstrated, however, that retropharyngeal lymph nodes as well as nodes in the mid and lower jugular and posterior triangle regions are rarely greater than 1 cm in diameter, except when they are pathologic. Consequently, a homogeneous, clearly defined nodal mass greater than 1.5 cm in diameter situated in the submandibular chain or jugulodigastric region or any such node greater than 1 cm in diameter situated in the remaining areas of the neck should be considered abnormal (Fig. 8–3). Final pathologic examination will reveal about 80% of these lymph nodes to be malignant.[14–18] Although these results are

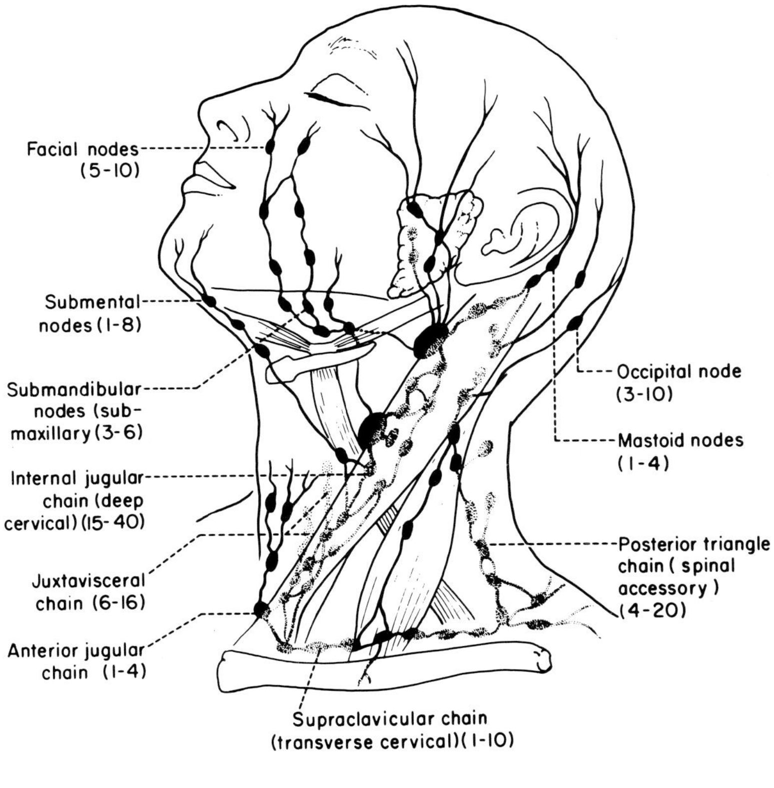

Figure 8–1. Diagram of the major superficial lymph node chains of the head and neck. The most commonly used nomenclature is given and any alternate names are in parentheses. The numbers refer to the number of lymph nodes present in each chain. (From Som.[1] Reprinted with permission.)

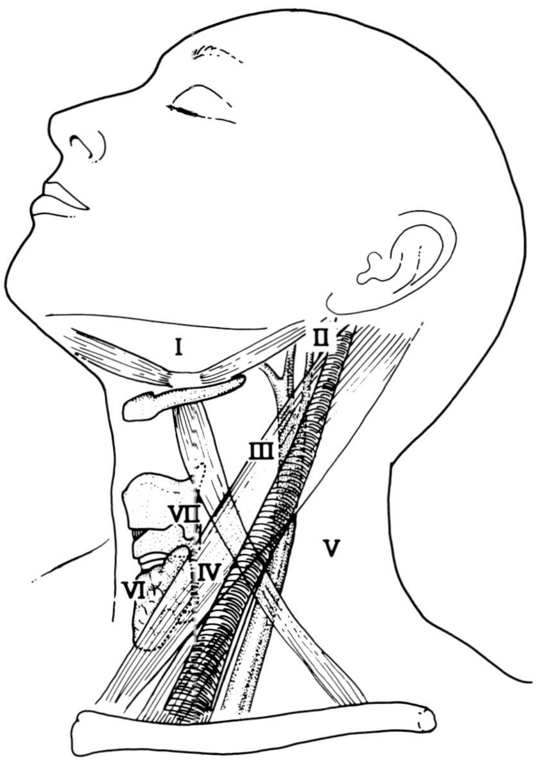

Figure 8–2. Diagram of the simplified nomenclature system. Levels II, III, and IV are all along the internal jugular chain of lymph nodes. See Table 8–1 for a description of each group of nodes. (From Som.[1] Reprinted with permission.)

essentially identical to those obtained by clinical examination, the scope of such examination is enhanced by the ability of imaging modalities to visualize lymph nodes that are inaccessible to physical examination, particularly in the retropharyngeal chain, tracheoesophageal groove, and posterior triangle or internal jugular chains lying immediately deep to the sternocleidomastoid muscle. Nonmalignant lymph nodes are "lima bean" or ovoid in shape, whereas metastatic lymph nodes are spherical.[1,7,19–22] Thus, a lymph node at the upper limits of normal size with spherical rather than ovoid shape may be suspected of being potentially malignant.

Table 8-1. Simplified Nodal Classification*

Level I	Submandibular and submental nodes
Level II	Internal jugular chain from the skull base to the level of the carotid bifurcation (hyoid bone)
Level III	Internal jugular chain from the carotid bifurcation to the level where the omohyoid muscle (cricoid cartilage) crosses the internal jugular vein
Level IV	Infraomohyoid portion of the internal jugular chain
Level V	The posterior triangle nodes
Level VI	Nodes related to the thyroid gland
Level VII	The tracheoesophageal groove nodes and superior mediastinal nodes

*From Som.[1] Reprinted with permission.

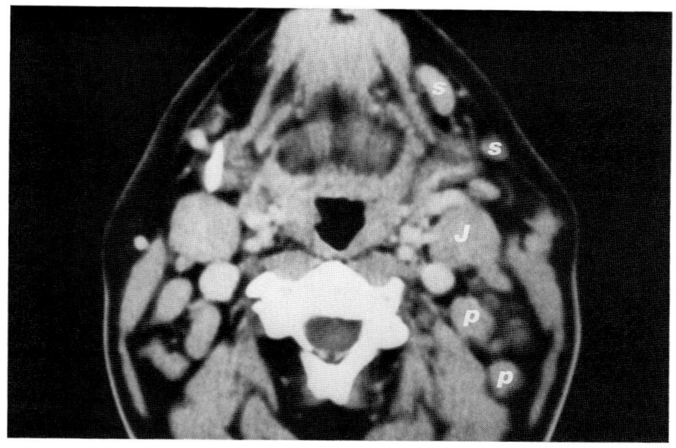

Figure 8–3. Axial postcontrast computed tomography scan reveals multiple bilateral submandibular (s), posterior triangle (p), and jugulodigastric (J) lymph nodes. They are all homogeneous and sharply outlined. They also do not exceed the size limits described in the text and therefore they all most probably represent hyperplastic lymph nodes.

Necrosis

Necrotic lymph nodes demonstrate central areas of decreased attenuation on the postcontrast CT scan (Fig. 8–4). Focal attenuation measurements taken in the necrotic region vary between 10 and 20 HU. Central necrosis must be differentiated from a site of fatty nodal replacement, which usually is peripherally located within the lymph node and has a lower attenuation. Such postinflammatory fatty replacement can almost always be differentiated from an area of central necrosis by visual assessment of the scan, without actually having to measure attenuation numbers (Fig. 8–5).[1,3,23]

Demonstration of a lymph node is significant because any

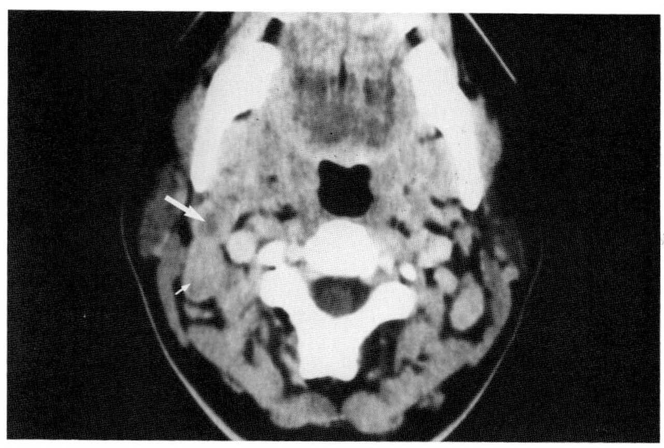

Figure 8–4. Axial postcontrast computed tomography scan reveals bilateral jugulodigastric and posterior triangle lymph nodes. On the left side, these nodes are small and homogeneous. On the right side, the jugulodigastric node (large arrow) is not enlarged, but the central region of the node has a lower attenuation (necrotic). The right posterior triangle node (small arrow) is both enlarged and minimally necrotic. These contained metastatic squamous cell carcinoma.

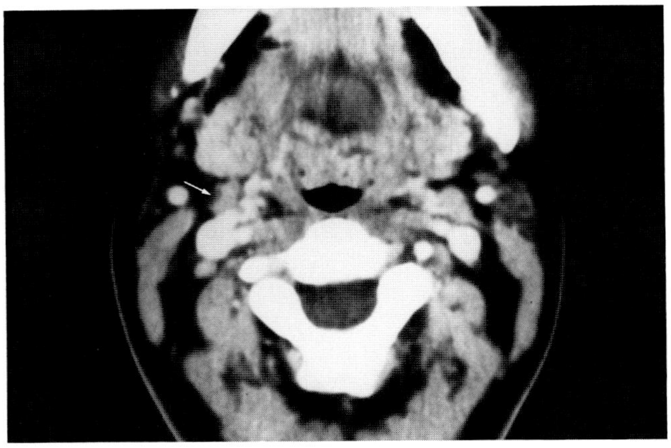

Figure 8–5. Axial postcontrast computed tomography scan reveals bilateral, nonenlarged jugulodigastric lymph nodes. On the right side, there is a small area of peripheral fatty replacement (arrow). This is usually easily distinguished from an area of central tumor necrosis (see Fig. 8–4).

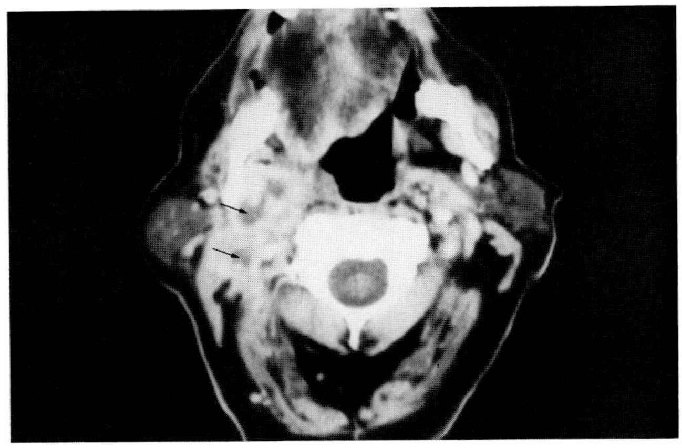

Figure 8–6. Axial postcontrast computed tomography scan reveals at least two necrotic lymph nodes on the right side. The central areas of necrosis (arrows) are surrounded by nodular, irregular, thickened, enhancing rims. The outer nodal contour is not sharp, indicating extranodal tumor spread. The right internal carotid artery cannot be identified, indicating that it is invaded by tumor.

necrotic lymph node, regardless of size, is pathologic. Thus, nonenlarged, nonpalpable necrotic lymph nodes will be recognized on the basis of imaging criteria, although undetectable by physical examination.

Intravenous Contrast Medium

Detection of necrosis is facilitated by administration of intravenous contrast medium prior to CT scanning because of minimal degrees of enhancement of the non-necrotic portions of the lymph node. Recognition of such nodes may be quite difficult on CT studies performed without contrast. Postcontrast CT scans also allow overall assessment of the degree of variation in nodal enhancement and provide a means of distinguishing lymph nodes from blood vessels. Consequently, it is recommended that all CT scans of the neck should be done as postcontrast examinations, unless a medical contraindication to the use of contrast medium exists.

Most hyperplastic lymph nodes have some degree of enhancement on postcontrast CT scans or have an attenuation similar to that of muscle. Marked enhancement of lymph nodes usually reflects either an acute inflammatory node or, less often, a lymphomatous node.

Differential Diagnosis

The necrotic areas in tumorous nodes are lower in attenuation than muscle and usually the margins of the central necrotic region are irregular and nodular in configuration (Fig. 8–6). Most often, such a CT appearance represents a node with metastatic squamous cell carcinoma; however, any type carcinoma or lymphoma can have a similar imaging appearance.

Although a uniformly thin, smooth-walled cystic mass is most often a benign cyst, this appearance can also be found with some metastatic lymph nodes; most often, metastatic papillary thyroid carcinoma with almost total central necrosis (Fig. 8–7). A thin, slightly enhancing rim around a central region of decreased attenuation that is slightly lower in density than that of muscle, but higher than that of classic necrosis, is most suggestive of a lymphomatous node (Fig. 8–8). Lymphomatous nodes are most often either minimally enhancing, isodense with muscle, or have slightly lower attenuation than muscle (with a thin, uniform, slightly enhancing outer rim). It is rare for lymphomatous nodes to have a central necrotic low attenuation region surrounded by thick, irregular walls, as is characteristic of metastatic squamous cell carcinoma. Occasionally, carcinoma can have an isodense non-necrotic imaging appearance that is similar to that of hyperplastic lymph node. Significant enhancement of a lymph node with metastatic carcinoma, however, is rare. Hyperplastic nodes are usually homogeneous in appearance and are most often either isodense with muscle or

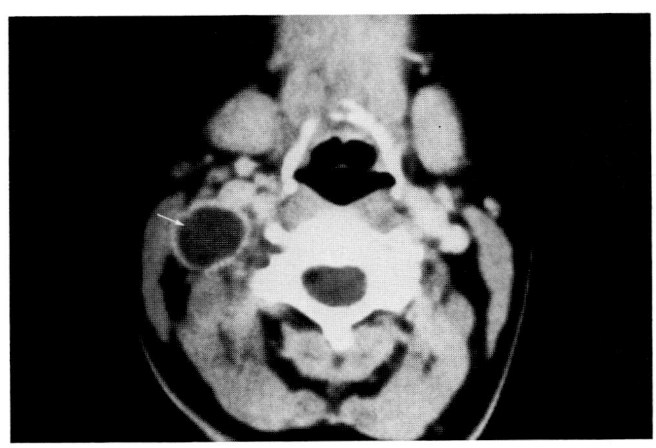

Figure 8–7. Axial postcontrast computed tomography scan reveals a right posterior triangle benign-appearing cystic mass (arrow). The central low attenuation region is surrounded by a thin, smooth, minimally enhancing rim. This was a metastatic node from a papillary thyroid carcinoma.

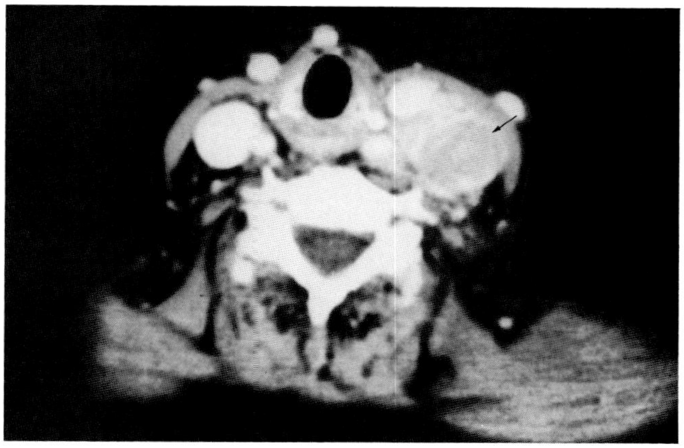

Figure 8–8. Axial postcontrast computed tomography scan reveals a large right posterior triangle lymph node (arrow). Despite its size, the node is not necrotic and there is a thin, uniform enhancing rim. This patient had lymphoma.

minimally enhancing. An aggressive nodal infection may develop an area of central necrosis mimicking the appearance of a metastatic carcinomatous node. However, the clinical presentation usually allows distinction between these entities. When multiple lymph nodes are present with some of them enhancing, some isodense with muscle and some truly necrotic, the most likely diagnosis is a granulomatous process such as tuberculosis (Fig. 8–9).[1,5,24]

Although these postcontrast CT scan nodal appearances represent the major trends for the various disease entities, these generalizations are unreliable for prediction of exact nodal histology characteristics based only on the CT appearance without correlation of other clinical information.

Extranodal Spread of Disease

A single staging system has finally been adopted by both the American Joint Committee on Cancer (AJCC) and the International Union Against Cancer (UICC).[25] This should allow for more accurate statistical comparisons to be made between American and European communities. In the new system, the concept of "fixation," previously utilized by the UICC to describe the N_3 category of nodes, was abandoned because of variability and subjectivity of interpretation by different observers.

The clinical finding of nodal "fixation" is caused by extracapsular spread of tumor that may have infiltrated the surrounding interstitial fat planes, vessels, nerves, and muscles. Although once thought to only occur in lymph nodes 3 cm or larger in diameter, it is now known that such extranodal extension occurs in 23% of lymph nodes smaller than 1 cm, 53% of lymph nodes 2 to 3 cm, and 74% of lymph nodes greater than 3 cm in diameter. This represents 60% of all lymph nodes less than 3 cm in diameter.[26,27] Many of these nodes, particularly with lesser degrees of extranodal extension, are still readily mobile on physical examination. CT imaging can identify most such lymph nodes by revealing an "unsharp" or infiltrating outer nodal contour, often associated with enhancement of the nodal rim (Fig. 8–10). A similar imaging appearance may be produced by previous surgery, irradiation, infection, or hemorrhage. Such conditions can often be discerned from the patient's history, and if present must be considered in diagnosis. If a previous "baseline" CT scan is available for comparison, interval widening of a prior zone of extranodal infiltration should be considered as evidence of progressive extranodal tumor spread. Extracapsular spread of tumor to the skull base or the ICA can usually be well demonstrated by imaging (Fig. 8–11). Coronal scans often best display the relationship of the tumor to the skull base and in this regard are most beneficial in helping plan surgical approaches and irradiation fields.

Calcification

Gross nodal calcification is unusual and is often associated with old tuberculosis. Smaller psammomatous nodal calcifications may be found in metastases from papillary thyroid cancer (Fig.

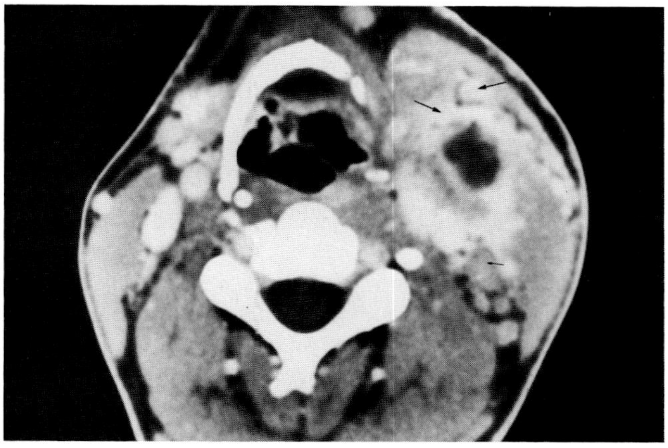

Figure 8–9. Axial postcontrast computed tomography scan reveals multiple lymph nodes on the left side. One node at this scan level is clearly necrotic, one or two adjacent nodes enhance (large arrows), whereas the nodes posteriorly (small arrow) are the same attenuation as muscle. This appearance is most suggestive of tuberculosis.

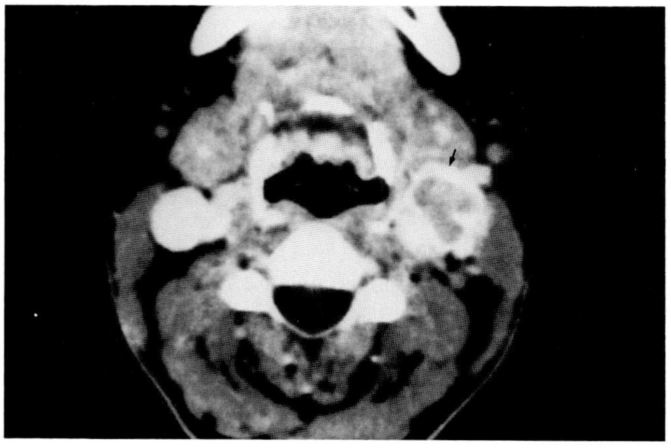

Figure 8–10. Axial postcontrast computed tomography scan reveals an enlarged left jugulodigastric lymph node with an enhancing rim (arrow) and a somewhat poorly defined outer contour. This metastatic squamous cell carcinoma node had extracapsular spread.

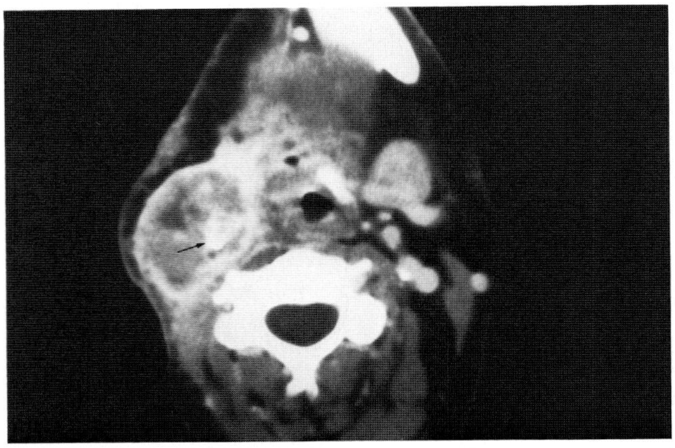

Figure 8–11. Axial postcontrast computed tomography scan reveals a large necrotic nodal mass on the right side with an enhancing "unsharp" nodal rim. Within the nodal mass, arteriosclerotic calcification in the internal carotid artery wall is seen (arrow). This patient had metastatic squamous cell carcinoma with extracapsular spread and complete encasement of the internal carotid artery.

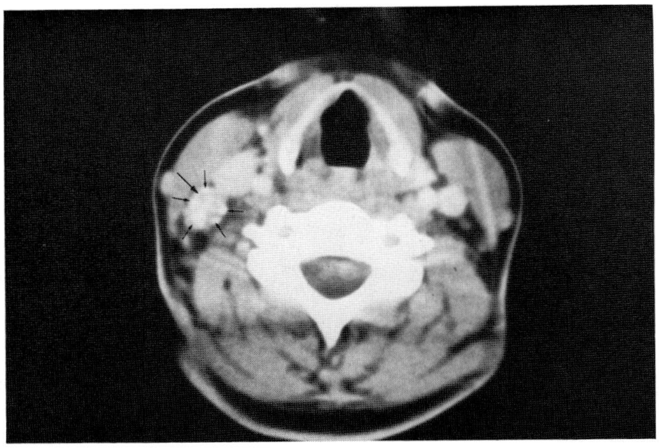

Figure 8–12. Axial postcontrast computed tomography scan reveals a right posterior triangle node (large arrow). Within the node are multiple small calcifications (small arrows) that were also identified on a noncontrast CT scan. This patient had metastatic papillary thyroid carcinoma.

8–12). Calcifications may also occur in metastases from a mucus-producing cancer, healed previously irradiated carcinomatous or lymphomatous lymph nodes, or, rarely, a healed aggressive infection.

Psammomatous calcification may often not be visualized on plain films, whereas CT produces a tenfold advantage over such films in detecting these small calcifications. In some cases of papillary carcinoma without either palpable lymphadenopathy or evident primary tumor, CT may provide the only evidence of the disease.

MAGNETIC RESONANCE IMAGING

Obstacles to Use

The recently developed modality of MRI provides new opportunities for accurate noninvasive evaluation of cervical nodes. Several obstacles, however, have yet to be surmounted completely. The most important of these arise from lack of conformity of the patient's habitus to the "coil," or sensor, that must surround the neck in order to record the image. Problems in this regard arise because most commerically available coils are designed for an individual with "average" proportions. Disparity between coil size and the neck, for example, in tall thin or short obese individuals produces degradation of MR images with obfuscation of much detail by background signal noise. This type of image degradation is also somewhat dependent on the strength of the magnetic field used. High-field (1.5 to 2.0 T) units, as well as midfield units ((0.5 T) depend considerably on coil-patient match for production of high-quality images. Only with low-field units (0.3 T range) can neck coils be more easily designed to correlate well with each individual's neck anatomy. The low-field units, however, produce the poorest quality T_2 weighted scans (see later). Optimal scans can be produced only with a 0.5 T or stronger MR scanner with good signal-to-noise ratio.

Three types of MR images are routinely obtained, determined primarily by the parameters of time to repetition (TR) and time to echo (TE). These parameters may be manipulated so that a short TR, short TE scan gives what is called T_1 weighted (T_1W) information. T_1W pictures are the clearest of the sequences used and usually best display the anatomy. A long TR, long TE scan gives T_2 weighted (T_2W) information. T_2W pictures are less clear than the T_1W images, but usually provide the best distinction between pathologic and normal tissues. Comparison of the T_1 and T_2 weighted signal intensities is utilized to discern information about the specific nature of a tissue (Fig. 8–13). A long TR, short TE scan is called a mixed or proton-density image and gives T_1W and T_2W information. These mixed images are often used to approximate the T_1W images, since in most cases they are more heavily T_1W than T_2W, particularly with higher field strength MRI units.[28]

Another obstacle encountered with current MRI technology is the length of time required for examination. Unlike CT, which can scan the entire neck from the skull base to the manubrium within 15 to 20 minutes in one continuous examination, MRI has several time-related problems. For the average patient, neck examination requires two or three contiguous, consecutive studies, each of which takes from 20 to 30 minutes and necessitates repositioning the patient as well as adjustment of scanning parameters. A complete MRI examination may, at present, take from ½ to 2 hours, depending on how many sequences and views (such as transverse, coronal, and sagittal) are used. Because MRI scans are more sensitive to motion artifact than are CT scans, the longer the MRI examination lasts, the more prone the patient is to move.

Cost is also a factor; MRI examinations are often twice as expensive as CT scan studies. The present result of these obstacles is that CT remains the preferred modality for initial imaging examination of the neck. MRI examination, limited if possible, may be employed to resolve specific problems left

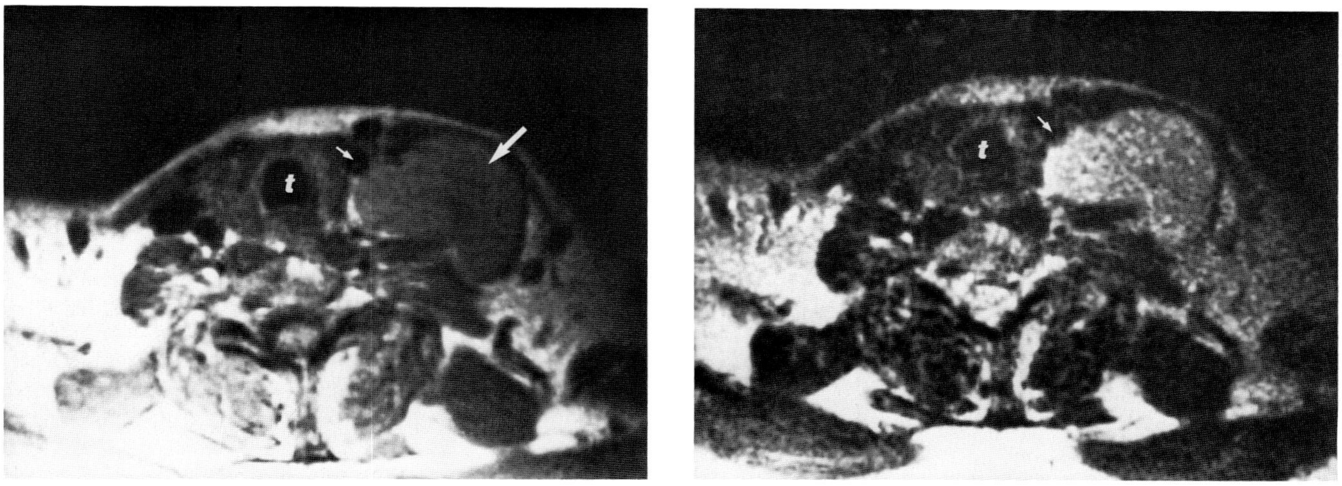

A B

Figure 8–13. Transverse T_1 weighted (T_1W) (A) and T_2 weighted (T_2W) (B) magnetic resonance scans. There is a large left posterior triangle lymph node (large arrow). The resolution is better and the anatomy is better appreciated on the T_1W scan. The T_2W scan is noisier in appearance, but better separates the mass from the adjacent muscles. This patient had lymphoma: (t) trachea, (small arrow) carotid artery.

unsolved by CT. With anticipated future improvements in technology, MRI may become the universally applied modality for evaluation of the neck in head and neck cancer.

Evaluation of Malignant Nodes

Additional problems with MR scans are related to the interpretation of lymph node pathologic changes. Lymph node invasion by cancer occurs in two stages. Initially, cancer cells enter a lymph node via the afferent vessels and lodge in the reticular meshwork of the marginal sinuses of the nodal cortex. Tumor cell proliferation results in invasion of the nodal medulla and blockage of lymph flow. During this stage, there is a dense accumulation of tumor cells within the lymph node, eventually resulting in propagation of tumor cells to other nodes. At a later stage, necrosis of the nodal medulla occurs.[1,14]

An MRI scan performed during the stage prior to necrosis will show, on all imaging sequences, an area of low-to-intermediate signal intensity within the node that corresponds to the area of dense, cellular tumor (Fig. 8–14). An MRI scan performed after necrosis of the lymph node has occurred reveals an area of low-to-intermediate T_1W signal intensity and a "bright" or high T_2W signal intensity corresponding to the fluid (water) filling the necrotic cavity (Fig. 8–15). If areas of tumor infiltration and necrosis are intermixed within a node, the result is an overall intermediate signal intensity on all imaging sequences (Fig. 8–16). As a general statement, any nonhomogeneous node demonstrated by MRI should be considered pathologic until proven otherwise.

On CT studies, malignant lymph nodes appear necrotic whether there is only tumor cell infiltration, actual necrosis, or a mixture of these states. Thus, all nodes that appear necrotic on CT are considered malignant. With MRI, however, metastatic nodes can vary in appearance and may not be identified as "necrotic" on the supposedly tissue-sensitive T_2W scans. At the present time, necrotic lymph nodes are more readily diagnosed by CT than by MRI.

Fine needle aspiration cytology, guided by either CT or MRI, may be employed to confirm malignancy in nonpalpable abnormal nodes demonstrated by imaging studies. Imaging-guided needle aspiration can also be used for evaluation of suspected tumor spread to the skull base or other regions.[29–32]

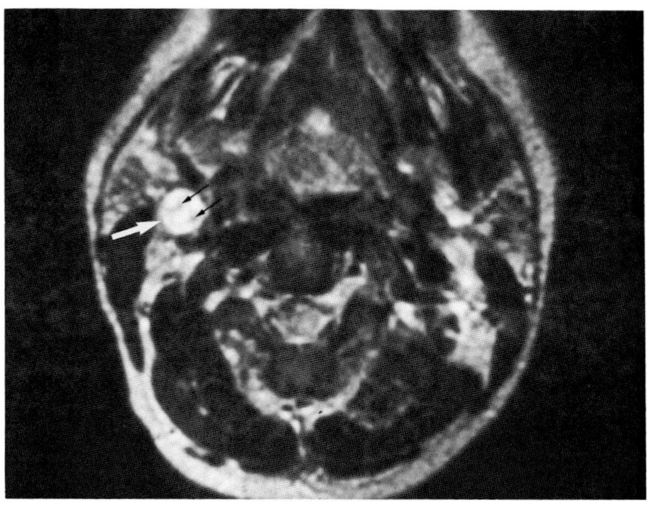

Figure 8–14. Transverse T_2 weighted (T_2W) magnetic resonance scan reveals a right jugulodigastric lymph node that has an overall high (bright) signal intensity (large arrow). Within the node are two small zones of low signal intensity (small arrows). This was a necrotic squamous cell carcinoma node and was totally necrotic in appearance on computed tomography scan.

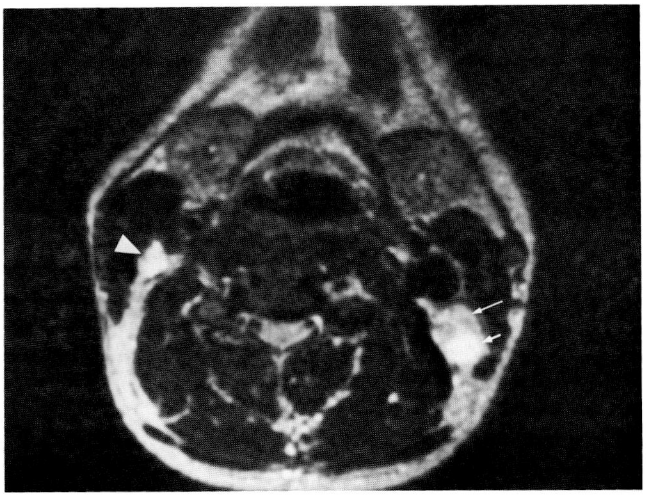

Figure 8–15. Transverse T_2 weighted (T_2W) magnetic resonance scan reveals a small right posterior triangle lymph node (arrowhead) that has a high (bright) signal intensity. In the left posterior triangle, there is an enlarged lymph node that has an area of both intermediate (large arrow) and high signal intensity (small arrow). Both of these metastatic squamous cell carcinoma nodes appeared totally necrotic on computed tomography scan.

EVALUATION OF THE PRIMARY TUMOR

The previous discussion has been devoted to the value of imaging studies for evaluation of cervical lymph nodes in patients with head and neck cancer. These advantages are enhanced by information gained by imaging the primary tumor.[33] Whether by displaying the true submucosal extension of a pharyngeal tumor, illustrating laryngeal cartilage invasion, or revealing subtle extralaryngeal tumor spread, information gained from imaging can lead to improved staging of disease and development of a more effective treatment plan.

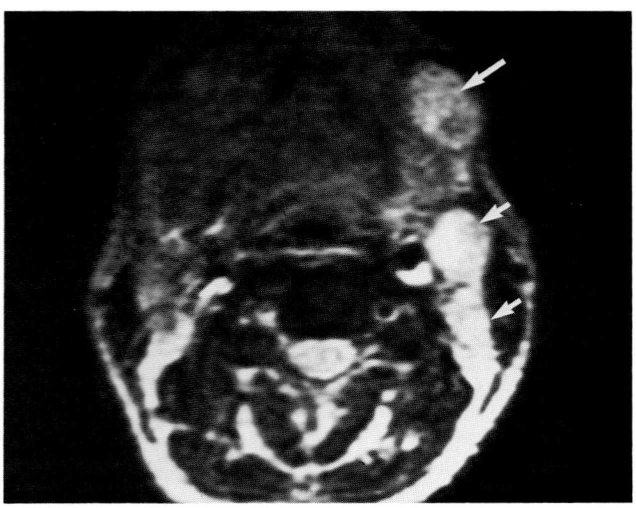

Figure 8–16. Transverse T_2 weighted (T_2W) magnetic resonance scan reveals an enlarged left submandibular lymph node with an overall intermediate signal intensity and one or two small areas of high signal intensity (large arrow). There are also enlarged left jugulodigastric and posterior triangle lymph nodes (small arrows) that have high signal intensity. All of these metastatic squamous cell carcinoma nodes appeared totally necrotic on CT scan.

CONCLUSIONS AND PROSPECTS

CT or MR scanning is of great value in pretreatment planning for the patient with head and neck cancer. Imaging may reveal the presence of cervical lymph node metastases, inapparent on physical examination, particularly in instances of single nonpalpable ipsilateral (N_1) or contralateral (N_{3c}) malignant nodes. Such discovery will clearly affect planned treatment as well as prognostication. With advancement in MRI technology, it appears inevitable that examination time will shorten, motion artifacts will present less of a problem, coil design will improve, and costs will decrease. Paramagnetic contrast agents have been developed that should add to the value of MRI studies, although their impact cannot, at present, be adequately assessed. Tagging of such agents with monoclonal antibodies is currently under investigation. In this age of continued dramatic medical advances, it can be hoped that such innovations will further improve both quantity and quality of information provided to the clinician by imaging techniques.

REFERENCES

1. Som PM. Lymph nodes of the neck. Radiology 1987;165:593–600.
2. Som PM, Biller HF. Computed tomography of the neck in the postoperative patient: radical neck dissection and the myocutaneous flap. Radiology 1983;148:157–60.
3. Mancuso AA, Maceri D, Rice D, Hanafee WN. CT of cervical lymph node cancer. Am J Radiol 1981;136:381–5.
4. Kuisk H. Cervical lymphography. In: Kuisk H, ed. *Technique of lymphography and principles of interpretation*. St. Louis; Green, 1971:156–62.
5. Reede DL, Bergeron RT. Computed tomography of cervical lymph nodes. In: Clause ME, Wallace S, eds. *Lymphatic imaging: lymphography, computed tomography, and scintigraphy*, 2nd ed. Baltimore: Williams & Wilkins, 1985:472–95.
6. Hajek PC, Salomonowitz E, Turk R, et al. Lymph nodes of the neck: evaluation with US. Radiology 1986;158:739–42.
7. Rouviere H. Lymphatic system of the head and neck. In: Tobias MJ, ed. *Anatomy of the human lymphatic system* (trans). Ann Arbor: Edwards Brothers, 1938:5–28.
8. Paff GH. *Anatomy of the head and neck*. Philadelphia: WB Saunders, 1973:221–8.
9. Taillens JP. Les adenopathies cervicales: essai d'une classification etiologique des adenites en fonction de leur localisation anatomo-topographique. Rev Med Suisse Romande 1962;82:259–80.
10. Hollingshead WH. *Anatomy for Surgeons, vol. 1, the head and neck*. New York: Hoeber-Harper, 1954:448–94.
11. Last RJ. *Anatomy regional and applied*, 6th ed. Edingburgh: Churchill Livingstone, 1978:376–8, 443–4.
12. Montgomery WW. *Surgery of the upper respiratory system*. Philadelphia: Lea & Febiger, 1971:75–87.
13. Shah JP, Strong EW, Spiro RH, Vikram B. Surgical grand rounds, neck dissection: current status and future possibilities. Clin Bull 1981;11: 25–33.
14. Mancuso AA, Harnsberger HR, Muraki AS, Stevens MH. Computed tomography of cervical and retropharyngeal lymph nodes: normal anatomy, variants of normal, and application in staging head and neck cancer. I. Normal anatomy. Radiology 1983;148:709–14.
15. Jinkins JR. Computed tomography of the craniocervical lymphatic

system: anatomical and functional considerations. Neuroradiology 1987;229:317–26.

16. Friedman M, Shelton V, Mafee M, Bellity P, Skolnik E. Metastatic neck diseases: evaluation by computed tomography. Arch Otolaryngol 1984;110:443–7.
17. Cinberg JZ, Silver CE, Molnar JJ, Vogl SE. Cervical cysts: cancer until proven otherwise. Laryngoscope 1982;92:27–30.
18. Stevens MH, Harnsberger HR, Mancuso AA. Computed tomography of cervical lymph nodes: staging and management of head and neck cancer. Arch Otolaryngol 1985;11:735–9.
19. Schuller DE. *Management of Cervical Metastasis in Head and Neck Cancer*. No. 82200. Washington, DC: American Academy of Otolaryngology, Head and Neck Surgery Foundation, 1982.
20. Lindberg R. Distribution of cervical lymph node metastases from squamous cell carcinoma of the upper respiratory and digestive tracts. Cancer 1972;29:1446–9.
21. Sako K, Pradier RN, Marchetta FC, Pickren JW. Fallibility of palpation in the diagnosis of metastasis of cervical nodes. Surg Gynecol Obstet 1964;118:989–90.
22. Kuisk H. Development, structure and function of the lymphatic system. In: Kuisk H, ed. *Technique of lymphography and principles of interpretation*. St. Louis: Green, 1971:5–14.
23. Mancuso AA, Harnsberger HR, Muraki AS, Stevens MA. Computed tomography of cervical and retropharyngeal lymph nodes: normal anatomy, variants of normal, and application in staging head and neck cancer. II. Pathology. Radiology 1983;148:715–23.
24. Reede DL, Bergeron RT. Cervical tuberculous adenitis: CT manifestations. Radiology 1985;154:701–4.
25. Beahrs OH, Henson DE, Hulter RVP, Myers MA. eds. Manual for Staging of Cancer, 3rd ed. Philadelphia: JB Lippincott, 1988:27–30.
26. Collins SL. Controversies in management of cancer of the neck. In: Thawley SE, Panje WR, eds. *Comprehensive management of head and neck tumors,* vol 2. Philadelphia: WB Saunders, 1987:1386–443.
27. Snow GB, Annyas AA, Van Slooten EA, Bartelink H, Hart AA. Prognostic factors of neck node metastases. Clin Otolaryngol 1982;7:185–92.
28. Bradley WG Jr. Pathophysiologic correlates of signal alterations. In: Brant-Zawadzki M, Normal D, eds. *Magnetic resonance imaging of the central nervous system*. New York: Raven Press, 1987:23–42.
29. Gatenby RA, Mulhern CB Jr, Strawitz L, Moldofsky PJ. Comparison of clinical and computed tomographic staging of head and neck tumors. AJNR 1985;6:399–401.
30. Gatenby RA, Mulhern CB Jr, Richter MP, Moldodsky PJ. CT-guided biopsy for the detection and staging of tumors of the head and neck. AJNR 1984;5:287–9.
31. Zornoza J. Percutaneous lymph node biopsy. In: Clause ME, Wallace S, eds. *Lymphatic imaging, lymphography, computed tomography, and scintigraphy,* 2nd ed. Baltimore, Williams & Wilkins, 1985:496–510.
32. Lufkin R, Teresi L, Hanafee W. New needle for MR-guided aspiration cytology of the head and neck. AJR 1987;149:380–2.
33. Som PM. An approach to tumors of the head and neck: the role of computed tomography in the staging and follow-up of patients. In: Margulis AR, Gooding CA, eds. *Diagnostic radiology*. San Francisco: University of California Press, 1985:347–52.

PART THREE

Radiation Therapy and Chemotherapy

9

Radiation Therapy in the Management of Early Laryngeal and Pyriform Sinus Cancer

William M. Mendenhall, James T. Parsons, Nicholas J. Cassisi, Scott P. Stringer, Rodney R. Million

This chapter will present the results of radiation therapy alone or combined with neck dissection for early squamous cell carcinoma of the larynx and pyriform sinus. The term "early" is somewhat ambiguous and, for the purpose of this chapter, an early lesion is defined as a primary lesion suitable for an attempt at cure by radiation therapy with surgery reserved for failure; immediate neck dissection may be a part of the initial plan in those patients with positive lymph nodes. Even a T_3 or T_4 lesion may be suitable for this strategy. Patients treated at the University of Florida are staged according to the 1983 recommendations of the American Joint Committee on Cancer (AJCC).[1] Patients who died within 2 years of treatment with the primary site continuously disease-free were excluded from the local control analysis. Likewise, patients who died within 2 years of treatment with the primary site and neck continuously disease-free were excluded from the analysis of disease control above the clavicles. All patients were eligible for a minimum of 2 years of observation, and all patients were included in the analyses of complications and survival. In most reports, local control is calculated as the number of patients with the disease controlled locally or regionally as a percentage of the total number treated, without restriction as to the minimum period of observation. This results in higher apparent rates of local-regional control than produced by our technique.

SUPRAGLOTTIC LARYNX

Selection of Treatment Modality

For purposes of treatment planning, patients may be considered to be in either an early or favorable group, suitable for radiation therapy or supraglottic laryngectomy, or an unfavorable group, often requiring total laryngectomy. Neck nodes are commonly involved and influence the overall treatment plan. Treatment of the primary lesion for the early group is either by external beam irradiation or supraglottic laryngectomy.[2,3] Total laryngectomy would rarely be indicated as the initial treatment for this group of patients and is reserved for those in whom such treatment fails.

Irradiation and supraglottic laryngectomy are both highly successful modes of therapy for early lesions. Approximately 50% of supraglottic laryngectomies performed at the University of Florida have been followed by postoperative radiation therapy because of either positive margins or neck disease.

Our guidelines for selection of supraglottic laryngectomy or radiation therapy will be outlined. The patient and family are sometimes instrumental in making the decision, often based on their own previous experience with surgery or radiation therapy.

Approximately half the patients seen in our clinic whose lesions are technically suitable for a supraglottic laryngectomy are not suitable for medical reasons (eg, inadequate pulmonary status or other major medical problems). These patients are treated by radiation therapy. Poorly motivated or elderly patients are not good candidates for supraglottic laryngectomy.

Analysis of local control by anatomic subsite within the supraglottic larynx shows no obvious difference in local control rates with radiation therapy when comparing similar stage lesions. Transglottic lesions are not suitable for supraglottic laryngectomy, but they may be managed by radiation therapy in favorable cases. Invasion of the preepiglottic space is not a contraindication to supraglottic laryngectomy or radiation therapy. Supraglottic laryngectomy is often favored for large, bulky infiltrative lesions.

The status of the neck often determines the selection of treatment of the primary lesion. Patients with clinically negative neck nodes at high risk for occult bilateral neck disease (eg, poorly differentiated carcinoma of the suprahyoid epiglottis with midline base of tongue involvement) may be treated by radiation therapy because of the ease of bilateral elective neck irradiation. Alternatively, supraglottic laryngectomy and bilateral conservation neck dissections may be done.

For patients with early-stage primary lesions but advanced neck disease (N_{2B} or N_3), combined treatment is frequently necessary to produce satisfactory control of the neck disease. In these cases the primary lesion is usually treated for cure by irradiation, with surgery added to the involved hemineck. If the same patients were managed by supraglottic laryngectomy, neck dissection, and postoperative irradiation, the radiation therapy portals would unnecessarily irradiate the primary site as well as the neck. When patients with early, resectable neck disease (N_1 or N_{2A}) have been treated surgically, postoperative irradiation is added only for specific indications, such as positive margins, multiple positive nodes, or extracapsular extension. We generally prefer to avoid routine high-dose preoperative or postoperative irradiation in conjunction with supraglottic laryngectomy, since this may produce marked, although transient, lymphedema of the remaining larynx. Robbins and coworkers from M.D. Anderson Hospital, however, have reported good results with combined supraglottic laryngectomy and postoperative irradiation for moderately advanced lesions.[4]

Treatment Technique

Patients are treated with parallel opposed fields to the primary lesion and upper neck (Fig. 9–1). The anterior border of the field is placed at or behind the anterior skin edge, and clothespins are used to pull as much tissue out of the field as possible to minimize postirradiation edema. The field size is reduced to avoid further irradiation of the spinal cord at approximately 4500 cGy, and, if necessary, an electron beam is used to treat the posterior cervical lymph node in the event of clinically positive neck nodes in this location (Fig. 9–2). The low neck is irradiated with an en face field using a small tapered midline block to minimize the risk of field overlap at the spinal cord (Fig. 9–3). Patients are treated with one or two fractions per day, 5 days a week, with a continuous course technique. The total doses recommended for various treatment schemes are listed in Table 9–1.

The clinically negative neck is irradiated electively, covering the jugulodigastric and midjugular areas bilaterally. The low neck is irradiated with a tight anterior field designed to treat the low jugular nodes.

Patients with one or two nodes that are less than 3 cm in diameter and located within the primary portals are treated with irradiation alone to the neck. Patients with more advanced neck disease are considered for neck dissection 4 to 6 weeks following irradiation. If it is necessary to perform bilateral neck dissections, they may be staged 3 to 4 weeks apart. The need to stage bilateral neck dissections may be less critical if modified or functional rather than standard radical neck dissections are planned.

Following treatment, patients are seen monthly for 1 year, every 2 months for the second year, every 3 months for the third year, every 4 to 6 months for the fourth and fifth years, and annually after 5 years. Chest roentgenograms are obtained every 6 to 12 months following treatment. If there is a question of a local recurrence on follow-up examination, a CT scan is obtained and direct laryngoscopy may be performed. It is unwise to perform deep biopsies of the larynx following irradiation unless a definite abnormality consistent with recurrent tumor is noted, because such biopsies may precipitate osteochondronecrosis that could result in laryngectomy. Occasionally, it may be very difficult to distinguish post-treatment changes from recurrent cancer, and if a patient has severe persistent edema and pain, laryngectomy may be necessary, even though the specimen may be negative for tumor on pathologic examination. This is particularly true after irradiation for a locally advanced lesion.

Results

The rates of disease control at the primary site with irradiation alone at the University of Florida are shown in Table 9–2. There is no difference in the local control rate as a function of site

A 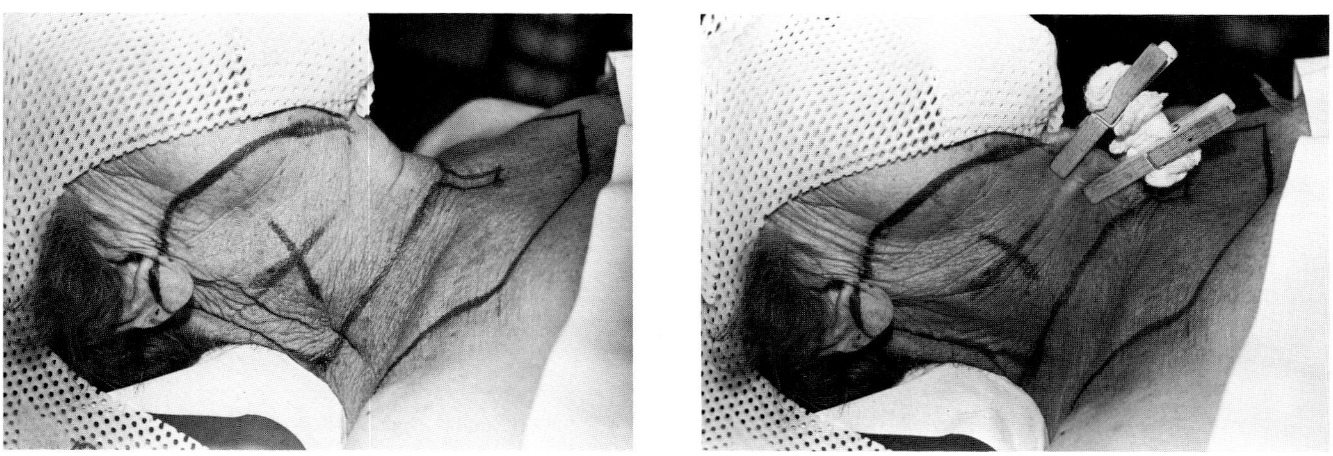 B

Figure 9–1. A: Patient in treatment position using a nonfilled low-temperature thermal plastic (polycaprolactone) face mask to immobilize the head. B: Clothespins are used to increase the amount of tissue spread anteriorly. (From Mendenhall et al.[35] Reprinted with permission.)

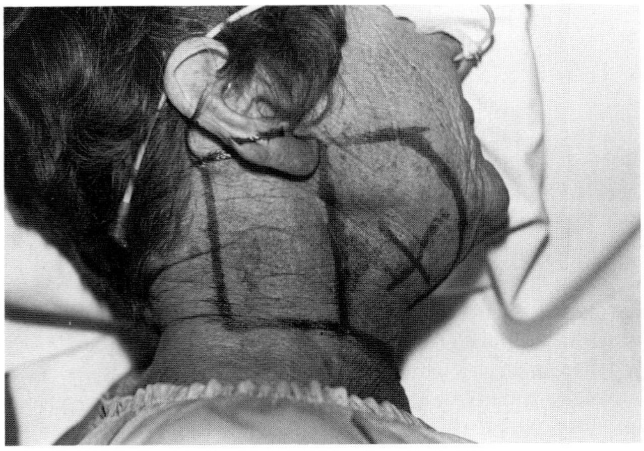

Figure 9–2. Posterior strip boost with electron beam after reducing the initial photon fields to avoid the spinal cord. The junction line is included for both the photon and electron portals. (From Mendenhall et al.[35] Reprinted with permission.)

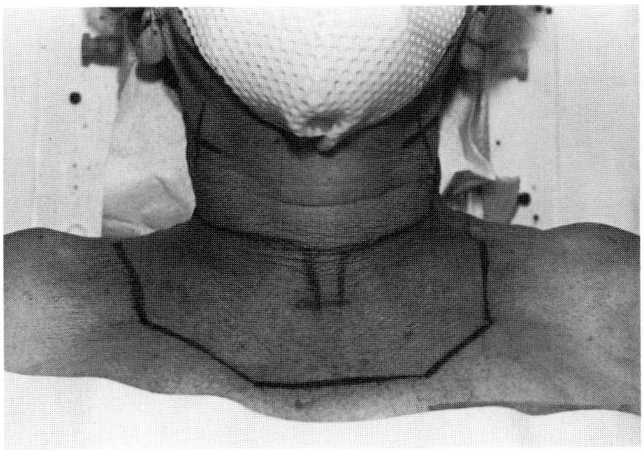

Figure 9–3. Low neck field with midline block. (From Mendenhall et al.[35] Reprinted with permission.)

within the supraglottic larynx. "Salvage" surgery, performed in 23 patients with local recurrence, was successful in 15 (65%).

Control above the clavicles refers to disease control at the primary site and in the neck. The rate of disease control above the clavicles as a function of AJCC stage is depicted in Table 9–3. Stage IV is stratified into IVA (T_{1-3}, N_{2-3A}) and IVB (T_4 and/or N_{3B}).[5]

The absolute and cause-specific (excluding intercurrent deaths) survival rates at 5 years are presented in Table 9–4.

Complications

During the course of irradiation, the patient experiences sore throat, loss of taste, and a variable degree of xerostomia, depending on how much of the parotid gland is irradiated. Approximately 10% of patients require a nasogastric feeding tube for nutritional support during treatment; it is very unusual to require an unplanned treatment interruption. If ^{60}Co is used, most patients develop dry desquamation of the skin within the treatment portals. Moist desquamation of the skin rarely occurs if care is taken to avoid tangential irradiation of the skin of the anterior neck. With advanced lesions, there is a small risk of

Table 9-1. Supraglottic Larynx Carcinoma: Dose Recommendations for Irradiation Alone to the Primary Lesion

STAGE	DOSE (cGy ONCE DAILY) *180 (cGy/Fraction)*	*200 (cGy/Fraction)*	DOSE (cGy TWICE DAILY; 120 cGy/FRACTION)
T1	6500	6000	No data
T2	7000	6400-7000	7440
T3	7000-7500	7000	7680
T4	7500	7000	7680

Table 9-2. Supraglottic Larynx: Local Control*† (129 Patients with 131 Lesions)

AJCC STAGE	LOCAL CONTROL AFTER RT‡	NO. SALVAGED/ NO. ATTEMPTED§	ULTIMATE LOCAL CONTROL
T1	13/13 (100%)	nd†	13/13 (100%)
T2	34/42 (81%)	3/7	37/42 (88%)
T3	25/41 (61%)	9/13	34/41 (83%)
T4	3/9	3/3	6/9

*Adapted with permission from Mendenhall et al.[9]

†Continuous-course irradiation, once or twice a day fractionation. Excludes 26 patients dead less than 2 years from treatment with primary site continuously disease-free.

‡RT: radiation therapy; nd: no data.

§Surgical salvage implies continuous local control 12 months or more following salvage procedure.

Table 9-3. Supraglottic Larynx: Control Above the Clavicles*† (129 Patients)

AJCC STAGE	CONTROL WITH INITIAL TREATMENT	NO. SALVAGED/ NO. ATTEMPTED	ULTIMATE CONTROL
I	8/8	nd‡	8/8
II	18/23 (78%)	4/5	22/23 (96%)
III	20/34 (59%)	8/10	28/34 (82%)
IVA	8/14 (57%)	2/4	10/14 (71%)
IVB	13/30 (43%)	4/8	17/30 (57%)

*Adapted with permission from Mendenhall et al.[9]
†Continuous-course irradiation, once or twice a day fractionation. Two patients with synchronous primary lesions were staged according to the more advanced lesion. Excludes 20 patients dead less than 2 years from treatment who remained continuously disease-free above the clavicles.
‡nd: no data.

laryngeal edema leading to airway compromise that would necessitate temporary tracheostomy.

Late side effects of irradiation include xerostomia and an increased risk of dental caries. This may be successfully managed with the use of fluoride carriers and periodic dental evaluation. Xerostomia is usually minimal to moderate, because only the tail of the parotid and part of the submaxillary gland are irradiated. Osteoradionecrosis of the mandible is rare, because only the angle of the mandible is included in the treatment field. Late complications may include severe laryngeal edema, osteochondronecrosis, and a remote risk of radiation myelitis. The risk of inducing a second malignancy is neglible.[6–8] Severe late complications developed in 9% of 129 patients treated at the University of Florida.[9]

GLOTTIC LARYNX

Treatment Selection

The goal of treatment is cure with the best functional result and the least risk of serious complications. For the purpose of treatment planning, patients may be considered to be in either an early group, where there is a high rate of cure with voice preservation, or a moderately advanced group, where the cure rate is still good but larynx preservation is possible only in 60 to 70% of cases. The early group may be treated initially with irradiation or, in selected cases, by partial laryngectomy. The moderately advanced group may be treated with radiation, with laryngectomy reserved for failure, or by total laryngectomy with or without radiation therapy.

Table 9-4. Supraglottic Larynx: Survival at Five Years*† (84 Patients)

STAGE	ABSOLUTE SURVIVAL	CAUSE-SPECIFIC SURVIVAL
I	2/6	2/2
II	10/20 (50%)	10/12 (83%)
III	9/20 (45%)	9/13 (69%)
IVA	4/9	4/6
IVB	7/29 (24%)	7/22 (32%)

*Adapted with permission from Mendenhall et al.[9]
†Continuous-course irradiation, once or twice a day fractionation. One patient with synchronous primary lesions was staged according to the more advanced lesion.

CARCINOMA IN SITU

This lesion may sometimes be controlled by "stripping" the cord. It is, however, difficult to exclude the possibility of microinvasion on these specimens. Recurrence is frequent, and the cord may become thickened and the voice hoarse with repeated stripping. Consequently, we have come to recommend irradiation much earlier for carcinoma in situ, realizing that most such patients would eventually come to this treatment and that earlier use of irradiation means a better chance of preserving a good voice.*

EARLY VOCAL CORD CARCINOMA

Early vocal cord cancer is defined as the subset of lesions that can be cured with larynx preservation in a substantial number of cases. In most centers, irradiation is the initial treatment prescribed for T_1 and T_2 lesions. Whereas hemilaryngectomy or cordectomy produces a comparable cure rate in selected instances, surgery is most often reserved for treatment of irradiation failures. There is limited short-term information available pertaining to the efficacy of laser excision.[10] The major advantages of irradiation over hemilaryngectomy or cordectomy are improved voice quality and avoidance of a major operation.[11] Voice after hemilaryngectomy usually remains hoarse; we tell the patient that the voice will be "as hoarse as it is now or even worse." Voice is usually improved by successful radiation therapy, although, occasionally there is no improvement or, uncommonly, deterioration. Another advantage is that irradiation is less expensive than a major surgical procedure.[12,13]

*Editor's note: The view taken here of the clinical significance of carcinoma in situ stands in marked contrast to the position outlined by Dr. Robert Fechner in Chapter 1. Both represent valid positions at the extremes of the spectrum of opinion regarding this lesion of unpredictable biologic behavior. A majority of clinicians at the present time would manage carcinoma in situ by an initial stripping procedure with close follow-up and repeat biopsy if indicated. Definitive treatment with irradiation or surgery is employed usually for lesions that recur after initial stripping. There are also differing opinions with regard to the significance of "microinvasion" demonstrated in biopsy specimens.

Hemilaryngectomy finds its major use as a salvage operation in suitable cases after irradiation failure.** Even if the patient has a local recurrence after a salvage hemilaryngectomy, there is a third chance in the form of total laryngectomy, which may still be successful.[14]

Verrucous lesions are reputed to be unresponsive to irradiation and, in some instances, to have been converted into invasive, often anaplastic, metastasizing lesions after unsuccessful irradiation. Hemilaryngectomy is recommended for early verrucous carcinoma of the glottis, but radiation therapy is recommended if the alternative is total laryngectomy. We have observed typical verrucous lesions that have disappeared with radiation therapy and not recurred. Burns and coworkers[15] have reported a similar experience. The patient must be advised of the risks when radiation therapy is used for verrucous carcinoma. Hemilaryngectomy is also used in patients who have had prior head and neck irradiation that prohibits further irradiation.

Fixed cord lesions (T_3) may be subdivided into relatively favorable and unfavorable lesions, the latter usually consisting of extensive bilateral disease associated with compromise of the airway. Lesions considered favorable for radiation therapy are confined mostly to one side of the larynx and are found in patients with satisfactory airway who are relatively easy to examine and may be relied on to appear for follow-up examinations. Some degree of supraglottic extension is nearly always present but does not, by itself, predict success or failure. Subglottic extension is frequently present. Subglottic extension of 1 cm or less did not affect the local control rate with twice a day irradiation; extension of more than 1 to 2 cm reduced chances of local control, but two patients were successfully treated with radiation therapy alone. Women have a better chance of cure overall and should be seriously considered for conservative treatment. The patient with a favorable lesion is advised of the alternatives of radiation therapy with surgical salvage or immediate total laryngectomy. The current local control rate at the University of Florida with voice preservation for 21 patients managed with twice a day radiation therapy is 67%, and 50% of local failures are salvaged.[16] The patient is advised that there may be a 5 to 10% reduction in the 5-year survival rate compared with the results of immediate total laryngectomy. The patient must be willing to return for follow-up every month for the first 2 years. He must understand that total laryngectomy may be recommended purely on clinical grounds because recurrent tumor is often deeply situated within the larynx and may be difficult to prove by biopsy, and that the risk of laryngeal osteochondronecrosis is about 5%.

The major difficulty in the use of irradiation for the more advanced lesions is in distinguishing between radiation edema and local recurrence during follow-up examinations. Progressive laryngeal edema, persistent throat pain, and fixation of a previously mobile vocal cord are frequently associated with recurrent neoplasm in the larynx, although an occasional patient with these findings will remain disease-free with long-term follow-up.

"Near total" laryngectomy has been used by a few surgeons in the treatment of fairly extensive but well-lateralized fixed-cord lesions.[17] A permanent tracheostomy is required because of the extent of mucosal resection of the larynx, but a useful voice may be retained.

Treatment Technique

Patients with T_1-T_2 vocal cord cancers are treated with limited fields covering the primary lesion; the neck is not electively irradiated. The patient is treated in the lateral decubitus position using stacked lead blocks to collimate the beam. At the University of Florida, ^{60}Co is used to treat essentially all patients with early vocal cord cancer; occasionally, a very obese patient is managed with high-energy x-rays.[18] The physician draws the portal lines on the patient each day, using anatomic landmarks to determine the field borders. A typical treatment field used to irradiate a T_1N_0 lesion involving the anterior two thirds of the true vocal cord is shown in Figure 9–4. The field borders may be modified according to the precise location of the tumor. If, for example, the tumor extended minimally onto the false vocal cord, the top of the field would be raised to the top of the thyroid notch. Patients are treated at 225 cGy per fraction; one fraction per day, 5 days a week, using continuous-course irradiation. The final tumor dose is as follows: T_{IS} or very early T_1 cancer, 5625 cGy in 25 fractions; T_1 and early T_2 cancer, 6300 cGy in 28 fractions; and late T_2 cancer, 6525 cGy in 29 fractions. At the University of Florida, most T_2 lesions are currently treated with twice a day irradiation ("hyperfractionation"), 120 cGy per fraction, to 7440 cGy total dose.

Patients with T_3 and early T_4 lesions are treated with parallel opposed fields covering the primary lesion and upper neck (Fig. 9–5). The field size is reduced once or twice during the course of treatment, and en face portal with a small midline tracheal block is used to irradiate the low neck. At the University of Florida, patients are treated with twice a day irradiation, 120 cGy per fraction, to a total dose of 7440 to 7680 cGy. For patients treated with once a day fractionation, the total dose is 7000 cGy at 200 cGy per fraction. If the reduced field is small, it may be possible to increase the dose per fraction to 225 cGy after the initial 4600 cGy has been delivered.

The follow-up policy for patients with true vocal cord cancer is the same as that previously outlined for patients with cancer of the supraglottic larynx.

Results

T_{IS}

Thirteen patients with carcinoma in situ of the glottic larynx have been treated with definitive irradiation at the University of Florida. One patient died of intercurrent disease within 2 years of treatment and is not evaluable for local control. Of the remaining 12 patients, local control with irradiation was ob-

**Editor's note: A perusal of the section on "Surgical Management of Early Laryngeal Cancer" in this book will reveal to the reader the wide variations in opinion and practice with regard to this statement. The chapter by Henry Shaw indicates that in Great Britain conservation surgery is employed almost exclusively for management of radiation failures, and only rarely as initial treatment. The same is true in many areas of Europe and Canada, as well as centers in the United States, such as the University of Florida. Nevertheless, at many United States institutions, there is a strong trend toward primary surgical treatment of selected "early" laryngeal cancers, as well as reluctance to employ such procedures for management of irradiation failures.

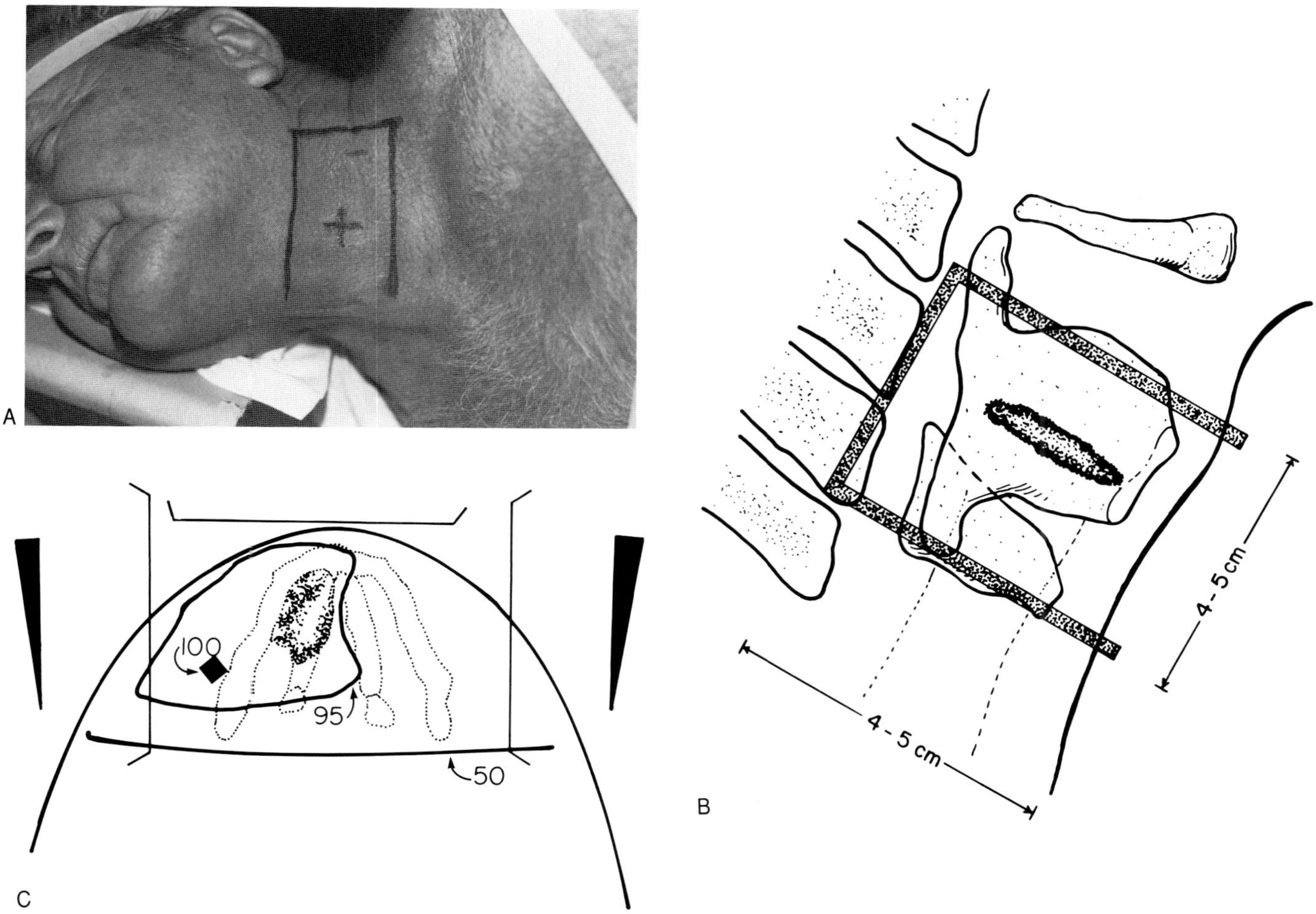

Figure 9–4. Patient with a T_1N_0 squamous cell carcinoma confined to the anterior two thirds of the vocal cord. **A:** Patient in the lateral "chicken-wing" position for treatment. **B:** Schematic diagram of the field, which extends from the middle of the thyroid notch to the bottom of the cricoid cartilage, 1 cm posterior to the cartilages and with 1 cm fall-off anteriorly. **C:** Computer-generated dosimetry; the dose is specified at the 95% isodose line. (A from Mendenhall et al.[18] Reprinted with permission. B and C from Million and Cassisi.[36] Reprinted with permission.)

tained in 11 of 12 (92%), with follow-up ranging from 2 to 16 years.[19] The patient who had a local recurrence was salvaged with a total laryngectomy and is alive and well 11.5 years following irradiation (7.5 years since salvage surgery).

T_1–T_2

Radiation therapy was used to treat 304 patients with invasive, previously untreated, T_1 and T_2 squamous cell carcinomas of the glottic larynx between 1964 and 1984 at the University of Florida.[20] All patients had been observed for at least 2 years, and 82% had a minimum 5-year follow-up. T_1 lesions were stratified into two groups based on whether the tumor involved one (T_{1A}) or both (T_{1B}) vocal cords. T_2 lesions were stratified based on vocal cord mobility: normal (T_{2A}) and impaired (T_{2B}). Lesions were also stratified according to the surgical procedure that would have been required to resect the lesion had the patient been treated initially by an operation (Table 9–5).[21,22]

The rates of local control after irradiation and ultimate local control, including patients successfully salvaged after local recurrence, are depicted in Table 9–6. Involvement of the anterior commissure did not adversely affect the likelihood of local control. Four patients who had not been suitable for hemilaryngectomy before radiotherapy later had a hemilaryngectomy for a local recurrence, and the surgical procedure was successful in two of four cases. The overall incidence of voice preservation, which includes as successes those patients salvaged from a local recurrence by hemilaryngectomy, is shown in Table 9–7. Voice preservation was achieved in 68 of 85 (80%) patients whose lesions would have required total laryngectomy had they been initially treated by operation.

The rate of freedom from neck node recurrence for patients with T_1–T_2 N_0 lesions treated with irradiation to the primary site only is shown in Table 9–8.[23] When the primary lesion was controlled, the rate of recurrent disease in the neck was 0% for T_1 lesions and 3% for T_2 lesions. When tumor recurred at the primary site, however, the rate of neck recurrence increased to 20% for T_1 tumors and 22% for T_2 lesions. Four of eight patients

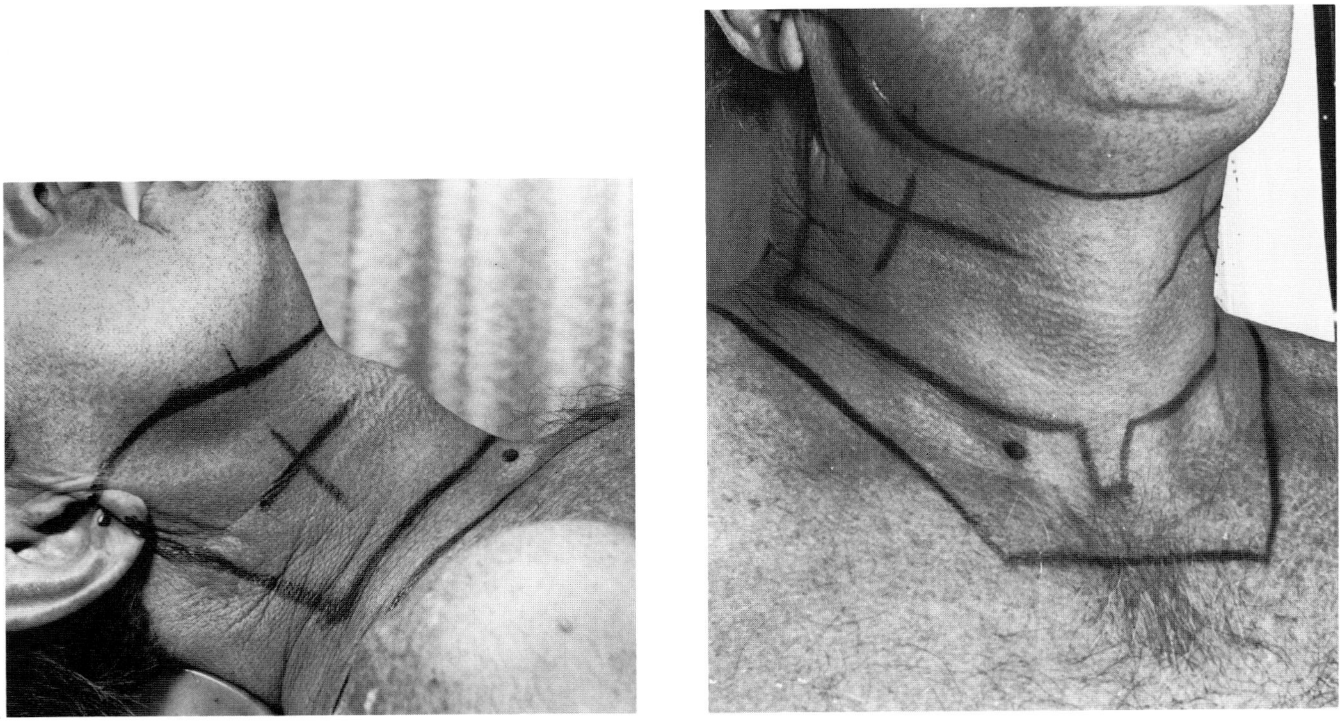

A B

Figure 9–5. Parallel opposed fields and anterior low neck field with tracheal block. A: Lateral view. B: Anterior view. (From Mendenhall et al.[24] Reprinted with permission.)

Table 9-5. T_1-T_2 Carcinoma of the Glottic Larynx: Definition of Subgroups

SUITABLE FOR	ANATOMIC EXTENT OF DISEASE
Cordectomy[21]	Lesion involving up to one entire true vocal cord, including the anterior commissure; mobility normal
Hemilaryngectomy[22]	Lesion involving up to one entire vocal cord and up to one third of the contralateral true cord. The lesion may extend into the subglottic space up to 1 cm anteriorly and 5 mm posteriorly. There may be minimal involvement at the vocal process and/or arytenoid. There may be reduced cord mobility
Total laryngectomy	More extensive disease than that stated above

Table 9-6. T_1-T_2 Carcinoma of the Glottic Larynx: Local Control—279 Patients* (No. Controlled/No. Treated)

STAGE	SUBGROUP†	SIZE	EXCLUDED‡	LOCAL CONTROL	NO. SALVAGED§/ NO. ATTEMPTED *Hemi-laryngectomy*	*Total Laryngectomy*	ULTIMATE LOCAL CONTROL
T_{1a}	C	<5 mm	1	12/12 (100%)	nd†	nd	12/12 (100%)
		5-15 mm	8	73/78 (94%)	3/4	0/1	76/78 (97%)
		>15 mm	2	45/50 (90%)	nd	4/5	49/50 (98%)
T_{1b}	HL	All	0	14/15 (93%)	nd	0/1	14/15 (93%)
	TL	All	2	15/16 (94%)	0/1	nd	15/16 (94%)
T_{2a}	HL	All	5	23/27 (85%)	nd	4/4	27/27 (100%)
	TL	All	2	27/38 (71%)	2/3	7/8	36/38 (95%)
T_{2b}	HL	All	3	13/18 (72%)	1/2	2/3	16/18 (89%)
	TL	All	2	18/25 (72%)	nd	4/6	22/25 (88%)

*Adapted with permission from Mendenhall et al.[20]
†C: suitable for cordectomy; HL: suitable for hemilaryngectomy; TL: suitable for total laryngectomy; n.d., no data.
‡Died within 2 years of treatment with the primary site continuously disease-free.
§Continuously disease-free at the primary site for 12 months or longer after salvage surgery.

Table 9–7. T_1-T_2 Carcinoma of the Glottic Larynx: Voice Preservation—304 Patients* (No. Patients with Voice Preservation/No. Treated)

STAGE	SUBGROUP†	SIZE	PROPORTION WITH VOICE PRESERVATION
T_{1a}	C	<5 mm	13/13 (100%)
		5-15 mm	83/86 (97%)
		>15 mm	47/52 (90%)
T_{1b}	HL	All	14/15 (93%)
	TL	All	17/18 (94%)
T_{2a}	HL	All	28/32 (88%)
	TL	All	31/40 (78%)
T_{2b}	HL	All	17/21 (81%)
	TL	All	20/27 (74%)

*Adapted with permission from Mendenhall et al.[20]
†C: suitable for cordectomy; HL: suitable for hemilaryngectomy; TL: suitable for total laryngectomy.

who developed recurrent disease in the neck were successfully salvaged by further treatments. Absolute and cause-specific survival rates are shown in Table 9–9.

T_3

Between 1965 and 1981, 68 patients with T_3 squamous cell carcinoma of the glottic larynx were treated with curative intent at the University of Florida by irradiation alone (22) or surgery with or without adjuvant irradiation (46). Of those patients treated surgically, seven received preoperative irradiation and 14 received postoperative radiation therapy. All patients were observed for at least 2 years, and 79% had a minimum 5-year follow-up. The rates of local control, control above the clavicles, and survival for the two treatment groups are listed in Table 9–10. There is no difference in the rates of ultimate local control, ultimate control above the clavicles, or survival between the two groups. Overall, 14 of 22 (64%) patients treated with irradiation alone retained a functional larynx compared with 1 of 46 (2%) patients treated with surgery with or without adjuvant irradiation.[24] The lesions treated by surgery were generally more advanced than those managed by radiation therapy.

Parsons et al[16] reported on 21 patients with T_3 squamous cell carcinomas of the true vocal cord treated between 1978 and 1986 with irradiation, using a twice a day fractionation schedule to total doses of 7440 to 7680 cGy. The rate of local control following irradiation was 67%; taking into account salvage surgery, there was only one failure above the clavicles among the 21 patients. Three died of distant metastasis. Five-year absolute and cause-specific survival rates were 59% and 81%, respectively.

A review of the literature as it pertains to T_3 glottic cancer that has been managed with irradiation alone is summarized in Table 9–11.[25–30]

Complications

During the course of irradiation, patients treated for T_1–T_2 glottic cancer will experience transient deterioration of voice, dry desquamation of skin within the treatment fields, and mild to moderate sore throat. Patients treated for T_3–T_4 lesions experience more pronounced sore throat, minimal xerostomia, and have a small chance of laryngeal edema necessitating a temporary tracheostomy.

The likelihood of long-term complications for patients with T_1–T_2 lesions is low (Table 9–12). Five of 304 patients (1.6%) developed moderate or severe treatment complications. The incidence was lower for T_1 lesions (1 of 184 or 0.5%) than for T_2 cancers (4 of 120, or 3%). Two patients developed complications that responded to conservative management: osteochondronecrosis in one patient and fat necrosis in the other. Three patients developed severe laryngeal edema requiring tracheostomy. One of these patients was thought to have local recurrence and underwent total laryngectomy with no tumor found in the specimen. Of the other two patients, the tracheostomy was temporary in one and permanent in the other.

Patients with T_3–T_4 carcinomas of the glottic larynx treated with irradiation alone experience acute effects secondary to treatment that are similar to those observed in patients irradiated for carcinoma of the supraglottic layrnx. Late complications include laryngeal edema that may necessitate tracheostomy and osteochondronecrosis that may result in laryngectomy. There is a remote risk of radiation myelitis. Parsons et al[16] reported two severe complications in a series of 21 patients with T_3 lesions treated with twice a day irradiation to total doses of 7440 to 7680 cGy. One patient with a T_3 N_{2B} tumor treated to 7680 cGy developed a cervical esophageal stricture necessitating esophageal dilations at 12, 16, and 24 months after treatment. The last dilation caused a perforation that closed spontaneously. The

Table 9–8. T_1-T_2 Carcinoma of the Glottic Larynx: Control of Disease in the Neck*† (No. Controlled/No. Patients Treated)

STAGE	PRIMARY SITE CONTINUOUSLY DISEASE-FREE	INITIAL CONTROL OF NECK DISEASE	NO. SALVAGED/ NO. ATTEMPTS	ULTIMATE CONTROL OF NECK DISEASE
T_1	Yes	160/160 (100%)	no data	160/160 (100%)
	No	8/10 (80%)	0/1	8/10 (80%)
T_2	Yes	73/75 (97%)	0/2	73/75 (97%)
	No	18/23 (78%)	4/5	22/23 (96%)

*Modified with permission from Mendenhall et al.[23]
†University of Florida data; patients treated October 1964 to December 1984; analysis, December 1987.

Table 9-9. T_1–T_2 Carcinoma of the Glottic Larynx: Five-Year Survival*†

STAGE	SUBGROUP‡	ABSOLUTE SURVIVAL	CAUSE-SPECIFIC SURVIVAL
$T_{1a}N_0$	C	107/122 (88%)	107/110 (97%)
$T_{1b}N_0$	HL	12/13 (92%)	12/12 (100%)
	TL	11/16 (69%)	11/12 (92%)
$T_{2a}N_0$	HL	16/23 (70%)	16/18 (89%)
	TL	27/34 (79%)	27/28 (96%)
$T_{2b}N_0$	HL	11/16 (69%)	11/13 (85%)
	TL	18/22 (82%)	18/20 (90%)

*Adapted with permission from Mendenhall et al.[20]
†Excludes three patients with synchronous primary head and neck cancers and one patient with clinically positive neck nodes at presentation.
‡C: suitable for cordectomy; HL: suitable for hemilaryngectomy; TL: suitable for total laryngectomy.

Table 9-10. T_3 Carcinoma of the Glottic Larynx: Results of Treatment*

PARAMETER	IRRADIATION ALONE	SURGERY ± ADJUVANT IRRADIATION
Local control after initial treatment	11/18 (61%)	31/37 (84%)
Ultimate local control	15/18 (83%)	33/37 (89%)
Control above clavicles after initial treatment	11/19 (58%)	31/39 (79%)
Ultimate control above the clavicles	15/19 (79%)	34/39 (87%)
Five-year absolute survival	8/15 (53%)	19/38 (50%)
Five-year cause-specific survival	8/12 (67%)	19/28 (68%)

*Adapted with permission from Mendenhall et al.[24]

Table 9-11. T_3 Carcinoma of the Glottic Larynx Treated with Irradiation Alone*

REFERENCE	INSTITUTION	NO. PATIENTS	MINIMUM FOLLOW-UP (YR)	LOCAL CONTROL (%)	ULTIMATE CONTROL AFTER SALVAGE SURGERY (%)
Harwood et al,[25] 1980	Princess Margaret Hospital	112	3	51	77
Wang,[26] 1987	Massachusetts General	70	4	36	57
Fletcher et al,[27] 1969	M. D. Anderson Hospital	17	2	77	No data
Skolyszewski and Reinfuss,[28] 1981	15 European centers	91	3	50	No data
Stewart et al,[29] 1975	Manchester, England	67	10	57	67
Mills,[30] 1979	Capetown, S.A.	18	2	44	78
Mendenhall et al,[24] 1984	University of Florida	13†	2	54	77
Parsons et al,[16] 1989	University of Florida	21‡	2	67	83

*Adapted with permission from Parsons et al.[16]
†Continuous-course, once a day treatment.
‡Continuous-course, twice a day treatment.

patient was alive and disease-free at 57 months, subsisting on a blenderized diet.

One patient, clinically free of disease after receiving 7680 cGy for a T_3 N_0 lesion, underwent direct examination of his larynx 6 weeks following irradiation, at which time multiple deep biopsies were obtained. This resulted in chondronecrosis and severe laryngeal edema that led to a laryngectomy 5 months later. The pathologic specimen was negative for tumor, and the patient was alive and disease-free at 84 months.

PYRIFORM SINUS

Treatment Selection

Lesions that are best suited for irradiation are T_1 and exophytic, low-volume T_2 cancers that do not involve the apex of the pyriform sinus and are associated with an adequate airway.[31] Although some of these lesions may be suitable for partial

Table 9–12. T_1-T_2 Carcinoma of the Glottic Larynx: Incidence of Moderate to Severe Complications: 304 Patients* (No. with Complications/No. Treated)

STAGE	SUBGROUP†	NO. PATIENTS	NO. WITH COMPLICATIONS
T_{1a}	C	151	1
T_{1b}	HL	15	0
	TL	18	0
T_{2a}	HL	32	0
	TL	40	2
T_{2b}	HL	21	1
	TL	27	1
Total	All	304	5 (<2%)

*Adapted with permission from Mendenhall et al.[20]
†C: suitable for cordectomy; HL: suitable for hemilaryngectomy; TL: suitable for total laryngectomy.

laryngopharyngectomy, combined resection of supraglottic larynx and pharyngeal wall often results in significant persistent aspiration of food and saliva. Irradiation may also be used for larger T_2 and early T_3 lesions that would otherwise require total laryngectomy. Poor pulmonary function is not a contraindication to irradiation as it is for conservation surgery, because chronic aspiration following irradiation is unlikely. Radical radiation therapy may be tried with limited success for patients with unfavorable T_2, T_3, or T_4 lesions who are medically inoperable or refuse surgery.

Treatment Technique

Patients are treated with continuous-course irradiation, one or two fractions per day, to the total doses outlined in Table 9–13.[32,33] The patient is treated in the supine position with parallel opposed fields, taking care to spare the skin of the anterior neck, if possible (Fig. 9–6). The fields are reduced once or twice during the course of treatment to minimize the volume of tissue treated to the final tumor dose. The low neck is irradiated through an en face field (Fig. 9–7). A neck dissection is added on an individualized basis following irradiation for nodes 3 cm or larger in diameter and in patients with multiple clinically positive neck nodes.[34]

Results

Between 1964 and 1984, 54 patients with previously untreated squamous cell carcinoma of the pyriform sinus were treated with irradiation with or without a neck dissection at the University of Florida.[32] All patients were observed for at least 2 years; 85% had at least 5 years of follow-up.

The rates of local control as a function of T stage are depicted in Table 9–14. Local control is excellent for T_1–T_2 lesions and falls off substantially for T_3–T_4 cancers. Seven patients underwent an attempt at surgical salvage for local recurrence; this was successful in four of the seven.

Control of local-regional (combined primary and neck) disease is shown in Table 9–15. A 75% rate of local-regional control was achieved for stage IV_A lesions (relatively early primary cancers associated with N_{2-3A} neck disease) following initial treatment. Five-year absolute and cause-specific (excluding intercurrent deaths) survival rates are listed in Table 9–16.

Complications

Acute side effects and complications secondary to treatment are similar to those described for patients with supraglottic laryngeal carcinomas. Late complications may include laryngeal edema necessitating tracheostomy, osteochondronecrosis, inability to swallow, and a remote risk of radiation myelitis. Six of 54 patients (11%) treated with irradiation developed a severe late complication.[32] Two patients developed laryngeal chondronecrosis, necessitating a total laryngectomy in one patient and permanent tracheostomy in the other. One patient developed severe laryngeal edema that required permanent tracheostomy. Another patient developed severe laryngeal edema; he subsequently underwent direct laryngoscopy and biopsy at another institution with equivocal findings, followed by total

Table 9–13. Pyriform Sinus Carcinoma Dose Guidelines*

STAGE	ONCE A DAY FRACTIONATION† (180 cGy/FRACTION)	TWICE A DAY FRACTIONATION† (120 cGy/FRACTION)
T_1	6000-6500 cGy	No data
T_2	6500-6800 cGy	7440-7680 cGy
T_3	7000 cGy	7680 cGy
T_4	7000 cGy	7680 cGy

*Adapted with permission from Mendenhall et al.[32]
†Continuous-course irradiation.

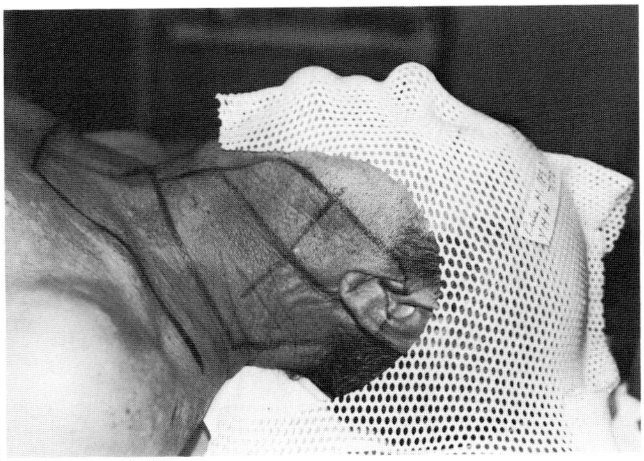

A

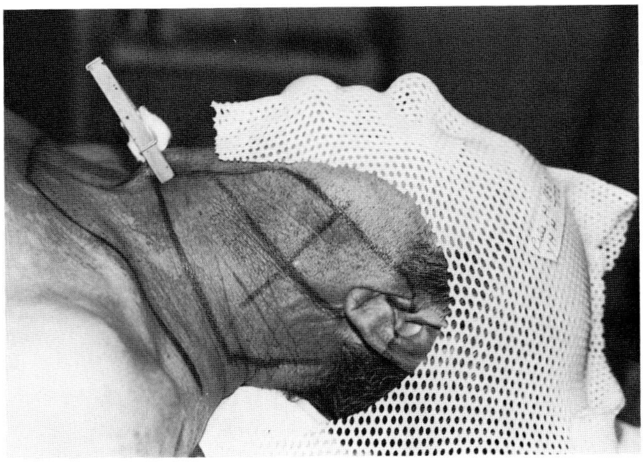

B

Figure 9–6. A: Primary treatment fields. B: With clothespin to increase amount of subcutaneous tissue spared anteriorly. (From Mendenhall et al.[32] Reprinted with permission.)

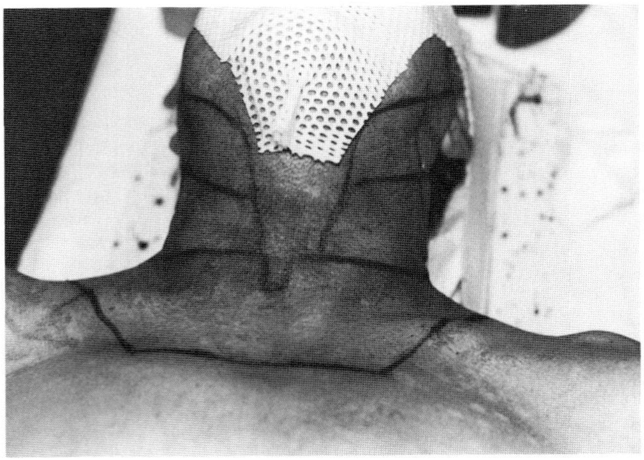

Figure 9–7. En face low neck field with midline tracheal block. (From Mendenhall et al.[32] Reprinted with permission.)

laryngectomy or partial pharyngectomy. The surgical specimen was negative for tumor. Other complications encountered were laryngeal edema requiring temporary tracheostomy, dysphagia necessitating temporary gastrostomy or parenteral hyperalimentation, and bilateral cranial nerve XII palsies. Neither patient who experienced severe postirradiation dysphagia had evidence of a stricture. It is possible that destruction of the pharyngeal constrictor muscles by tumor and subsequent scarring following irradiation may account for the dysphagia.

CONCLUSIONS

Radiation therapy constitutes an effective form of therapy for initial management of most early (T_1–T_2) carcinomas of the larynx and pyriform sinus. It may also be the preferred treatment for more advanced lesions in selected instances, as well as for patients who refuse or present unacceptable risks for surgery.

Table 9-14. Pyriform Sinus Carcinoma: Local Control* (No. Controlled/No. Treated)

STAGE	EXCLUDED†	LOCAL CONTROL WITH RADICAL RT‡	NO. SALVAGED/ NO. ATTEMPTS	ULTIMATE CONTROL
T_1	2	8/9	0/0	8/9
T_2	10	15/20	3/4	18/20
T_3	2	2/5	1/2	3/5
T_4	2	0/4	0/1	0/4

*Modified with permission from Mendenhall et al.[32]
†Died within 2 years of treatment with the primary site continuously disease-free.
‡RT: radiation therapy.

Table 9–15. Pyriform Sinus Carcinoma: Control Above the Clavicles* (No. Controlled/No. Treated)

MODIFIED AJCC STAGE	EXCLUDED†	CONTROL WITH INITIAL TREATMENT	NO. SALVAGED/ NO. ATTEMPTS	ULTIMATE CONTROL
I	0	1/1	0/0	1/1
II	1	5/6	1/1	6/6
III	3	5/10	1/2	6/10
IVA	6	12/16	1/2	13/16
IVB	2	1/9	0/2	1/9

*Adapted with permission from Mendenhall et al.[32]
†Died within 2 years of treatment with the primary site and neck continuously disease-free.

Table 9–16. Pyriform Sinus Carcinoma: Five-Year Survival* (No. Alive/No. Treated)

MODIFIED AJCC STAGE	ABSOLUTE SURVIVAL	CAUSE-SPECIFIC SURVIVAL
I	1/1	1/1
II	3/5	3/3
III	5/13	5/8
IVA	7/17	7/12
IVB	2/10	2/8

*Adapted with permission from Mendenhall et al.[32]

Radiation produces comparable cure rates to those achieved by surgical treatment of early laryngeal carcinoma, and treatment failures may often be salvaged by conservation surgery. The functional results of radiation therapy, particularly with regard to voice and deglutition, are superior to those achieved with conservation surgery. Radiation therapy produces minimal complications when employed for treatment of early laryngeal cancer; more severe complications occur after treatment of advanced lesions. Recognition or biopsy proof of recurrent tumor after failed radiation therapy may be difficult and biopsy may produce osteochondronecrosis. Postirradiation laryngectomy may be indicated on the basis of clinical findings.

REFERENCES

1. American Joint Committee on Cancer. *Manual for Staging of Cancer,* ed. 2. Philadelphia: JB Lippincott, 1983:37–42.
2. Weems DH, Mendenhall WM, Parsons JT, et al. Squamous cell carcinoma of the supraglottic larynx treated with surgery and/or radiation therapy. Int J Radiat Oncol Biol Phys 1987;13:1483–7.
3. Million RR, Cassisi NJ, Parsons JT, Mendenhall WM. Radiation therapy in the management of carcinoma of the larynx. In Fried MP, ed. *The Larynx: a multidisciplinary approach.* Boston: Little, Brown, 1988:557–89.
4. Robbins KT, Davidson W, Peters LJ, Goepfert H. Conservation surgery for T_2 and T_3 carcinomas of the supraglottic larynx. Arch Otolaryngol Head Neck Surg 1988;114:421–6.
5. Mendenhall WM, Parsons JT, Million RR, et al. A favorable subset of AJCC stage IV squamous cell carcinoma of the head and neck. Int J Radiat Oncol Biol Phys 1984;10:1841–3.
6. Kogelnick HD, Fletcher GH, Jesse RH. Clinical course of patients with squamous cell carcinoma of the upper respiratory and digestive tracts with no evidence of disease 5 years after initial treatment. Radiology 1975;115:423–27.
7. Seydel HG. The risk of tumor induction in man following medical irradiation for malignant neoplasm. Cancer 1975;35:1641–5.
8. Parker RG, Enstrom JE. Second primary cancers of the head and neck following treatment of initial primary head and neck cancers. Int J Radiat Oncol Biol Phys 1988;14:561–4.
9. Mendenhall WM, Parsons JT, Stringer SP, et al. Carcinoma of the supraglottic larynx: a basis for comparing the results of radiotherapy and surgery. Head Neck 1990;12:204–9.
10. Haraf DJ, Weichselbaum RR. Treatment selection in T_1 and T_2 vocal cord carcinoma. Oncology 1988;2(10):41–7.
11. Urken ML, Biller HF. Management of early vocal cord carcinoma. Oncology 1988;2(4):48–59.
12. Mittal B, Rao DV, Marks JE, Ogura JH. Comparative cost analysis of hemilaryngectomy and irradiation for early glottic carcinoma. Int J Radiat Oncol Biol Phy 1983;9:407–8.
13. Million RR, Sigal MC. Cost of management of head and neck cancer. In: Million RR, Cassisi NJ, eds. *Management of head and neck cancer: a multidisciplinary approach.* Philadelphia: JB Lippincott, 1984: 647–9.
14. Biller, HF, Barnhill FR Jr, Ogura JH, Perez CA. Hemilaryngectomy following radiation failure for carcinoma of the vocal cords. Laryngoscope 1970;80:249–53.
15. Burns HP, van Nostrand AWP, Bryce DP. Verrucous carcinoma of the larynx. Management by radiotherapy and surgery. Ann Otol Rhinol Laryngol 1976;85:538–43.
16. Parsons JT, Mendenhall WM, Mancuso AA, Cassisi NJ, Stringer SP, Million RR. Twice-a-day radiotherapy for T_3 squamous cell carcinoma of the glottic larynx. Head Neck 1989;11:123–8.
17. Pearson BW. Woods RD, Hartman DE. Extended hemilaryngectomy for T_3 glottic carcinoma with preservation of speech and swallowing. Laryngoscope 1980;90:1950–61.
18. Mendenhall WM, Parsons JT, Million RR, Fletcher GH. T_1–T_2 squamous cell carcinoma of the glottic larynx treated with radiation therapy: relationship of dose-fractionation factors to local control and complications. Int J Radiat Oncol Biol Phys 1988;15:1267–73.
19. Mendenhall WM, Parsons JT, Million RR, Cassisi NJ. The article reveiwed (commentary). Oncology 1988;2(4):59–61.
20. Mendenhall WM, Parsons JT, Stringer SP, Cassisi NJ, Million RR. T_1–T_2 vocal cord carcinoma. A basis for comparing the results of radiotherapy and surgery. Head Neck Surg 1988;10:373–7.
21. Neel HB, Devine KD, DeSanto LW. Laryngofissure and cordectomy for early cordal carcinoma: outcome in 182 patients. Otolaryngol Head Neck Surg 1980;88:79–84.
22. Biller HF, Ogura JH, Pratt LL. Hemilaryngectomy for T_2 glottic cancers. Arch Otolaryngol 1971;93:238–43.
23. Mendenhall WM, Parsons JT, Brant TA, et al. Is elective neck treatment indicated for T_2N_0 squamous cell carcinoma of the glottic larynx? Radiother Oncol 1989;14:199–202.
24. Mendenhall WM, Million RR, Sharkey DE, Cassisi NJ. Stage T_3 squamous cell carcinoma of the glottic larynx treated with surgery and/or radiation therapy. Int J Radiat Oncol Biol Phy 1984;10:357–63.
25. Harwood AR, Beale FA, Cummings BJ, Hawkins NV, Keane TJ,

Rider WD. T_3 glottic cancer: an analysis of dose time-volume factors. Int J Radiat Oncol Biol Phys 1980;6:675–80.
26. Wang CC. Radiation therapy of laryngeal tumors: curative radiation therapy. In Thawley SE, Panje WR, eds. *Comprehensive management of head and neck tumors*. Philadelphia: WB Saunders, 1987:906–19.
27. Fletcher GH, Lindberg RD, Jesse RH. Radiation therapy for cancer of the larynx and pyriform sinus. EENT Digest 1969;31:58–67.
28. Skolyszewski J, Reinfuss M. The results of radiotherapy of cancer of the larynx in six European countries. Radiobiol Radiother 1981;22:32–43.
29. Stewart JG, Brown JR, Palmer MK, Cooper A. The management of glottic carcinoma by primary irradiation with surgery in reserve. Laryngoscope 1975;85:1477–84.
30. Mills EED. Early glottic carcinomas: factors affecting radiation failure, results of treatment and sequelae. Int J Radiat Oncol Biol Phys 1979;5:811–7.
31. Mendenhall WM, Parsons JT, Devine JW, et al. Squamous cell carcinoma of the pyriform sinus treated with surgery and/or radiotherapy. Head Neck Surg 1987;10:88–92.
32. Mendenhall WM, Parsons JT, Cassisi NJ, Million RR. Squamous cell carcinoma of the pyriform sinus treated with radical radiation therapy. Radiother Oncol 1987;9:201–8.
33. Parsons JT, Mendenhall WM, Cassisi NJ, et al. Hyperfractionation for head and neck cancer. Int J Radiat Oncol Biol Phys 1988;14:649–58.
34. Mendenhall WM, Million RR, Cassisi NJ. Squamous cell carcinoma of the head and neck treated with radiation therapy: the role of neck dissection for clinically positive neck nodes. Int J Radiat Oncol Biol Phys 1986;12:733–40.
35. Mendenhall WM, Million RR, Cassisi NJ. Squamous cell carcinoma of the head and neck treated with radiation therapy: analysis of treatment parameters and results. Int J Radiat Oncol Biol Phys 1984;10:2223–30.
36. Million RR, Cassisi NJ. Larynx. In: Million RR, Cassisi NJ, eds. *Management of head and neck cancer: a multidisciplinary approach*. Philadelphia: JB Lippincott, 1984:340–1.

10

Definitive Radiation Therapy in the Management of Advanced Laryngeal Cancer

Bryan Eggert, Lawrence W. Davis

Most advanced laryngeal cancer is treated surgically, either alone or in combination with radiation therapy. Radiation therapy for the treatment of advanced disease is usually reserved for patients with surgically unresectable tumors, those who are not surgical candidates because of associated medical conditions, or those who refuse surgery. As a result, the number of patients treated with definitive radiation therapy and reported in the literature is much smaller than in surgical series. Results of treatment of extensive primary tumors of all sites in the head and neck or advanced nodal disease by radiation therapy are generally poor. Therefore alternative treatment programs are being investigated, primarily within National Cancer Institute supported clinical cooperative groups. Since the total number of patients diagnosed each year with advanced head and neck malignancies and entered into clinical studies is relatively small, meaningful progress in treatment must be derived from data on the treatment of advanced tumors from all head and neck sites. Consequently, the value of alternative methods of radiation therapy for the treatment of advanced laryngeal primaries must be judged on the basis of results of treatment from all head and neck sites.

CONVENTIONAL RADIATION THERAPY

Radiation therapy techniques and doses used vary among different authors and institutions. Fletcher[1] recommends 60 Gy in 6 weeks followed by an additional 10 to 15 Gy in 7 to 10 days using reduced fields; so-called "boost" techniques. Mendenhall et al[2] treat the initial field to 46 Gy using 2 Gy fractions daily and then, using reduced fields, delivers 22.5 to 24.75 Gy in 2.25 Gy fractions. Total doses range from 68.50 Gy in 33 fractions to 70.75 Gy in 34 fractions. At the Princess Margaret Hospital in Toronto, patients usually receive 50 to 55 Gy in 20 to 26 fractions.[3]

Reported results using definitive irradiation also vary (Table 10–1). Wang[4] reported a 5-year disease-free survival rate of 25% for patients with T_3 primary tumors. Similar results were reported by Lederman[5] who reviewed the treatment of T_3N_0 and T_4N_0 primaries and found a 26% 10-year survival rate. Other reports, however, show more favorable results. Harwood et al[6] reported results of treatment of 112 patients with $T_3N_0M_0$ glottic carcinoma with radical radiation. Five-year control was achieved by radiation alone. Of the 55 who had a recurrence, 48 had a partial or total laryngectomy. Sixty-five percent of these were cured by surgery, thus producing overall local control rate of 76% and 3-year survival rate of 68%.

Harwood et al[7] also reported the results of treatment of T_4 tumors. Thirty-nine patients were staged T_4N_0, and four had palpable neck disease. Local control was accomplished in 53% of patients with radiation alone. Three recurrent T_4N_0 tumors were salvaged with surgery, producing an overall 60% control rate.

Harwood et al demonstrated a significant dose response effect with almost a twofold improvement in local control when a nominal standard dose of greater than 1700 rets (equivalent to approximately 55 Gy in 24 fractions) was used. In their series, complications of radiation were exceedingly rare, occurring in only one instance of T_3 tumor and less than 1% of the T_4 tumors.

Similar findings were reported by Mendenhall et al[2] in their review of 68 patients treated at the University of Florida. Twenty-two were treated with definitive radiation. Four of six failures were successfully salvaged with surgery for overall control rate of 83%.

Karim et al[8] in Amsterdam reported results of treatment of 137 patients. Definitive radiation followed by salvage surgery resulted in a local disease-free rate of 85% at 3 years. Moderate to severe complications occurred in 14 of 38 patients following surgery. A significant dose-response effect was also noted by Karim et al. Over 50% of tumors recurred when doses were less

Table 10–1. Result of Radiation Therapy in Advanced Laryngeal Carcinoma

REFERENCE	STAGE	NO. PATIENTS	LOCAL CONTROL (%) *RT* only*	LOCAL CONTROL (%) *+Surgery +RT*	SURVIVAL (%)
Wang, 1974		70			57
Harwood et al,[6] 1980	T_3N_0	112	51	76	68
Mendenhall et al,[2] 1984	T_3	22	61	83	53
Karim et al,[8] 1987	T_3T_4	137	67	85	56
Harwood et al,[3] 1979	T_4	43	53	60	49

*RT: radiotherapy.

then 72 Gy. This led to the use of doses as high as 78 Gy in their series in an attempt to eradicate local disease.

In spite of some favorable results using planned definitive radiation therapy with surgery reserved for salvage, this treatment program has not had general acceptance in the United States. One argument against this approach is the often cited high morbidity incurred from a surgical procedure performed in a heavily irradiated area. In Karim et al's series, 14 of 38 patients developed moderate to severe complications following salvage surgery. Harwood et al,[3] however, reported an "acceptable" morbidity following surgery. One reason for the reduced morbidity reported by Harwood et al may be the loser dose used.

There is evidence that the acute effects and the late morbidity of radiation alone are not excessive. Careful attention to the fields and appropriate field reductions can further maximize the probability of local control and minimize late sequelae.[9] Preservation of voice following primary radiation has been favorable; approximately 50% of patients can be expected to retain a satisfactory voice.[6,7]

RADIATION THERAPY MODIFIERS

The efficacy of x-radiation is oxygen dependent. At a cellular level x-radiation generates free radicals that in the presence of oxygen can permanently bind to DNA.[10] As tumors increase in size, they outgrow their blood supply and become oxygen deficient. Zones of hypoxic cells develop that are thought to be radioresistant and responsible for a large proportion of local failures following radiation therapy.

Adjuvant radiosensitization is predicated on the ability of various agents selectively to enhance the effect of radiation on hypoxic cells without contributing to increased normal tissue toxicity (Tables 10–2, 10–3). As early as 1953, Gray et al[11] demonstrated that hyperbaric oxygen was an effective sensitizer to radiation in animal models. In 1964 Henk et al[12] initiated a controlled randomized trial testing the efficacy of adding hyperbaric oxygen to conventional radiation. Two hundred ninety-four patients with malignancies arising in various head and neck sites were accrued, including 34 with laryngeal carcinoma. Because of the difficulties associated with treating patients in a hyperbaric chamber, an unconventional fractionation scheme using fewer but larger fractions of radiation was utilized in the group receiving hyperbaric oxygen (35 Gy given in 10 fractions over 3 weeks). Overall recurrence-free rates at 5 years were superior in the group treated under hyperbaric oxygen. A trend toward improved local tumor control was noted in the patients with laryngeal carcinoma treated with hyperbaric oxygen; 64 versus 49%, but this was not statistically significant. In addition, the group treated with hyperbaric oxygen had a much higher incidence of laryngeal complications.

In an attempt to reduce local toxicity, Henk and Smith[13] undertook a second randomized trial. Once again, tumors arising from a variety of head and neck sites were treated, including a number with T_3 and T_4 laryngeal primary lesions. Compared to the first trial, a 10% dose reduction was used in those patients with carcinoma of the larynx who were randomized to treatment with hyperbaric oxygen. This dose reduction resulted in complications similar to the control group, which had been treated with radiation alone (60 Gy in 30 fractions). Two-year actuarial local recurrence-free rates were statistically superior among the hyperbaric group; 80 versus 39%. However, in spite of these improvements, the trial has been criticized because of the unconventional fractionation schedule used for the patients treated with hyperbaric oxygen. Henk and Smith did compare this fractionation schedule to the longer, conventional one and found no difference in local tumor control.

Table 10–2. Radiation Modifiers Based on Oxygen Effect

Hyperbaric oxygen breathing
Carbogen breathing
Nitroimidazoles
Metronidazole
Misonidazole
SR-2508
Other sensitizers
Perfluorochemical emulsions

Table 10–3. Clinical Trial Results: Radiation Modifiers

MODIFIER	LOCAL CONTROL (%) *Experimental Treatment*	LOCAL CONTROL (%) *Conventional Treatment*
Hyperbaric oxygen	64	49
Hyperbaric oxygen	80	39
Carbogen	51	51
Misonidazole	22	26

Treating patients with hyperbaric oxygen is a time-consuming procedure and strict precautions are necessary to prevent injuries to patients and staff.[13] To circumvent these problems, carbogen breathing during irradiation has been investigated. Carbogen is a mixture of 95% oxygen and 5% carbon dioxide and produces a higher circulating oxygen tension. It also induces systemic vasodilation with elevation of the blood pressure. Theoretically, these changes should result in increased oxygen delivery to hypoxic tumor cells. This approach was partially validated in animal models[14] but failed in later randomized clinical trials.

The Radiation Therapy Oncology Group (RTOG) conducted a study in which 254 patients with advanced primary tumors of the head and neck region were included (T_{3-4} N_{0-3}).[15] Patients were "randomized" to either conventional radiation alone or conventional radiation plus carbogen breathing. No improvement in local tumor control or survival was seen in the carbogen group, including the subgroup of patients with T_3 and T_4 carcinoma of the larynx.

The early hyperbaric oxygen trials produced evidence of improved local control in laryngeal carcinoma with the use of radiation modifiers. However, these improvements were not as pronounced with bulkier head and neck primary tumors. Henk et al[12] postulated that in large tumors the proportion of hypoxic cells is greater and the blood flow is inadequate, so that a residue of viable hypoxic tumor cells remains despite the increased oxygen tension in the blood. This led to investigation of hypoxic cell radiation sensitizers that could diffuse to central hypoxic areas without being metabolized by the intervening, more metabolically active tissues.

Metronidazole (Flagyl) was one of the earliest compounds tested.[16] Although displaying activity as a radiation sensitizer, its efficacy, in therapeutic doses, was limited by severe nausea and vomiting as well as neurotoxicity. Structural analogues of metronidazole followed, which were either less toxic or had greater sensitizing capacities. Misonidazole, a more potent sensitizer, has been studied in patients with advanced carcinoma of the head and neck region.

The RTOG conducted a pilot study (78-02) utilizing misonidazole as an adjuvant to radiation for patients with T_3 and T_4 carcinomas of the oral cavity, oropharynx, or hypopharynx.[17] Results were encouraging, for 67% of patients completing treatment had complete response. However, a Phase III trial failed to confirm these results.[18] The RTOG Phase III trial involved 306 patients, 73% of whom had T_3 and T_4 primaries. Patients were randomized to conventionally fractionated radiation with or without misonidazole. Analysis of multiple endpoints including primary tumor clearance and local-regional control at 2 years showed no benefit for the misonidazole-treated group.

Doses of misonidazole greater than those given in the Phase III trial produce both central and peripheral nervous system toxicity. Newer compounds such as SR-2508 and SR-2555 have been developed. They are equal to misonidazole in efficacy as hypoxic cell sensitizers but are less neurotoxic. The higher doses thus obtained may lead to better hypoxic cell sensitization.

The RTOG currently is conducting a randomized trial utilizing the hypoxic cell sensitizer SR-2508. Patients with T_3 or T_4 squamous cell carcinomas of the head and neck region receive either conventional radiation or conventional radiation plus SR-2508 given three times per week. This trial is in its early phase of patient accrual and no results are available.

NEUTRON THERAPY

Neutron therapy has been proposed as a possible alternative to conventional photon irradiation. Neutrons have two distinct biologic advantages. First, they are much more effective against hypoxic cells, since their efficacy does not depend on the presence of cellular oxygen. Second, unlike photons, which are much more useful against actively dividing rather than resting cells, neutrons are cell cycle independent. In the past, the main disadvantage of neutron therapy was poor tissue penetration of the beam, since initial units were modified physics machines based in laboratories. Current hospital-based units produce beams similar in penetration to photon beams from low energy accelerators (4 to 6 MV).

Stone[19] pioneered neutron irradiation for head and neck primary tumors in the late 1930s and early 1940s. At that time, only limited data existed on the radiobiologic properties of neutrons. He assumed, incorrectly, that equivalent doses of photons and neutrons would yield comparable clinical results. Neutrons, however, have a much greater "relative biological effectiveness." Thus, doses equivalent to those employed in photon therapy cause much greater biologic damage. As a result, many patients, treated in the early years of neutron therapy, were severely overdosed.

For the next two decades, clinical interest in neutron therapy ceased. During the interim, however, a number of radiobiologic studies were performed on cell cultures and animals. In this manner various biologic properties as well as commensurate physical dose reductions were identified.

The potential clinical advantages of neutron therapy, as well as recognition of the pitfalls in Stone's work, inspired new clinical investigations, primarily by Catterall and his/her group[20] at the Hammersmith Hospital in London. In 1977, these investigators reported the results of a prospective randomized trial in patients with advanced head and neck malignancies. A total of 107 patients were included with T_3 and T_4 primary tumors. The patients were randomized to receive treatment with either 15.60 Gy of neutrons given in 12 fractions over 4 weeks or 45.40 to 68.40 Gy of photons given in 4 to 6 weeks. After 2 years, there was a 55% recurrence rate in the photon-treated patients versus 1% with neutrons. However, the neutron-treated patients had a greater number of complications, particularly in the larynx and oropharynx. Despite these favorable results, the Hammersmith trial has been criticized because the photon group was treated at several different institutions, with varying doses, and without strict control of treatment technique. In addition, the average dose of photons was lower than the biologic equivalent of that used for the neutron group.

In 1977, Duncan and coworkers[21] began a randomized trial in Edinburgh. A total of 168 patients were recruited, all of whom had advanced tumors of the oral cavity, oropharynx, larynx, and hypopharynx. In contrast to the Hammersmith study, there were no differences in local control (Table 10–4). Moreover, at 2 years, the local disease-free survival was significantly better in the photon group. These differences persisted when patients

Table 10-4. Medical Research Council Neutron Studies

	HAMMERSMITH (%)		EDINBURGH (%)	
	Neutrons	*Photons*	*Neutrons*	*Photons*
Complete regression	77	43	70.6	77.5
Local control (2 yr)	76	19	29.4	41.3
Complications	14	3	24	13

were analyzed on a stage by stage basis. Notably, patients with carcinoma of the larynx had a significantly poorer survival than the photon-treated patients. Late radiation morbidity was approximately equal in both groups.

There were several differences in the conduct of the Hammersmith and Edinburgh trials. In Edinburgh, all patients were treated at the same facility with a fractionation schedule identical for both photon- and neutron-treated patients—20 fractions delivered over 4 weeks. At Hammersmith, the controls were treated at the referring hospital using their conventional technique. The neutron-treated patients received 12 fractions of neutrons delivered over 4 weeks.

The National Cancer Institute has supported the investigation of neutron therapy in the United States. Studies are conducted by the Neutron Therapy Collaborative Working Group (NTCWG), which has completed randomized trials studying neutrons as definitive therapy in patients with advanced head and neck cancer. The first study included 40 patients with advanced tumors.[22] Patients were randomized to receive either photons (66 to 74 Gy in 6 to 8 weeks) or neutrons using an equivalent dose and overall time but delivered in four fractions per week. The majority of the patients had T_3 and T_4 primary tumors of the oropharynx, oral cavity, hypopharynx, and supraglottic larynx. Overall the distribution was similar to the Edinburgh series; however, the results were quite different. The NTCWG found superior complete response and 2-year survival rates in the neutron group. This was achieved with similar complication rates to the photon group.

A second NTCWG trial (78-08) investigated the potential benefit of a "boost" using neutrons (Table 10–5).[23] All patients received an initial 45 to 50 Gy of large field photon irradiation. Patients were randomized to either a 25 to 30 Gy boost with photons or an equivalent boost with neutrons. It was believed that this combination would maximize the beneficial effects of neutrons on hypoxic cells while minimizing morbidity. Although efficacy of a neutron "boost" appeared theoretically plausible, the study of 115 patients failed to demonstrate any improvement in complete response or control of local disease at 2 years. The neutron group also had an increased incidence of severe late reactions.

In analyzing available data, it is difficult to determine if neutron therapy is superior to photon treatment. Some of the conflicting results probably lie in the wide range of neutron doses and fractionation schemes employed. Also of note is the wide variability in local control rates seen in the photon control arms. These ranged from 17% in the first NTCWG trial to 77.5% in the Edinburgh group. This may reflect treatment techniques or the result of differences in study populations. Subset analysis in those studies is difficult because of the small sample sizes.

Current NTCWG studies may answer these questions. The current neutron therapy units used in the United States trial are hospital-based machines with features similar to low energy linear accelerators. Therefore, treatment techniques are more comparable between the photon- and neutron-treated patients. Also, the favorable results of the Hammersmith trial suggest that a shortened fractionation schedule may contribute to improved results with neutrons. As a result, the NTCWG initiated a study to determine the maximum tolerated dose using 12 fractions given over 4 weeks. On the basis of the findings of that study, a Phase III randomized trial has been started comparing 20.4 Gy of neutrons given in 12 fractions over 4 weeks to 70 Gy of photons given in 35 fractions over 7 weeks. Patients are currently being accrued for this protocol and no results have yet been reported.

ALTERED FRACTIONATION SCHEDULES

Conventional fractions of 1.8 to 2.0 Gy and schedules of one daily treatment were developed empirically, and the maximum tolerated dose for normal structures with acceptable complication rates was determined on the basis of clinical experience. Although acceptable control rates are achieved for smaller tumors, the control rates obtained with conventional dose and treatment regimens for larger, more advanced tumors remain

Table 10-5. Neutron Therapy Collaborative Working Group Studies

	DEFINITIVE RADIATION (%)		"BOOST" (%)	
	Neutrons	*Photons*	*Neutrons*	*Photons*
Complete regression	52	17	60	64
Local control (2 yr)	25	0	20	31
Complications	18	33	16	7

Table 10-6. Altered Fractionation: Local-regional Control with Radiation Therapy

REFERENCE	NO. PATIENTS	FRACTION SIZE*	TOTAL DOSE (Gy)	LOCAL CONTROL (%)
Lee et al[24]	30	4 Gy/day	44-52	61
Percarpio and Fischer[25]	35	4 Gy/day	40-48	33†
Weissberg et al[26]	30	4 Gy/day	44	66†
Medini et al[29]	15	1.1 Gy/bid	75	53
Marcial et al[30]	187	1.2 Gy/bid	60	52
Million et al[31]	57	1.2 Gy/bid	74-81	
			T_3	81
			T_4	10/38‡
Gray[33]	48	1.8 Gy/tid	59.4	56
Knee et al[32]	53	1.8 Gy/day + 1.2-1.5 biw/tiw	70	65
Wang et al[34]	106	1.6 bid split	65	66
Wang et al[35]	321	1.6 bid	64	59

*bid twice daily; tid: three times daily; biw: twice weekly; tiw: three times weekly.
†Control of primary with or without control of neck.
‡Doses <74.4 Gy = 10%; >76 Gy = 38%.

unsatisfactory. Investigators have altered the standard programs in an attempt to improve tumor control rates (Table 10–6).

Lee et al[24] and Percarpio and Fischer[25] have reported encouraging results with a scheme using 4 Gy daily for 10 to 13 treatments. Both reported small numbers of patients with advanced malignancies of the head and neck region. Lee et al's series included both untreated and previously treated patients, nine of whom also received concomitant misonidazole, a hypoxic cell radiation sensitizer. The previously untreated patients had an initial local control rate of 61%, and there was no instance of severe, late radiation morbidity. Percarpio and Fischer also reported no later morbidity in their patients, but the results at 1 year of 33% disease-free survival versus 0% for a randomized, conventionally treated control group was not a statistical improvement.

A later randomized trial at Yale, however, failed to demonstrate any benefit for this treatment regimen.[26] Sixty-four patients, primarily with stage IV disease, were randomized to receive either 4 Gy per day for a total dose of 44 Gy in 2 to 3 weeks or 2 Gy per day for a total dose of 60 to 70 Gy in 6 to 7 weeks. The distribution of T and N stages, primary site, age, and sex were comparable. Although tumor regression was more rapid with the larger fractions, there was no difference in local-regional tumor control or in disease-free survival.

Radiobiologic concepts have become increasingly important in the design of other fractionation schedules. As a result, two related modes of therapy, hyperfractionation and accelerated fractionation, have emerged. The biologic basis of both have been described.[27,28]

Hyperfractionation utilizes smaller fraction sizes given more than once per day to total doses equal to or higher than conventional fractionation in the same overall time. Experimental data indicate that late responding, radiation dose limiting tissues tolerate higher total doses when the individual fraction sizes are reduced. It is postulated that tumors do not display this differential effect with fraction size so that the higher overall doses achieved will result in greater cell kill in the tumor and improved local control.

Medini et al[29] treated 15 patients with advanced squamous cell carcinoma of the head and neck region utilizing two daily fractions to a total dose of approximately 75 Gy. At the completion of therapy, 53% of the patients had total regression of their primary tumor and 60% (most with N_2 and N_3 adenopathy) had total regression of their neck disease. This was accomplished without any increase in local morbidity.

The RTOG conducted a Phase III trial comparing twice daily hyperfractionation of 1.2 Gy per fraction to a total dose of 60 Gy with conventional fractionation to a total dose of 66 to 73.8 Gy.[30] Analysis of multiple endpoints including initial tumor clearance, and 1- and 2-year tumor control failed to show any difference between the two groups. Based on more recent clinical experience, the RTOG study can be criticized because of the low total dose given with the hyperfractionation schedule. Despite this low total dose, however, control rates were comparable to the conventional fractionation schedule.

Million et al[31] demonstrated that while T_3 tumors were well controlled with hyperfractionated schedules with total doses of 74.4 Gy, only one of ten T_4 tumors responded to total doses of this size. Dose escalations as high as 76.8 to 81 Gy were necessary to produce improvements in local control rates for T_4 tumors. These high doses did not result in increased complications or any increase in morbidity following surgical salvage.

Another altered fractionation schedule currently under study is accelerated fractionation. Accelerated fractionation utilizes fraction sizes and total doses similar to conventionally fractionated regimens. As more than one fraction is delivered each day, the total dose of radiation is delivered in a shorter period of time. Acute reactions are typically more severe but late reactions are theoretically equivalent to conventional techniques. Since the radiation is delivered in a shorter period, there should be less tumor growth during treatment and an improved chance for local control. The technique has merit for rapidly growing tumors.

Knee et al[32] at the M.D. Anderson Hospital examined 53 patients with advanced head and neck primary tumors. Forty-one had rapidly growing, previously untreated tumors and the remainder had early, rapidly growing recurrences after surgery. Overall, there was a 65% 2-year local-regional control rate. Similar results have been obtained by others even when there was no selection for rapidly growing tumors. Gray[33] at Wellington Hospital advocated a scheme that delivered 1.8 Gy three times per day on a Monday-Wednesday-Friday basis. He accumulated 48 patients with locally advanced head and neck primary tumors. Fifty-six percent achieved complete resolution of tumor. Late sequelae were rare; however, acute complications, particularly mucositis, were common.

The resultant brisk mucositis is often the acute limiting factor in the delivery of accelerated fractionation. Wang et al[34,35] has circumvented this problem by introducing a planned 2-week break after the 12th treatment day. This permits mucosal healing. Irradiation is then continued on a twice daily basis to a total dose of 64 to 65 Gy. T_3 and T_4 supraglottic lesions as well as T_3 and T_4 tumors in other head and neck sites have shown a statistically significant improvement in local control compared with institutional historical controls. The 2-week break extends treatment time, but the overall duration of treatment is still more than a week shorter than the 1.8 Gy/day conventional regimen. Nonetheless, some argue that the treatment break can provide a "window" where tumor cells can repopulate. Certainly, studies utilizing conventional fractionation with and without treatment breaks have shown that such interruptions produce inferior results.[36]

Other techniques of accelerated fractionation include delivering daily treatments with conventional-sized fractions and then on predetermined days delivering a concomitant "boost" to a smaller field that encompasses the tumor and excludes as much normal mucosa as possible. This technique was utilized by Knee et al.[32] In this group, only three patients required treatment breaks for severe mucosal reactions, whereas local control rates were approximately the same.

The RTOG is studying altered fractionation schedules. Phase II studies have been conducted to determine the maximum tolerated hyperfractioned dose that can be delivered. If indicated, this schedule will subsequently be tested in a Phase III trial. A current protocol is evaluating an accelerated fractionation schedule for Phase III testing.

CONCLUSIONS

Definitive radiation therapy is an option for patients with advanced carcinoma of the larynx who by choice or for medical reasons cannot be operated on. A significant proportion of such patients may be cured and can retain a useful voice. Investigative programs are in progress that may improve the results of definitive radiation therapy; however, increased patient accession and subsequent analysis of current studies will be required to determine the benefit, if any, of these programs.

REFERENCES

1. Fletcher GH. *Textbook of radiotherapy,* 3rd ed. Philadelphia: Lea & Febiger, 1980:345.
2. Mendenhall WM, Million RR, Sharkey DE, Cassisi NJ. Stage T_3 squamous cell carcinoma of the glottic larynx treated with surgery and/or radiation therapy. Int J Radiat Oncol Biol Phys 1984;10:357–63.
3. Harwood AR, Hawkins NV, Beale FA, Rider WD, Bryce DP. Management of advanced glottic cancer: a 10 year review of the Toronto experience. Int J Radiat Oncol Biol Phys 1979;5:899–904.
4. Wang CC. Treatment of glottic carcinoma by megavoltage radiation therapy and results. AJR 1974;130:157–63.
5. Lederman M. Radiotherapy of cancer of the larynx. J Laryngol Otol 1970;84:867–96.
6. Harwood AR, Beale FA, Cummings BJ, et al. T_3 glottic cancer: an analysis of dose time-volume factors. Int. J Radiat Oncol Biol Phys 1980;6:675–80.
7. Harwood AR, Beale FA, Cummings BJ, et al. $T_4N_0M_0$ glottic cancer: an analysis of dose-time volume factors. Int. J Radiat Oncol Biol Phys 1981;7:1507–12.
8. Karim ABMF, Kralendonk JH, Njo KH, et al. Radiation therapy for advanced ($T_3T_4N_0$-N_3N_0) laryngeal carcinoma: the need for a change of strategy: a radiotherapeutic viewpoint. Int J Radiat Oncol Biol Phys 1987;13:1625–33.
9. Niederer J, Hawkins NV, Rider WD, Till JE. Failure analysis of radical radiation therapy of supraglottic laryngeal carcinoma. Int J Radiat Oncol Biol Phys 1977;2:621–9.
10. Hall EJ. *Radiobiology for the radiologist,* 3rd ed. Philadelphia: JB Lippincott, 1988:141.
11. Gray LH, Conger AD, Ebert M, et al. The concentration of oxygen dissolved in tissues at the time of irradiation as a factor in radiotherapy. Br J Radiol 1953;26:638–48.
12. Henk JM, Kunkler PB, Smith CW. Radiotherapy and hyperbaric oxygen in head and neck cancer: final report of the first clinical trial. Lancet 1977;2:101–3.
13. Henk JM, Smith CW. Radiotherapy and hyperbaric oxygen in head and neck cancer: interim report of second clinical trial. Lancet 1977;2:104–5.
14. Inch WR, McCredie GA, Kruuv J. Effect of breathing 5% carbon dioxide and 95% oxygen at atmospheric pressure on tumor radiocurability. Acta Radiol (Ther) 1966;4:17–25.
15. Rubin P, Hanley J, Keys HM, et al. Carbogen breathing during radiation therapy: the Radiation Therapy Oncology Group study. Int J Radiat Oncol Biol Phys 1979;5:1963–70.
16. Urtasun RC, Coleman CN, Wasserman TH, Phillips TL. Clinical trials with hypoxic cell sensitizers: time to retrench or time to push forward? Int J Radiat Oncol Biol Phys 1984;10:1691–6.
17. Fazekas JT, Goodman RL, McLean CJ. The value of adjuvant misonidazole in the definitive irradiation of advanced head and neck squamous cancer: an RTOG pilot study (#78-02). Int J Radiat Oncol Biol Phys 1981;7:1703–8.
18. Fazekas J, Pajak TF, Wasserman T, et al. Failure of misonidazole-sensitized radiotherapy to impact upon outcome among stage III-IV squamous cancers of the head and neck. Int J Radiat Oncol Biol Phys 1987;13:1155–66.
19. Stone RS. Clinical experience with fast neutron therapy. Am J Roentgenol Radium Ther 1948;59:771–85.
20. Catterall M, Bewley DK, Sutherland I. Second report on a randomized clinical trial of fast neutrons compared with X or gamma ray treatment of advanced cancers of the head and neck. Br Med J 1977;1:1642.
21. Duncan W, Orr JA, Arnott SJ, et al. Fast neuron therapy for squamous cell carcinoma in the head and neck region: results of a randomized trial. Int J Radiat Oncol Biol Phys 1987;13:171–8.
22. Griffin TW, Davis R, Henderickson FR, et al. Fast neutron radiation therapy for unresectable squamous cell carcinomas of the head and neck: the results of a randomized RTOG study. Int J Radiat Oncol Biol Phys 1984;10:2217–21.
23. Maor MH, Schoenfeld DA, Hendrickson FR, et al. Evaluation of a neutron boost in head and neck cancer: results of the randomized RTOG trial 78-08. Am J Clin Oncol 1986;9:61–6.
24. Lee DJ, Wharam MD, Kashima H, Order SE. Short course high fractional dose irradiation in advanced and recurrent head and neck cancer. Int J Radiat Oncol Biol Phys 1979;5:1829–32.
25. Percarpio B, Fischer JJ. Irradiation of advanced head and neck cancer with large daily fractions. Radiology 1976;121:489–90.
26. Weissberg JB, Son YH, Percarpio B, Fischer JJ. Randomized trial of conventional versus high fractional dose radiation therapy in the

treatment of advanced head and neck cancer. Int J Radiat Oncol Biol Phys 1982;8:179–85.

27. Withers RH. Biologic basis for altered fractionation schemes. Cancer 1985;55:2086–95.
28. Thames HD, Peters LJ, Withers HR, Fletcher GH. Accelerated fractionation vs hyperfractionation: rationales for several treatments per day. Int J Radiat Oncol Biol Phys 1983;9:127–38.
29. Medini E, Rao Y, Kim T, Jones TK, Levitt SH. Radiation therapy for advanced head and neck squamous-cell carcinoma using twice-a-day fractionation. Radiology 1980;134:531–2.
30. Marcial VA, Pajak TF, Chang C, et al. Hyperfractionated photon radiation therapy in the treatment of advanced squamous cell carcinoma of the oral cavity, pharynx, larynx, and sinuses, using radiation therapy as the only planned modality: (preliminary report) by the Radiation Therapy Oncology Group (RTOG). Int J Radiat Oncol Biol Phys 1987;13:41–7.
31. Million RR, Parsons JT, Cassisi NJ. Twice-a-day irradiation techniques for squamous cell carcinomas of the head and neck. Cancer 1985;55:2096–9.
32. Knee R, Fields RS, Peters LJ. Concomitant boost radiotherapy for advanced squamous cell carcinoma of the head and neck. Radiother Oncol 1985;4:1–7.
33. Gray AJ. Treatment of advanced head and neck cancer with accelerated fractionation. Int J Radiat Oncol Biol Phys 1986;12:9–17.
34. Wang CC, Blitzer PH, Suit HD. Twice-a-day radiation therapy for cancer of the head and neck. Cancer 1985;55:2100–4.
35. Wang CC, Suit HD, Blitzer PH. Twice-a-day radiation therapy for supraglottic carcinoma. Int J Radiat Oncol Biol Phys 1986;12:3–7.
36. Parsons JT, Bova FJ, Million RR. A reevaluation of split course technique for squamous cell carcinoma of the head and neck. Int J Radiat Oncol Biol Phys 1980;6:1645–52.

11

Postoperative Irradiation in the Management of Laryngeal Cancer

Bhadrasain Vikram

Even when all gross tumor has been removed surgically, many patients, particularly those with advanced laryngeal cancer, suffer relapse in the local-regional area. This is due to unrecognized, subclinical extensions of tumor beyond the area of resection. Careful analysis of the patterns of failure following seemingly adequate initial surgical treatment has indicated the need for additional treatment to prevent such relapses. In some cases this might be additional surgery, whereas in others the morbidity of further or more extensive surgery makes it undesirable or unacceptable. As discussed elsewhere in this book, radiation therapy alone has had some degree of success in the management of laryngeal cancer, particularly in the early stages. This demonstrated effectiveness, coupled with the recognition that subclinical deposits of cancer can be eradicated by relatively modest doses of irradiation, has led to the increasing application of postoperative radiation therapy in larynx cancer in recent years.

When postoperative radiation therapy is delivered by megavoltage equipment using careful technique, morbidity is relatively low.[1] The short-term side effects include pharyngeal mucositis and odynophagia. If a significant amount of salivary tissue has to be irradiated, however, xerostomia can be a long-term problem, with potentially devastating effects on dentition unless careful and conscientious dental hygiene is practiced and supplemented by topical fluoride applications. In order to determine whether a given patient should be subjected to this potential morbidity, the following should be considered:

1. How high is the risk of relapse without postoperative radiation therapy?
2. How effective is radiation therapy in decreasing this risk?
3. If no radiation therapy is given, and the patient relapses, what are the chances of salvage treatment being successful in the preservation of life or function or both?

In the discussion to follow we shall consider these issues in the context of tumor control in cervical lymph nodes as well as the primary site.

MANAGEMENT OF CERVICAL LYMPH NODES

Clinically Negative Neck Nodes

NEED FOR POSTOPERATIVE RADIATION THERAPY

It has been shown that occult metastatic disease in the cervical lymph nodes is present in a significant proportion of patients with supraglottic laryngeal carcinoma, even those who presented with T_1 or T_2 primary tumor and N_0 in the neck.[2–4] When the T_1 or T_2 primary tumor was treated by supraglottic or total laryngectomy, and no treatment was given to the cervical lymph nodes, 29% of the patients subsequently had a relapse with recurrence in the neck. For patients with T_3 and T_4 primary tumors and N_0 in the neck, as many as 49% of the patients had a relapse in the neck.[3]

Even when unilateral neck dissection was performed electively, the subsequent relapse rate in the neck was far from negligible; Levendag et al[2] found essentially no difference in the relapse rate between those patients who had a unilateral radical neck dissection electively and those who had no elective treatment to the neck. This was due partly to unrecognized contralateral metastases and partly to relapses within the ipsilateral dissected neck. Marks et al[4] noted that among those patients who had elective unilateral radical neck dissection, the contralateral neck accounted for 75% of relapses.

Because of the high incidence of bilaterality or contralaterality of cervical nodal metastases in supraglottic laryngeal carcinoma, elective bilateral neck dissections might be more accurate in identifying occult disease than unilateral radical neck dissections. No data regarding the accuracy of staging by this approach are as yet available in the literature.

The situation is different in the glottic larynx, where the incidence of cervical nodal metastases from T_1 and T_2 primary tumors is very low; therefore elective treatment to the cervical lymph nodes is rarely indicated. For patients with T_3 and T_4

glottic primary tumors, however, the situation is not too dissimilar to that described for supraglottic carcinomas, and similar considerations should apply.

EFFECTIVENESS OF POSTOPERATIVE RADIATION THERAPY

In striking contrast to the high relapse rate in the neck among patients with supraglottic laryngeal cancer who received no elective treatment to the neck are the low relapse rates among patients who received elective irradiation to both sides of the neck (Table 11–1).[5–7] Doses of the order of 5000 cGy in 5 weeks are required in order to sterilize occult disease in the N_0 neck. In many cases the primary site can be easily shielded from irradiation while still adequately irradiating the cervical lymph nodes.

It might be possible to all but eradicate mortality from early supraglottic laryngeal carcinoma by eliminating relapses in the N_0 neck with the application of elective bilateral irradiation.[5]

RECOMMENDATIONS

All patients with N_0 supraglottic larynx cancer should receive postoperative radiation therapy to both sides of the neck electively, unless bilateral neck dissections have been performed. In the latter case, if no metastases are found in the cervical lymph nodes, radiation therapy is not indicated. If metastatic lymph nodes are present, postoperative irradiation should be given, as described later. It must be pointed out, however, that in such cases it is generally more difficult to shield the primary site from irradiation and that the combination of partial laryngectomy, bilateral neck dissections, and postoperative radiation therapy can result in persistent edema of the remaining larynx.

Clinically Metastatic Neck Nodes

NEED FOR POSTOPERATIVE RADIATION THERAPY

Nearly one-half of the patients with metastases in the cervical lymph nodes, treated by radical neck dissection alone, subsequently develop recurrence in the dissected neck. The patients with metastases at multiple levels, or with extracapsular extension of tumor, were at especially high risk.[8,9] In addition, as discussed earlier, the incidence of relapse in the contralateral neck is significant in all stages of supraglottic laryngeal cancer and in the advanced stages of glottic laryngeal cancer.

EFFECTIVENESS OF POSTOPERATIVE RADIATION THERAPY

Recent data suggest that postoperative irradiation following radical neck dissection markedly decreases the incidence of relapse in the dissected neck (Table 11–2).[10–12] For maximum effectiveness, postoperative irradiation should be started within 6 weeks after surgery. A longer delay might be deleterious in terms of the probability of tumor control, and also necessitates a higher dose of irradiation with a greater likelihood of complications.[10]

RECOMMENDATIONS

Most, if not all, patients with metastatic cervical lymph nodes should receive postoperative radiation therapy to both sides of the neck to a dose of 5000 cGy in 5 weeks. If there has been a delay of more than 6 weeks prior to the start of irradiation, the dose should be increased to at least 6000 cGy in 6 weeks.[13]

MANAGEMENT OF THE PRIMARY SITE

T_1 or T_2 Primary Tumors

NEED FOR POSTOPERATIVE RADIATION THERAPY

If the primary tumor has been treated surgically with satisfactory resection margins, the likelihood of local recurrence is small. In such cases there is no need for postoperative radiation therapy. If the margins of resection are unsatisfactory, the likelihood of local recurrence is much greater and additional treatment is indicated. It is of interest, however, that Bauer et al[14] found relatively few local recurrences in patients with early stage vocal cord cancer who were treated by partial laryngectomy even when the margins of resection were unsatisfactory. In selected cases, therefore, observation might be a reasonable option if the patient is reliable for follow-up, is easy to examine; particularly if another voice-preserving operation, rather than total laryngectomy, might be possible in the event of local recurrence. In general, though, most surgeons regard unsatisfactory margins as an indication for additional treatment, either surgical or radiotherapeutic.[15]

When postoperative radiation therapy is given following partial or total laryngectomy for T_1 and T_2 carcinomas of the supraglottic or glottic larynx, the likelihood of local recurrence should be extremely low, but published data are sparse in early stage disease.

RECOMMENDATIONS

No radiation therapy is indicated when a T_1 or T_2 primary tumor has been treated surgically and the margins of resection are satisfactory. When margins are unsatisfactory, postoperative radiation therapy would generally appear to be indicated except in selected cases, as already discussed. The volume irradiated

Table 11–1. Relapse Rates in the Cervical Lymph Nodes After Elective Irradiation to the N_0 Neck in Early Stage Supraglottic Larynx Cancer

REFERENCE	RELAPSE RATE (%)
Harwood et al[5]	4
Ghossein and Batain[6]	6
Fletcher[7]	3

Table 11–2. Relapse Rates in the Cervical Region after Radical Neck Dissection and Elective Postoperative Irradiation in Advanced Larynx Cancer

REFERENCE	RELAPSE RATE (%)
Vikram et al[10]	13
Amdur et al[11]	6
Bartelink et al[12]	20

should include the residual larynx and adjacent pharynx to a dose of the order of 6000 cGy in 6 weeks. As pointed out earlier, this might leave the patient with persistent laryngeal edema. In my experience, however, this has never been sufficiently severe as to require total laryngectomy.

T3 or T4 Primary Tumors

NEED FOR POSTOPERATIVE RADIATION THERAPY

If the margins of resection are unsatisfactory, the likelihood of local recurrence is high and additional treatment is indicated. Even with satisfactory margins, however, the risk of local recurrence among patients with advanced primary tumors is far from negligible and postoperative radiation therapy is generally indicated.

EFFECTIVENESS OF POSTOPERATIVE RADIATION THERAPY

Several recent studies suggest that postoperative radiation therapy is highly effective in preventing local recurrence following partial or total laryngectomy (Table 11–3).[11,16,17]

RECOMMENDATIONS

Most, if not all, patients with T_3 or T_4 primary tumors should receive postoperative radiation therapy to the residual larynx, if any, and the adjacent pharynx. The dose required is 5000 cGy in 5 weeks if margins were satisfactory and 6000 cGy in 6 weeks if margins were unsatisfactory.

Postoperative Radiation Therapy After Salvage Laryngectomy

Patients who were treated initially by radiotherapy for laryngeal cancer, but have persistent or recurrent tumor in the larynx, are often treated by salvage laryngectomy. The likelihood of long-term tumor control after salvage laryngectomy depends on the extent of disease, subglottic extension, nodal metastases, and other factors.[18] Many surgeons, and even some radiation oncologists, assume that due to the prior irradiation postoperative radiation therapy has no place in the management of patients treated by salvage laryngectomy. In general, it is indeed true that re-irradiation carries a higher risk of radiation-related complications. In the case of salvage laryngectomy, however, if the clinical or pathologic findings are ominous, it might still be possible to deliver effective postoperative radiation therapy without a prohibitive risk of complications. The two structures of greatest concern in irradiation of the neck are the spinal cord and the larynx. The larynx is, of course, no longer present after salvage laryngectomy. In addition, the usual techniques for treating stage I and stage II glottic or supraglottic laryngeal cancer deliver minimal irradiation to the spinal cord. Because of these factors, it is often possible to deliver adequate doses of radiation to the peristomal (electrons are very useful in this regard) and the cervical nodal regions with low likelihood of complications. Careful beam shaping and precise dosimetry are of the utmost importance when delivering postoperative irradiation following salvage laryngectomy.

Table 11-3. Relapse Rates at the Primary Site after Resection and Elective Postoperative Irradiation in Advanced Laryngeal Cancer

AUTHOR	RELAPSE RATE (%)
Amdur et al[11]	7
Vikram et al[16]	10
HNCP[17]	3

TECHNICAL CONSIDERATIONS

Patients who require postoperative radiation therapy are most commonly treated by photon beams from cobalt-60 or low energy linear accelerator (4 to 6 MVP) photons. Electron beams are useful for selective boosting of certain areas. The most common technique involves treating the upper part of the neck through parallel opposing lateral portals (the beam is shaped by customized blocks to protect the oral cavity, brainstem, and so on), whereas the lower part of the neck is treated through a single anterior en face portal with shielding to protect the lungs. If the primary site is to be irradiated, it is generally included in the upper neck portals. If the primary site is to be shielded from radiation, however, it is included in the lower neck portal and a midline shield is employed to protect it.

Those patients whose primary tumor extends outside the larynx to involve the hypopharynx are at risk for occult metastatic disease in the retropharyngeal lymph nodes. In such patients the field of radiation is extended superiorly to the base of the skull in order electively to irradiate those lymph nodes. Similarly, those patients whose primary tumor involves the subglottic region are at risk for occult metastases in the pretracheal and paratracheal lymph nodes, and the field of irradiation must include these lymph nodes as well. Both the retropharyngeal and the paratracheal lymph nodes are also electively irradiated in those patients who present with extensive cervical nodal metastases, stages N_2 or N_3.

Stomal recurrence following total laryngectomy is common in patients with advanced laryngeal cancer. Adequate elective irradiation of the stomal and peristomal regions can virtually eliminate this as a cause of failure. It is important to recognize that the usual technique of postoperative radiation therapy as already described might underdose the stomal mucocutaneous suture line region, unless adequate buildup material ("bolus") is employed to circumvent the surface-sparing characteristic of megavoltage photon irradiation. A plastic laryngectomy tube admirably serves the purpose as buildup material and should always be used during such radiation therapy.

REFERENCES

1. Fletcher GH. Clinical dose response curves of human malignant epithelial tumors. Br J Radiol 1973;46:1–12.
2. Levendag P, Sessions R, Vikram B, et al. The problem of neck relapse in early supraglottic larynx cancer. Cancer 1989;63:345–8.
3. Shah JP, Tollefsen HR. Epidermoid carcinoma of the supraglottic larynx: the role of neck dissection in initial surgical treatment. Am J Surg 1974;128:170–5.

4. Marks JE, Freeman RB, Ogura JH. Carcinoma of the supraglottic larynx. AJR 1979;132:255–60.
5. Harwood AR, Beale FA, Cummings BJ, et al. Management of early supraglottic laryngeal carcinoma by irradiation with surgery in reserve. Arch Otolaryngol 1983;109:583–5.
6. Ghossein NA, Bataini P. The role of radiotherapy in the treatment of neck metastases from head and neck cancer. In: Wolf GT, ed. *Head and neck oncology,* Boston: Martinus Nijhoff, 1984:169–97.
7. Fletcher GH. The place of irradiation in the management of head and neck cancers. Semin Oncol 1977;4:375–80.
8. Strong EW. Preoperative radiation and neck dissection. Surg Clin North Am 1969;49:271–6.
9. Johnson JT, Myers EN, Bedetti CD, et al. Cervical lymph node metastases: incidence of extracapsular carcinoma. Arch Otolaryngol 1985;111:534–7.
10. Vikram B, Strong EW, Shah JP, Spiro R. Failure in the neck following multi-modality treatment for advanced head and neck cancer. Head Neck Surg 1984;6:724–9.
11. Amdur RJ, Parsons JT, Mendenhall WM, et al. Postoperative irradiation for squamous cell carcinoma of the head and neck: an analysis of treatment results and complications. Int J Radiat Oncol Biol Phys 1989;16:25–36.
12. Bartelink H, Breur K, Hart G, et al. The value of postoperative radiotherapy as an adjuvant to radical neck dissection. Cancer 1983;52:1008–13.
13. Vikram B, Strong EW, Shah JP, et al. Elective postoperative radiation therapy in stages III and IV epidermoid carcinoma of the head and neck. Am J Surg 1980;140:580–4.
14. Bauer WC, Lesinski SG, Ogura JH. The significance of positive margins in hemi-laryngectomy specimens. Laryngoscope 1975;85: 1–13.
15. Looser KG, Shah JP, Strong EW. The significance of positive margins in surgically resected epidermoid carcinoma. Head Neck Surg 1978;1:107–111.
16. Vikram B, Strong EW, Shah JP, Spiro R. Failure at the primary site following multimodality treatment in advanced head and neck cancer. Head Neck Surg 1984;6:720–3.
17. Head and Neck Contracts Program. Adjuvant chemotherapy treatment for advanced head and neck carcinomas: Final report of the Head and Neck Contracts Program. Cancer 1987;60:301–31.
18. Million RR, Cassissi NJ. *Management of head and neck cancer: a multidisciplinary approach*. Philadelphia: JB Lippincott, 1984:79–86.

12

Chemotherapy in the Management of Advanced Laryngeal Cancer

John F. Ensley, Fillippo de Braud, Julie A. Kish, Efstathios Tapazoglou, Muhyi Al-Sarraf

The larynx is the most common site of all squamous cell carcinomas (SCC) of the head and neck. These tumors are categorized at diagnosis on the basis of parameters that reflect their natural history, treatment outcome, and prognosis: size and location of the tumor, adjacent structures involved, and the degree of tumor metastases to regional lymph nodes. Tumors of the glottis tend to present as relatively small lesions and are less likely than other laryngeal tumors to metastasize to regional lymph nodes due to the lack of submucosal lymphatics underlying these structures.[1] Symptoms produced by involvement of the vocal cords and restriction of the airway often result in the detection of these lesions at an early stage. Tumors of the supraglottic larynx (false vocal cords, epiglottis, and aryepiglottic folds), on the other hand, frequently present with advanced disease consisting of large tumors and regional metastases that are often bilateral. Symptoms produced by these lesions occur late and reflect the advanced degree of the tumor growth.

Early (T_{1-2}) lesions of the larynx may be successfully treated in most patients with definitive radiation, conservation surgery, or radiation followed by salvage surgery. In most instances, these early lesions may be treated successfully without the loss of voice or problems with deglutition. Nevertheless, it is important to remember that even for early lesions of the glottis, failure rates in some large series have approached 25 to 40% following radiation and salvage surgery.[2] For T_3 and larger lesions of the larynx, total laryngectomies are nearly always required either for removal of tumor or prevention of problems associated with chronic aspiration. Failure rates for T_3 lesions of the glottis have been reported to approach 60 to 70% following radiation and salvage surgery.[2]

Patients with locally advanced stages III and IV disease, especially those with nodal involvement, usually have very poor prognosis. Resectable, locally advanced cancers are commonly treated with surgery and postoperative radiotherapy. For unresectable or inoperable lesions, the traditional therapy has been total radiation treatment that resulted in a very poor outcome.

The addition of systemic chemotherapy to conventional modalities currently employed for potentially curable laryngeal cancer has two major rationales.[3–5] If patients with early to moderately advanced lesions that are destined to fail conventional therapy could be identified pretherapeutically, clinical trials could be designed to test the benefit of adding chemotherapy to their treatment plans.[6,7] It is hoped that such strategies might result in the reduction of tumor recurrence rates and improved survival in this group of patients with laryngeal cancers. Previous studies that have been reported as prospective randomized trials[8–17] in advanced SCC of the head and neck (SCCHN) have been flawed by improper clinical and statistical design.[5,18] Adjuvant chemotherapy trials in patients with negative resection margins, such as the current Head and Neck Cancer Intergroup Study, which includes patients with laryngeal cancers, are sentinel studies in this regard.

A second and equally important application of systemic chemotherapy for the treatment of these diseases is in those groups of patients with laryngeal cancers in which cure may be achieved with conventional therapy, but with the resulting loss of natural speech or other serious functional deficits. Salvage laryngectomies become necessary in as many as 25% of patients with T_2 glottic carcinomas and are required in nearly all patients presenting with T_3 lesions.[19] Therapeutic strategies that include aggressive combination chemotherapy regimens have been designed for laryngeal preservation, and clinical trials that employ them, are currently being conducted at several institutions.[20–22]

Traditionally, patients with metastatic or recurrent SCCHN have been entered in Phase II chemotherapy trials. Patients with metastatic or recurrent laryngeal tumors usually comprise a minor component of Phase II clinical trials in patients with SCCHN.[23] More recently, such patients have been placed in trials that compare combination chemotherapy regimens,[24] but chemotherapy trials in this tumor as a single site have not been conducted until very recently. Previously untreated, advanced, unresectable tumors of the larynx and supraglottic structures are conventionally treated with radiotherapy alone, which usually results in treatment failure or tumor recurrence.[2,19] Results of aggressive chemotherapy with effective combinations have resulted in impressive overall and complete response (CR) rates in neoadjuvant trials of advanced, unresectable SCCHN.[25–28] These trials have also included patients with cancers of the larynx, but this site is usually a minor component of these studies. Regardless of the site, when CRs are accompanied by eradication of microscopic disease (50% of CR) in patients with advanced, unresectable SCCHN, long-term disease-free survival has resulted.[29–32] Currently, a number of combination chemotherapy regimens[26–29] and concurrent chemotherapy-radiation regimens[33] are employed as neoadjuvant therapy in such advanced tumors. Studies are currently ongoing to define the upper limits of efficacy of such regimens, with acceptable toxicity and patient tolerance.[5,10,34,35] At present, patients with advanced, unresectable stages III and IV laryngeal carcinomas should be subjects for such experimental studies because of the dismal outcome expected with conventional treatment.[2,25–28]

Before discussing the role of chemotherapy in patients with laryngeal cancers, it is important to mention the prognostic factors that will influence the outcome in these patients. In locally advanced and previously untreated cancers, the most important factors are the stage of the cancer, especially the nodal status, and the subsite of the primary cancer. Other factors may be of importance, including the performance status of the patients, type of chemotherapy, number of courses, as well as the incidence and type of response to chemotherapy.

In patients with recurrent or metastatic cancers, important prognostic factors include: performance status, location of the active disease (local-regional versus systemic), size of the tumor mass (minimal versus bulky), bone erosion, response, and type of response to chemotherapy.

It is important that chemotherapy be given in adequate doses and with proper frequency and intensity. As surgeons require the resection of all gross tumor with adequate and negative margins, and the radiotherapists require an adequate dose with the proper port, medical oncologists must administer chemotherapy of sufficient quantity and quality to meet standards of adequacy.

CHEMOTHERAPY FOR ADVANCED RESECTABLE LARYNGEAL CARCINOMA

The overall results of definitive treatments of surgery and radiotherapy in patients with resectable and locally advanced head and neck cancers have been poor. The 5-year overall survival for surgery with either preoperative or postoperative adjuvant radiotherapy in large and cooperative group series is about 30%. Cancers arise in the larynx in about one third of the patients in these reports. Usually the results in patients with laryngeal cancers are somewhat better compared with other sites, such as the oropharynx or oral cavity, even when corrected for stage. Patients with glottic carcinoma usually had better survival compared with those patients with supra- or subglottic regions. Many of the living patients may have recurrent disease, which is beyond hope of cure or long-term salvage.

Most of the patients died either of persistent disease or recurrence in local-regional sites despite negative margin at the time of surgical resection and the addition of postoperative adjuvant radiotherapy to eradicate microscopic disease. Fewer than 20% of the patients with recurrence develop systemic metastases, particularly in the lungs, bone, or liver. Patients who survive free of disease for 2 years face the risk of second primary cancers in the head and neck area, lung, or esophagus, which increases with the passage of time because of exposure to the same etiologic agents.

The development of effective and safe combination chemotherapy, which has been tested in patients with unresectable or inoperable locally advanced head and neck cancer (Tables 12–1, 12–2), has led to the investigation of the same chemotherapy in patients with resectable laryngeal cancers. Most of the induction or "proto-" (prior to surgery or radiation therapy) chemotherapy trials demonstrated the greatest activity employing combinations of cisplatin with other agents. In the absence of prospective and randomized clinical trials, the current consensus is that cisplatin and 5-fluorouracil (5-FU) 120 hour infusion given in three courses is the most active combination that has been

Table 12-1. Complete and Overall Response Rate to Cisplatin-Containing Regimen in Previously Untreated Locally Advanced Head and Neck Cancer: Wayne State University Experience*

		NO. PATIENTS		RESPONSE (%)			
AGENTS†	NO. OF SERIES	*Range*	*Total*	*CR Range*	*CR Total*	*Overall Range*	*Overall Total*
C	3	22-30	80	0-4	1	3.5-40	28
CB	9	16-291	557	0-24	8	37-81	51
CB (V or O)	8	14-85	396	0-32	16	58-93	74
CBM	21	10-107	798	0-48	19	46-89	68
CBM (V or O)	5	21-130	328	0-35	18	48-86	63
CF	16	16-108	666	4-54	29	38-100	75
Other	14	7-162	466	0-36	21	10-100	71

*Data extracted from Al-Sarraf[27,36] and Taylor.[37–39]
†C: cisplatin; B: bleomycin; V: vincristine; O = vincristine (Oncovin); M: methotrexate; F: 5-fluorouracil.
‡Thirty-two percent of the patients had improved disease with 25 to 49% response.

Table 12–2. Overall and Complete Response Rates to Induction Chemotherapy According to Site in Patients with Previously Untreated Head and Neck Cancer: Wayne State University Experience

SITE	NO. PATIENTS	CR (%)	OVERALL (%)
Tongue	45	42	89
Oral cavity	33	30	88
Larynx	23	39	83
Pyriform sinus	22	23	82
Tonsil	21	52	90
Pharynx	17	39	88
Unknown primary	3	0	33

investigated to date. The mean clinical CR in collective series was about 27%, with a range of 4 to 54% regardless of stage of disease or nodal involvement (Table 12–1).[27,36–39] More than 50% of patients with clinical CR to cisplatin and 5-FU infusion had no disease found after radical surgical resection or multiple biopsies.[32] In addition, many tumors that demonstrated partial response (PR) to this regimen were found histologically negative after surgery or repeated biopsies. The overall survival reported in nonrandomized trials of the combined modality therapy using induction chemotherapy with cisplatin and 5-FU infusion were statistically better than with other cisplatin combinations.[29] Patients who achieved clinical and, especially, histologic CR were found to have increased survival, compared with those with lesser response to chemotherapy, regardless of the type and sequence of the definitive therapy of surgery or radiation.[29] This has led to three major areas and goals of randomized clinical trials in resectable head and neck cancers in general and in patients with laryngeal cancers in particular.

Induction Chemotherapy

At least two major randomized trials were conducted and completed utilizing cisplatin combinations before surgery, followed by radiotherapy, in patients with resectable head and neck cancers. In the National Cancer Institute (NCI) Head and Neck Contract trial activated in 1978,[8] one course of cisplatin and bleomycin was given before definitive treatment and results were compared with the same standard therapy of surgery and postoperative irradiation. The overall response rate to one course of the combination of cisplatin and bleomycin was less than 50%, and the CR rate was less than 5%. The results of this randomized trial were negative for reasons that seem fairly obvious. The clinical CR rate of less than 5% and histologic CR a fraction of this number would not be expected to produce an impact on this disease, or the effect would be so small that thousands of patients on each arm would be required to produce a statistically detectable difference.[5] In addition, use of only a single course of chemotherapy, in what was most likely a less than maximally active combination, could account for the negative results. This study did confirm that patients with stage III disease had statistically significant better survival than patients with stage IV disease. The same was true for patients with cancer of the larynx as opposed to patients with oropharyngeal carcinomas, and patients with good performance status in contrast with those with poor performance status.

The second prospective randomized trial of induction chemotherapy was the Southwest Oncology Group (SWOG 8006) protocol.[40] In the investigational arm, cisplatin was combined with three other agents (bleomycin, vincristine, methotrexate) to be administered on an outpatient schedule every 3 to 4 weeks for three courses, before surgery, followed by radiotherapy. The control group was to have the same surgery and postoperative radiotherapy. The clinical CR rate to this regimen was greater than 20%. Despite the higher CR rate, no statistical differences were found between the two groups and the study was terminated early, after about 100 patients had been entered on each arm. Although no differences were found on early evaluation, patients entered in this study should be reevaluated at 4 or more years after treatment to see if any effect appears at that time.

Another major and probably the most important factor in analyzing the SWOG study, and the experiences from other pilot trials from single institutions or the cooperative group, is the issue of the timing and sequence of chemotherapy as part of the combined treatment approach. When chemotherapy is given first, about 35% of all patients treated, and about 50% of those who achieve clinical CR, will refuse surgery. This may affect the outcome of the clinical trial and may cause an imbalance in the randomized group. A second and possibly more important issue is the theoretical question of why should shrinking the disease that the surgeon is going to remove in any case change the overall outcome of these patients. In addition, the surgical resection may not be the same for patients with no clinical disease remaining after chemotherapy as for patients who had not been treated preoperatively. It is important to mention that the investigation of induction chemotherapy will continue for the purpose of obtaining a more effective and safer combination in patients with unresectable cancer, and for laryngeal and voice preservation in resectable cancer.

Chemotherapy After Surgery and Before Radiotherapy

Because of the problems inherent with induction chemotherapy in patients with resectable head and neck cancer, timing and sequence of chemotherapy as part of combined modality therapy were investigated.[41,42] Both radiotherapy and chemotherapy were found to increase in effectiveness in inverse proportion to the size of the tumor mass under treatment. This was particularly true against microscopic disease. Since most recurrences in resectable head and neck cancers occur at local and regional sites because of persistent microscopic disease, adjuvant therapies are being tested postoperatively. Three possible sequences of administration of chemotherapy after surgery can be considered; after postoperative radiotherapy, concurrent with postoperative radiotherapy, or following surgery and before radiation treatment. Information obtained in 1980 indicates that giving chemotherapy after radiotherapy is hampered by very poor patient compliance. A regimen of chemotherapy of three courses of cisplatin and 5-FU infusion after surgery and before radiotherapy was investigated at Wayne State University in patients with locally advanced but resectable head and neck cancers.[37] When the feasibility of such combined modality treatment was established, the same trial was activated on the cooperative group level to further confirm such feasibility and acceptance.[38,43] At the end of this pilot study, the Radiation Therapy Oncology Group (RTOG) activated a prospective randomized protocol. One arm consisted of standard treatment with surgery and postoperative radiotherapy; the other arm was surgery followed by chemotherapy followed by radiation treatment (RTOG 8322). All patients had resectable stages III and IV cancers of the head and neck, including those arising in the larynx. All had confirmed negative resection margins. Patients were then stratified by pathologic T and N stage, site, performance status, and institution. With the establishment of the Head and Neck Intergroup, this trial was adopted as the first national study for this group (#0034). This protocol had a successful accrual of patients and registration closed in July, 1989. No analysis has yet been performed at this early date.

Chemotherapy in Preservation of Voice and the Larynx

During the early investigation of feasibility and effectiveness of induction chemotherapy at Wayne State University, the discovery was made that response to cisplatin combination therapy predicted further response to radiotherapy; absence of response to chemotherapy (less than PR) was usually associated with similar lack of response to subsequent radiation treatment, and dismal outcome.[44] This important observation was confirmed by other investigators and led our group to offer those patients with resectable head and neck cancers, particularly those who refused surgery because of the need for total laryngectomy, chemotherapy prior to the start of radiation treatment. Responders underwent radiotherapy; nonresponders to induction chemotherapy were offered surgery again. The first ten patients with stage III and early stage IV cancers of the larynx were part of this group. Nine patients who had good response to the combination of cisplatin-based chemotherapy were subsequently treated with radiotherapy and were still alive at 5 years. One patient with T_3 glottic carcinoma did not respond to chemotherapy but continued to refuse surgery. This patient failed to respond to radiotherapy, had salvage laryngectomy and is alive at 5 years. In a pilot study by Jacobs et al[21] patients with advanced, resectable SCCHN, including laryngeal carcinomas, were treated with an initial three courses of 5FU and cisplatin and assessed by endoscopy and biopsy for response. Patients with negative biopsies were treated with definitive radiotherapy alone, whereas patients with positive biopsies underwent definitive resections followed by radiotherapy. Twelve of 30 patients achieved histologically CRs and were treated with radiation alone. The remainder underwent surgical resection and irradiation. Overall and relapse-free survival for the entire group at 2 years was 53% and 52%, respectively. For the 12 patients (40%) treated without surgery, the overall and relapse-free survival was 70 and 60%, respectively.

A retrospective review of the clinical outcome of 131 patients from Wayne State University with laryngeal carcinoma who were treated with and without combination chemotherapy and had minimal follow-up of 5 years was performed.[36] The results indicate that patients with equivalent degrees of disease (TNM categories) treated with aggressive combination chemotherapy initially have the same overall survival as patients treated with standard surgery and radiotherapy. Importantly, a significant number (36%) of the group treated with initial combination chemotherapy (all stage IV) have remained disease-free without laryngectomies (Table 12–3).

Recently, studies have been designed to achieve maximal preservation of larynges in advanced but resectable tumors of the larynx.[20–22] Such studies utilize all three modalities employed in the treatment of SCCHN: chemotherapy, radiotherapy, and salvage surgery. A pilot study at the Boston Veterans Medical Center addressed this same question in patients with advanced laryngeal carcinomas. Data presented during the 1988 meeting of the American Society of Clinical Oncology for 36 patients with advanced laryngeal or paralaryngeal carcinomas (primarily stages III and IV) demonstrated laryngeal preservation in 34 of 36 patients.[22] Nineteen of 34 patients achieved disease-free status, and 13 patients (36%) remain alive and disease-free with only 7 of 23 (30%) of the subsequent deaths due to local recurrence. Median survival for the whole group was 23 months.

Preliminary studies such as these indicate that approximately one third of patients who otherwise would require laryngectomy may benefit from clinical trials directed toward laryngeal pres-

Table 12–3. Results of Treatments in Patients with Locally Advanced Laryngeal Cancer with Minimal Follow-up of 5 Years: Wayne State University Experience

		STAGE III*				STAGE IV			
TREATMENT*		*No. Patients*	*NED*	*DWD*	*DNDR*	*No. Patients*	*NED*	*DWD*	*DNDR*
Surgery		18	5	5	8	7	1	2	4
Radiotherapy		12	1	4	7	8	—	8	—
S + RT		25	10	6	9	13	—	8	5
	Total	55	16	15	24	28	1	18	9
			29%	27%	44%		4%	64%	32%
CT + RT		6	3	2	1	12	2	8	2
CT + S + RT		14	5	3	6	16	2	10	4
	Total	20	8	5	7	28	4	18	6
			40%	25%	35%		14%	64%	21%

*NED: alive, no evidence of disease; DWD: dead with disease; DNDR: dead, not disease related; S: surgery; RT: radiotherapy; CT: chemotherapy.

ervation through the use of systemic chemotherapy. A national, randomized, prospective clinical trial within the Veterans Administration Hospitals in the United States, which addresses larynx preservation in patients with advanced, resectable, laryngeal cancers, has been initiated as a direct result of such preliminary pilot data. Patients with advanced but resectable stages III and IV carcinomas of the larynx are randomized to standard therapy (total laryngectomy and radiotherapy) or an experimental arm consisting of three courses of 5-FU and cisplatin initial therapy. Following chemotherapy, endoscopy and biopsy are performed to assess degree and completeness of response. Good responders, including those with CRs who have negative biopsies, are then treated with definitive radiation alone. Those with no response to the initial two courses of chemotherapy undergo total laryngectomy followed by radiation. This protocol accrued very well and was recently closed. The results of early analysis of this important prospective trial were presented recently, confirming the excellent response clinically and histologically to the combination of cisplatin and 5-FU infusion. Also, in about 61% of the patients, no laryngectomy was done. With median follow-up of about 17 months, the 2-year overall survival of the two groups was identical. It is too early to reach a final and more definite conclusion about this study, but it has led the way for further investigations in this area in the near future. Ultimately, long-term follow-up and analysis of patients entered into such studies may help define characteristics of subsets of patients with laryngeal carcinomas that are destined to fail conventional therapy, and other groups that may be candidates for laryngeal preservation strategies.

Table 12-4. Agents Used in Chemotherapy and Radiotherapy for Patients With Locally Advanced Head and Neck Cancer: Wayne State University Experience

I. Single
- A. Methotrexate
- B. Hydroxyurea
- C. Bleomycin
- D. 5-Fluorouracil (5-FU)
- E. Cisplatin
- F. Carboplatin

II. Combination
- A. Bleomycin, vincristine, and methotrexate
- B. Bleomycin and methotrexate
- C. Bleomycin, doxorubicin, and 5-FU
- D. Bleomycin and cyclophosphamide
- E. Bleomycin, cyclophosphamide, and vincristine
- F. 5-FU and mitomycin C
- G. 5-FU and cisplatin
- H. 5-FU (L) and cisplatin
- I. Cisplatin, vincristine, bleomycin
- J. Cisplatin and ifosfamide
- K. 5-FU and hydroxyurea
- L. 5-FU, methotrexate, mitomycin C

Unresectable Locally Advanced Laryngeal Cancer

The standard treatment for patients with locally unresectable or inoperable head and neck cancers, including those of laryngeal origin, has been definitive radiotherapy. Although generally good local disease control is often achieved with this modality, disease-free and overall survival tends to be poor. In most of the large or randomized series, fewer than 25% of patients are alive with or without disease at 2 years. These poor results have led to investigation of addition of chemotherapy to radiation treatment. Induction chemotherapy (discussed earlier) was usually given to patients with unresectable disease. Other investigations include the concurrent use of chemotherapy and radiotherapy (Table 12–4). The interest in trials using concurrent chemotherapy and radiotherapy began in the 1960s. At that time, three available agents demonstrated to have activity in head and neck tumors were methotrexate, 5-FU, hydroxyurea, and later bleomycin. Alone or in combination these agents were used with radiotherapy. These drugs were administered before or during radiation treatment. The overall response to the combination of chemotherapy and radiotherapy was higher than with radiation alone, but unfortunately the incidence of local side effects with these agents, especially oral and oropharynx mucositis, also increased. This led to a compliance problem, a delay in therapy, or refusal of treatment. In most of the studies, including the randomized trials, no differences in overall survival were reported.

With the introduction of cisplatin in the mid-1970s as an active agent against this disease, and since cisplatin was not known to produce stomatitis or mucositis, the combination of cisplatin concurrent with radiotherapy was investigated in the early 1980s in patients with unresectable cancers.[33] At least four dose schedules of cisplatin were used (Tables 12–5, 12–6).[37–39] At Wayne State University, a small pilot study employed cisplatin 100 mg/m^2 on the day of radiotherapy and every 3 to 4 weeks for three courses during radiation treatment. The tolerance and side effects of this combination were acceptable. In 1981, this led to the activation of a similar pilot trial in the RTOG (RTOG 8117) for patients with unresectable or inoperable head and neck cancers, including patients with carcinoma of the larynx. The acute and subacute toxicities were acceptable and reversible. The clinical CR rate was excellent (70%). Obtaining CR was the most important prognostic factor influencing overall survival of these patients. Good CR rate was obtained in both sexes and stages (III or IV), regardless of nodal involvement, morphologic differentiation, or site of primary cancer. The results of this important trial were updated recently, with minimal follow-up of 4 years on every patient, and compared to identical patients treated with radiotherapy alone in the RTOG. There were no differences with regard to the incidence of delayed local-regional side effects between patients who received concurrent chemotherapy and radiotherapy or those who had radiation treatment alone. The incidence of complete disease clearance, disease-free and overall survival was better in the chemotherapy and radiotherapy group. No statistical analyses were performed because this was not a prospective randomized trial and the comparison was made to an historical control.

A randomized trial comparing radiotherapy to chemotherapy and radiotherapy using cisplatin 20 mg/m^2 weekly was activated on the intercooperative group level for patients with unresectable head and neck cancers, including laryngeal carcinomas. No prospective stratification was performed in this trial. Patient entry to this protocol was completed and closed more than a year

Table 12-5. Response to Concurrent Cisplatin and Radiotherapy in Patients With Untreated Head and Neck Cancer: Wayne State University Experience*

REFERENCES	AGENT	DRUG SCHEDULE	NO. PATIENTS	RESPONSE (%)	
				CR†	*Overall*
Snyderman, 1986	Cisplatin	15 mg/m^2 D1-5	36	25	81
Slotman, 1986	Cisplatin	20 mg/m^2, D1-4	18	72	89
Zerillo, 1986	Cisplatin	20 mg/m^2/wk	16	75	100
McDonald, 1987	Cisplatin	10-20 mg/m^2 D1-5	38	18	82
Tobias, 1987	Cisplatin	10 mg/day	16	56	100
Chang, 1988	Cisplatin	20 mg/m^2 days 1-4	43	49	98
Wheeler, 1988	Cisplatin	40 mg/m^2 days 1-5	17	100	100
Eisenberger, 1988	Carboplatin	60-100 mg/m^2/wk	22	45	77

*Data extracted from Taylor.[37-39]
†CR: complete response.
‡Preoperative.

ago. Early analysis showed significant difference in overall response rate for the chemotherapy and radiotherapy arm, but no difference in overall survival between the two groups. It is important to note that until we have at least 2 years minimal follow-up on each patient, no final or definite conclusion can be reached about this trial or any study in unresectable head and neck cancers. Efforts to continue to improve on the effectiveness and safety of chemotherapy and radiotherapy are underway.

CONCURRENT CHEMOTHERAPY AND RADIOTHERAPY AFTER SURGERY OR CHEMOTHERAPY

Once the feasibility of concurrent chemotherapy and radiotherapy as the primary treatment of patients with unresectable and locally advanced head and neck cancer was established, this regimen was investigated postoperatively in resectable patients with stage IV cancers and positive surgical margins, and in unresectable patients who were nonresponders to induction chemotherapy.[45,46]

The feasibility of postoperative chemotherapy and radiotherapy using cisplatin 100 mg/m^2 for three courses was established on the institution level and is now being confirmed in the RTOG for the possibility of including such treatment in future protocols for treatment of resectable tumors.

Initially, concurrent chemotherapy and radiotherapy were investigated in patients with unresectable cancer who were nonresponders to induction chemotherapy, due to the poor results of radiation alone in these patients. CRs were achieved in 37% and the rest of the patients had PR after chemotherapy and radiotherapy. In patients with CR, the overall survival was improved. Because of such excellent results in these patients with an overall dismal outlook, chemotherapy and radiotherapy are being investigated in all patients, not on protocols, who refused surgery, or who had unresectable disease treated initially with induction chemotherapy.

RECURRENT AND METASTATIC LARYNGEAL CANCERS

Patients with recurrent or metastatic cancers of the larynx not amenable to surgery or radiotherapy are usually treated with systemic chemotherapy as part of a pilot study or a randomized trial for head and neck cancer patients.[26,27] Many active single agents and combination chemotherapy have been tested in these patients. Various prognostic factors were found to influence the response rate and type of response to this chemotherapy, in addition to influencing the duration of response and overall

Table 12-6. Complete Response Rate to Concurrent Cisplatin and Radiotherapy According to Site in Unresectable Patients With Previously Untreated Head and Neck Cancer: Wayne State University Experience

SITE	NO. PATIENTS	COMPLETE RESPONSE	
		No.	*%*
Oropharynx	51	37	73
Nasopharynx	28	26	93
Oral cavity	23	13	57
Hypopharynx	8	3	38
Larynx	8	7	88
Paranasal sinus	8	6	75

Table 12-7. Response to Chemotherapy According to Site in Patients With Recurrent Head and Neck Cancer: Wayne State University Experience

SITE	NO. PATIENTS	RESPONSE (%)
Pharynx	37	27
Tongue	32	28
Oral cavity	28	25
Larynx	25	16
Tonsil	20	20
Salivary glands	16	18
Total	158	23

Table 12–8. Overall Response Rate and Complete Response to Cisplatin and 5-Fluorouracil Infusion in Patients With Recurrent Head and Neck Cancer: Wayne State University Experience*

REFERENCES	NO. EVALUABLE PATIENTS	RESPONSE (%)	
		CR†	*Overall*
Kish, 1984	30	27	70
Rowland, 1984, 1986	32	16	56
Creagan, 1984	20	—	25
Sridher, 1984	20	17	72
Kish, 1985	18	22	72
Dasmahapatra, 1985	18	—	11
Amrein, 1985	39	18	46
Raymond, 1985	16	Not stated	75
Fosser, 1985	21	19	62
Mercier, 1987	20	5	35
Parades, 1988	60	7	33
Vallicioni, 1988	41	15	37
Airaldi, 1988	30	17	57
Choksi, 1988	21	10	24
Vokes, 1988	21	5	48

*Data extracted from Al-Sarraf[27,36] and Taylor.[37-39]
†CR: complete response.

survival of these patients.[7] Without the achievement of a CR with chemotherapy, particularly with negative biopsies, the overall survival of these patients remained very poor. The duration of response to most of these agents is about 3 to 4 months, with overall survival of 6 to 8 months. With the investigation of cisplatin and 5-FU infusion in patients with recurrent and/or metastatic cancers at Wayne State University, the overall response rate was about 70% and the CR rate was 20%. Most of the patients who achieved CR to this combination are alive and well without further treatment for more than 4 years. Most of the series reporting the use of cisplatin and 5-FU infusion confirmed the results obtained at the single institution (Tables 12–7, 12–8).[27,36–39] Efforts are underway to continue to improve the activity and safety of these agents in patients with recurrent cancer (Tables 12–8, 12–9).[27,36–39]

CONCLUSIONS

Advanced squamous cell cancers of the larynx and supraglottic area are not cured by conventional therapy in most cases. Smaller tumors (T_{1-3}) may be cured with radiation or combina-

Table 12–9. Overall Response Rate and Complete Response to Cisplatin Combination in Patients With Recurrent Head and Neck Cancer: Wayne State University Experience*

REFERENCES	AGENT†	NO. PATIENTS	RESPONSE (%)	
			CR‡	*Overall*
Dimery, 1986	CFM	48	8	44
Veronesi, 1988	CFB	18	8	27
Vogl, 1986	CFMB	46	4	50
Stewart, 1986	C, Ara-C	26	4	42
Bernstein, 1986	C, Ara-C	17	0	13
Powell, 1988	C, Ara-C	15	0	7
Coninx, 1986	C, VP-16	40	0	20
Creagan, 1987	CB, VP-16	15	7	40
Varela, 1988	CB, VP-16, MPC	31	23	45
Takasugi, 1986	C, MGBG	31	6	35
Jaske, 1986	CA	23	9	26
Creagan, 1986	CAMC	15	?	47
Natale, 1987	C, DCM	30	20	43
Chamvergue, 1988	CMBV	107	1	28

*Data extracted from Al-Sarraf[27,36] and Taylor.[37-39]
†C: cisplatin, F: 5-fluorouracil; M: methotrexate; B: bleomycin; Ara-C: cytosine arabinoside; VP-16: etoposide; P: prednisone; MGBG: methylglyoxal bis (guanylhydrazone); A: doxorubicin (Adriamycin); C: cyclophosphamide; D: daunorubicin; V: vincristine.
‡CR: complete response.

tions of radiation and surgery, but may recur with an unacceptably high frequency, particularly with T_{2-3} lesions. In addition, many patients cured with conventional therapy do so at a high cost in terms of loss of natural voice or swallowing problems, or both.

System chemotherapy has demonstrated effectiveness in producing impressive tumor reduction. The application of such therapy may prove to be of clinical benefit in three groups of patients with laryngeal carcinomas: (1) adjuvant trials for patients with early tumors who may be identified as high risk for recurrence following conventional therapy; (2) neoadjuvant trials for patients who otherwise require total laryngectomies with conventional therapy; (3) patients with advanced, unresectable metastatic or recurrent laryngeal carcinomas who are currently incurable with conventional therapy.

Investigations are currently underway that examine the application of systemic chemotherapy in these three groups. The results of these trials may aid in identifying patient populations with laryngeal cancer who will benefit from addition of systemic chemotherapy to their treatment.

REFERENCES

1. Lederman M. Cancer of the larynx. Part I: Natural history in relation to treatment. Br J Radiol 1971;44:569–78.
2. Goffinet DR, Eltringhan JR, Glatsein E, Bagshaw MA. Carcinoma of the larynx. Results of radiation therapy in 213 patients. Am J Roentgenol Radium Ther Nucl Med 1973;117:553–64.
3. Ensley JF, Kish JA, Al-Sarraf M. The development of optimum induction chemotherapy for advanced head and neck cancer: the Wayne State University experience. In: Jones SE, Solmon SE, eds. *Adjuvant therapy of cancer,* vol. V. Philadelphia: BC Decker, 1987:353–62.
4. Ensley JF, Kish J, Tapazaglou E, Al-Sarraf M. Strategies for improvements in complete response rates with adjuvant combination chemotherapy in advanced head and neck cancer (SCC of H&N). In: Jones SE, Solmon SE, eds. *Adjuvant therapy of cancer,* vol. V. Philadelphia: BC Decker, 1987:101–11.
5. Ensley JF, Kish J, Tapazaglou E, et al. The justification and strategies for the continued intensification of induction regimens in patients with advanced, untreated head and neck cancer. In: Olf, Carey T, eds. *Head and neck oncology research.* Proceedings of the Second International Head and Neck Research Conference. Amsterdam: Kugler Publishers, 313–321.
6. Ensley JF, Maciorowski, Kish JA, Al-Sarraf M. The significance of pretreatment identification of prognostically important subgroups of squamous cell cancer of the head and neck. In: Jacobs J, Al-Sarraf M, Crissman J, Valeriote F, eds. *Scientific and clinical perspective of head and neck cancer management strategies for cure.* New York: Elsevier, 1987:35–56.
7. Ensley JF, Kish JA, Al-Sarraf M. The pretherapeutic identification of prognostically important parameters predictive of tumor response in squamous cell cancers of the head and neck. In: Vogl S, ed. *Head and neck cancer.* New York Churchill Livingstone, 1988:109–24.
8. Adjuvant chemotherapy for advanced head and neck squamous carcinoma: Final report of the Head and Neck Contracts Program. Cancer 1987;60:301–11.
9. Schuller DE, Wilson H, Hodgson S, et al. Preoperative reductive chemotherapy for stage III and IV operative epidermoid carcinoma of the oral cavity, oropharynx, hypopharynx, or larynx, phase III, A Southwest Oncology Group Study. International Conference on Head and Neck Cancer, Baltimore, MD, July, 1984:48.
10. Taylor SG, Applebaum E, Showel JL, et al. A randomized trial of adjuvant chemotherapy in head and neck cancer. J Clin Oncol 1985;3:672–9.
11. Holoye PY, Grossman TW, Toohil RJ, et al. Randomized study of adjuvant chemotherapy for head and neck cancer. Otolaryngol Head Neck Surg 1985;93:712–7.
12. Stell PM, Dalby JE, Strickland P, et al. Sequential chemotherapy and radiotherapy in advanced head and neck cancer. Clin Radiol 1983;34:463–7.
13. Price LA, Hill BT. Safe and effective combination chemotherapy without cisplatinum for squamous cell cancers of the head and neck. Cancer Treat Rep 1981;65:149–54.
14. Martin M, Mazeron JJ, Glaubinger D, et al. Neo-adjuvant polychemotherapy of head and neck cancer: preliminary results of a randomized study. Proc Am Soc Clin Oncol 1986;5:141.
15. Fazekas JT, Sommer C, Kramer S. Adjuvant intravenous methotrexate or definitive radiotherapy alone for advanced cancers of the oral cavity, oropharynx, supraglottic larynx or hypopharynx. Int J Radiat Oncol Biol Phys 1980;6:533–41.
16. Petrovich Z, Block J, Kuisk H. et al. A randomized comparison of radiotherapy with a radiotherapy-chemotherapy combination in stage IV carcinoma of the head and neck. Cancer 1981;47:2259–64.
17. Collin FF, Ansfield FJ, Brandenburg JH, et al. Combined therapy in advanced head and neck cancer: a randomized study. Head Neck Cancer 1972;114:83–8.
18. Ensley J, Kish J, Tapazoglou E, et al. An intensive, five course alternating combination chemotherapy induction regimen employed in patients with advanced, unresectable head and neck cancer. J Clin Oncol 1988;6:1147–53.
19. Lustig RA, MacLean CJ, Hanks GE, Kramer S. The patterns of care outcome studies: results of the national practice in carcinomas of the larynx. Int Radiat Oncol Biol Phys 1984;10:2357–62.
20. Hong WK, O'Donaghue GM, Sheetz S, et al. Sequential response patterns to chemotherapy and radiotherapy in head and neck cancer: potential impact of treatment in advanced laryngeal cancer. Prog Clin Biol Res 1985;201:191–7.
21. Jacobs C, Goffinet DR, Goffinet L, et al. Chemotherapy as a substitute for surgery in treatment of advanced resectable head and neck cancer. Cancer 1987;60:1178–83.
22. Karp D, Carter R, Vaughan C, et al. Voice preservation using induction chemotherapy (CT) plus radiation therapy in advanced head and neck cancer: long term follow-up. Proc Am Soc Clin Oncol 1988;24:152.
23. Kish J, Ensley J, Al-Sarraf M. Clinical results of chemotherapy in recurrent head and neck carcinoma. In: Jacobs J, Al-Sarraf M, Crissman J, Valeriote F, eds. *Scientific and clinical perspective of head and neck cancer management strategies for cure.* New York: Elsevier 1987:199–211.
24. Forastiere A, Metch B, Keppen M, et al. Randomized comparisons of cisplatinum (CDDP) + 5-fluorouracil (5-FU) vs. carboplatinum (CBP) + 5-FU vs. methotrexate in advanced squamous cell carcinomas of the head and neck. Proc Am Soc Clin Oncol 1989:25.
25. Nahum AM. Overview of chemotherapy of cancer of the larynx. In: Alberti PW, Bryce DP, ed. *Workshops from the Centennial Conference on Laryngeal Cancer.* New York: Appelton-Century-Crofts 1976: 172–9.
26. Al-Sarraf M. Chemotherapeutic strategies in squamous cell carcinoma of the head and neck. CRC Crit Rev Oncol Hematol 1984;1:323–55.
27. Al-Sarraf M. Head and neck cancer. Chemotherapy concepts. Semin Oncol 1988;15:70–85.
28. Al-Sarraf M, Kish J, Ensley JF. Current progress in head and cancer: the Wayne State University Experience. In: Jacobs J, Al-Sarraf M, Crissman J, Valeriote F, eds. *Scientific and clinical perspective of head and neck cancer management strategies for cure.* New York: Elsevier, 1987:13–34.
29. Rooney M, Kish J, Jacobs J, et al. Improved complete response rates and survival in advanced head and neck cancer after three course induction therapy with 120 hour 5-fluorouracil infusion and cisplatinum. Cancer 1985;56:1123–8.
30. Ensley J, Kish JA, Jacobs J, et al. Incremental improvements in median survival associated with degree of response to adjuvant chemotherapy in patients with advanced squamous cell cancer of the head and neck. In: Jones SE, Solmon SE, eds. *Adjuvant therapy of cancer,* vol IV. Orlando: Grune & Stratton, 1984:117–25.
31. Schwert R, Jacobs J, Crissman J, et al. Improved survival in patients with advanced head and neck cancers achieving a complete response to induction chemotherapy. Proc Am Soc Clin Oncol 1983;2:159.
32. Al-Kourainy K, Kish J, Ensley J, et al. Achievement of superior

survival for histologically negative versus histologically positive clinical complete responders to cisplatinum combination in patients with locally advanced head and neck cancer. Cancer 1987;59:233–8.

33. Al-Sarraf M, Pajak TF, Marcial VA, et al. Concurrent radiotherapy and chemotherapy with cisplatin in inoperable squamous cell carcinoma of the head and neck. RTOG study. Cancer 1987;59:259–65.
34. Kish J, Ensley J, Jacobs J, et al. Evaluation of high dose cisplatinum and 5-fluorouracil infusions as initial therapy in advanced squamous cell cancers of the head and neck. Cancer. In press.
35. Greenberg B, Ahmann F, Gerwal H, et al. Neoadjuvant therapy for advanced head and neck cancer with allopurinol modulated high dose 5-fluorouracil and cisplatinum. Proc Am Soc Clin Oncol 1985;21:571.
36. Al-Sarraf M. Chemotherapeutic management of head and neck cancer. Cancer Met Rev 1987;6:181–98.
37. Taylor SG. IV. Head and neck cancer. In: Longo DL, Chabner DA, eds. *Cancer Chemotherapy and Biological Respiratory Modifiers*. Elsevier Science Publishers, 1987:226–38.
38. Taylor SG. IV. Head and neck cancer. In: Longo DL, Chabner DA, eds. *Cancer Chemotherapy and Biological Respiratory Modifiers*. Elsevier Science Publishers, 1987:210–21.
39. Taylor SG. IV. Head and neck cancer. In: Longo DL, Chabner DA, eds. *Cancer Chemotherapy and Biological Respiratory Modifiers*. Elsevier Science Publishers, 1989.
40. Schuller DE, Metch B, Mattox D, Stein DW, McCracken JD. Preoperative chemotherapy in advanced resectable head and neck cancer: final report of the Southwest Oncology Group. Laryngoscope 1988;98:1205.
41. Al-Sarraf M, Kinzie J, Jacobs J, et al. New way of giving chemotherapy as part of multi-disciplinary treatment for patients with head and neck cancers. Preliminary report. Proc Am Assoc Cancer Res 1982;23:134.
42. Al-Sarraf M, Pajak T, Laramore G. Timing of chemotherapy as part of definitive treatment for patients with advanced head and neck cancer. An RTOG study. Proc Am Soc Clin Oncol 1985;4:137.
43. Jacobs JR, Pajak TF, Al-Sarraf M, et al. Chemotherapy following surgery for head and neck cancer. A Radiation Therapy Oncology Group Study. Am J Clin Oncol 1989;12:185–9.
44. Ensley JF, Jacobs JR, Weaver A, et al. The correlation between response to cisplatinum combination chemotherapy and subsequent radiotherapy in previously untreated patients with advanced squamous cell cancers of the head and neck. Cancer 1984;54:811–4.
45. Ensley J, Ahmad K, Kish J, et al. Improved response to radiation and concurrent cisplatinum (CACP) in patients with advanced head and neck cancers (SCCHN) that failed induction chemotherapy. Proc Am Soc Clin Oncol 1989;8:168.
46. Ensley J, Ahmad K, Kish J, et al. Feasibility and toxicity of concurrent administration of cisplatinum and radiotherapy post-operatively in patients with head and neck cancers (SCCHN). Proc Am Soc Clin Oncol 1989;8:172.

PART FOUR

Surgical Treatment of Early Laryngeal Cancer

13

Technical Aspects of Conservation Surgery

Carl E. Silver

The following chapters on surgical management of early cancer of the larynx have been written by distinguished contributors who emphasize their experience and philosophy with regard to indications and results in management of particular tumors. Although technical aspects of some operative procedures are discussed in relative detail, others are not. While the primary purpose of this volume is to capture the varying opinions and controversies contributing to the current status of management of laryngeal cancer, I, as editor, believe that a discussion of the basic techniques of partial laryngectomy would serve as a reference, helping the nonsurgeon as well as the surgeon in training to grasp the nature of various procedures and modifications discussed in subsequent chapters.

One of the major features of current surgical treatment of laryngeal cancer has been the advent of "conservation surgery" for oncologically adequate excision of tumor with preservation of the essential functions of the larynx. The feasibility of this surgery is based on the tendency of many laryngeal tumors to remain confined within various compartments of the larynx during early stages of development and on the fact that relatively healthy people are capable of adapting to the loss of substantial portions of the larynx while retaining ability to breathe, swallow, and speak. Details of the anatomic, embryologic, and historic basis of this type of surgery are discussed in various succeeding chapters.

Conservation surgery, or partial laryngectomy, is approached in the vertical or horizontal plane according to the location of the tumor. Thus, a vertical approach (such as laryngofissure and hemilaryngectomy) is employed for glottic tumors, whereas supraglottic tumors are approached horizontally (supraglottic subtotal laryngectomy). Because surgical exploration may reveal extension of tumor beyond the limits estimated preoperatively, consent for total laryngectomy should be obtained prior to attempted conservation surgery.

In this section, I will discuss techniques of partial laryngectomy for glottic carcinoma, supraglottic carcinoma, and hypopharyngeal tumors. Since endoscopic management, with or without laser, is covered adequately in Chapters 14 and 15, this aspect of surgical management will not be addressed.

PARTIAL LARYNGECTOMY FOR GLOTTIC CARCINOMA

Glottic carcinoma, the most common laryngeal neoplasm, occurs predominately in males. Tumors usually arise on the anterior half of the vocal cord and extend most commonly in an anterior and inferior direction. Posterior extension onto the vocal process of the arytenoid occurs less often, and initial involvement of the posterior commissure is rare. As the tumor spreads laterally and inferiorly, the thyroarytenoideus muscle is invaded and eventually vocal cord fixation occurs. Although the lateral thyroid cartilage is resistant to tumor invasion, as tumor extends inferiorly the cricothyroid junction is penetrated and tumor extends readily into perilaryngeal tissue. The thyroid cartilage is vulnerable to invasion in the anterior midline. The tendency for extralaryngeal spread and cartilage invasion places limitations on the applicability of conservation surgery to sufficiently advanced tumors.

Lymphatic metastases do not commonly occur with glottic carcinoma confined to the endolarynx. Once tumor has traversed the cricothyroid membrane, however, the frequency of lymph node metastasis increases significantly.

Laryngofissure (Cordectomy via Thyrotomy)

Laryngofissure is suitable for carcinoma confined to the mobile portion of the vocal cord without deep invasion. A lesion suitable for such resection and the technique of cordectomy via thyrotomy is outlined in Figure 13–1. After placement of a transverse skin incision and development of skin flaps suitable to expose the larynx, a tracheotomy tube is inserted through the second tracheal ring. The prelaryngeal muscles are separated in the midline and retracted sufficiently to expose the laryngeal

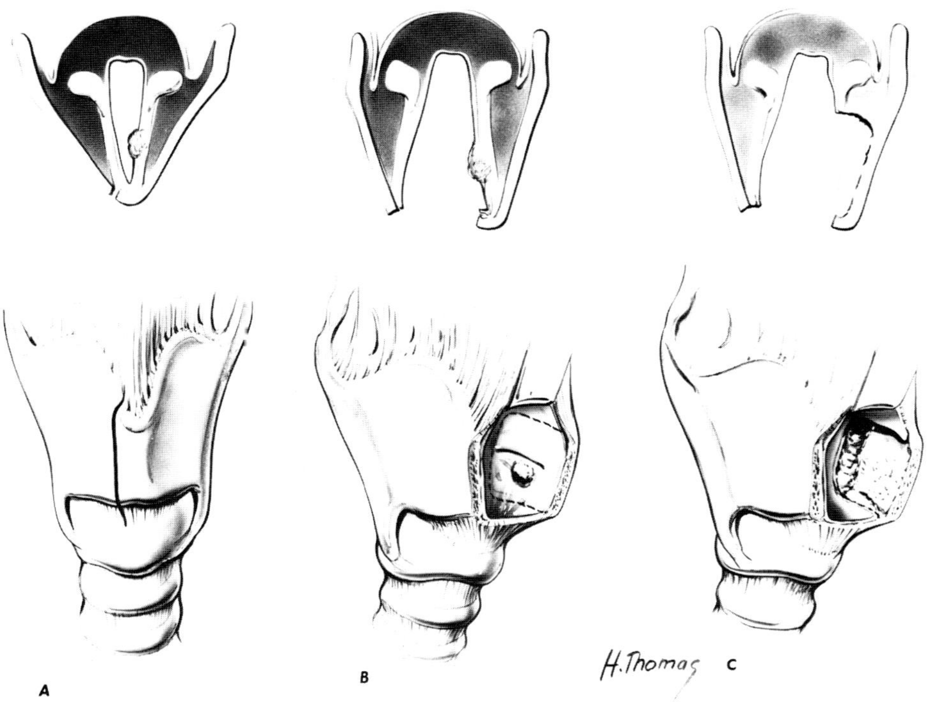

Figure 13–1. Laryngofissure. (From Silver.[22] Reprinted with permission.)

prominence and midportions of thyroid and cricoid cartilages and cricothyroid membrane. An oscillating saw is used to make a vertical thyrotomy incision near the midline on the side opposite the tumor (Fig. 13–1A), and the larynx is entered through a small horizontal incision in the cricothyroid membrane. This incision is extended upward through the laryngeal mucosa in order to transect the contralateral vocal cord 2 or 3 mm posterior to the commissure (Fig. 13–1B). The resection is outlined superiorly above the false vocal cord, inferiorly at the lower border of thyroid cartilage, and posteriorly immediately anterior to the vocal process of arytenoid. Incisions are deepened through mucosal and muscular layers to the inner aspect of the thyroid cartilage, and the portion of tissue to be resected is separated from the inner aspect of the thyroid cartilage as far posteriorly as the vocal process (Fig. 13–1C). The specimen is liberated with the posterior vertical incision, best made with a curved scissors.

When the resulting mucosal defect is permitted to heal by granulation and reepithelialization, a "pseudocord" of scar tissue develops, which may be reasonably effective in duplicating the function of the resected vocal cord. Techniques employed to improve voice have included subperichondrial resection of the anterior half of the thyroid cartilage to facilitate "collapse" of the resected side and approximation of vocal cords, or interposition of a bipedicled flap of sternohyoid muscle into the defect as described by Bailey.[1] The latter may be particularly useful in restoring intralaryngeal bulk if the resection has been extended to include part of the arytenoid or the contralateral side.

Cure rates reported for laryngofissure during the past 40 years have ranged from 60 to almost 100%. Differing results are accounted for by variations in indications for the procedure and depending on whether the patients in particular reported series consisted mainly of radiation failures. When indications for this procedure are limited to those already outlined, cure rates greater than 90% are consistently obtainable. It is most important, in dealing with radiation failures, to employ this procedure only for lesions that would have been suitable prior to irradiation.

Anterior Frontal Partial Laryngectomy ("Anterior Commissure Technique")

As glottic carcinomas progress, they tend to extend anteriorly across the commissure and onto the contralateral vocal cord. In many cases, this extension is superficial and involves only a few millimeters of the contralateral cord. When such lesions are treated surgically, a vertical midline segment of thyroid cartilage should be included. If an adequate margin can be assured by excision of no more than a third of the contralateral vocal cord, the contralateral side may be resurfaced by suturing a flap of preserved external perichondrium to the cut margin of the contralateral cord. The ipsilateral side is permitted to granulate, without surgical resurfacing, as with laryngofissure.

A more difficult problem is presented by a tumor that crosses the anterior commissure to involve significant portions of both vocal cords. Adequate surgical resection requires removal of a vertical midline segment of thyroid cartilage plus major portions of both vocal cords. Such a lesion is depicted in Figure 13–2A. Although resections of this nature present no particular technical problem, the surgical defects following resection are quite formidable. Usually, only the mucosa of the posterior commissure remains in the endolarynx. A variety of reconstructive techniques have been employed, including skin grafts, skin flaps, perichondrium, and muscle flaps. The technique described by Som and Silver[2] in 1968 avoids the need for

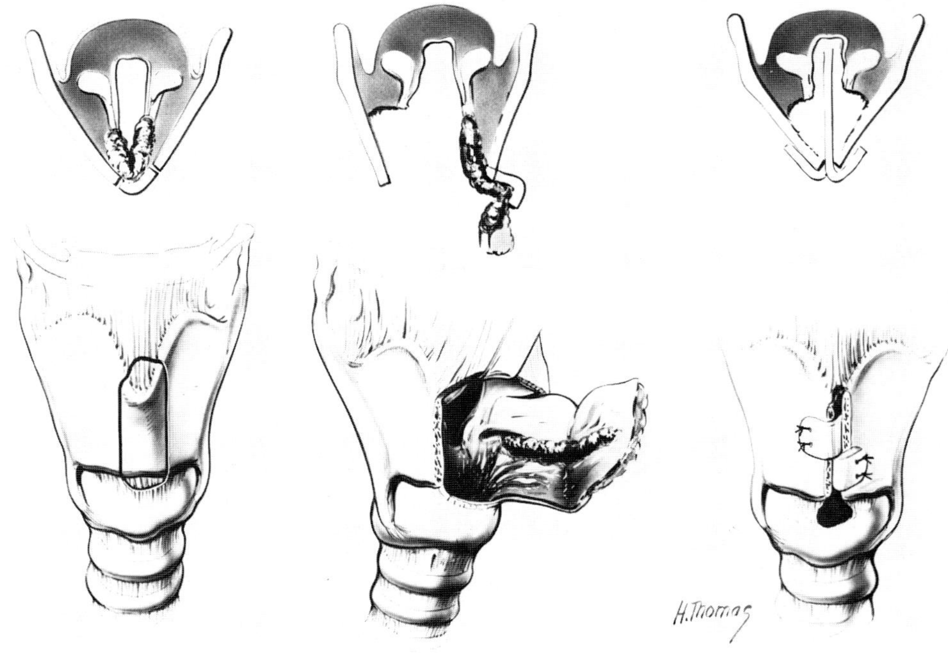

Figure 13–2. Anterior commissure partial laryngectomy. (From Silver.[22] Reprinted with permission.)

intralaryngeal resurfacing by utilizing a temporary midline partition, as developed by McNaught[3] for treatment of laryngeal web. This simple measure produces satisfactory airway and voice.

The resection is approached in a similar manner as laryngofissure, except that bilateral vertical thyrotomy incisions are made (Fig. 13–2A). The endolaryngeal tissue is separated subperichondrially from the thyroid alae bilaterally as far as the vocal processes of the arytenoids. The laryngeal lumen is entered through the inferior cricothyroid membrane anteriorly, and the mucosa retracted with a small hook as the incision extends posteriorly on the side of lesser involvement and ascends vertically through mucosa and muscle, passing just anterior to the vocal process of arytenoid. Accurate assessment of the extent of tumor involvement prior to entering the larynx is essential in order to avoid compromising the resection margin at this point. As exposure is gained, the superior horizontal incision on that side is carried back toward the anterior commissure and through the thyrohyoid membrane. The mobilized portion of the specimen can now be retracted forward (Fig. 13–2B) affording an excellent view of the endolarynx and the tumor. Resection of the specimen is completed by circumscribing mucosa and muscle appropriately around the tumor. If necessary, the resection may be extended to include the arytenoid on the side of greater involvement as well as the upper half of anterior cricoid cartilage.

Following resection, a prosthesis is inserted to partition the larynx (Fig. 13–2C). A semirigid silicone rubber "keel" of the McNaught type may be employed, as shown here. This type of prosthesis is secured to the thyroid cartilage and requires a small second operation, 6 weeks after insertion, for removal. A more flexible silicone rubber sheet, which can be removed endoscopically, may be used instead.

The results of anterior frontal partial laryngectomy in several series reported in the literature are compiled in Table 13–1.[2,4,5] Three-year cure in 111 of 157 (71%) cases was reported.

Vertical Hemilaryngectomy

The procedure shown here is a conventional vertical "hemilaryngectomy" performed for glottic carcinoma with extension posteriorly to involve the vocal process and anterior surface of the arytenoid, or with involvement of the floor of the ventricle laterally with infiltration of the thyroarytenoideus muscle. Limitation of vocal cord motion, including complete fixation in some cases, may be present. Suitability for hemilaryngectomy is determined mainly by the degree and location of subglottic extension. Conventional hemilaryngectomy is possible if subglottic extension does not exceed 8 to 9 mm anteriorly or 5 to 6 mm posteriorly. Cases in which vocal cord fixation is due simply to the bulk of the tumor are also amenable to resection by hemilaryngectomy. Hemilaryngectomy is not feasible, however, when vocal cord fixation is due to involvement of the cricoarytenoid joint.

Following transverse skin incision, elevation of skin flaps, and tracheostomy, thyrohyoid and sternothyroid muscles are separated from the oblique line of the thyroid ala, exposing its

Table 13-1. Results of Anterior Frontal Partial Laryngectomy

SERIES	YEARS	STAGE	RESULTS
Som and Silver[2]	3	T_2	26/38 (68%)
Kirchner and Som[4]	4	T_2	40/58 (69%)
Sessions et al[5]	3	T_1-T_2	45/61 (74%)
Total			111/157 (71%)

anterior two thirds. Because the posterior third of the ala will be used to reconstruct the laryngeal vestibule, the inferior constrictor muscle is left attached. Vertical thyrotomy incisions are made on the contralateral side near the anterior commissure, as for laryngofissure, and on the side to be resected, at the junction of middle and posterior thirds of the ala (Fig. 13–3A). After ligation and division of superior laryngeal vessels and nerves, and avulsion of the cricothyroid joint, the posterior third of the thyroid ala is separated from the underlying pyriform sinus mucosa.

The laryngeal interior is exposed by retracting the ipsilateral hemilarynx outward while mucosa is incised inferiorly and superiorly through the cricothyroid and thyrohyoid membranes (Fig. 13–3B). As resection proceeds posteriorly, the inferior mucosal incision should rise slightly to the level of the cricoarytenoid joint and ascend vertically in the posterior midline, between the arytenoids, transecting the interarytenoideus muscle. In order to avoid incision of the postarytenoid mucosa while dividing the muscle, a finger or instrument is inserted into the hypopharynx, placing the tissues under moderate tension. The mucosal incision is now continued from the posterior midline superiorly along the aryepiglottic fold to join the incision in the thyrohyoid membrane. A finger in the pyriform sinus permits palpation and stabilization of the cricoarytenoid joint while it is transected, and helps avoid injury to the pyriform sinus mucosa while the specimen, including arytenoid cartilage, is dissected from its outer surface.

Figure 13–3C shows the specimen, including arytenoid cartilage, removed with pyriform sinus preserved. The pyriform sinus mucosa will be advanced anteriorly to resurface the hemilarynx. When this procedure was originally described, no further reconstruction was performed. This resulted in a defect in the posterior vestibule, predisposing the patient to aspiration. Younger patients could adapt to this defect, but older individuals could not, thus imposing a limitation on utility of the procedure. Various techniques, subsequently developed, for glottic and vestibular reconstruction employed cartilage, muscle, and other tissues and were helpful in restoring deglutatory function as well as voice. On our service, reconstruction with a portion of preserved posterior thyroid cartilage, pedicled on the

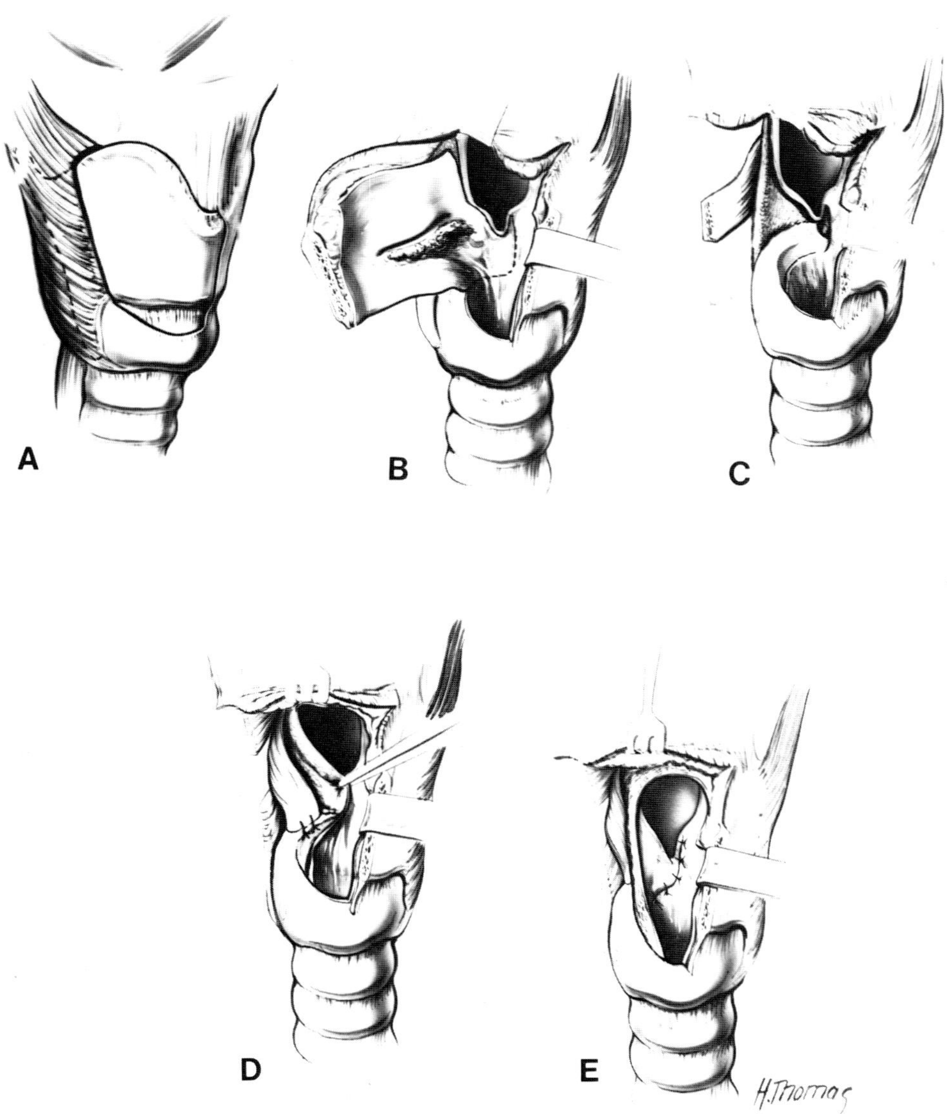

Figure 13–3. Hemilaryngectomy. (From Silver.[22] Reprinted with permission.)

inferior constrictor muscle, has been preferred and has reduced morbidity from hemilaryngectomy, particularly in older individuals.

Reconstruction is commenced by excising the upper and lower portion of the posterior thyroid ala that has been left attached to inferior constrictor muscle. The middle portion of this cartilage will be used for reconstruction. The cartilage "flap" is sutured to the cricoid rostrum, providing replacement for the resected arytenoid (Fig. 13–3D). This provides bulk to restore the laryngeal vestibule as well as the glottis, assisting postoperative deglutition and phonation. The endolarynx is now resurfaced by advancement of hypopharyngeal mucosa, including the preserved pyriform sinus (Fig. 13–3E). Prior to advancing the mucosa, the cut edge of aryepiglottic fold should be thinned by removing remaining cartilaginous and ligamentous material. This will facilitate mobility of mucosa and avoid creation of an obstructive flap of tissue within the lumen. Hypopharyngeal mucosa is sutured to the cut edge of subglottic mucosa as far anteriorly as possible, covering the cartilage flap and resurfacing most of the hemilarynx. The anterior edge of mucosa is sutured to the preserved sternohyoid muscle, and the prelaryngeal muscles reapproximated in the midline to complete closure of the endolarynx. There is usually insufficient mucosa to resurface completely the anterior larynx, but this heals well by secondary intention.

The results of vertical hemilaryngectomy for T_2 and T_3 glottic tumors from several series reported in the literature are summarized in Table 13–2. Overall results indicate approximately 82% cure rates for T_2 carcinoma and 64% for T_3.[6–13] Biller and Lawson[14] have extended the indications for vertical hemilaryngectomy to include lesions with posterior subglottic extension exceeding the limitations already described. An oversized thyroid cartilage flap is employed to replace the resected portion of cricoid cartilage, as well as the arytenoid. The authors reported 2-year survival in 10 of 15 patients treated with this technique.

Table 13–2. Results of Vertical Hemilaryngectomy

SERIES	YEARS	STAGE	TUMOR FREE
Ogura et al[6]	3	T_2	45/55 (82%)
Som[7]	3	T_2	79/105 (75%)
	3	T_3	15/26 (58%)
Mohr et al[8]	5	T_2	25/27 (93%)
	5	T_3	5/5 (100%)
Bauer et al[9]	5	T_3	12/18 (67%)
Leroux-Robert[10]	5	T_2	187/215 (87%)
	5	T_3	55/95 (58%)
Skolnik et al[11]	5	T_2	23/32 (72%)
	5	T_3	2/5 (40%)
Biller et al[12]	5	T_2	23/33 (70%)
Kessler et al[13]	2	T_3	23/27 (85%)
Total		T_2	382/467 (82%)
		T_3	112/176 (64%)

SUPRAGLOTTIC CARCINOMA

Supraglottic (Horizontal) Subtotal Laryngectomy

Supraglottic carcinomas, confined to the endolarynx, tend to be exophytic, well-differentiated, and circumscribed, with "pushing" rather than infiltrating margins. These lesions rarely extend inferiorly to involve the glottis and rarely invade thyroid cartilage, although they frequently infiltrate the preepiglottic space. Such involvement is confined above the anterior commissure, and the entire preepiglottic space is effectively resected by supraglottic laryngectomy. A smaller number of supraglottic carcinomas with infiltrating rather than "pushing" borders are usually poorly differentiated, tend to be transglottic, and are rarely amenable to supraglottic laryngectomy.

Supraglottic subtotal laryngectomy (SSL) is indicated for supraglottic carcinomas that do not involve the vocal cord or thyroid cartilage. The procedure may be extended superiorly to include resection of various portions of the hypopharynx and base of the tongue. Inferiorly, even when the lesion appears grossly to be close to the vocal cord, several millimeters of uninvolved ventricular mucosa are usually found in the resected specimen and constitute an adequate margin of resection. Both arytenoids may be preserved, thus preserving vocal cord mobility, for resection of lesions confined to the laryngeal surface of the epiglottis and anterior portion of the false vocal cord. Lesions that extend further posteriorly to approach or involve the arytenoid require inclusion of the arytenoid in the resected specimen. After removal of the arytenoid, fixation of the vocal cord in the midline, by suture to the cricoid cartilage, is necessary in order to restore glottic competence.

A transverse cervical incision is made at the level of the midthyroid cartilage, extended appropriately if simultaneous neck dissection is to be performed. After insertion of a tracheostomy tube through the second tracheal ring, infrahyoid muscles are transected close to their insertions on the hyoid bone and reflected inferiorly as far as necessary to expose the upper half of the ipsilateral thyroid ala as well as anterior portion of the contralateral side. Suprahyoid muscles are severed from their insertions on the ipsilateral greater cornu as well as the body of the hyoid bone (Fig. 13–4A). The junction of body and contralateral greater cornu of the hyoid bone are transected and external perichondrium is dissected from the ipsilateral and anterior contralateral thyroid alae and reflected downward as far as the estimated location of the vocal cord (in a male, half the anterior height of the thyroid cartilage; in a female, the upper third). The thyroid cartilage is transected horizontally along the line of reflection of the flap. In cases in which the valleculae are known to be free of tumor, the hypopharynx is entered, as shown by incising the laryngeal wall superior to the hyoid bone, immediately anterior to the epiglottis. As this incision is enlarged, the epiglottis is secured with a suture and retracted forward into the pharyngeal opening (Fig. 13–4B). Further enlargment of the pharyngotomy permits exposure of the entire supraglottis, as far posteriorly as the arytenoids (Fig. 13–4C).

Resection of the supraglottis is commenced by incising the aryepiglottic fold, first on one side, then the other, immediately in front of the arytenoids (Fig. 13–4D). Each incision extends inferiorly into the ventricle and then anteriorly through the ventricular mucosa immediately above the vocal cord. Supraglottic mucosa should be resected close to the vocal cord on either side, even if the area is widely free of tumor, because

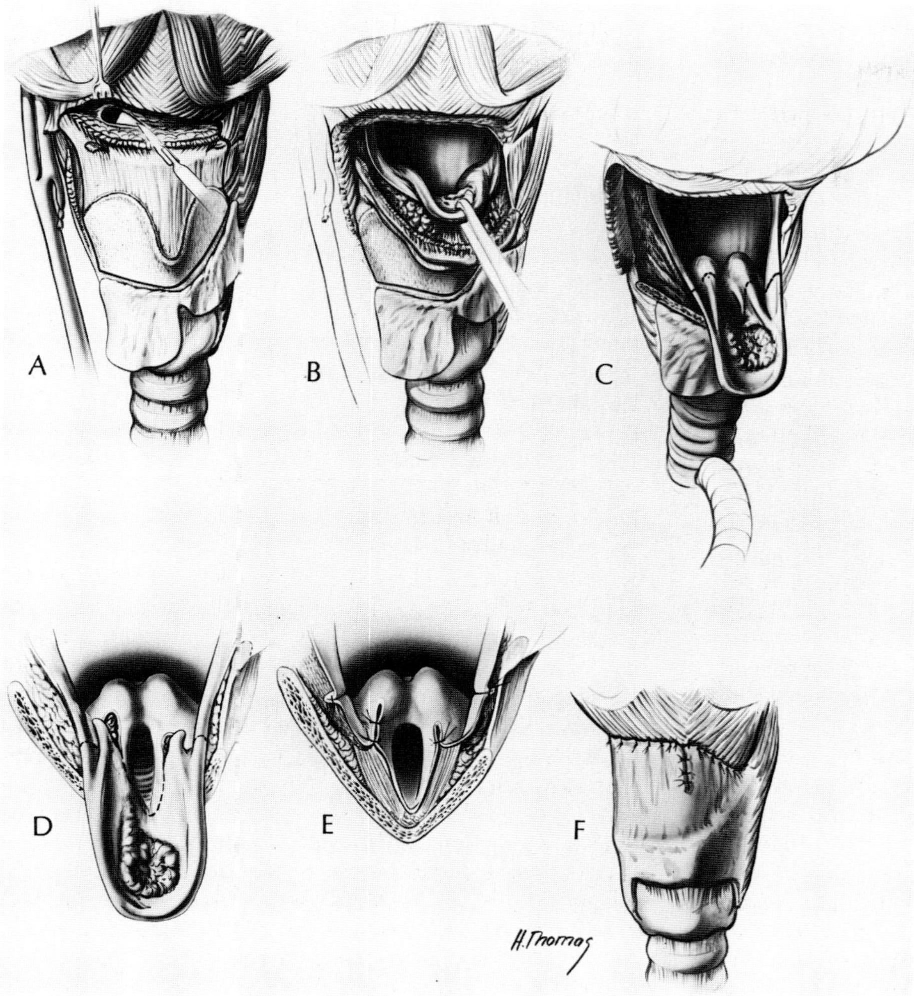

Figure 13–4. Supraglottic subtotal laryngectomy. (From Silver.[22] Reprinted with permission.)

excessive supraglottic mucosa, remaining after resection, is of little value in closure and tends to become edematous, causing postoperative glottic obstruction. The resection proceeds through the ventricles until the mucosa immediately above the anterior commissure has been transected. The mucosa incisions are carried through the full thickness of the larynx as they are made, corresponding externally with the previously placed cartilage cuts.

After removal of the specimen, a cricopharyngeal myotomy is performed and a nasogastric tube inserted. Reconstruction is commenced by suturing the cut edges of the pyriform sinus and supraglottic mucosa to each other (Fig. 13–4E). The hypopharyngeal defect is now closed by direct suture as far anteriorly as possible. As the region of the resected supraglottis is approached, it is no longer possible to repair the hypopharynx by direct approximation of mucosal edges. The previously created perichondrial flap is sutured to the cut edge of the base of the tongue in order to repair the supraglottic defect (Fig. 13–4F). This repair is reinforced by suturing the preserved infrahyoid muscles to the suprahyoid and inferior constrictor muscles.

SSL for treatment of endolaryngeal supraglottic carcinoma produces survival rates virtually the same as for total laryngectomy, consistently ranging from approximately 75 to 90%, varying mostly according to length of follow-up. Results of some of the larger reported series are summarized in Table 13–3.[15–20]

Subtotal Laryngectomy

The procedure of subtotal or "three-quarter" laryngectomy has been employed by various authors for treatment of selected cases of supraglottic carcinoma with downward vertical extension on the ipsilateral side to involve the vocal cord. The vertical

Table 13-3. Results of Supraglottic Subtotal Laryngectomy

SERIES	YEARS	PATIENTS	TUMOR FREE (%)
Ogura et al[15]	3	177	76
Bocca et al[16]	5	467	75
Som[17]	5	75	68
Burnstein and Calcaterra[18]	2	41	90
Maceri et al[19]	2	25	80
Robbins et al[20]	5	34	89

resection has been extended to include portions of the cricoid cartilage. This subject is discussed in detail by Friedman and Katsantonis in Chapter 18.

The major problems involved with such extensive partial laryngectomy include proper selection of patients and reconstruction. The latter must maintain the diameter of the glottic region and restore glottic competence. Use of the contralateral superior cornu of thyroid cartilage for this purpose is described in Chapter 18. Biller and Lawson[21] employ the posterior portion of ipsilateral thyroid cartilage pedicled on the inferior constrictor muscle to replace the resected vocal cord and cricoid. The technique is similar in concept to the other applications of pedicled posterior thyroid cartilage described before (Fig. 13–5).

HYPOPHARYNGEAL TUMORS

Some localized hypopharyngeal tumors may be treated by conservation procedures. Tumors confined entirely to the pharyngeal wall may be resected without involving the larynx; other lesions are managed by extended partial laryngectomy. The entire supraglottis, except for one arytenoid, various amounts of the base of tongue, and one pyriform sinus with adjacent pharyngeal wall may be excised with preservation of laryngeal function. The procedures demonstrated here are based on the "lateral pharyngotomy" approach employed for SSL. The term "partial pharyngolaryngectomy" (PPL) is often used to describe such procedures.

Partial Pharyngolaryngectomy For Superior Hypopharyngeal Tumors

Suitable lesions for this approach are confined predominantly to the valleculae and lingual surface of the epiglottis, should be less than 3 cm in diameter, and should not infiltrate extensively into the base of the tongue. Lesions involving both valleculae with extension to the circumvallate papillae cannot be treated by conservation surgery.

Mobilization of the larynx, development of the perichondrial flap, and bone and cartilage cuts are similar to those described for treatment of supraglottic carcinoma but may include the upper halves of both thyroid alae and the entire hyoid, if necessary. The pharynx is entered through the ipsilateral pyriform sinus and the incision enlarged superiorly, permitting exposure of the base of the tongue. This incision is continued onto the base of the tongue, allowing a 2 cm margin of normal mucosa around the tumor (Fig. 13–6). It is important to preserve at least one lingual artery. The remainder of the procedure is the same as for supraglottic carcinoma (Fig. 13–7).

Closure of the hypopharyngeal defect is accomplished with the perichondrial flap, as described for SSL, but is more difficult because of resection of the base of the tongue. Suspension of the larynx from the mental area by heavy polygalactin sutures (Fig. 13–8) will minimize the surgical defect and relieve tension on the suture line. Elevation of the larynx in this manner helps restore the normal "hyomandibular" apparatus and may assist in postoperative deglutition.

Partial Pharyngolaryngectomy for Pyriform Sinus Tumors

Pyriform sinus carcinomas are suitable for PPL if the true cord and arytenoid are freely mobile without gross tumor involvement, the apex of the pyriform sinus is uninvolved, and there is no thyroid cartilage invasion.

Bone and cartilage cuts are similar to SSL, modified for increased exposure of the pyriform sinus. The hypopharynx is entered in the valleculae or through the posterolateral pharyngeal wall. The pyriform sinus is retracted outward, exposing the tumor (Fig. 13–9), and the resection proceeds inferiorly beneath the tumor and through the cricoarytenoid joint, vocal process, and ventricle (Figs. 13–10, 13–11). The remainder of the operation is similar to SSL. Sufficient mucosa usually remains to achieve closure with local tissue. Lesions large enough to need a pedicled cutaneous or myocutaneous flap for closure require total or near-total laryngectomy for adequate resection and postoperative function.

Posterolateral Pharyngeal Wall

The lateral pharyngotomy approach may be employed for excision of tumors of the posterolateral pharyngeal wall not in continuity with the larynx. Suitable lesions may extend from above the cricopharyngeus to the level of the tip of the epiglottis or slightly higher.

The thyrotomy is made in a slightly oblique vertical direction over the posterior third of ala and extends through the junction of body and greater cornu of the hyoid bone (Fig. 13–12). The hypopharynx is entered superiorly and mucosal incision extended laterally and inferiorly to expose posterolateral pharyngeal wall and tumor. The lesion is circumscribed with a safe margin of uninvolved mucosa (Fig. 13–13). The method of hypopharyngeal repair varies according to the extent of resection. Primary closure may be possible by mobilization and direct approximation of pharyngeal tissue. Larger defects have been repaired with a split-thickness skin graft placed on the prevertebral muscles, rotated to close the defect (Fig. 13–14). More extensive defects may be repaired with myocutaneous flaps, or various free flaps of skin or jejunum.

CONCLUSIONS

The descriptions given of basic techniques of partial laryngectomy and PPL are of those procedures and approaches that have been employed on my service. Perusal of the succeeding chapters will indicate variations in approach and technique by the contributors. Nevertheless, the basic definitions and surgical objectives are similar.

In all applications of partial laryngectomy, careful selection of patients is of paramount importance. Considerable adaptation is required, particularly in recovery of deglutitory function after removal of large portions of the larynx. Such procedures are not suitable for patients with chronic neurologic or respiratory problems and should be considered with great caution for aged patients who may find adaptation difficult. Indeed, a patient may lead a more comfortable life following uncomplicated total extirpation of the larynx than after a functionally unsuccessful

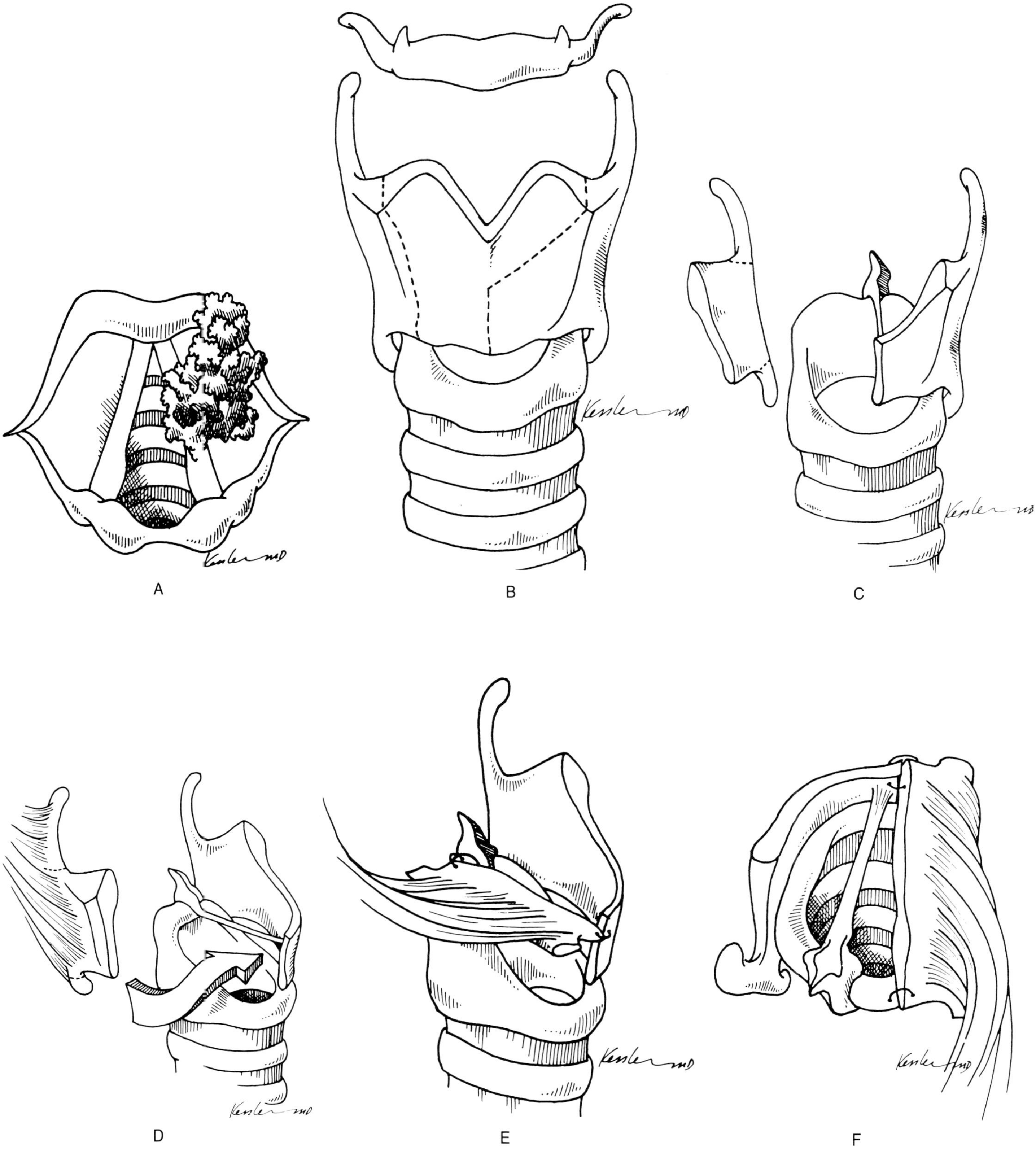

Figure 13–5. Subtotal laryngectomy (courtesy of Dr. H.F. Biller): A: supraglottic carcinoma with involvement of right vocal cord. B: cartilage cuts. (From Biller and Lawson.[21] Reprinted with permission.) C: specimen removed. Remaining portions of laryngeal framework demonstrated. D: right posterior thyroid cartilage pedicled on inferior constrictor muscle. (From Biller and Lawson.[21] Reprinted with permission.) E: cartilage flap advanced into right glottic defect. (From Biller and Lawson.[21] Reprinted with permission.) F: position of replaced vocal cord. (From Biller and Lawson.[21] Reprinted with permission.)

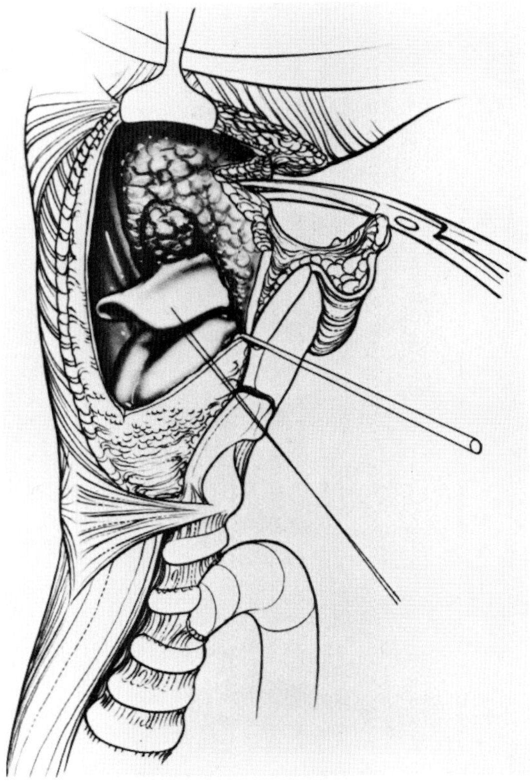

Figure 13–6. Partial pharyngolaryngectomy for superior hypopharynx. (From Silver.[23] Reprinted with permission.)

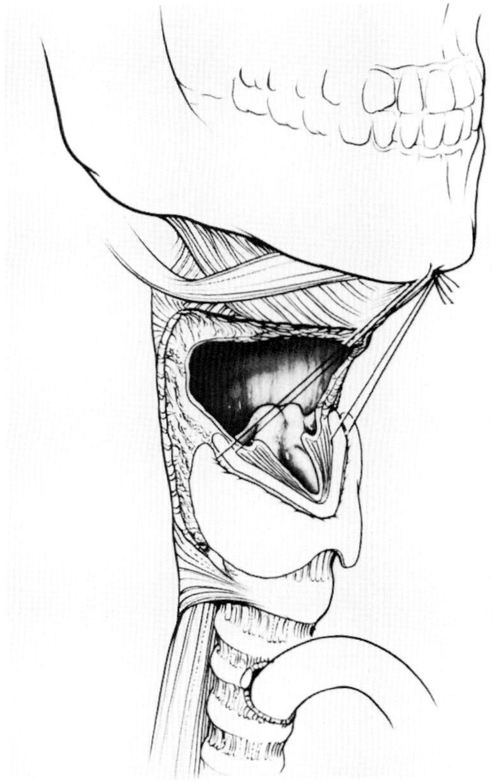

Figure 13–8. Partial pharyngolaryngectomy for superior hypopharynx (continued). (From Silver.[23] Reprinted with permission.)

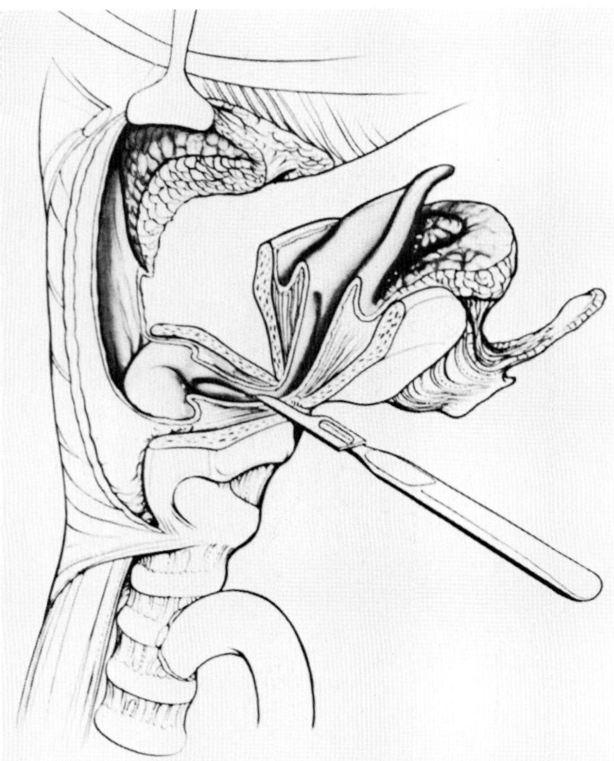

Figure 13–7. Partial pharyngolaryngectomy for superior hypopharynx (continued). (From Silver.[23] Reprinted with permission.)

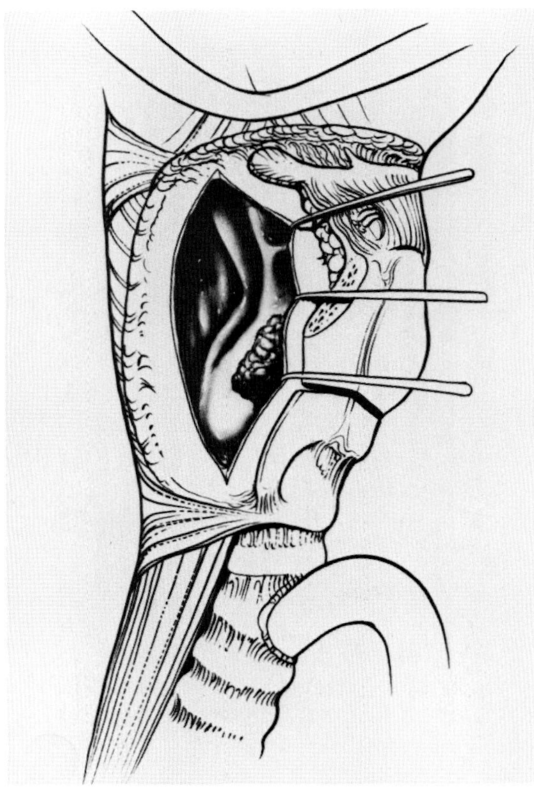

Figure 13–9. Partial pharyngolaryngectomy for pyriform sinus lesion. (From Silver.[23] Reprinted with permission.)

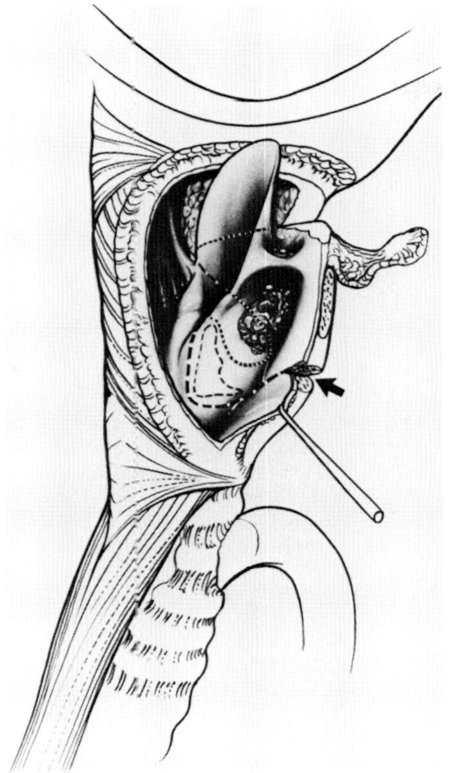

Figure 13–10. Partial pharyngolaryngectomy for pyriform sinus lesion (continued). (From Silver.[23] Reprinted with permission.)

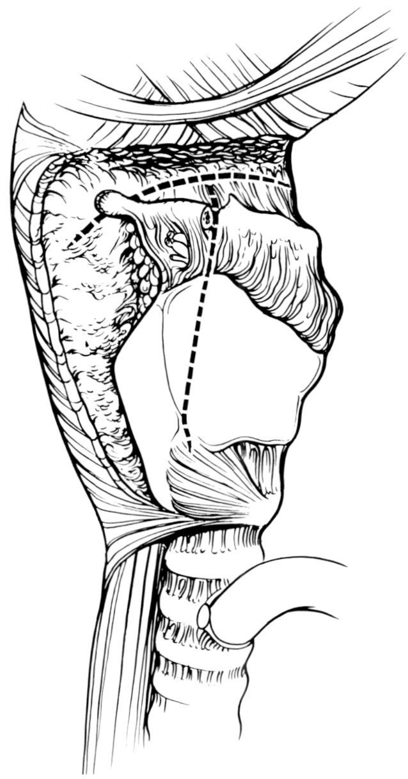

Figure 13–12. Partial pharyngolaryngectomy for posterolateral pharyngeal wall. (From Silver.[23] Reprinted with permission.)

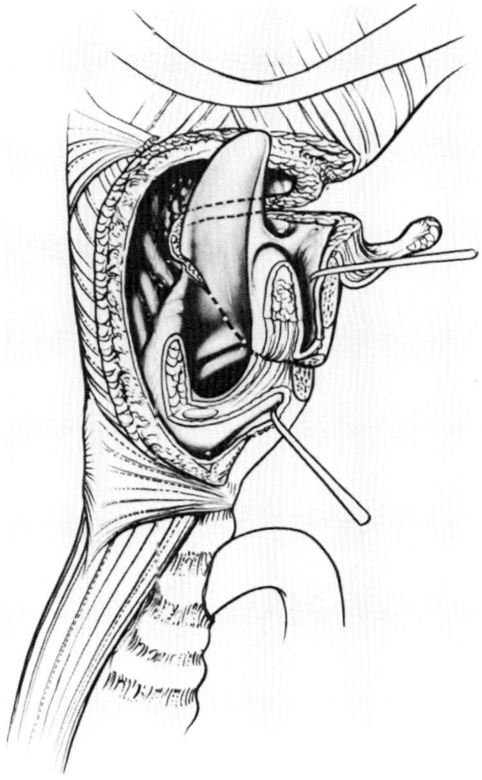

Figure 13–11. Partia pharyngolaryngectomy for pyriform sinus lesion (continued). (From Silver.[23] Reprinted with permission.)

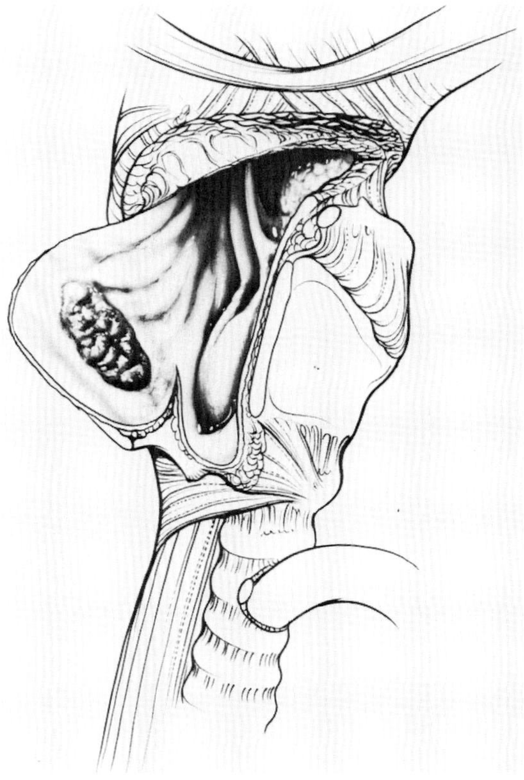

Figure 13–13. Partial pharyngolaryngectomy for posterolateral pharyngeal wall (continued). (From Silver.[23] Reprinted with permission.)

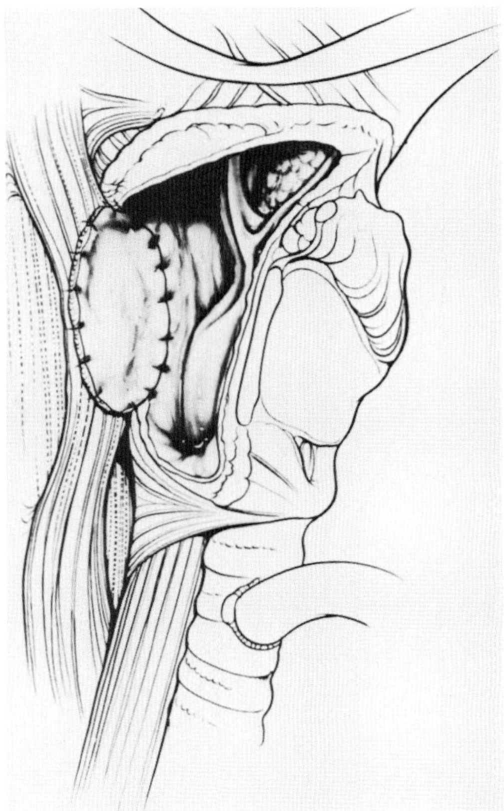

Figure 13–14. Partial pharyngolaryngectomy for posterolateral pharyngeal wall (continued). (From Silver.[23] Reprinted with permission.)

"conservation" operation with attendant chronic aspiration of food and saliva.

The question of relative indications for conservation surgery and radiation therapy and the appropriateness of conservation surgery for salvage of irradiation failure has been left for discussion by other contributors to this volume. With regard to the latter issue, however, it is of importance to recognize the generally accepted maxim that conservation surgery may be employed after radiation failure only for those lesions that were suitable for such resection prior to treatment.

Above all, the patient's chance of cure must not be compromised by an attempt to preserve laryngeal function for a tumor too large for adequate resection by partial laryngectomy. When employed skillfully, for properly selected patients and tumors, conservation surgery affords a most effective and humane method for management of curable laryngeal cancer.

REFFERENCES

1. Bailey BJ. Glottic reconstruction after hemilaryngectomy: bipedicle muscle flap laryngoplasty. Laryngoscope 1975;85:960–77.
2. Som ML, Silver CE. The anterior commissure technique of partial laryngectomy. Arch Otolaryngol 1968;87:42.
3. McNaught RC. Surgical correction of anterior web of the larynx. Laryngoscope 1950;60:264–72.
4. Kirchner J, Som ML. The anterior commissure technique of partial laryngectomy: clinical and laboratory observations. Laryngoscope 1975;85:1308.
5. Sessions DG, Ogura JH, Fried MP. The anterior commissure in glottic carcinoma. Laryngoscope 1975;85:1624–32.
6. Ogura JH, Sessions DG, Spector GJ. Analysis of surgical therapy for epidermoid carcinoma of the laryngeal glottis. Laryngoscope 1975;85:1522–30.
7. Som ML. Cordal cancer with extension to vocal process. Laryngoscope 1975;85:1298–307.
8. Mohr RM, Quenelle DJ, Shumrick DA. Verticofrontolateral laryngectomy. Indications, techniques and results. Arch Otolaryngol 1983;109:384–95.
9. Bauer WC, Lesinski SG, Ogura JH. The significance of positive margins in hemilaryngectomy specimens. Laryngoscope 1975;85:1–13.
10. Leroux-Robert J. A statistical study of 620 laryngeal carcinomas of the glottic region personally operated upon more than five years ago. Laryngoscope 1975;85:1440–52.
11. Skolnik EM, Yee KF, Wheatley MA, et al. Carcinoma of the laryngeal glottis: therapy and end results. Laryngoscope 1975;85:1453–66.
12. Biller H, Ogura J, Pratt L. Hemilaryngectomy for T_2 glottic cancers. Arch Otolaryngol 1971;93:238–43.
13. Kessler DJ, Trapp TK, Calcaterra TC. The treatment of T_3 glottic carcinoma with vertical partial laryngectomy. Arch Otolaryngol Head Neck Surg 1987;113:1196–9.
14. Biller HF, Lawson W. Partial laryngectomy for vocal cord cancer with marked limitation or fixation of the vocal cord. Laryngoscope 1986;96:61–4.
15. Ogura JH, Session DG, Spector GJ. Conservation surgery for epidermoid carcinoma of the supraglottic larynx. Laryngoscope 1975;85:1808–15.
16. Bocca E, Pignataro O, Oldini C. Supraglottic laryngectomy: 30 years of experience. Ann Otol Rhinol Laryngol 1983;92:14–18.
17. Som ML. Conservation surgery for carcinoma of the supraglottis. J Laryngol Otol 1970;84:655–78.
18. Burnstein FD, Calcaterra TC. Supraglottic laryngectomy: series report and analysis of results. Laryngoscope 1985;95:833–6.
19. Maceri DR, Lampe HB, Makielski KH, et al. Conservation laryngeal surgery—a critical analysis. Arch Otolaryngol 1985;111:361–5.
20. Robbins KT, Davidson W, Peters LJ, Goepfert H. Conservation surgery for T_2 and T_3 carcinomas of the supraglottic larynx. Arch Otolaryngol Head Neck Surg 1988;114:421–6.
21. Biller HF, Lawson W. Partial laryngectomy for transglottic cancers. Ann Otol Rhinol Laryngol 1984;93:297–300.
22. Silver CE. Surgical management of neoplasms of the larynx hypopharynx and cervical esophagus. Curr Prob Surg 1977;14(9):1–63.
23. Silver CE. *Surgery for Cancer of the Larynx*. New York: Churchill Livingstone, 1981.

14

Early Carcinoma of the Larynx

Lawrence W. DeSanto, Charles W. Vaughan

We have neither trained nor practiced together. In the late 1970s and early 1980s we were participants in a series of annual courses on "Microscopic Laryngoscopy." At that time, radiation therapy was the generally accepted "treatment of choice" for early cancers of the larynx; in particular, early glottic cancers. As we came to appreciate the precision that resulted from the brilliant light and magnification afforded by "microscopic laryngoscopy," we became aware that the single therapeutic approach of irradiation was overly limited. It ignored the fact that a spectrum of early cancers exists, that the single therapeutic approach creates its own set of new problems, and that new knowledge and technology demand new thinking.

We, from separate ends of the country and from two different types of practices, began and continue to conduct a dialogue and, at times, a debate concerning treatment of early laryngeal cancers. This chapter summarizes our consensus and points out our differences.

The one theme we share enthusiastically is that multiple options exist for the treatment of early (T_1) cancers. We also agree that the T_1 stage includes such a broad range of lesions that there cannot be one treatment that is optimal for every lesion. Management of these growths requires lesion definition, analysis of options, awareness of consequences, communication between patient and physician, estimates of probable outcomes, and precise execution of treatment.

NATURE OF THE DISEASE

The most common early laryngeal cancers are those of the glottis. Early supraglottic cancers are seen but are proportionately far less common in North America than glottic cancer. Most of this discussion will be about early glottic cancer. Glottic cancer differs from supraglottic cancer in that, since voice can be altered by a small growth on the phonating surface of a vocal cord, symptoms occur earlier. The cords are devoid of lymphatics, so neck metastases are not common. We can treat small growths with a low probability of regional or distant metastasis.

End results depend on effectiveness of treatment of the primary lesion. Since few people die from early glottic cancer, issues other than death become more relevant than with other sites in the head and neck. These are, in particular, voice "quality" and a low recurrence rate as a result of successful outcome of initial treatment. Other important factors are the cost of treatment; the patient's occupation, general health, reliability to follow-up, and distance from treatment facility, and, in particular, the patient's preference.

Carcinomas of the larynx are almost always squamous cell cancer. They develop after exposure to carcinogens in tobacco. The carcinogens' effects are dose dependent, additive, irreversible, and require time for expression. If a carcinogen is widely distributed, its effects are widely expressed because all cells exposed to a carcinogen become unhealthy and, given enough time, will become cancerous.[1] The term "field cancerization" is employed by most workers in this area to describe this phenomenon.[2]

Because the process of carcinogenesis is not reversible, an "unhealthy" mucosa is not made healthy when a mass of cancer cells in that field is destroyed or removed, no matter how wide the margin. A patient may be cured of his or her cancer, but, similar to sun-induced skin cancer, if the patient lives long enough, further tobacco-induced cancers can be expected in the diseased mucosa. In addition, radiation therapy cannot sterilize the epithelium or make it "healthy" and prevent further cancerization.[3,4]

DEFINITIONS

An early glottic cancer is defined as one that is limited to a single site within the larynx and has not fixed a vocal cord. A cancer that fixes a vocal cord is not an early cancer. The laryngologic pioneers understood, to a degree, the importance of cordal fixation, although its scientific basis came later with studies of sections of whole larynges. An early primary cancer can occasionally be advanced-stage disease if it has metastasized.

The glottis is made up of the true vocal cords and the anterior and posterior commissures. Unfortunately, there is no agreement on the definition of these structures. Ogura and Mallen[5] defined the glottis as extending to a line 1 cm inferior to the free edge of the vocal cord (but then we have to agree on what the free edge of a curved structure is). Kirchner and Som[6] stated that the cord extends to the superior border of the cricoid cartilage. The International Union Against Cancer (UICC) classification does not define cordal limits at all.[7] The 1988 American Joint Committee for Cancer Staging and End Results Reporting[8] (AJC) made a futive attempt: "The lower boundary [of the glottis] is the horizontal plane 1 cm below the apex of the ventricle." The upper border of the glottis is that same apex of the ventricle. There is no easy way to find the apex of the ventricle in the living person. In Europe, the ventricular surface of the cord is considered a supraglottic structure; in the United States, it remains part of the glottis; and in Canada, it is part of both. Precise definition may not be particularly important when dealing with early cancers. Stell and Morton,[9] for example, reviewed 185 cases staged as T_1 glottic cancer that were treated with appropriate radiation therapy. They were subdivided into those arising from the vocal cords, those parts of the glottis not included in the UICC definition, and those affecting the upper and lower surfaces of the cords where classification may be in doubt. The outcome of each group was similar. This suggests that our concern for precision is unimportant in the early stage. These findings do suggest that the T_2 classification may overestimate a tumor's potential if ventricular and minimal involvement below the cordal edge result in a tumor being staged as T_2.

The anterior boundary of the cords is the anterior commissure. Posteriorly, the boundary is the posterior commissure, including the part of the arytenoid between the cordal muscle and the posterior commissure (even though the arytenoids are specifically defined as part of the supraglottis in the AJC system). Much attention, but not much importance, is given in the definition of the anterior commissure as to whether it is a plane or a point.

An early glottic cancer (T_1) is defined as that tumor that is confined to one or both true vocal cords with normal cordal mobility (the concept of partial mobility is not considered in either the AJC or UICC systems). The T_1 classification implies that the tumor has not invaded, or has minimally invaded, the underlying muscle or conus elasticus and thus does not interfere with mobility or expose the lymphatics. Kirchner[10] states that "[T_1 lesions] associated with normal vocal cord mobility do not penetrate the conus elasticus, nor do they invade the underlying thyro-arytenoid muscle." Kirchner's collection of cordectomy, hemilaryngectomy, and laryngectomy specimens studied by whole-organ serial sections contained 12 T_1 glottic cancers, half verrucous tumors. None penetrated the conus or vocal ligament. Vaughan's unpublished experience with transoral excisional biopsy specimens is different. As many as 20% of T_1 glottic cancers with normal cordal mobility invaded the conus or beyond. These cancers have the potential to enter the lymphatic system and carry the risk of cervical metastasis. Theoretically, a cancer that has penetrated to the conus elasticus and beyond, and yet not affected cordal mobility, has the biologic potential of a cancer that has fixed or nearly fixed a cord. In contrast, a cancer that is exophytic can produce cordal fixation by its bulk, and thus be recorded as a T_3 cancer. With no invasion, such a lesion has the biologic potential of a more obvious T_1 lesion.

The point is that the glottic T_1 stage encompasses a wide spectrum of tumors that may vary from tiny to rather large. We prefer to think that depth of invasion and, to a lesser degree, size are more important than are imperfect estimates of site of origin. Also, we believe that treatment planning rests more on clinical and histopathologic assessment than on stage definition.

If all T_1 glottic cancers are to be managed with a single modality of therapy, these subtleties are not important. On the other hand, we believe that the previously described properties of various T_1 glottic cancers are of importance and permit considerable precision in selecting treatment options. In our opinion, uniform therapy for each point on the spectrum can result in overtreatment of some and undertreatment of others.

GROWTH OF EARLY LESIONS

One concept of how cancers grow is that for some reason a single cell breaks free of the organism's reproductive restraints and expands concentrically until some biologic barrier deflects the growth pattern. This is probably simplistic. More realistic is the idea of a field dedifferentiation from orderly to uncontrolled growth. The mental image of a rusting part of an automobile comes to mind. The first rust bubble is only the initial manifestation of field decay.

Most glottic cancers are initially visible on the cord itself rather than at the commissures. The logic of this is that the cord makes up the major part of the glottis, whereas the anterior commissure is smaller. Cancers first seen posteriorly are rare, although this may be related to the fact that anterior cord lesions cause early symptoms, whereas more posteriorly situated tumors must be larger in order to be noticed.

If a cord is mobile and a cancer involves the ventricular surface of the cord or the undersurface, it is still considered cordal and treated as such.

The distinction between normal cord motion, impaired motion, and fixation is not always easy. In some instances there will be disagreement within a group of observers or the same observer will make different judgments at different times. When there is doubt about mobility, the only reliable determinant that a lesion is biologically a T_1 cancer or a higher stage is histologic data about muscle invasion. The reason for this is that the surgical options are distinctly different for mobile cord lesions and fixed cord lesions and the intellectual machinations that accompany the concept of "partial fixation" or "partial mobility" invite treatment planning errors.

BASIS OF TREATMENT PLANNING

Whole larynx section studies form the infrastructure for treatment planning for cancers on mobile cords. Kirchner and Som[6] observed that true cord fixation indicates deep invasion. They correlated survival with whole larynx section studies and observed that anterior subglottic extension is less of an impediment to conservation surgery than posterior subglottic extension.

The risk of conservation surgery in the fixed cord situation is explained by Kirchner's studies. With cordal fixation, cancer can extend beyond the larynx by growing around the lower end of the thyroid cartilage, invading cartilage, or spreading subglottically by microscopic invasion.

EVALUATION OF THE PATIENT

Mirrors and Scopes

Evaluation begins in the office with the old diagnostic tools of indirect visualization. The mirrors, flexible fiberoptic instrument, and rigid laryngoscopic telescope are all used as needed. For obvious superficial growths, such as the one depicted in Figure 14–1, office instruments alone will permit an option discussion prior to confirming the impression by excisional biopsy. If a single lesion is easily seen, both cords visualized from front to back, and the cord is unequivocally mobile, the lesion will be histologically confirmed as a true T_1 cancer.

It must be appreciated that the naked eye cannot always make a histologic diagnosis that differentiates an invasive cancer from other epithelial disorders, such as dysplasia, keratosis, atypia, and the myriad other terms used to describe epithelial changes that are not clearly invasive cancer.

Video Laryngoscopy

Video laryngoscopy is a new concept that will find its place in diagnosis and treatment planning. One of us (L.W.D.) uses video recordings primarily for patient education during the treatment planning and option discussion. It is helpful to be able to share the concept of the lesion with the patient by using the video.

Panendoscopy

Some laryngologists (including C.W.V.) believe that microlaryngoscopy and panendoscopy are needed in all patients with early cancers. L.W.D. does not perform panendoscopy in all cases. Careful office examination of the entire upper aerodigestive system with the office tools as well as selective bronchoscopy and esophagoscopy seems adequate. With office endoscopy more available, the old concept of rigid panendoscopy is being replaced by newer technology.

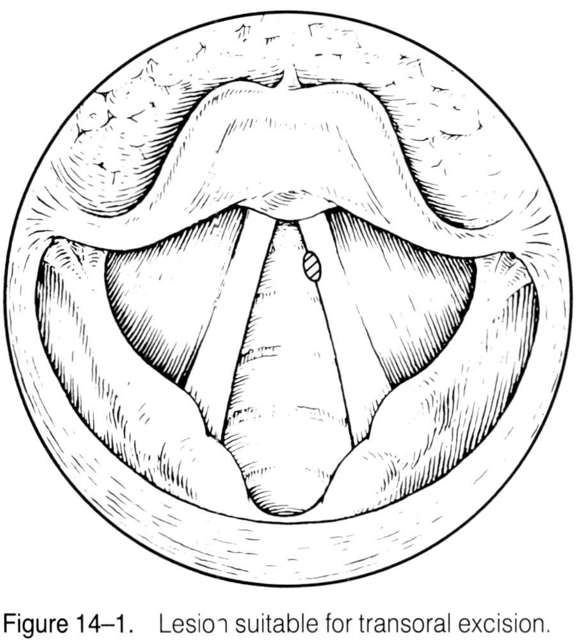

Figure 14–1. Lesion suitable for transoral excision.

Microscopic Laryngoscopy and Excisional Biopsy

The notion underlying "microscopic" laryngoscopy as a diagnostic procedure is that the cords are examined with 6×, 10×, and 20× magnification and the examiner can directly visualize surface limits and satellite cancer, palpate the cords with instruments, evert the cords or view the subglottis with telescopes, and then perform what one hopes will be an excisional biopsy. This concept, popularized by Vaughan and colleagues,[11] shifts some responsibility for margin control from the pathologist to the laryngologist. An excisional biopsy is attempted by grasping the cord with a cup forceps and placing tension on the cord by pulling it toward the midline. Limiting cuts are then made anteriorly and posteriorly and the tumor, with an appropriate amount of underlying cord, is separated from the patient. The carbon dioxide laser is ideal for this procedure but it can be accomplished with scalpel, microscissors, or even cutting cautery. Vaughan then recommends that the cordal wound be examined under high magnification to look for residual cancer. With 20× magnification, it is thought that cancer aggregates as small as 100 cells can be seen and confirmed with frozen sections of biopsy specimens. Further excisions can then be effected as necessary, stopping only when all tumor has been removed, or it is determined that all cannot be removed endoscopically. The excised specimen is then oriented and submitted to the pathologist so all margins can be studied with fixed pathologic sections. This approach considers most early glottic cancers suitable for endoscopic excisional biopsy; those where the margins are not free of tumor are re-treated with radiation, whereas those with free margins are followed without further treatment.

A variation of this approach, favored by L.W.D., is to limit excisional biopsy to only that subgroup of patients in whom excisional biopsy alone is predicted to be adequate for treatment on the basis of office and laryngoscopic examination. That subgroup has been defined by laryngologists, experienced in endoscopic surgery for cancer,[12–14] as those small and superficial cancers located on the free edge of a clearly mobile cord. The anterior and posterior commissures must be uninvolved and precise three-dimensional exposure must be attained through the laryngoscope. Cancers that do not meet these standards are simply biopsied and then are treated either with irradiation or partial vertical operation; the choice is based on other criteria. The adequacy of the excisional biopsy is determined at frozen section study and confirmed by fixed sections. Limiting the procedure to only those patients for whom success is almost certainly assured has been demonstrated by the reports of practitioners of this approach to verify safety.

TREATMENT OPTIONS FOR EARLY GLOTTIC CANCER

As implied by the previous discussion, we believe there are three options for treating early glottic cancer: (1) endoscopic removal, already mentioned; (2) some form of partial vertical laryngectomy; and (3) external fractionated radiation. Each has its place and no option exists to the exclusion of another. Advocacy of a single option as exclusive treatment for all early glottic cancers is controversial.[15]

Endoscopic Surgery

Endoscopic destruction or removal of selected early cancers is an alternative as old as laryngology itself. Frankel was cited by Okada[16] as a proponent of the concept before the beginning of this century. The surgeons of the early days rejected the concept because they thought it to be uncertain and they lacked the instruments and experience of laryngoscopy. Their oncologic concepts were derived from abdominal surgery and the idea of treating cancer through a tubular instrument was unacceptable. Lynch,[13] New and Dorton,[14] and Lillie and DeSanto[12] carried the concept through this century, although in many quarters the idea is not accepted, is unappreciated, or rejected as unsound. Modern instrumentation with improved laryngoscopes, illumination, magnification, and surgical lasers have enhanced our ability to treat selected early cancers endoscopically. The key to this treatment option, however, is in the premise that there is a range of severity of the early growths and with selection some can be destroyed or removed through the laryngoscope.

This concept has been vitalized by the experience of Stutsman and McGavran,[17] Vaughan et al,[18] and Lillie and DeSanto.[12] Each has recognized that some patients who undergo open cordectomy after laryngoscopic biopsy do not have cancer in the cordectomy specimen because it had been removed by the biopsy. The percentage of such cases may be as high as 20%. It is likely that a similar percentage of patients who undergo radiation therapy after biopsy do not have cancer at the beginning of their treatments, for the same reason. These patients are usually cured.

In over 200 suitable lesions treated by L.W.D. and colleagues, of which 100 were invasive and the rest in situ cancer, there were only six local recurrences and each of these was re-treated through the laryngoscope. Two patients required total laryngectomy for recurrent disease years later. There were no deaths. The procedure can often be performed on an outpatient basis or with only 1 day in the hospital. Tracheotomy is not needed.[19] The term "stripping" has been used for this type of treatment, but that is imprecise. It implies that the biopsy is the treatment. What is actually done can vary from surface electrocautery to surface laser destruction or actual transoral cordectomy. What is done depends on the lesion, but it is more than "stripping."

As already noted, there are two attitudes toward the endoscopic approach. At the Mayo Clinic, this modality is employed in precise situations, depending on lesion size, location, and exposure as well as pathologic control; the decision is made by a surgical pathologist in the operating area who is experienced in quick frozen section management of margins.

The other approach, popularized by Vaughan and the Boston group,[11,18] is the endoscopic excisional biopsy concept. Here, a lesion on a mobile cord undergoes excisional biopsy using the laser, and the specimen is oriented and submitted to the pathologist for microscopic study. If the margins are clear, that is all that is done. If the margins are not clear, something else (usually radiation) is added. The differences in these approaches are not great and hinge more on how one uses the pathologist (frozen section versus fixed section) than on any conceptual difference. Our selective approach implies that by enforcing rigid selection criteria one can anticipate the pathologist's confirmation of free margins by restricting the use of the technique to small midcordal cancers. The second difference is that our group will often proceed to an open operation if the margins are insecure or exposure is inadequate or they will simply obtain a biopsy specimen and proceed to radiation therapy in this situation if the patient so prefers.

Partial Laryngectomy for Early Glottic Cancer

There are several controversial issues regarding partial operations for early glottic cancer.[19] Are the operations obsolete, and if they are not, which procedures are appropriate? In reading the literature one finds that the preponderance of articles on early glottic cancers involves radiation therapy. There are a few references to conservation operations and they generally conclude that partial operations do relieve most patients of the cancer.[10,18,20,21] The effectiveness of such basic operations as the "fissure" in eliminating properly selected cancers has been known for many years.[22] The procedure has stood the test of time and the indications are clearly defined. The modifications and refinements are easy to understand. Some think a procedure as old as the laryngofissure and cordectomy is obsolete. We think differently. We fail to see how such a basic procedure can be obsolete. In our practices the laryngofissure with cordectomy is the main open operation for cordal cancer. The appropriate lesion is the cancer on a mobile cord. The procedure can be used for small growths that cannot be removed endoscopically because of limitation of laryngoscopic exposure as well as for larger tumors that extend from the anterior commissure to the vocal process of the arytenoid.

The concept of cordal mobility is fundamental to a safe cordectomy. If the affected cord moves, cordectomy is feasible. Variations are appropriate for cancers that involve the anterior commissure. The variations are not different operations but rather simple technical adjustments to accommodate the removal of specific cancers. Cancers with fixed vocal cords cannot be safely removed by laryngofissure. These lesions have extended laterally, down or up, to a degree that renders the fissure operation inadequate for complete removal.

Neel et al[23] documented our recent experience with laryngofissure and cordectomy. They noted four local recurrences in 188 patients; three of these were for surgical salvage of a radiation failure. Two patients died of cancer. We continue to look at this old operation as a reference standard to which other treatments should be compared in all dimensions of the problem, including cost as well as cure rates. We do not believe it is the treatment of choice for every early cancer, but it is one option.

The laryngofissure operation removes only soft tissue from within the larynx. There are variations (Figs. 14–1 to 14–5). The anterior commissure modification takes a small vertical strip of thyroid cartilage in the front. Multiple descriptive terms have been applied to what to us are simple variations of a basic operation. Bailey and Biller's text talks about three basic types of partial vertical operations and several modifications to

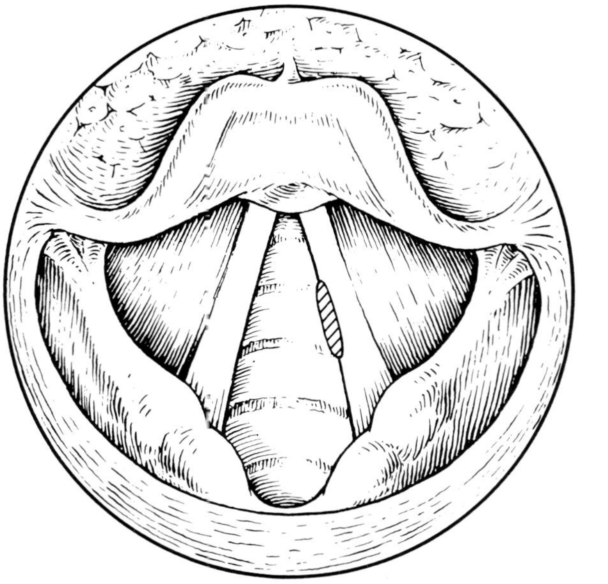

Figure 14–2. Even larger lesions can be accommodated by this approach.

these.[24] These variations should be understood as part of the basic infrastructure, but to think of these modifications as distinct operations seems unduly restrictive. If there is cord mobility in a patient with a vocal cord cancer, then some sort of partial operation is possible, with the laryngofissure-cordectomy the most often used operation. Any variation is determined by the situation and with the pathologist's assistance.

Other Observations on the Laryngofissure

There are articles in the literature that define size limitations for partial vertical operations, such as the laryngofissure and cordectomy: "laryngofissure. . .is limited to a carcinoma of 1 to 5 mm in size on the free edge of the membranous vocal cord at its middle one-third" and "subglottic extension must not exceed 2 to 3 mm" for the operations that remove some thyroid cartilage.[24] These guidelines are well-intended but ignore the whole section infrastructure of conservation surgery. They seem to us to be unnecessarily restrictive. If the meaning of cord mobility is kept in mind and a skilled pathologist is used to control margins, we belived a much more flexible approach is possible and the scope of the laryngofissure can be broadened to include cancers along the entire cord, cancers that go onto the ventricular surface or below to the subglottic cord, and even cancers up to and including the commissure. The entire true, false, and subglottic mucosa is removable via the laryngofissure. In cases with anterior commissure involvement, the operation can be adapted to accommodate that presentation without doing a formal hemilaryngectomy.

Hemilaryngectomy

There is another operation called the vertical hemilaryngectomy, which by definition includes one thyroid cartilage ala (Fig. 14–6). This operation really has little place in the treatment of the ordinary early glottic cancer because there is little oncologic benefit from removing a thyroid cartilage ala in the presence of cordal mobility. Voice is poorer than after the fissure operation and stenosis is possible. The hemilaryngectomy seems occasionally suited for carefully selected glottic cancers of a more advanced stage with some cordal fixation and the rare instance in which the cord is mobile but the cancer extends back onto the arytenoid. In this situation the posterior vertical cut on the thyroid cartilage permits the cord to "pop" forward by flattening out the pyriform sinus and allows a safer mucosal cut behind the arytenoid. The hemilaryngectomy operation for cancers of mobile cords gives the extra margin where it is least needed—laterally. Cancer simply cannot spread too far laterally and still leave a mobile cord. Some references to hemilaryngectomy in the literature may actually be using that term synonymously with laryngofissure, but that is not precise.

Reconstruction After Partial Vertical Operations

After laryngofissure and cordectomy, we do not perform any reconstruction other than attempting to pull the remaining cord forward to whatever will be the anterior commissure. The reconstruction with muscle pedicles or flaps may actually handicap voice quality and it certainly makes follow-up more

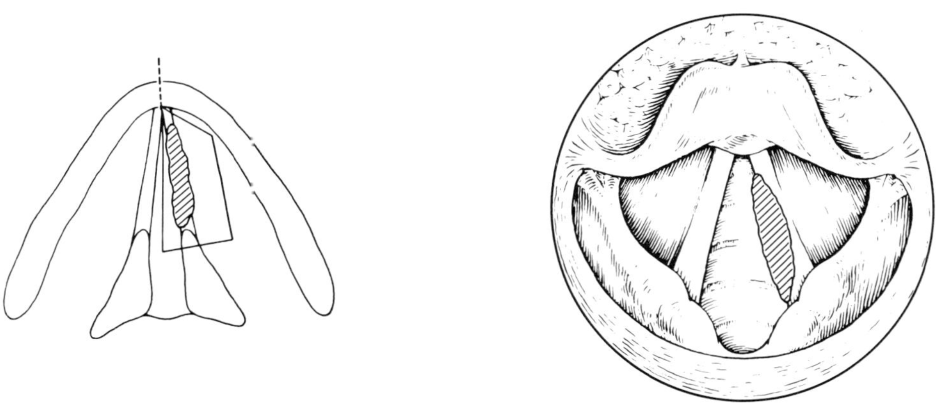

Figure 14–3. The basic laryngofissure for open cordectomy. The "usual" operation.

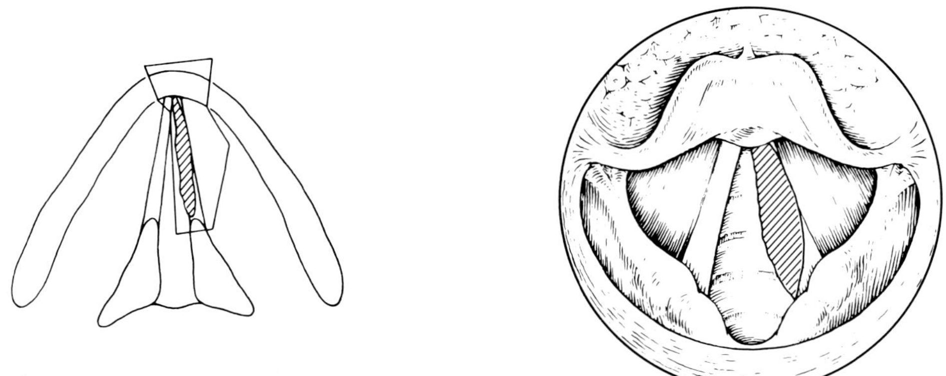

A

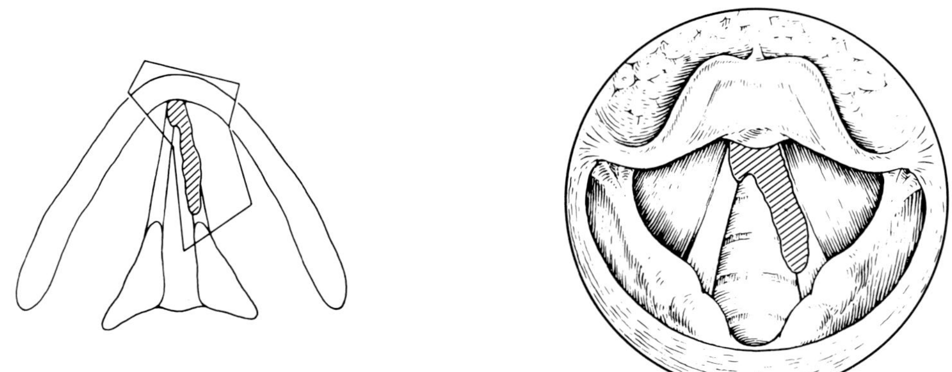

B

Figure 14–4. A and B: The so-called "frontal lateral" operation as a variation of the basic operation for tumor that extends to anterior commissure.

complicated. Within 3 to 6 months after cordectomy, the surgical wound fills in and epithelializes. After a year or so, it is often difficult to be sure which cord was removed. Voice is usually altered. The degree of alteration varies from a soft breathy voice to a near-normal voice. Few of our patients demand a perfect voice and those who do are not interested in a surgical option. One of the advantages of the laryngofissure-cordectomy is that vocal quality is relatively predictable and usually satisfactory compared with the hemilaryngectomy or fissure with reconstruction, without oncologic compromise, if the basic criteria are enforced. It is a simple procedure, without flaps or cartilage alterations. Convalescence is rapid, with decannulation achieved within a few days.

Nearly 70% of L.W.D.'s patients, when offered the choice of radiation therapy or cordectomy, with an implied altered voice, select the operation after they are presented with the options and their consequences. This preference may be a regional phenomenon.

Radiation for Early Glottic Cancer

Radiation therapy for early glottic cancer is an acceptable option. When the procedure is successful, the early voice quality is usually satisfactory. Some have questioned the long-term voice quality in the overall population treated because of either laryngeal edema or late tissue atrophy. We recommend

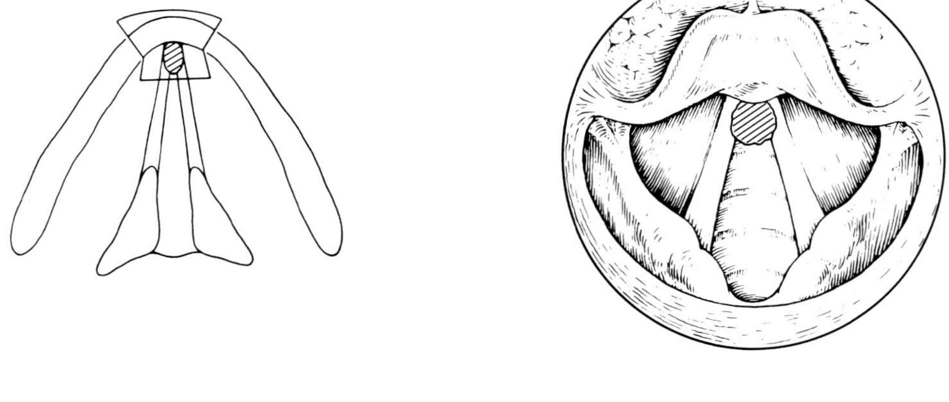

Figure 14–5. The anterior commissure variation for those rare tumors that start and stay at the anterior commissure.

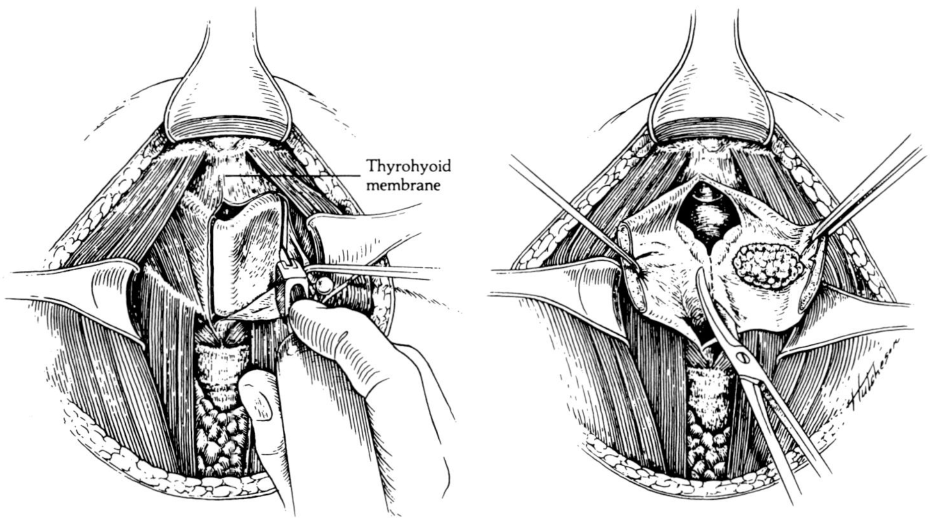

Figure 14–6. Hemilaryngectomy. This differs from the basic operations in that the entire thyroid ala is removed. This operation is rarely used for early glottic cancer. (From DeSanto.[35] Reprinted with permission.)

radiation therapy for some early glottic cancers but not for all of them. The patients whose growths can be removed transorally at biopsy are not treated with radiation. To do so would expose the patient to the consequences and cost of radiation without providing any benefit. These cancers have already been removed at the biopsy before the start of radiation therapy. The fact that some patients who do not have cancer are being given radiation therapy is not fully appreciated.

Mendenhall et al,[15] in making their case for radiation for all early glottic cancers, cite 140 (50%) of 279 early lesions treated by radiation as small lesions (less than 15 mm), of which 130 were cured. The advocates of excisional biopsy point out that most of these could be treated endoscopically and some would not have cancer at the start of radiation because the cancer was removed with the biopsy specimen.

The issue of cost is also raised when comparing treatment options; radiation is cited as a less expensive option compared to partial vertical laryngectomy. Vaughan et al[11] did a cost comparison in 1985 dollars of the various options at the teaching hospitals in Boston. Factoring in the cost of biopsy, which all patients require, and including loss of time, but neglecting cost of lodging for out-of-town patients, they found the cost of radiation and open surgery to be about the same, whereas excisional biopsy was considerably less expensive.

Voice quality is the final comparison. Little of scientific value has ever been done to compare voice quality overall between the treatment options. One is left with subjective feelings and personal biases. Our impression after treating a large group of patients using all options is that none of the options leaves a "perfect" voice over the long term. The voice after either form of cordectomy varies from near-normal in a small percentage to a poor voice in another group of about 20%. The rest of the voices are somewhere between "normal" and "poor" and none are perfect. Our bias is that the person with vocal cord cancer, who insists on an unaltered voice, is asking more than our technology can deliver. He is best handled by a review of reasonable options and allowed to select his own treatment.

One of the problems with voice comparison is the confusion that exists between the place for hemilaryngectomy versus simple cordectomy. A true hemilaryngectomy alters the voice more than a simple cordectomy in most patients. It is our contention that hemilaryngectomy represents excessive treatment for the T_1 glottic cancer. If a cancer needs, for oncologic purposes, a hemilaryngectomy, then it is not a T_1 glottic cancer.

Other Considerations About Radiation Versus Surgery

A cancer that develops in an epithelial field such as the larynx is the first manifestation of a field disease. Approximately 10 to 15% of patients with glottic cancer who survive the first treatment will develop a second upper aerodigestive system cancer. The treatment of the first cancer should not make the later treatment more difficult or preclude options for the second treatment when probability of survival of the first is high. Because we know that most patients treated for early vocal cord cancers will be cured, the possibilities of later disease must be considered, and our options should not be exhausted.

Age becomes a variable to be considered in choosing radiation therapy or open surgery. For example, a 40-year-old with early glottic cancer might gain a greater long-term benefit from laryngofissure than radiation, not because excision would be more likely successful, but because he has many years to live and can develop another cancer for which radiation might be a preferred option. An epithelial field is not made healthier by radiation, and a long-range view of the field disease is necessary. An older patient, on the other hand, might have radiation recommended because he would not face the same risk of a second cancer as a younger patient.

On the basis of these principles for treatment selection, approximately 25% of L.W.D.'s patients with early glottic cancer receive external fractionated radiation, 20% have transoral treatment, and the remainder undergo some form of partial laryngectomy. C.W.V. finds that up to 50% of his patients can be treated with transoral excision and the rest are usually treated with radiation. In many instances, the exact choice is made by the patient after a careful review of the options.

Control Bias

The three major options—radiation therapy, partial vertical laryngectomy (fissure and cordectomy), and transoral excision—produce control rates that are said to be similar.[15] We believe there is some statistical skewing that is inherent because of staging errors. Some lesions stated as T_1 invade muscle or the conus elasticus and are actually biologic T_3 cancers.

A biopsy is implied in all patients treated with radiation therapy and some of the lesions so treated are small enough to have been removed by the biopsy. In the end, the biologic T_3 lesions undertreated by radiation therapy are probably balanced by the group without tumor that are overtreated. Cordectomy produces a surgical specimen for pathologic examination, so staging is more precise. Control rates after excisional biopsy should be reliable because an accurate assessment of tumor extent, and therefore accurate staging, is obtained by this option.

In our opinion, the only valid way to compare results of surgery and irradiation is in initial success rate. Lumping together first treatment plus salvage treatment and reporting only patients alive at the end of some period is inappropriate for early glottic cancer.

It should not be surprising that the control rate of T_1 glottic cancer, adequately treated by any means, is not 100%, when one considers that all of the glottic mucosa has been altered by exposure to the carcinogens in tobacco, but all is not removed. The development, in time, of further cancers in mucous membrane adjacent to areas already treated is the expected norm.[25]

Other Considerations

Because the reported control rates are about the same for treatment by radiation therapy, by cordectomy, and by excisional biopsy, the choices among them should be based on other criteria; many have already been discussed.

NEEDS AND ABILITIES OF THE PATIENT

All patients differ in their attitudes toward themselves, their disease, and life in general. This factor and medical problems—especially recent myocardial infarction, the presence of mental deterioration, general health and ability to undergo any treatment, and some abnormalities of body configuration—can make some treatment options impossible to carry out. Distance from the treatment facility, the amount of time the patient is willing to give to treatment, his or her occupation, and his or her preference are other variables to consider.

PATIENT BIAS

Many patients are quite sophisticated with regard to medical matters. They may have read or heard about others with similar cancers, how they were treated, and their outcomes. They may have developed strong opinions on the form their own treatment should take. It is wise to respect such bias when possible and to communicate clearly why such bias cannot be respected when the patient's attitude is incompatible with the treatment planner's perception of the problem.

Some patients have had earlier cancers successfully treated. The methods used and the results (morbidity and presence or absence of tumor) influence present options.

The ability of a physician to provide each option with equal skill is rare. The most skillfully used option usually is the most successful. The patient deserves to know the physician's biases too.

INTRAEPITHELIAL NEOPLASIA

The diagnosis of intraepithelial neoplasia or carcinoma in situ of the larynx is recognized, but there is a lack of consensus on the frequency of this condition, its oncologic implications, and the histologic criteria for the diagnosis of carcinoma in situ and other precursor conditions.

It is useful to think of the early epithelial changes as a spectrum of epithelial response to irritants. The most benign end of the spectrum is surface keratosis with orderly epithelial maturation and absence of cellular atypia. This change is innocent and probably reversible. Next are mucosal changes with intraepithelial cellular abnormalities of variable nuclear size and staining and associated cellular maturation abnormalities that represent dysplasia. Dysplasia can be mild, moderate, or severe. The distinctions are based on individual judgment. Severe epithelial changes with surface keratinization and cellular atypia probably represent the transition zone to true neoplasia. Crissman and Fu[26] demonstrated that these epithelial changes are associated with aneuploid DNA content consistent with neoplastic transformation. The structural abnormalities within the epithelium include individual cell keratin (dyskeratosis) and, rarely, extracellular keratin pearls, cellular atypia with nuclear variations, typical and atypical mitosis, and a loss of the orderly pattern of nuclei. There is an increase in number of nuclei and the nuclear arrangement is more random.

Carcinoma in situ is the next step on the spectrum. There is no evidence of epithelial differentiation, no surface keratinization, and mitosis at all levels of epithelium. The basal layer of cells is no longer seen but the basement membrane is not breached. This finding in the larynx is rarely found alone but can be seen in association with severe keratosis and microinvasive or grossly invasive cancer. Whether all cancers go through an in situ phase or whether invasive cancer can arise de novo is not known. That the various pathologic states can coexist, that they represent a larynx at risk for more serious problems, and that the entire field is at risk is undisputed.

Microinvasive cancer is the next region of the spectrum. The definition of microinvasive cancer is a focus of invasive cancer arising from the surface or submucosal gland epithelium. Penetration of the basement membrane by infiltrating carcinoma represents the best criterion for defining early invasive cancer.[27] Much of what is known about microinvasive cancer and in situ cancer comes from gynecologic pathology research.

The clinical implications of the keratosis-dysplasia-in situ-microinvasive spectrum are not settled. There do seem to be some useful principles. One of these is the concept of a field disorder and the implication that when one treats a segment of that field for a surface lesion the treatment should not harm the rest of the field, the treatment should not preclude further treatment, and the treatment of the abnormality should be effective for the part treated. The implication of this principle is that unless the epithelial degradation is reversible by elimination of the noxious stimuli, then the field will be at risk as long as the patient lives or the larynx is in place.

The treatments used for what is called in situ or microinvasive cancer are radiation and endolaryngeal removal or destruction. Doyle and Flores[28] championed the use of radiation for so-called in situ cancer and reported good results with few recurrences. The problem with radiation for these early epithelial changes is that a biopsy precedes the radiation and much, most, or all of the growth may be removed with the biopsy specimen so the radiation is redundant. The other concern is that the radiation cannot discriminate between the diseased epithelium and the rest. Another unhealthy stimulus applied to an already sick epithelium for a nonfatal condition is a short-term expedient that is a long-term threat. Whether radiation cures or does not cure in situ or microinvasive cancer is not the issue. Radiation seems excessive and potentially harmful.

The conceptual comparison of the laryngeal dysplasia-microinvasive cancer spectrum to oral cavity malignant and premalignant lesions is useful. A multicentric oral cancer syndrome is well-recognized. Small superficial lesions that vary in histologic appearance from dysplasia to early invasive cancer are treated, but radical excision or radical radiation is not usually employed. Rather, the lesions are selectively destroyed as they are discovered, with full awareness that treating one lesion will not prevent the next nor will it make the epithelial field healthier. As much is done with whatever destructive tool as seems best. Some lesions are excised, some are vaporized with a laser, a few are frozen, and others are desiccated with electrocautery. Vigilant follow-up is pursued in recognition of the field nature of the problem. These same options are used in the larynx. Selective laser destruction is used today because it is technically easy. Before the laser was available, electrocautery did just as adequate a job. The tool is less important than the concept that intraepithelial premalignant or early malignant lesions can be just as successfully treated in the larynx as in the oral cavity by selective complete destruction or removal. Our review of 200 early lesions called microinvasive in situ carcinoma (not atypia or dysplasia) found no deaths, six recurrences, and two lost larynges over a 20-year period by using endoscopic removal or destruction only.[12] Others have reported similar results.[7]

Is it really important what words the pathologists use to classify these dysplasias and early cancers? *There is no good evidence that such semantics are of importance.* Completely removed or destroyed dysplasia or atypia is no more likely to cause the patient harm than a lesion of the same location and size called carcinoma in situ that is likewise adequately treated. The use of the term "carcinoma" with the in situ lesions might imply a more ominous condition than actually exists. The gynecologist's term "intraepithelial neoplasia" might be more descriptive without the implications attached to the words "cancer" and "carcinoma."

EARLY SUPRAGLOTTIC CANCER

The Problem

Early supraglottic cancer is a different problem from glottic cancer in several ways. Diagnosis is more difficult because symptoms are not obvious. Only vague throat discomfort or otalgia may occur, or the patient may be asymptomatic. Because of their tendency to invade the preepiglottic space, supraglottic cancers have a third dimension that is invisible at laryngoscopy so that an apparently early lesion may be more advanced than it appears.[29] The third dimension is anterior to the preepiglottic space.[29] Lymph node metastases occur in approximately 20% of T_1 and 30% of T_2 primary cancers.[30]

Treatment Options

There are four options for treating early supraglottic cancers: (1) supraglottic laryngectomy, (2) total laryngectomy, (3) radical radiation for cure with surgical salvage, or (4) the near-total laryngectomy.

Supraglottic laryngectomy is an oncologically valid treatment supported by studies of sections of whole larynx, with a few exceptions such as high-grade tumors.[29] The local recurrence rate, less than 2%, is comparable to that after total laryngectomy.[30,31] The operation has been tested over time. The surgical block includes the hidden third dimension. Voice quality is usually good. The operation seems an ideal way to treat early supraglottic cancers.

Unfortunately, not every patient can tolerate the operation. Elderly and debilitated patients and those with poor pulmonary function fare poorly because of chronic aspiration. In these situations another option is needed. Total laryngectomy is better tolerated by these patients because separation of the respiratory system from the upper digestive system makes recovery more likely. There appears here to be a place for the so-called near-total laryngectomy as a compromise when the patient is physiologically unsuited for the supraglottic operation. The compromise accepts a permanent tracheotomy but keeps a small internal, lung-powered shunt between the pulmonary air source and the gullet for phonation. The precise place for this in-between option is not a settled issue nor are the local control rates or failures caused by aspiration settled. L.W.D. has employed this procedure effectively for treatment of supraglottic carcinoma.[32]

The radiate and watch option is a controversial subject.[30] This concept is supported mostly by those who are uncomfortable or unfamiliar with the supraglottic partial and near-total options. There is no doubt that some patients can be cured of T_1 and T_2 supraglottic cancers and keep their larynx. The big problem is that there is much less predictability compared with early glottic cancers because staging is not precise. The hidden third dimension and the tangential laryngoscopic view of supraglottic cancers make precise staging difficult. Computed tomographic scanning does not give microscopic information. Epiglottic cancers may invade cartilage quickly and may be protected there from otherwise lethal radiation. The issue today is: are we saving larynges or are we losing lives by radiating early supraglottic cancers? A secondary question is: is it wise to treat four, five, or even seven people twice (those that fail) to save three, four, or even seven out of ten larynges?

It would be easier to endorse the radiate and watch concept if the salvage effort could be a supraglottic partial operation or even the near-total option. The reality is that recurrence is difficult to detect after radiation and the true nature of the recurrence is often appreciated only with the onset of cordal fixation or airway obstruction. Even when the lesion is detected early, the less than total operations become oncologically unsafe and practically dangerous because of healing problems, cartilage necrosis, and stenosis.

We are afraid that patients who accept the radiate and watch option in an effort to avoid an operation or to save a glottic voice are substituting hope of an improbable event for reality. We think more larynges and perhaps lives are lost than should be with this approach.*

Some early cancers on the free edge of the epiglottis can be safely excised through the laryngoscope. Care must be taken in the selection of the endoscopic approach for supraglottic cancer. Microscopic pathologic clearance must be certain.

THE NECK IN EARLY CANCER

With early glottic cancer, the risk of neck metastasis is small and the need to treat the neck infrequent. This is not controversial. The few early glottic cancers that metastasize are probably best treated as the situation arises. Any elective or "prophylactic" treatment to the neck, when the probability of metastasis is less than 10% or even 20%, is excessive.

The problem of neck metastasis in early supraglottic cancer is real and is perhaps the major unsolved issue in the management of cancer of the larynx. The problem is multiplied because both sides of the neck are at risk.

Scenarios of Neck Presentation in Supraglottic Cancer

There are four scenarios that exist for the neck with early supraglottic cancer: (1) Both sides of the neck are uninvolved by palpation; (2) one side of the neck has palpable nodes suspicious for metastatic cancer and that side is the side of the primary cancer if there is a prominent side; (3) both sides of the neck have palpable nodes that are suspicious for cancer; and (4) the side opposite the primary lesion has palpable nodes suspicious for cancer.

The clinical situation determines the options. In the first scenario the options are to do nothing to either side of the neck, or to do something to one side (but which side?). The second scenario mandates doing something to the suspect side and then making a decision about the other. The third and fourth scenarios mandate treating both sides of the neck.

We recognize that elective treatment in the first scenario, whether radiation or neck dissection, delivered to the pathologically negative neck is of no oncologic benefit to the patient. The information acquired from histologic evaluation of the neck node specimen is of value in staging and prognostication; thus, dissection of a pathologically negative neck should not be considered an unnecessary procedure.

We usually elect to perform neck dissection in early supraglottic cancer, except for small tumors high on the suprahyoid epiglottis. We ask the pathologist to screen the nodes while we do the supraglottic resection or laryngectomy or near-total operation and then we make a decision about the other side of the neck. If the screening shows no metastasis, the contralateral side is not dissected; if positive, then bilateral dissections may be performed, particularly if the primary tumor traverses the midline. The issue of what kind of dissection, as well as other controversies regarding management of the neck, are beyond the scope of this discussion.

The option of simply waiting to see if metastases develop in the clinically negative neck is attractive when one realizes that in 70 to 80% of the patients nothing will happen. Bocca et al[33] have been interested in the fate of those who do develop a delayed metastasis in an untreated neck, as have we.[34] Bocca et al estimate about a 20% attrition in survival probability in those patients who have delayed neck metastasis treated by neck dissection. We agree with that estimate. Death in this subgroup is caused both by cervical disease as well as a higher incidence of distant metastasis. For those reasons, we prefer elective neck treatment to at least one side of the neck in all but the early cancers high on the epiglottis. The treatment is usually a neck dissection with preservation of the accessory nerve. Elective radiation therapy of the neck in a patient with surgically treated cancer is, in our opinion, unnecessary.

CONCLUSIONS

The management of early cancer of the larynx requires option analysis, consequence communication, probability estimates, and treatment execution. These actions can be performed by computers but are better accomplished by physicians in an office with the patient and his family. Protocols preclude options and are best avoided. There is no "treatment of choice" for early laryngeal cancer. There are options, consequences, and probabilities.

*Editor's note: These opinions obviously differ sharply with those expressed by other contributors to this volume. Mendenhall et al (Chapter 9) have treated a large series of early supraglottic lesions with irradiation, as has the group at the M.D. Anderson Hospital (Chapter 17). Mancuso (Chapter 7) has demonstrated minimal degrees of preepiglottic space and cartilage invasion with sophisticated imaging techniques that are thought not to preclude successful radiation therapy. Nevertheless, the opinions presented by DeSanto and Vaughan are in conformity with the experience of many surgeons and must be weighed heavily in choice of therapy by individual practitioners for individual patients.

REFERENCES

1. Incze J, Vaughan CW Jr, Lui P, et al. Premalignant changes in normal appearing epithelium in patients with squamous cell carcinoma of the upper aerodigestive tract. Am J Surg 1982;144:401–5.
2. Slaughter DP. Multicentric origin of intraoral carcinoma. Surgery 1946;20:133–46.
3. Gillis TM, Incze J, Strong MS, et al. Natural history and management of keratosis, atypia, carcinoma in situ, and microinvasive cancer of the larynx. Am J Surg 1983;146:512–6.
4. Hellquist H, Lundgren J, Olofsson J. Hyperplasia, keratosis, dyplasia and carcinoma in situ of the vocal cords—a follow-up study. Clin Otolaryngol 1982;7:11–27.
5. Ogura JH, Mallen RW. Carcinoma of the larynx: diagnosis and treatment. Postgrad Med 1963;34:493–8.
6. Kirchner JA, Som ML. Clinical significance of fixed vocal cord. Laryngoscope 1971;81:1029–44.
7. Harmer MH. *TNM classification of malignant tumors,* 3rd ed. Geneva: International Union Against Cancer, 1978.
8. *Manual for Staging of Cancer*. Chicago: American Joint Committee, 1978:27–48.

9. Stell PM, Morton RP. What is the glottis? In: Wigant ME, Steiner W, Stell PM, eds. *Functional partial laryngectomy: conservation surgery for carcinoma of the larynx*. Berlin: Springer-Verlag, 1984:76–9.
10. Kirchner JA. The systems of UICC and AJC for staging of laryngeal carcinoma. In Wigand ME, Steiner W, Stell PM, eds. *Functional partial laryngectomy: conservation surgery for carcinoma of the larynx*. Berlin: Springer-Verlag, 1984:69–74.
11. Vaughan CW, Hicks JH, DeSanto LW. Options in the treatment of early laryngeal carcinoma. Am Acad Otolaryngol Instruction Course Monograph 1988:1511.
12. Lillie JC, DeSanto LW. Transoral surgery of early cordal carcinoma. Trans Am Acad Ophthalmol Otolaryngol 1973;77:92–6.
13. Lynch RC. Intrinsic carcinoma of the larynx, with a second report of cases operated on by suspension and dissection. Trans Am Laryngol Assoc 1920;42:119–124.
14. New GB, Dorton HE. Suspension laryngoscopy in the treatment of malignant disease of the hypopharynx and larynx. Proc Staff Meet Mayo Clin 1941;16:411–6.
15. Mendenhall WM, Parsons JT, Stringer SP, et al. T_1–T_2 vocal cord carcinoma: a basis for comparing the results of radiotherapy and surgery. Head Neck Surg 1988;10:373–7.
16. Okada W. The treatment and prognosis of carcinoma of the larynx. Trans Am Laryngol Assoc 1922;44:162–81.
17. Stutsman AC, McGavran MH. Ultraconservative management of superficially invasive epidermoid carcinoma of the true vocal cord. Ann Otol Rhinol Laryngol 1971;80:507–12.
18. Vaughan CW, Strong MS, Shapshay SM. Treatment of T_1 and in situ glottic carcinoma: the transoral approach. Otolaryngol Clin North Am 1980;13:509–13.
19. DeSanto LW. The options in early laryngeal carcinoma. N Engl J Med 1982;306:910–2.
20. Brandenburg JH, Rutter SW. Residual carcinoma of the larynx. Laryngoscope 1977;87:224–35.
21. Meyer-Breiting E, von Ilberg C. Behandlungsergebnisse der Chirurgie fruher Stimmbandkarzinome. HNO 1981;29:41–6.
22. Jackson C, Jackson CL. *Cancer of the larynx*. Philadelphia: WB Saunders, 1939.
23. Neel HB III, Devine KD, DeSanto LW. Laryngofissure and cordectomy for early cordal carcinoma: outcome in 182 patients. Otolaryngol Head Neck Surg 1980;88:79–84.
24. Bailey BJ. Glottic carcinoma. In: Bailey BJ, Biller HF, eds. *Surgery of the larynx*. Philadelphia: WB Saunders, 1985:257–78.
25. Vaughan CW, Homburger F, Shapshay SM, Soto E, Bernfeld P. Carcinogenesis in the upper aerodigestive tract. Otolaryngol Clin North Am 1980;13:403–12.
26. Crissman JD, Fu YS. Intraepithelial neoplasia of the larynx: a clinicopathologic study of six cases with DNA analysis. Arch Otolaryngol Head Neck Surg 1986;112:522–8.
27. Sedlis A, Sall S, Tsukada Y, et al. Microinvasive carcinoma of the uterine cervix: a clinical-pathologic study. Am J Obstet Gynecol 1979;133:64–74.
28. Doyle PJ, Flores AD. Treatment of carcinoma in situ of the larynx. J Otolaryngol 1977;6:363–7.
29. McDonald TJ, DeSanto LW, Weiland LH. Supraglottic larynx and its pathology as studied by whole laryngeal sections. Laryngoscope 1976;86:635–48.
30. DeSanto LW. Cancer of the supraglottic larynx: a review of 260 patients. Otolaryngol Head Neck Surg 1985;93:705–11.
31. Coates HL, DeSanto LW, Devine KD, Elveback LR. Carcinoma of the supraglottic larynx: a review of 221 cases. Arch Otolaryngol 1976;102:686–9.
32. DeSanto LW, Pearson BW, Olsen KD. Utility of near-total laryngectomy for supraglottic, pharyngeal, base-of-tongue, and other cancers. Ann Otol Rhinol Laryngol 1989;98:2–7.
33. Bocca E, Pignataro O, Oldini C, Cappa C. Functional neck dissection: an evaluation and review of 843 cases. Laryngoscope 1984;94:942–5.
34. DeSanto LW, Magrina C, O'Fallon WM. The second side of the neck in supraglottic cancer. Otolaryngol Head Neck Surg. In press.
35. DeSanto LW. Resection of the larynx and the pharynx for cancer. In: Nyhus LM, Baker RJ, eds. *Masters of Surgery*, vol 1. Boston: Little, Brown, 1984:215–35.

15

Laser Management of Laryngeal Cancer

Stanley M. Shapshay, Elie E. Rebeiz

Since the introduction of the carbon dioxide (CO_2) laser for microlaryngeal applications by Strong and Jako in 1972,[1] the use of this modality for the treatment of patients with laryngeal cancer has been somewhat controversial. The CO_2 laser has gained widespread acceptance for the management of benign laryngeal lesions, such as recurrent respiratory papillomatosis and polypoid changes and polyps of the vocal cords. Early reports by Strong et al,[2] however, that described the use of the CO_2 laser for laryngeal cancer were met with skepticism. Questions that were raised included the following: Can cancer be controlled safely by vaporizing the tumor? How can the pathologist determine specimen margins that have been "burned" or "cooked" by the laser? Does the laser destroy vocal cord tissue and permanently impair the voice? Does the radiotherapy provide a better voice after treatment than laser excision?

Experience collected during the past 15 years has proved the CO_2 laser to be a precise surgical tool, particularly when coupled to an operating microscope with a variable spot size micromanipulator. When good operative technique is used, surrounding tissue damage at the margins of laser excision is only 50 to 100 μm. In fact, a narrow zone of laser-induced char at the margins of the specimen marks the edges of excision for the pathologist. Minimal surrounding tissue trauma and reduced edema and scarring with the use of the laser have resulted in excellent vocal cord function. Voice quality is comparable to that after radiotherapy alone, although controlled studies are needed to compare laser excision with radiotherapy on a prospective basis.

As with any new technology, however, initial enthusiasm for the CO_2 laser may have resulted in overextension of its application. Laser excisions of vocal cord lesions that involve the anterior commissure and at times a few millimeters of the opposite vocal cord have resulted in a high incidence of tumor recurrence.[3] The laser has also been applied inappropriately in management of T_2 cancinomas associated with ventricular or subglottic extension. To some enthusiasts, the laser appeared not merely as another, albeit unique, surgical tool, but rather to possess magical qualities.

Patients with laryngeal cancer sometimes seek laser treatment as an alternative to standard therapy, such as radiotherapy or the classic surgical techniques of open partial and total laryngectomy. The laryngologist is often pressured by the patient or family to extend the indications for laser treatment in order to avoid surgery that would result in loss of voice and formation of a stoma. The surgeon who uses the laser is viewed as having the most modern technology and techniques available; once again, the patient believes that the laser is associated with mysterious and wonderful qualities. Thus, the clinician is tempted to use the laser to "chase" the tumor margins deep into the vocalis muscle toward the thyroid cartilage perichondrium. Extensive resection of T_1 vocal cord tumor is then justified by frozen section margins and random deep biopsy specimens after the lesion has been removed.

The laser should be used as part of a multimodality treatment environment, which presently includes radiotherapy, open partial laryngectomy, extended "three-quarter" laryngectomy, the "gold-standard" of total laryngectomy, and, most recently, the possibility of induction chemotherapy followed by planned radiotherapy. This chapter will discuss the indications, contraindications, and techniques for application of the laser in the treatment of patients with laryngeal cancer, including our experience at the Lahey Clinic from 1982 to 1989.

CHOICES OF LASER TECHNOLOGY

Presently, several types of lasers can be used in the larynx, including the CO_2, neodymium: yttrium-aluminum-garnet (Nd:YAG) with contact tip, argon, and potassium titanyl phosphate (KTP/532) lasers. Because it is beyond the scope of this chapter to review the soft tissue interaction and basic physics of all these lasers, only a summary will be presented.

The CO_2 laser, with a wavelength of 10.6 μm, has the most precise soft tissue interaction. This wavelength is almost completely absorbed into soft tissue, transferring light energy into heat energy and vaporizing water content. Minimal forward and back scatter of the laser beam permits the clinician to predict visible effects instantly. The CO_2 laser cannot, however, be handled through fiberoptic devices and must be coupled directly to the operating microscope with an articulated arm of mirrors. Although this method is clumsy, delivery systems have been improved vastly during the past 15 years, permitting the clinician to apply the laser with microprecision when laser impact diameters of 300 μm (0.3 mm) are used with the 400 mm lens on the operating microscope. With 16× magnification, the clinician has a noncontact microprecise technique of incising or ablating soft tissue, with minimal surrounding tissue damage. Hemostasis of capillary bleeding makes this an ideal surgical instrument for use on the vocal cords, which are not highly vascular.

In distinction of the CO_2 laser, the Nd:YAG wavelength of 1.06 μm is deeply penetrating to soft tissue beyond the surface effect. Thus, the clinician is not able to visualize immediately the full extent of tissue destruction. The power density of the Nd:YAG laser is maximal below the tissue surface, making it difficult to control in a noncontact fashion. The Nd:YAG laser with contact tips, however, allows a more predictable precise destruction of soft tissue. The disadvantage of this technique, however, is the reliance on the surgeon's freehand dexterity as opposed to the precise control available with the CO_2 laser coupled to a micromanipulator system. A noncontact technique is preferred so that the effects of the laser on tissue can be controlled visually. Hemostasis is satisfactory with contact Nd:YAG application and is comparable to that of the CO_2 laser.

The argon laser, with a wavelength of 458 to 515 μm, has the advantage of delivery through either a fiberoptic or micromanipulator system. The disadvantage of the argon laser (and also of the KTP/532 laser) is its selective absorption for pigmented tissue, particularly hemoglobin. When applied on nonpigmented tissue, some scatter occurs, although somewhat less than with the Nd:YAG laser used in a noncontact mode. A better cutting effect can be obtained by contact application; however, the precision of the argon laser, particularly in the larynx, is not equal to that of the CO_2 laser delivered with microspot application. For these reasons, we prefer to use the CO_2 laser with a variable spot micromanipulator system for endoscopic management of laryngeal tumors.[4]

EXCISIONAL BIOPSY WITH THE CO_2 LASER

Endoscopic management of laryngeal neoplasia presupposes adequate laryngoscopic exposure with a wide bore laryngoscope. In approximately 10 to 20% of our patients, the larynx has been difficult to expose because of a narrow dental arch, large tongue, previous neck surgery, or radiotherapy-induced tissue contracture. A typical example of a difficult laryngoscopy might occur with examination of an obese patient with a short thick neck, underdeveloped mandible, and full dentition. Difficulty with neck flexion can also be encountered during laryngoscopy on patients with cervical arthritis, which is prevalent in patients with rheumatoid arthritis and in elderly patients.

We usually prefer to use the Dedo-Jako laryngoscope with an anterior commissure design (Pilling Company, Fort Washington, PA) or the Kleinsasser laryngoscope of similar design (Karl Storz Endoscopy-America, Inc., Culver City, CA). Although we first attempt to place the largest possible laryngoscope for the best exposure, only approximately 60% of patients can tolerate this type of instrument. We also prefer the Boston University gallows suspension system (Pilling Company, Fort Washington, PA), which requires a specially adapted laryngoscope. Once the suspension is in place, the entire table can be moved in various positions without changing exposure. The Boston University system also prevents torquelike movement on suspension, which is seen with the Lewy system.

The lesions most suitable for transoral excisional biopsy with the CO_2 laser are hyperkeratosis, dysplasia, carcinoma in situ, and early invasive squamous cell (T_1) carcinoma. Again, the CO_2 laser is not a magical tool for this type of surgical treatment because a similar procedure can be performed using "cold" microsurgical techniques in which microscissors and microforceps are employed. The advantage of using the laser is noncontact microprecision in a bloodless field. The potential disadvantage is a thermal effect, which for superficial lesions, such as keratosis and dysplasia, puts an extra burden on the clinician with regard to the need for meticulous technique. Undoubtedly, the excision of tissue by thermal effects, such as with laser or cautery, results in slower wound healing than with nonthermal surgical treatment.

Laryngeal Keratosis

After adequate laryngeal exposure, excess mucus is suctioned or blotted dry with a laryngeal cottonoid. Using 25× magnification on the operating microscope, the larynx is examined carefully with the aid of fine microlaryngeal probes and mirrors to inspect the undersurface of the vocal cord and anterior commissure subglottic region. The false vocal cords are also retracted to expose the ventricular surfaces. Toluidine blue (2%) is used to identify any areas of increased nucleic acid content.[5] A cottonoid strip, saturated with toluidine blue, is applied liberally to the vocal cord surfaces. After 5 seconds, a suction-irrigation microlaryngeal instrument is employed for vigorous irrigation of excess toluidine blue from the vocal cords with approximately 20 ml of saline. Care should be taken to avoid abrasion of the vocal cord surfaces, because the abraded areas will absorb the dye. A positive stain with toluidine blue is deep purple rather than the lighter blue stain that adheres to normal respiratory epithelium on the false cords and subglottis. Toluidine blue staining permits the clinician to distinguish areas of severe dysplasia and carcinoma in situ from areas of more benign keratosis. Toluidine blue supravital staining is used for all mucosal dysplastic processes. Submucosal tumor will not stain with this technique. Supravital staining alerts the clinician to areas of dysplasia that may be multicentric, thereby permitting biopsy of appropriate sites.

Keratotic areas should be excised completely through the mucosa without exposing the vocalis muscle. The operating microscope is then switched to an optimum 16× magnification, and the CO_2 laser microspot is used to outline the lesion in a 0.1 second pulsed mode (Fig. 15–1A,B). Approximately 2 W of energy at 0.1 second exposures is used with the 300 μm spot

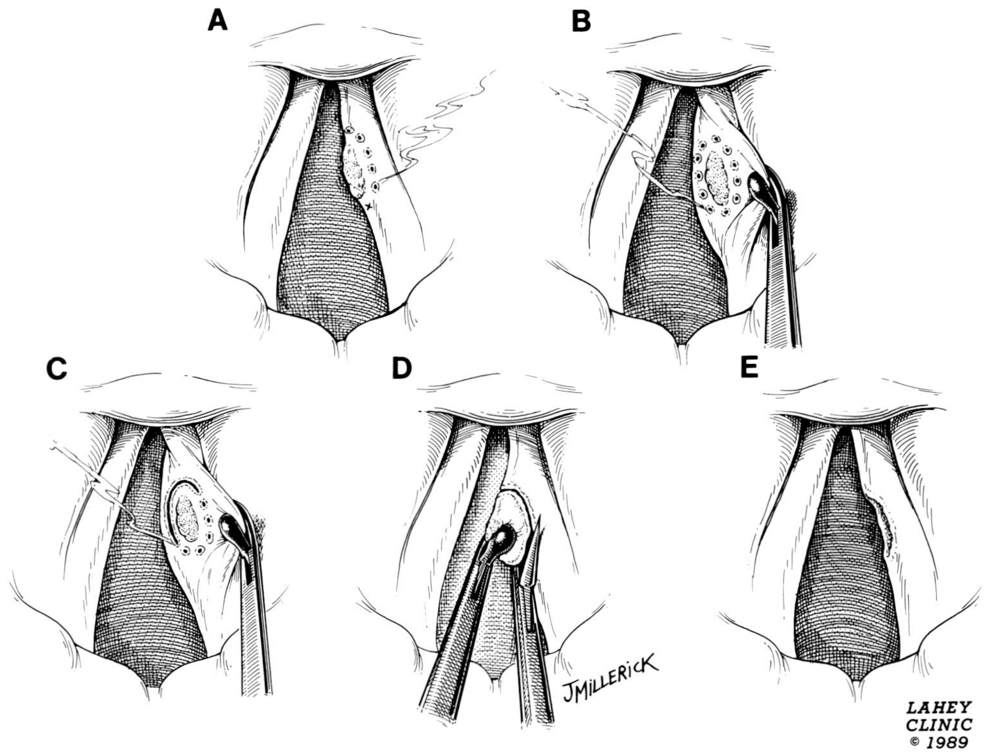

Figure 15–1. The carbon dioxide microspot is used to outline a vocal cord lesion on the superior surface of the vocal cord (A) and on the inferior surface (B). C: laser incision through the mucosa along the outline. D: medial retraction of the lesion during dissection with microscissors. E: mucosal defect after removal. (Printed by permission of Lahey Clinic.)

size. Once the depth of excision is reached with the outlining technique, the keratotic area separates from the surrounding tissue (Fig. 15–1C). A 1 mm laryngeal forceps is used to grasp the keratotic area, and a straight 1 mm laryngeal scissors is used to free the specimen from its base (Fig. 15–1D,E) This cold technique is preferred for the base of the specimen to diminish the heat effect near the vocalis muscle in order to preserve better vocal cord function. Because the specimen is very thin, minimal heat coagulation is desired, particularly at the base and margins of the specimen.

Dysplasia

Basically, the same technique, just described, for excisional biopsy of hyperkeratosis is used for dysplasia of varying severity. The only differences for dysplastic lesions are a slightly larger margin of excision around the lesion of approximately 1 to 2 mm and excision of the full thickness of epithelium through Reinke's space (Fig. 15–2A). This slightly thicker specimen is justified because dysplasia is usually a full-thickness epithelial change. Again, we prefer to outline the lesion by using an intermittent pulse mode technique and then switching to cold microlaryngeal instruments with 1 mm distal working ends to diminish thermal effects. The laser provides a bloodless operative field, incising the vocal cord surface and preparing the specimen for resection with scissors. Frozen section margins are desirable but not absolutely necessary. Often, wide-field dysplasia exists, making it difficult to obtain clear margins. In patients with field changes indicative of cancer, it is most important not to miss an area of early invasive carcinoma or carcinoma in situ. Toluidine blue staining techniques help to detect these changes.

Carcinoma in Situ

For lesions identified as carcinoma in situ, a more thorough excision exposing the vocalis muscle is necessary. A 2 to 3 mm margin around the tumor is obtained, and the lesion should be oriented carefully for the pathologist for the determination of frozen section margins. A full-thickness specimen should be obtained, because the pathologist needs to determine any invasion of the basal epithelial membrane (Fig. 15–2B). A shallow specimen often results in a biopsy report in which invasion cannot be determined. When this microprecise technique is used, both vocal cords can be treated simultaneously, taking care not to strip the epithelium from the anterior commissure. We prefer not to employ the traditional "cord stripping" technique, because this usually results in an uneven epithelial excision through Reinke's space, sometimes missing submucosal tissue.

Early Invasive (T_1) Carcinoma

Strict criteria of endoscopic excision need to be emphasized when managing early invasive carcinoma with the laser. The lesion should be a minimally invasive mid to anterior vocal cord

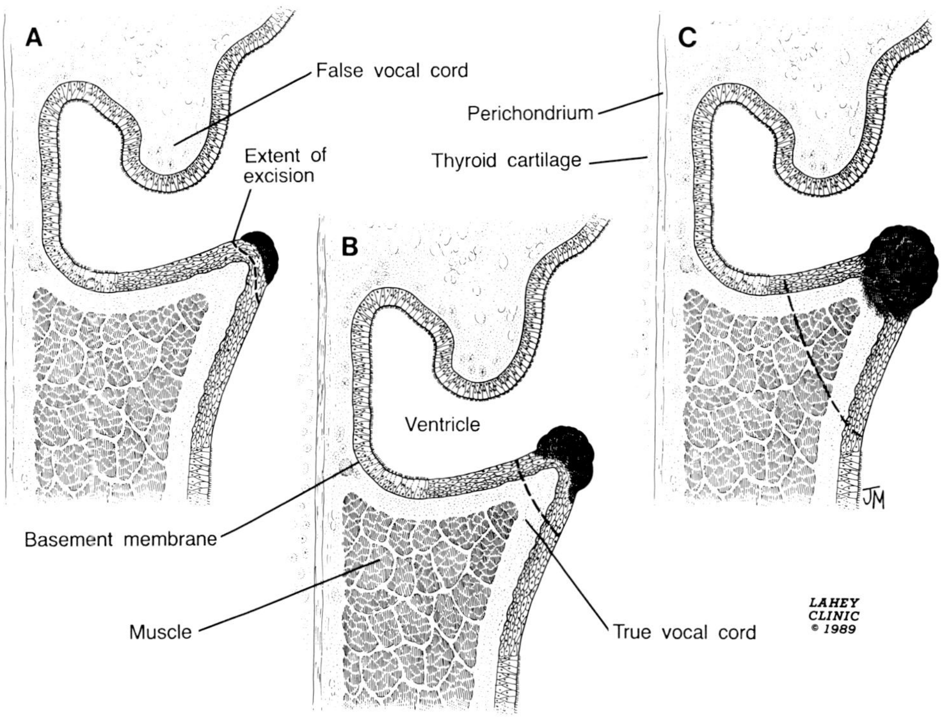

Figure 15–2. A: superficial laser excision of benign lesion of the true vocal cord; excision does not include basement membrane. B: line of excision through Reinke's space for carcinoma in situ includes basement membrane for histologic assessment of invasion. C: laser biopsy of invasive squamous cell carcinoma includes vocalis muscle to rule out cancerous invasion. (Printed by permission of Lahey Clinic.)

squamous cell carcinoma that does not involve the anterior commissure, vocal process, or supraglottic or subglottic larynx. A minimal degree of involvement, 1 to 2 mm, along the floor of the ventricle is permissible; however, any extension of tumor beyond this makes lateral control of excision more difficult. Full vocal cord mobility should be present, which indicates minimal invasiveness of the carcinoma. An anterior commissure tumor should not be excised, because the distance between the tumor and the thyroid perichondrium is narrow, making it difficult to obtain secure margins. If the tumor extends into the anterior commissure region, recurrence is likely with any endoscopic technique.

Endoscopic excision of an early vocal cord carcinoma demands meticulous technique. After careful exposure is obtained, constant tension upon the specimen is mandatory, using well-placed upbiting microlaryngeal forceps. Adequate evacuation of laser plume, preferably with a laser smoke evaluation system, is crucial. The lesion should be outlined with a margin of at least 2 to 3 mm of healthy surrounding tissue (Fig. 15–2C). The laser spot impact diameter is then increased from 300 μm to approximately 800 μm. A pulsed mode is used to diminish heat effects on the tumor margins as well as to diminish postoperative heat-induced swelling and subsequent scarring. Six to 8 W of energy is used in a pulsed 0.1 second exposure, although longer pulses of 1 second can be used with adequate tension on the specimen. Once removed, the specimen is hand carried to the pathologist by the clinician or a designated assistant for proper orientation of appropriate margins. The specimen is pinned to a strip of moist nonadherent dressing (Telfa) to avoid contraction. Longitudinal serial sections are taken for adequate margin orientation and sampling. If the margins are insecure or too close, laser excision is repeated, using the base as the deep margin. We do not obtain random deep biopsy specimens as margin controls, because such specimens are indeed random, and their orientation may be lost. A negative random deep biopsy may give the clinician a false sense of security. Close cooperation in joint review of histologic specimens and margins by the clinician and the pathologist is necessary for successful treatment.

PITFALLS AND PROBLEMS OF LASER EXCISIONAL BIOPSY

The most common problem in laser excisional biopsy is the use of excessive laser energy. This can occur when the wattage used is excessive or, more commonly, when an abrupt laser excision is performed using continuous laser exposure, resulting in excessive heat coagulation damage to the specimen. Another common error is the use of inadequate tension on the specimen, resulting in heat coagulation and difficult histologic recognition of margins. With larger T_1 vocal cord tumors and in patients who have undergone subtotal cordectomy as a salvage procedure after failed radiotherapy, orientation may be lost when the specimen is obtained. The most common mistake is to extend the excision deep into the subglottic larynx, a situation in which depth perception is lost with larger specimens that are difficult to retract (Fig. 15–3). Constant reorientation of the anatomy and

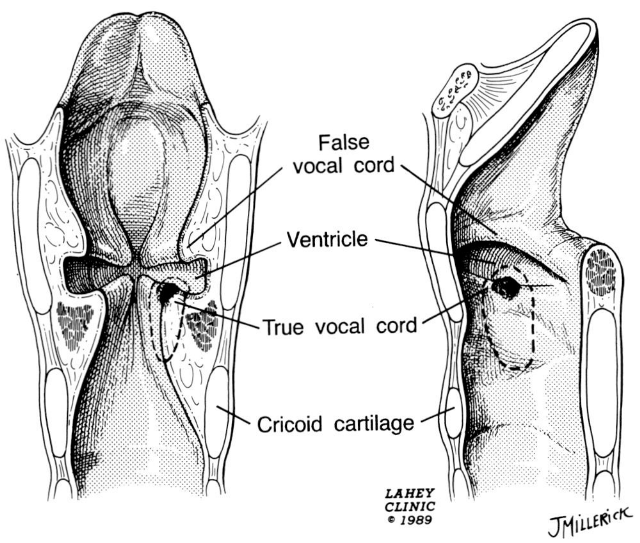

Figure 15–3. Laser excision of neoplastic lesion of true vocal cord; excision extends into subglottic space. (Printed by permission of Lahey Clinic.)

position of the specimen is necessary. Subtotal cordectomy is not an easy endoscopic procedure for the less experienced clinician.

OTHER USES OF THE CARBON DIOXIDE LASER FOR LARYNGEAL CANCER

Diagnosis and Staging

The uniqueness of having a microprecise surgical tool such as the CO_2 laser in a relatively bloodless operative field has generated the concept of "biologic staging." During the performance of an excisional biopsy, the clinician is sometimes surprised by the depth of tumor extension. Using the operating microscope at 16× magnification, and at times at 25×, the clinician can determine definite invasion of the vocalis muscle. Invasion is sometimes deeper than that expected on a clinical basis because vocal cord mobility may be unimpaired. From a biologic standpoint, this would appear to upgrade the tumor from a minimal T_1 vocal cord carcinoma to a somewhat more aggressive T_1 vocal cord carcinoma. In this situation, although the clinical staging does not change, the clinician may decide not to "chase" the tumor deep into the vocalis muscle, because vocal cord function may be less impaired if radiotherapy is chosen as the definitive treatment modality.

In other instances, a lesion involving the anterior commissure may be managed by an excisional biopsy with the laser, only to find with greater magnification on the operating microscope that thyroid cartilage has been invaded by the tumor. The lesion can then be staged correctly as a T_4 squamous cell carcinoma when, clinically, a T_1 lesion had been suspected.

Because computed tomographic scanning does not determine invasion of thyroid cartilage with any accuracy, particularly at the anterior commissure, endoscopic diagnosis can be very valuable. We use the CO_2 laser as an excisional or biopsy tool for more accurate determination of the depth of tumor invasion. Open surgical techniques can then be planned for the patient with an anterior commissure lesion that involves the thyroid cartilage, and radiotherapy can be chosen for the patient with a lesion deeply invasive into the vocalis muscle, where tumor control and vocal cord function are prime considerations.

Cytoreduction or Tumor "Debulking"

An attractive, although not proven concept, is to use the microlaryngeal laser to reduce tumor burden before definitive radiotherapy. This is most desirable in the management of bulky tumors, particularly when the depth of invasion is not easy to determine clinically. Whether the reduction of cancer cells before radiotherapy increases its effectiveness, has any deleterious effects on the voice, or slows the deliverance of radiotherapy is unknown. In our practice, tumor reduction or debulking is performed routinely, because there have not appeared to be any deleterious effects on the voice or any delay in treatment. Patients are usually happy with some improvement in their voice. Even with possible delay in initiating radiotherapy, a satisfactory airway is maintained with adequate voice. A prospective randomized study comparing this technique of tumor reduction with radiotherapy alone would be of interest.

Salvage Treatment With the Laser for Recurrent Tumor After Radiotherapy

Although endoscopic salvage treatment with the laser for recurrence of tumor after radiotherapy is an attractive concept, in reality, this is a most difficult and somewhat risky technique. If the recurrent tumor is superficial and has been detected at an early stage, it is worthwhile to attempt a salvage technique with the laser. We prefer a subtotal cordectomy for tumor control, again, with careful orientation and preparation of the specimen for the determination of margins. Unfortunately, recurrences of tumor after radiotherapy may be multicentric, and nests of tumor cells may be hidden between areas of radiation-induced fibrosis. In these situations, it is extremely difficult for the clinician to judge the margin of endoscopic excision. In a series reported by Blakeslee et al[6] the rate of control of tumor recurrence after radiotherapy was only 50%. Unfortunately, if the clinician is deluded into thinking that there is good margin control after laser excision, a deep nest of tumor cells hidden from detection may result in a fixed vocal cord later. If hidden tumor is not detected as a relatively early recurrence, the fixed cord places the patient in great jeopardy necessitating salvage by total laryngectomy.

Avoidance of Tracheotomy Before Total Laryngectomy

Endoscopic laser excision is a most useful technique for the management of an advanced vocal cord carcinoma presenting as an exophytic airway-obstructing tumor. Although this is not a common situation, debulking such a tumor, which is usually associated with supraglottic or subglottic extension and vocal cord fixation, can present an airway emergency. When the patient can be intubated with a small (5 to 5.5 mm) laser-resistant endotracheal tube, the laser can be used to debulk the obstructing tumor, thereby avoiding tracheotomy as a preliminary stage before laryngectomy. Debulking the tumor theoretically reduces the possibility of stomal recurrence, although this has not been definitively proven as an etiologic factor. Certainly, the infection associated with preliminary tracheotomy is best avoided before laryngectomy. This technique can only be used when the patient can be intubated, usually while awake, with a small endotracheal tube.

Once the majority of the tumor in the anterior portion of the larynx is removed with the laser, a Venturi jet ventilation system is placed on the laryngoscope. Extubation of the endotracheal tube is helpful for exposure of the subglottic and posterior larynx. Occasionally, hemostasis may be a problem with more vascular tumors, necessitating intermittent spot cautery of large blood vessels.

Palliation

Although not a common situation, elderly patients, often in the ninth decade, can present with recurrence of laryngeal cancer after radiotherapy. Endoscopic laser palliation is an attractive treatment modality to maintain an airway and some voice and to delay the use of a tracheotomy for as long as possible. Laser treatment for palliation is also useful for patients who present very high medical risk for open partial or total laryngectomy after failed radiotherapy. In a series of five patients on our service, all in the ninth decade, this endoscopic approach proved to be very useful.

CARBON DIOXIDE LASER TREATMENT OF SUPRAGLOTTIC CARCINOMA

In most patients, the abundant lymphatic system in the supraglottic larynx dictates the choice of treatment for a primary tumor of the neck. Supraglottic T_1 and T_2 cancers are usually considered to be in the same category because early T_1 tumors are discovered only rarely. Radiotherapy is an excellent choice of treatment for patients with these tumors because both the primary cancer and high-risk lymph nodes are treated simultaneously. Selected patients with T_2 supraglottic carcinomas are best managed by open supraglottic partial laryngectomy techniques and modified neck dissections, depending on the extent of neck node metastasis. In rare situations, a small T_1 epiglottic carcinoma involving the suprahyoid portion of the epiglottis, rim of the arytenoepiglottic fold, or both, can be treated by endoscopic laser excisional techniques. In our experience, only four patients have had tumors in this category and were cured by laser treatment. Extension of laser excision for a patient with a T_2 lesion or larger T_1 carcinoma is indicated only when the patient has refused other standard treatment modalities. Laser excision may be performed, however, in a patient who has a limited tumor recurrence in the supraglottis after radiotherapy. We have treated two such patients who used their voice professionally by performing endoscopic laser supraglottic partial laryngectomy or extended epiglottidectomy, preserving sensory innervation to the larynx. This concept can be extended to poor medical risk patients with accessible supraglottic tumors that have recurred after radiotherapy. Endoscopic supraglottic partial laryngectomy is associated with a decreased risk of aspiration when compared with open partial techniques, especially when they are employed after radiotherapy, and can be attempted in selected patients. Once again, the "gold standard" of cancer control and safety—total laryngectomy—should always be considered.

LAHEY CLINIC SERIES, 1982 TO 1987

Forty-six patients were referred for laser excision of early vocal cord carcinomas from 1982 to 1987 (Table 15–1). Patients with carcinoma in situ or dysplasia were excluded from the series. Follow-up ranged from 2 to 6 years, with a mean of 3.5 years. Twenty-five patients with small T_1 vocal cord carcinomas were treated with endoscopic laser excisional techniques. Twenty of these patients had no previous therapy, and five patients had radiotherapy 2 to 6 years before referral. This latter group most probably had second primary carcinomas in the same region, which were newly staged as T_1 vocal cord carcinomas. All patients met the previously described criteria for laser excision.

Thirteen patients had laser excisional biopsy for large T_1 vocal cord carcinomas. These patients had invasive squamous cell carcinoma leading deeply into the vocalis muscle but without limitation of mobility. Clinically, the tumors were still classified as T_1 vocal cord carcinomas, although biologically they were classified as T_3 carcinomas because of deep vocalis muscle invasion. Complete tumor removal in these patients would have necessitated a subtotal vocal cordectomy. Thus, radiotherapy was chosen as the definitive therapy, with minimal delay between laser excision and irradiation. Nine patients had involvement of the anterior commissure, and three patients had involvement of the full length of the vocal cord. One patient had a bilateral vocal cord invasive squamous cell carcinoma.

Eight patients had laser therapy for T_2 vocal cord carcinomas. Excisional biopsy with the CO_2 laser was used for accurate staging of the tumor and reduced tumor bulk. Deep vocalis muscle invasion or extension into the ventricle or subglottic larynx was noted. Seven patients underwent subsequent radiotherapy, and one patient who refused radiotherapy underwent a partial laryngectomy.

Tumor control was achieved in 18 of the 20 (90%) patients with small previously untreated vocal cord carcinomas. Control of disease was achieved by laser excisional therapy in all five patients who had previous radiotherapy and presented with a probable second vocal cord carcinoma. Excellent control of disease with combined laser excision and radiotherapy was achieved in the 13 patients who presented with larger, more invasive T_1 vocal cord carcinomas. No additional morbidity was associated with radiotherapy after laser excisional biopsy.

The eight patients with T_2 vocal cord carcinomas underwent laser excision as a staging and debulking therapy before definitive treatment. After accurate staging of their tumors, seven patients underwent radiotherapy. Five (71%) of these patients have had no evidence of recurrent tumor. Total laryngectomy was performed for salvage in two patients in whom radiotherapy failed. Currently, these patients are free of tumor. One patient refused radiotherapy, underwent open partial laryngectomy, and is free of tumor 3 years after surgery. None of the 46 patients

Table 15-1. Laser Management of 46 Early Vocal Cord Carcinomas*

GROUP	NO. PATIENTS	STAGE OF TUMOR		PREVIOUS TREATMENT	EXTENSION OF TUMOR	INITIAL TREATMENT	NO. OF FAILURES	CONTROL RATE (%)	DEFINITIVE TREATMENT	COMPLICATIONS
		Clinical	*Biologic*							
1A	20	T_1	T_1	None	None	Laser excision	2/20	90	Radiotherapy	None
1B	5	T_1	T_1	Radiotherapy	None	Laser excision	0	100		None
2A	9	T_1	T_3	None	Vocalis muscle, anterior commissure	Radiotherapy	0	100		None
2B	3	T_1	T_3	None	Vocalis muscle, full length of vocal cord	Radiotherapy	0	100		None
2C	1	T_1	T_3	None	Vocalis muscle, bilateral vocal cords	Radiotherapy	0	100		None
3A	7	T_2	T_2	None	Ventricle or subglottis	Radiotherapy	2/7	71	Total laryn-gectomy	None
3B	1	T_2	T_2	None	Ventricle or subglottis	Partial laryn-gectomy	0	100		None

*Follow-up was 2 to 6 years.

in this series had persistent cancer on completion of their definitive therapies. No complications, specifically chondritis or chondronecrosis, resulted from the use of the CO_2 laser or radiotherapy.

CONCLUSIONS

When treating patients with laryngeal cancer, clinicians should consider the potential for multiple sites of origin and the possibility of regional metastases with more invasive squamous cell carcinomas. They should also take into consideration the effects of treatment on the voice, swallowing, and the sphincteric function of the larynx to prevent aspiration. Fortunately, advanced surgical and reconstructive techniques are available, in addition to modern laser technology.

Since its introduction in the early 1970s, the surgical laser has been incorporated into reliable microprecise instruments. Radiotherapeutic techniques have also advanced, providing excellent cure rates, particularly for patients with early laryngeal cancer, and excellent preservation of vocal cord function. The head and neck oncologist must base his or her therapeutic choice on the patient's specific needs and requirements in a multidisciplinary treatment environment.

REFERENCES

1. Strong MS, Jako GJ. Laser surgery in the larynx. Early clinical experience with continuous CO_2 laser. Ann Otol Rhinol Laryngol 1972;81:791–8.
2. Strong MS, Jako GJ, Vaughan CW, et al. The use of CO_2 laser in otolaryngology: a progress report. Trans Am Acad Ophthalmol Otolaryngol 1976;82:595–602.
3. Krespi YP, Meltzer CJ. Laser surgery for vocal cord carcinoma involving the anterior commissure. Ann Otol Rhinol Laryngol 1989;98:105–9.
4. Shapshay SM. Laser applications in the trachea and bronchi: a comparative study of the soft tissue effects using contact and noncontact delivery systems. Laryngoscope 1987;97(7 Pt 2 Suppl 41):1–26.
5. Strong MS, Vaughan CW, Incze J.Toluidine blue in diagnosis of cancer of the larynx. Arch Otolaryngol Head Neck Surg 1970;91:515–9.
6. Blakeslee D, Vaughan CW, Shapshay SM, et al. Excisional biopsy in the selective management of T_1 glottic cancer: a three-year follow-up study. Laryngoscope 1984;94:488–94.

16

Vertical Partial Laryngectomy

Rose M. Mohr

The vertical partial laryngectomy has also been termed vertical hemilaryngectomy (VHL),[1] verticofrontolateral laryngectomy,[2] and extended verticofrontolateral laryngectomy.[3] The first VHL was performed by Billroth in 1875 or 1878 depending on which historical source is examined.[4–6] The procedure was then modified by Gluck[7] in 1912 and popularized by Hautant[8] in the 1930s. The Hautant operation involved excising an anatomic half of the larynx with the creation of a pharyngostome and laryngostome that was later closed with skin flaps. Later in the 1930s, Hautant further modified the procedure to permit one stage execution, although tracheotomy decannulation was rarely achieved.

Goodyear[9] in 1949 used an endolaryngeal glass rod for stenting purposes and improved the frequency of tracheal decannulation. Over the ensuing years, numerous modifications of the procedure have been developed. The major contributors include Norris,[1,3] Som,[10] Ogura and Biller.[11]

The multitude of procedural variations and the number of modifications are indicative of the complexities of this field, which requires maturity in preoperative endoscopy and appropriate surgical skills. Familiarity with the whole-organ serial section studies of Tucker,[12] Norris and Tucker,[13] and Kirchner,[14–19] as well as the injection studies of Pressman et al,[20] and the embryology of the larynx is necessary for the surgeon to develop a logical basis for utilizing the various VHL procedures.

INDICATIONS

VHL is indicated for selected T_1 through T_3 glottic carcinomas.[2,21] These lesions can be invasive squamous cell or verrucous carcinomas. VHL may be employed for primary treatment or for surgical salvage of radiation failures. Lesions staged T_2 because of ventricular invasion with invasion of the undersurface of the false cord or subglottic extension (lesions that extend more than 1 cm below the midportion of the ventricle) or lesions staged T_3 (vocal cord fixed) that are deeply invasive and transglottic are not amenable to VHL without adding some other mode of therapy (Fig. 16–1). Surgery for these more advanced lesions should be followed by radiation therapy because there is a 40% recurrence rate when they are treated with VHL alone.[2]

Most clinically staged T_3 transglottic lesions will be found on pathologic examination to have framework invasion or extralaryngeal spread and are thus truly T_4 primary tumors,[15,18] which should be treated by total laryngectomy rather than VHL. There is controversy as to whether the extended supraverticofrontolateral near total laryngectomy described by Pearson et al[22] would be adequate for this situation.*

Therefore, the indications for VHL, employed without adjuvant therapy are as follows: (1) T_1 carcinoma of the glottis, with maximum limits of tumor extension as demonstrated in Figure 16–1; (2) T_2 carcinoma of the glottis with vocal cord motion impairment; and (3) T_3 carcinoma of the glottis, with minimal vocalis muscle invasion, with fixation of the vocal cord caused mainly by the bulk of the tumor.

THE PROCEDURE

It is feasible to remove the glottic lesion with one entire half of the thyroid cartilage, with or without the arytenoid, as well as 1 cm of the contralateral side, and the upper half of the cricoid cartilage (Fig. 16–2). Further extension of the resection would require permanent tracheotomy for adequate airway. The more extensive VHL procedures require glottic reconstruction. I prefer to employ strap muscle to recreate the neocord with advancement of pyriform sinus mucosa in order to resurface the hemilarynx and prevent aspiration.[1,2,23] Numerous variations of this reconstruction have been described using epiglottis, strap muscle, posterior thyroid cartilage, and other tissues.[24] When VHL is extended to its limits, the lateral pharyngotomy approach affords better exposure for resecting subglottic structures and opposite cord margins (Figs. 16–3, 16–4). For these larger lesions, entry through the cricothyroid membrane is less pre-

*Editor's note: This subject is discussed in detail in Chapter 24.

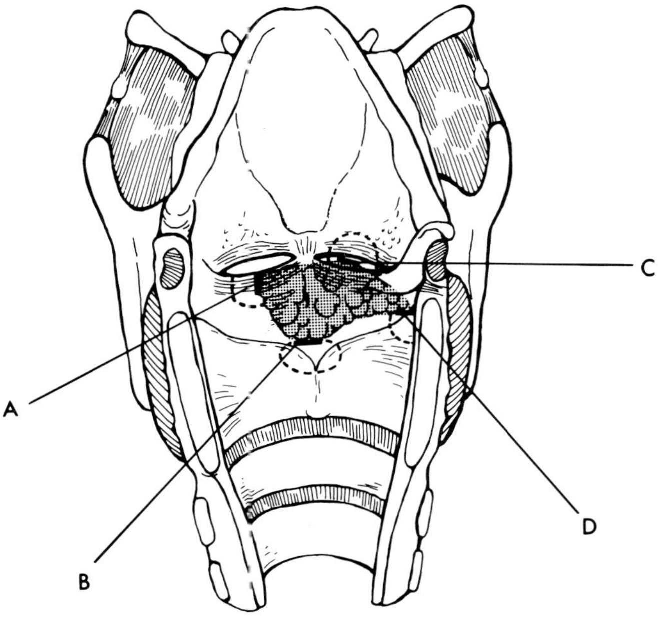

Figure 16–1. Lesions *not* amenable to vertical partial laryngectomy (VHL). A: extension beyond one third of opposite cord (risk of glottic stenosis). B: greater than 10 mm of anterior or midcordal subglottic extension (risk of T_4 through cricothyroid membrane). C: extension beyond midventricle (risk of thyroid cartilage invasion). D: more than 5 mm of posterior subglottic extension (risk of cricoid invasion or tracking into pyriform sinus). Subglottic extension is measured from the midportion of the ventricle. The lesion depicted is the maximum size amenable to VHL. (From Mohr et al.[2] Reprinted with permission.)

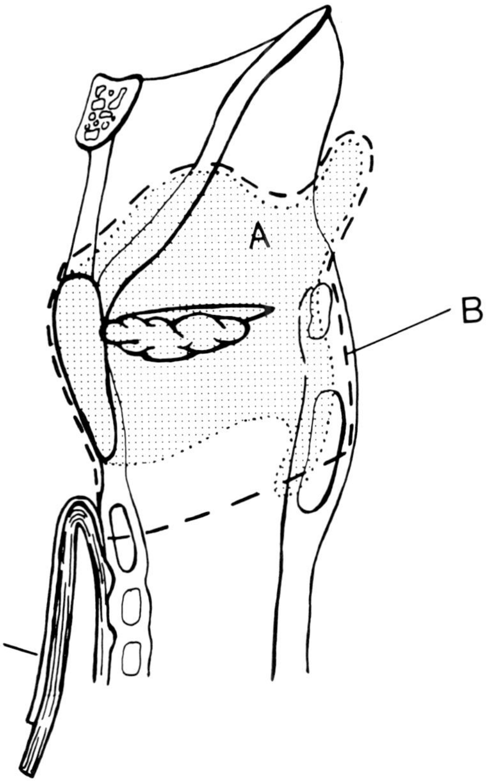

Figure 16–2. Maximum limits of thyroid and cricoid cartilage removal. A: thyroid cartilage. B: maximum limits of cartilage resection (up to 1 cm beyond midline and upper half of the ipsilateral cricoid hemisphere). C: perichondrium adherent to inner aspect of strap muscles. (From Mohr et al.[2] Reprinted with permission.)

cise. With small lesions that are well defined on one cord, any approach is acceptable and the procedure as described by Silver,[24] Montgomery,[25] and Lore[26] of entering the cricothyroid membrane is technically very easy.

If thyroid or cricoid cartilage or cricothyroid membrane invasion is found, total laryngectomy is indicated with voice restoration. Consent for possible total laryngectomy should be obtained in all patients prior to VHL.

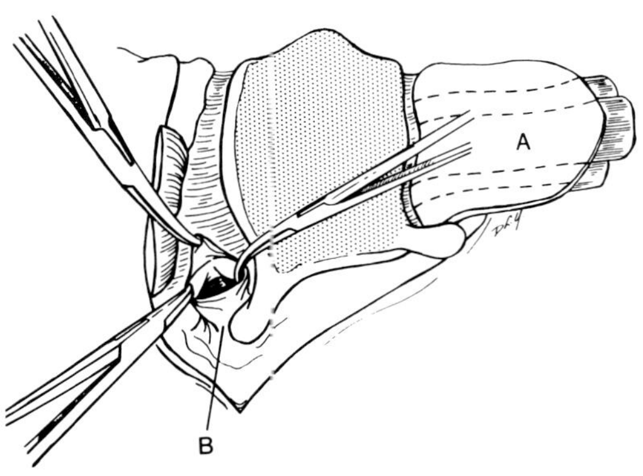

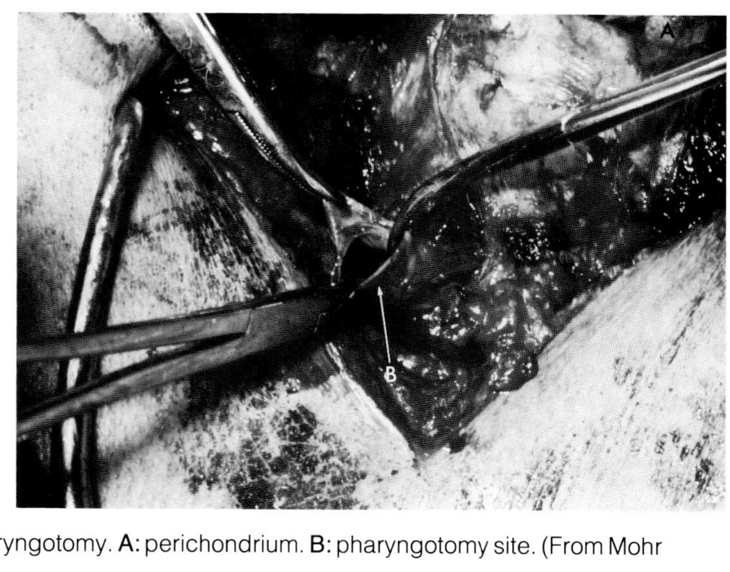

Figure 16–3. Entry through anterolateral pharyngotomy. A: perichondrium. B: pharyngotomy site. (From Mohr et al.[2] Reprinted with permission.)

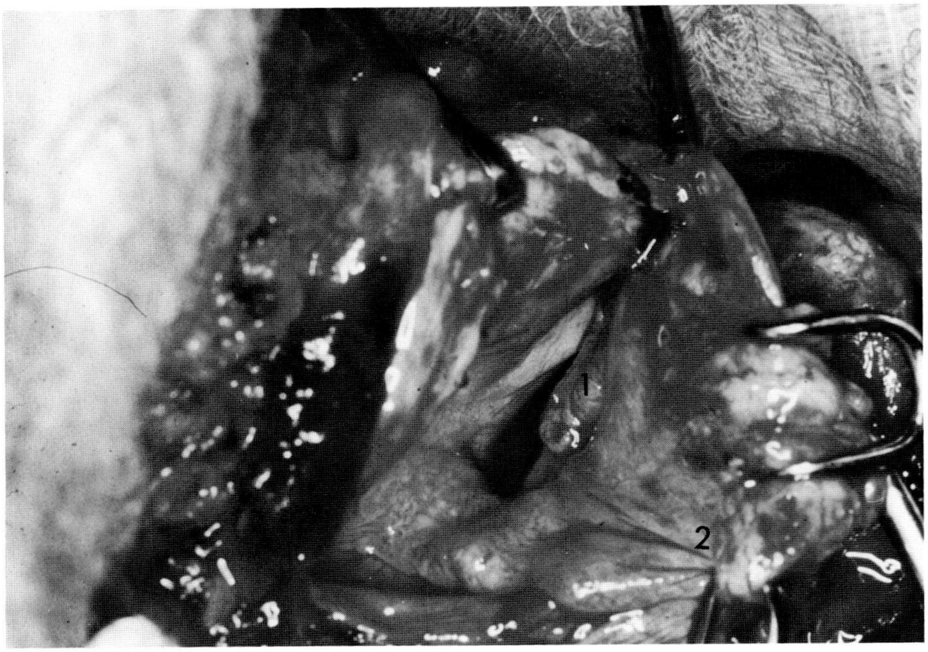

Figure 16–4. View upon entry. 1: the lesion; 2: pyriform sinus mucosa. (From Mohr et al.[2] Reprinted with permission.)

ENDOSCOPY AND BIOPSY OF GLOTTIC CARCINOMA

The previously alluded to endoscopic skill and familiarity with pathologic anatomy are required for proper staging and evaluation of glottic carcinoma. We employ a Hollinger "anterior commissure" laryngoscope in order to view and palpate the larynx gently. Endoscopic telescopes, microscopes, and flexible fiberoptic instruments are important adjuncts to examination. The telescope is particularly valuable for evaluation of subglottic involvement. General anesthesia with muscle relaxants and control of the airway with a small caliber endotracheal tube, which will not obstruct vision, permit optimal endoscopic examination.

Laryngeal tumors cannot be adequately evaluated by suspension laryngoscopy alone. During suspension, the laryngeal anatomy is distorted by stretching, and if the laryngoscope is not placed properly the ventricle may be obliterated. Suspension microlaryngoscopy should be used for biopsy if needed after initial examination with smaller, more maneuverable instruments. Although the large laryngoscopes used for suspension tend to obliterate certain features of pathologic anatomy, they do provide better light and binocular vision for precise and adequate biopsies.

Biopsy of a lesion in anticipation of partial laryngectomy should be in an inauspicious area, rather than at a margin,[2,23] for surgical judgments at the time of VHL can be altered by inflammatory reaction at the biopsy site. Since only a 1 mm margin is acceptable in VHL, preoperative biopsies to determine marginal involvement are counterproductive.

Complete panendoscopic examination is not recommended, because the incidence of synchronous primary tumors, approximately 10%,[2] is relatively low with glottic carcinoma and current methods of preliminary examination, including fiberoptic endoscopy and imaging procedures, afford adequately comprehensive evaluation.

DIAGNOSTIC IMAGING STUDIES

Although direct visualization usually provides more helpful information than do imaging studies, high resolution computed tomography and magnetic resonance imaging with axial, coronal, and sagittal views can be helpful with supraglottic, preepiglottic, or subglottic extension.* The combination of endoscopic study of the lesion and knowledge of whole organ serial section studies coupled with the diagnostic imaging studies was reported by Kirchner[18] to have reduced the incidence of diagnostic understaging of tumors from 40 to 22%.

PATHOLOGY AND RECURRENCE RATES

Since resection margins are very close, the specimen must be oriented for the pathologist by the surgeon so that false-positive or false-negative margins do not occur. I prefer, in addition, to take biopsies from tissues remaining in situ after removal of the hemilarynx. These include specimens from the entire subglottic mucosal margin and the opposite vocal cord or any other close

*Editor's note: In Chapter 7, Mancuso has demonstrated the enormous increase in diagnostic capability afforded by dedicated study of images produced by the most advanced equipment. Nevertheless, examination of the larynx by visualization of its mucosal aspect remains the primary means of clinical and preoperative evaluation. Dr. Mohr reflects the current practical experience of most clinicians working with available techniques.

margins (Fig. 16–5). This will provide better assurance of negative margins than full reliance on evaluation of the removed portion of the larynx. Surgical specimens are submitted for frozen and permanent sections.

When VHL is performed after failed radiation therapy, extensive frozen section margin evaluation is necessary. Ogura et al[27,28] have studied positive margins; when they are present, recurrence is more likely. Recurrence is more common in patients who have had VHL for supraglottic or subglottic extension.[2,30,31] If positive margins are confirmed by consultation with the pathologist, the patient should receive additional therapy. Positive margins after conservation surgery for radiation failure mandate a completion laryngectomy. Nonirradiated patients may be treated with postoperative radiation therapy or completion laryngectomy, depending upon various factors.

Recurrences after VHL tend to result in advanced lesions. I would suspect this is related to late presentation. Patients with VHL have a breathy voice and recurrences are often not recognized because voice and airway are not affected until the tumor is large. Reconstructive methods that create intralaryngeal bulk in order to improve voice may further impair detection of recurrent tumor. This is one reason why I prefer to employ the thin pyriform sinus mucosa for resurfacing. Any recurrence after VHL should be considered and treated as stage T_4. The incidence of stomal recurrence is high after completion laryngectomy for failed VHL, possibly because of the advanced stage of the tumors.[29,30]

VOICE

Voice after VHL is inferior to the voice after radiation therapy for early glottic lesions. Perhaps the poorest vocal function occurs when the larynx has been resurfaced by stented skin grafts; these patients have such a patulous airway that severe air wasting occurs. The multitude of reconstructions described, including pyriform sinus mucosa, muscle, epiglottis, thyroid cartilage, strap muscles, and digastric tendon, all serve to improve voice after VHL.[24–26] There is, however, no single optimal method of reconstruction.

Reconstruction should allow for visualization of the remaining laryngeal structures and some attempt should be made to create a neocord. Careful attention must be paid to reattaching the remnant of opposite vocal cord, creating the anterior commissure of the neocord at a slightly higher level than the remnant cord. The epiglottis must be secure in some fashion so that good postoperative visualization of the endolarynx is possible. Reconstruction, with pyriform sinus mucosa, the method that I prefer, is demonstrated in Figures 16–6, 16–7, and 16–8.[2,30]

ANTERIOR COMMISSURE INVASION

Anterior commissure invasion does not preclude radiation therapy, nor does it dictate the need for VHL. The anterior commissure is not any more readily invaded than any other part of

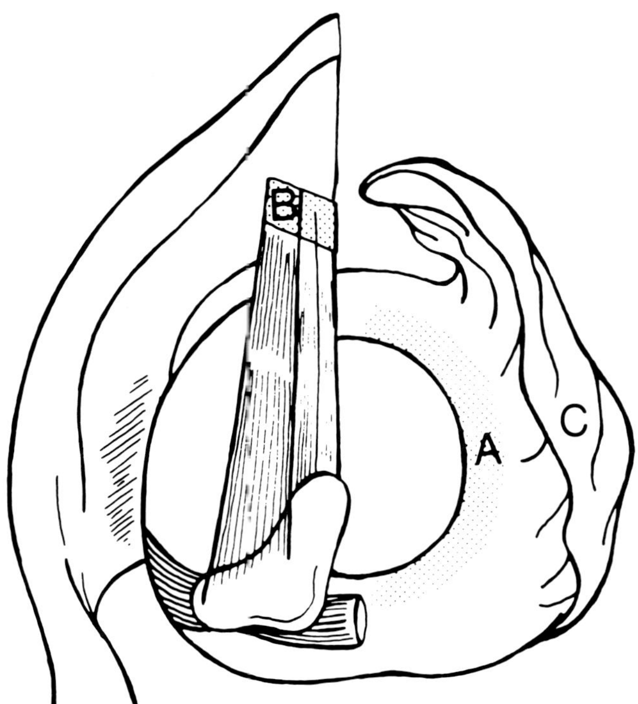

Figure 16–5. Recommended biopsies from patient. A: entire subglottic margin. B: opposite cord. C: pyriform sinus mucosa. (From Mohr et al.[2] Reprinted with permission.)

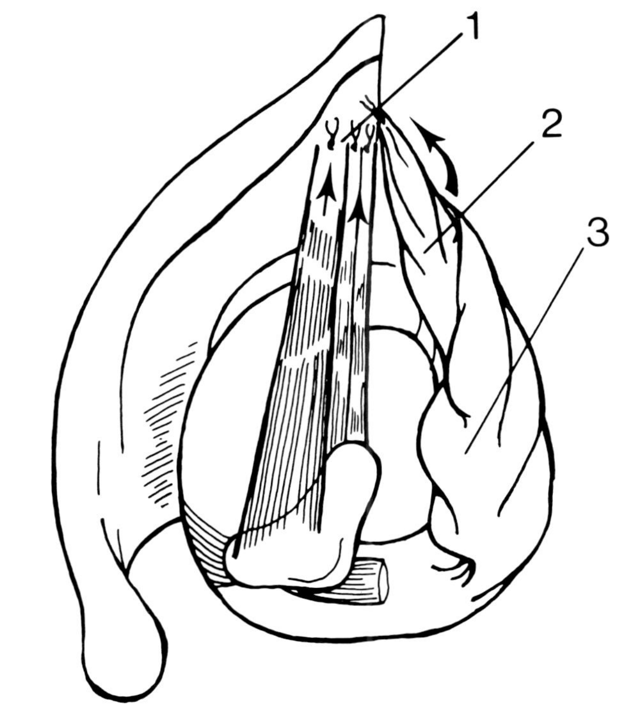

Figure 16–6. Recreating the anterior commissure. 1: reattachment of remnant cord to anterior commissure area; 2: insertion of neocord (pyriform sinus) slightly above new anterior commissure (allows for neocord retraction)—the arytenoid is removed and pyriform sinus drapes across posterior commissure area to prevent aspiration. (From Mohr et al.[2] Reprinted with permission.)

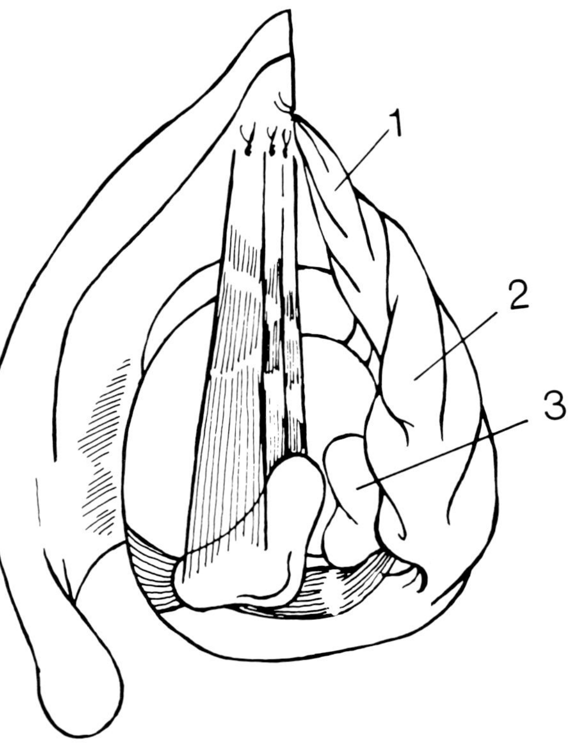

Figure 16–7. Reconstruction with pyriform sinus, arytenoid saved: 1: neocord from pyriform sinus; 2: redundant hypopharyngeal mucosa used to close pharyngotomy; 3: arytenoid, which tends to be herniated into airway—occasionally requiring arytenoidectomy to allow removal of tracheal tube. (From Mohr et al.[2] Reprinted with permission.)

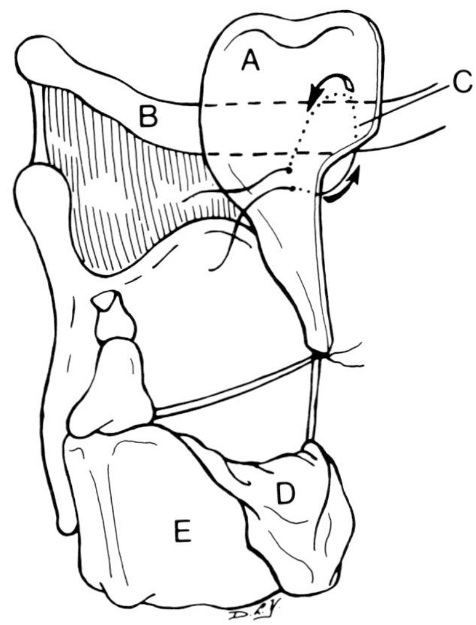

Figure 16–8. Reattaching the epiglottis to improve postoperative view of the endolarynx. (From Mohr et al.[2] Reprinted with permission.)

the larynx. It is the pattern of the tumor at the anterior commissure or laterally in the ventricle that may indicate thyroid cartilage invasion. If a tumor extends from the vocal cord onto the lower portion of the epiglottis at the anterior commissure, then the risk for cartilage invasion is extremely great.[18]

MANAGEMENT OF ASPIRATION

Postoperative aspiration of food and saliva can be minimized by reconstruction. If aspiration is a chronic problem, various methods may be employed to minimize glottic incompetence. Teflon injections in the neocord are not particularly rewarding because scarring prevents efficacious distribution of the injected material. If there is sufficient residual thyroid cartilage, the imbrication procedure of Liu et al[31] would seem a more acceptable way of medializing the neocord to improve voice. Following more extended resections, it may be necessary to overclose the glottis to prevent aspiration. Silastic or cartilage shims are a consideration if there is any cartilage left to hold them. Significant aspiration can, on occasion, require completion laryngectomy. However, this is very rare. Most patients can compensate by head position changes during swallowing or by utilizing swallowing techniques found effective for patients after horizontal supraglottic laryngectomy.[2]

RADIATION THERAPY AS AN ALTERNATIVE

Cure rates achieved by modern radiotherapy are comparable to those of VHL (90 to 95%) for early glottic lesions.[2,24,32] With proper tissue compensation, "wedging" and "dewedging," the entire larynx can receive a uniform, adequate dose. Pure glottic lesions, regardless of their anterior commissure extent can be cured without severe radiation complications.[2,27,33]

There is some controversy regarding the ability to perform partial laryngectomy after radiation. This has been proven by many authors to be a viable surgical option (78% cure) for selected glottic recurrences.[2,23,34] If recurrence is submucosal and extensive, then, of course, total laryngectomy would be required.

The question remains, then, should VHL be performed as the primary mode of treatment for early glottic cancer? Most radiation oncologists would say "no." They say the voice is better after radiation therapy and that patients can be salvaged with partial laryngectomy or total laryngectomy. I agree with them in most cases. Radiation-induced tumors are of some concern. Lawson and Som[35] reported occurrence of new primary carcinomas within the irradiated field in 9% of cases as opposed to 3.9% of patients treated by surgery alone. The second primaries occurred 5 to 25 years after completion of the radiation therapy. Thus, in the younger age group, fear of this occurrence would provide an impetus toward the choice of surgical treatment. I recommend surgery for all patients 40 years of age or younger.

Some glottic recurrences after radiation therapy do not require VHL. Many patients who have early or small recurrences can be treated successfully with laser surgery. Radiation therapy should be discussed with the patient as an alternative to VHL during preoperative counseling.

WHO, THEN, SHOULD HAVE THE PROCEDURE?

In my opinion, operative treatment of early vocal cord carcinoma is indicated with little question in patients up to age 40 years who have pure glottic lesions not amenable to vocal cord stripping or to laser therapy. Lesions that traverse the anterior commissure or extend into the anterior commissure do not lend themselves to laser therapy. T_2–T_3 glottic lesions with subglottic or supraglottic extension should, in my opinion, receive combined therapy of VHL followed by radiation therapy, or, alternatively, radiation therapy with surgery for salvage.

The choice of the therapy is dependent on the patient's response to the presentation of the potential consequences of VHL, VHL followed by radiation, or radiation alone. The sophistication of patients today requires that we give them alternatives and describe the pros and cons of each treatment. I do not think VHL should be performed for T_1 lesions even if there is anterior commissure involvement. Modern radiotherapy is a viable alternative for patients who are over age 40 years.

CONCLUSIONS

VHL is a satisfactory method of treating pure glottic carcinoma with preservation of voice and other laryngeal functions. Radiation therapy offers a suitable, and often preferable, alternative for treatment of early glottic lesions. A disadvantage of VHL is the difficulty in detection of recurrent tumor at an early stage. This is minimized by modern diagnostic techniques, as well as avoidance of bulky reconstructive techniques. Radiation therapy may predispose to second primary cancers within the irradiated field and should be avoided in young patients.

Although irradiation may leave the patient with a better voice than VHL, this factor is secondary to other considerations in selection of therapy. Voice after partial laryngectomy is generally serviceable, and, for most patients, satisfactory. A complex decision-making process, in which the patient should participate, is involved in choosing appropriate therapy for glottic carcinoma in each individual case.

The reference list for this discussion, although limited, is recommended to help the reader make informed decisions concerning glottic carcinoma that may be managed by VHL and its various extensions and reconstructions.

ACKNOWLEDGMENT

The author wishes to acknowledge the assistance of Dolores Fishbein, secretary, for her invaluable help preparing this manuscript and Donna Youmans for her superb illustrations.

REFERENCES

1. Norris CM. Role and limitations of vertical hemilaryngectomy. Can J Otolaryngol 1975;4:426–31.
2. Mohr RM, Quenelle DJ, Shumrick DA. Vertico-frontolateral laryngectomy (hemilaryngectomy). Indications, technique, and results. Arch Otolaryngol, 1983;109 384–95.
3. Norris CM. Technique of extended fronto-lateral partial laryngectomy. Laryngoscope 1958;68 1240–50.
4. Thomson StC, Colledge L. *Cancer of the Larynx*. New York: Macmillan, 1930:136.
5. Billroth T. Cited by Quinn HJ. Hemilaryngectomy: indications and a standardized technique. South Med J 1969;62:1031–5.
6. Schwartz AW. Dr. Theodore Billroth and the first laryngectomy. Ann Plast Surg 1978;1:513–6.
7. Gluck W. Hemilaryngectomy. In: Kirschner M, Lautenschlager A, Kleinschmidt O, eds. *Operative surgery*, vol. 3. Philadelphia, JB Lippincott, 1937:394–405.
8. Hautant A. Ma technique de l'hemilaryngectomie: ses resultats. Otorhinolaryngol Int 1930;5:217–24.
9. Goodyear HM. Hemilaryngectomy, method of maintaining satisfactory airway and voice. Ann Otol Rhinol Laryngol 1949;58:581–5.
10. Som ML. Hemilaryngectomy: a modified technique for cordal carcinoma with extension posteriorly. Arch Otolaryngol 1951;54:524–33.
11. Biller HF, Ogura JH, Pratt LL. Hemilaryngectomy for T_2 glottic cancers. Arch Otolaryngol 1971;93:238–43.
12. Tucker GF. Some clinical inferences from the study of serial laryngeal sections. Laryngoscope 1963;73:728–48.
13. Norris CM, Kuo BF, Tucker GF, Pitser WF. A correlation of clinical staging, pathological findings and five year end results in surgically treated cancer of the larynx. Ann Otol Rhinol Laryngol 1970;79:1033–48.
14. Kirchner JA. One hundred laryngeal cancers studied by serial section. Ann Otol Rhinol Laryngol 1969;78:678–709.
15. Kirchner JA, Som ML. Clinical significance of fixed vocal cord. Laryngoscope 1971;81:1029–44.
16. Kirchner JA. Two hundred laryngeal cancers: patterns of growth and spread as seen in serial section. Laryngoscope 1977;87:474–82.
17. Kirchner JA. Pathways and pitfalls in partial laryngectomy. Ann Otol Rhinol Laryngol 1984;93:301–5.
18. Kirchner JA. What have whole organ sections contributed to the treatment of laryngeal cancer? Ann Otol Rhinol Laryngol 1989;98: 661–7.
19. Pillsbury HRC, Kirchner JA. Clinical vs. histopathologic staging in laryngeal cancer. Arch Otolaryngol 1979;105:157–9.
20. Pressman JJ, Simon MB, Monell C. Anatomical studies related to the dissemination of cancer of the larynx. Trans Am Acad Ophthalmol Otolaryngol 1960;64:628–38.
21. *Manual for Staging for Cancer*, 3rd ed. American Joint Committee on Cancer, 1988:43–4.
22. Pearson BW, Woods RD, Hartman DE. Extended hemilaryngectomy for T_3 glottic carcinoma with preservation of speech and swallowing. Laryngoscope 1980;90:1950–61.
23. Norris CM, Peale AR. Partial laryngectomy for irradiation failure. Arch Otolaryng 1966;84:112–6.
24. Silver CE. Conservation surgery for glottic carcinoma. In: Silver CE, ed. *Surgery for Cancer of the Larynx*. New York: Churchill Livingstone, 1981:83–121.
25. Montgomery WW. Subtotal laryngectomy for carcinoma of the larynx. In: Montgomery WW, ed. *Surgery of the upper respiratory system*. Philadelphia: Lea & Febiger, 1973:514–27.
26. Lore JM. Partial laryngectomy. In: Lore JM, ed. *An atlas of head and neck surgery*, 3rd ed. Philadelphia: WB Saunders, 1988:894–911.
27. Myers EM, Ogura JH. Completion laryngectomy. Otolaryngol Head Neck Surg 1979;87:342–50.
28. Lee F, Perlmutter S, Ogura JH. Laryngeal radiation after hemilaryngectomy. Laryngoscope 1980;90:1534–9.
29. Myers EM, Ogura JH. Stomal recurrences: a clinicopathological analysis and protocol for future management. Laryngoscope 1979;89:1121–8.
30. Som ML. Cordal cancer with extension to vocal process. Laryngoscope 1975;85:1298–1307.
31. Liu C. Ward PH, Pleet L. Imbrication reconstruction following partial laryngectomy. Ann Otol Rhinol Laryngol 1986;95:567–71.
32. Million RR, Cassisi NJ. *Management of head and neck cancer. A multidisciplinary approach*. Philadelphia: JB Lippincott, 1985:351–8.
33. Parsons JT, Mendenhall WM, Mancuso AA, et al. Twice-a-day radiotherapy for T_3 squamous cell carcinoma of the glottic larynx. Head Neck 1989;11:123–28.
34. Biller HF, Barnhill FR, Ogura JH, Perez CA. Hemilaryngectomy following radiation failure for carcinoma of the vocal cords. Laryngoscope 1970;80:249–53.
35. Lawson W, Som M. Second primary cancer after irradiation of laryngeal cancer. Ann Otol 1975;84:771–5.

17

Treatment of Cancer of the Supraglottic Larynx

Helmuth Goepfert, Norris Lee, Charles D. Wendt, Lester J. Peters

Treatment of carcinoma of the supraglottic larynx should be selected not only to eradicate the cancer cost effectively but also, to preserve or restore laryngeal function. It should also encompass counseling and education likely to lead to habit and life-style changes that will reduce patients' exposure to environmental carcinogens and the probability of subsequent primary tumors of the upper aerodigestive tract. If total ablation of the larynx is necessary, phonation should be restored or another adequate means of communication established.

For a treatment team to give the maximum benefit to the patient, whether treated by surgery, irradiation, or a combination of both, the surgeon must understand the basic principles of radiation therapy, and, correspondingly, the radiotherapist should be familiar with the essentials of the surgical techniques employed in the management of cancer in this location.[1,2] As new modalities, such as neoadjuvant chemotherapy or biologic response modification, are employed and clinical research protocols are developed to test their merit, the purpose and risk-benefit ratio of any deviation from the best possible standard should be kept clearly in mind.

The most common histologic type of malignant tumor in the larynx is squamous cell carcinoma, with its histologic variations and degrees of differentiation. Spindle cell carcinomas and verrucous carcinomas are rare.[2] Salivary gland cancers occur in this area.[3] Oat cell carcinomas, soft tissue sarcomas, and chondrosarcomas are encountered but are extremely rare.[4]

The relative incidence of supraglottic versus glottic carcinoma in the larynx varies from 18 to 60%. In certain areas of the world there is a predominance of glottic carcinoma, but in other geographic locations supraglottic cancer prevails. Within the larynx, only relatively advanced tumors will spread in a caudal direction beyond the laryngeal ventricle into the paraglottic space or through the anterior commissure into the subglottic space, but invasion of the preepiglottic space and the base of the tongue by moderately advanced and very advanced lesions is well documented.[6,7] Most cancers of the supraglottic larynx arise on the epiglottis, specifically the infrahyoid portion.[8] The patterns of growth and spread of supraglottic larynx carcinomas depend on where the cancer arises and the contiguous sites involved in tumor progression. Except for small lesions of the false cords or the aryepiglottic folds, most cancers in this area involve a midline structure, and lymphatic spread is bilateral. The submucosa of the supraglottic larynx is permeated by a rich plexus of interconnecting lymphatic vessels with efferent channels to both sides. The tributaries of this plexus collect in channels that flow laterally in the submucosa of the pyriform sinus and exit through the thyrohyoid membrane together with the internal branch of the superior laryngeal nerve and the superior laryngeal artery and vein. The first echelon lymph nodes are the ones distributed about the carotid bifurcation and the midjugular lymph nodes. Over half of patients will have clinically positive nodes at the time of diagnosis, and the incidence of occult or subclinical metastatic cancer is between 30 and 50%.[9–11] Because of this propensity toward lymph node invasion, the management of primary tumors in the supraglottic larynx must be integrated with the treatment of clinically obvious, as well as subclinical, cancer in the regional lymph nodes.[9,12–14] The incidence of lymph node metastasis varies for the subsites of primary tumor growth in the supraglottic larynx.[15]

PATIENT EVALUATION

Comprehensive management of cancer of the supraglottic larynx requires thorough evaluation of the site of origin and a search for routes of local extension and spread.[1,2] Physical examination is complemented with appropriate imaging studies to define the submucosal boundaries of cancer at the primary site and the regional lymph nodes. The flexible fiberoptic endoscope has facilitated direct visualization of the hypopharynx and larynx. Videotape recording of fiberoptic endoscopy allows dynamic examination of the location and extent of cancer and is a valuable tool for objective documentation of treatment during radiation therapy or neoadjuvant chemotherapy. In addition, this technology creates a record of progress of rehabilitation of laryngeal function after conservation surgery.

Computed tomography (CT) is the preferred imaging technique for evaluation of laryngeal cancer.[2,16] This method allows determination of the extent of local disease, imaging of submucosal structures, and identification of cancer spread to regional lymph nodes. Prior to the advent of CT scanning, imaging of the larynx was done primarily by contrast laryngography, multiplanar tomography, and xeroradiography.[17,18] Such imaging techniques have been largely replaced by CT scanning with contrast enhancement and, lately, by magnetic resonance imaging. We recommend that imaging studies be done prior to the biopsy to avoid the distortion produced by the intervention and subsequent edema.

Cancer originating in the suprahyoid epiglottis usually presents as an exophytic growth and is seldom infiltrating or destructive. It may extend through surface spread into the vallecula and the adjacent pharyngeal wall. In contrast, cancer originating in the infrahyoid epiglottis has easy access through the epiglottic cartilage into the preepiglottic space and by contiguous growth may extend into the false cords or aryepiglottic folds in a caudal direction. Occasionally, cancer of this location may grow through the anterior commissure into the subglottic area and invade the thyroid cartilage. The amount of invasion of the preepiglottic space must be determined; in our opinion, it is not a contraindication for either partial laryngeal surgery or, if limited, for treatment by radiation therapy.

Cancer arising on the false cords or in the laryngeal ventricle may extend into the paraglottic space and the preepiglottic space and through the submucosal tissue planes into the pyriform sinuses. Cancers originating on the aryepiglottic fold can grow laterally into the pyriform sinus and may be difficult to differentiate from tumors arising in this area. The vallecula may be superficially invaded by cancers arising in the suprahyoid epiglottis or may be invaded secondarily by tumor growing out of the preepiglottic space. This latter circumstance usually portends a more advanced tumor. Vocal cord mobility can be difficult to document if the bulk of the tumor obstructs the view. The subtle distinctions between mobile, partially fixed, and fixed cords require visualization by an experienced examiner, sometimes by repeated examinations through a fiberoptic laryngoscope.

The character of the patient's voice is a subtle and sensitive indicator of both cord mobility and tumor invasion of this structure. We find that carefully listening to the patient's voice as different vowels are phonated is extremely helpful. Appropriate imaging of the larynx is the best means of determining preepiglottic space invasion and/or tumor break through the thyroid cartilage. Lateral soft tissue roentgenograms or xerograms of the neck allow for delineation of tumor in both its superior and inferior extensions.[17]

Staging of cancer in the supraglottic larynx is done according to the American Joint Committee on Cancer (AJCC) criteria for both the primary site and the regional lymph nodes.[19]

It is mandatory to test cardiopulmonary function of a patient with cancer in this location, especially if conservation surgery is contemplated.[2] Cancer of the supraglottic larynx occurs primarily in heavy cigarette smokers. Long-term smokers usually have various degrees of chronic obstructive pulmonary disease and, frequently, signs and symptoms of arteriosclerosis in different organs. The presence of significant pathologic abnormalities in any parenchyma should have a definite influence on the selection of treatment for these patients. We consider that a patient who can sustain a brisk walk up a flight of stairs or who has little or no difficulty with day-to-day activities may not require objective determination of spirometry or other pulmonary function testing. If there is doubt, spirometry should be done; if forced expiratory volume in 1 second is less than 50 to 60% of predicted normal, under the most optimal conditions, such a patient may not be capable of withstanding the chronic aspiration of food and saliva likely to follow any type of conservation surgery. A different treatment option should be chosen; we would consider this individual "unfit" for conservation surgery.

An evaluation of possible concomitant second primary tumors should be done in a cost-effective manner. Finally, the wishes and desires of the patient need to be respected in any treatment decision.

SELECTION OF TREATMENT

Figure 17–1 provides an outline of the algorithm we currently follow in selection of treatment for each T stage. Treatment

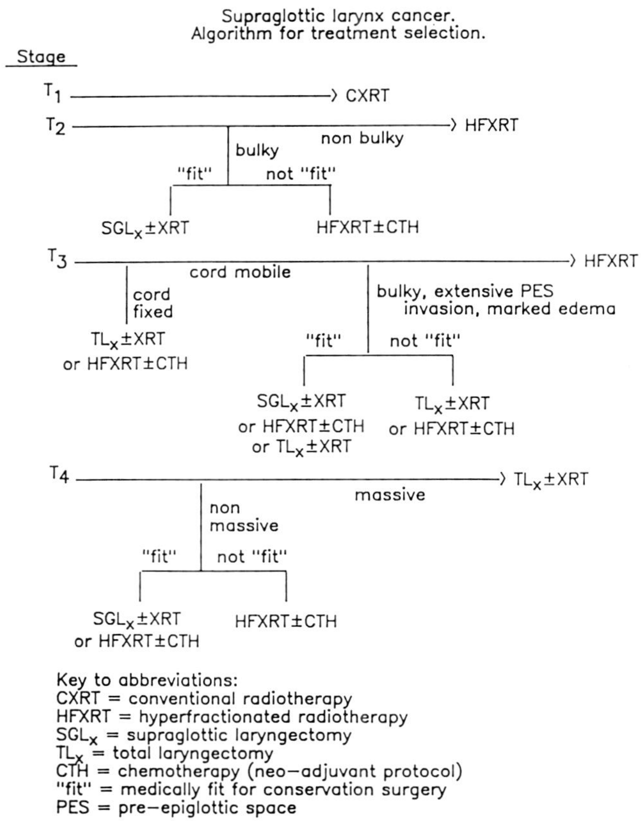

Figure 17–1. Algorithm for treatment selection of supraglottic larynx cancer. (From Lee et al.[26] Reprinted with permission.)

options include surgical resection, partial or total laryngectomy, radiation therapy, and, depending on the clinical situation, sequential use of both methods for treatment of the primary or neck disease. In addition, experimental treatment with neoadjuvant chemotherapy to "downstage" the primary tumor is available under a strict clinical protocol. Table 17–1 summarizes the methods of treatment of all patients with supraglottic cancer seen at the University of Texas, M.D. Anderson Cancer Center (MDACC) between 1974 and 1987.

Radiation therapy and conservation surgery are both effective therapeutic approaches for control of early supraglottic cancer.[2] Over the years, improvements in diagnostic capabilities and changing trends in combined surgical and radiotherapy treatment plans have evolved. All patients with supraglottic cancer should be evaluated by both the radiotherapist and the surgeon prior to treatment. In addition, we recommend dental evaluation whenever radiation therapy is part of the treatment plan. If the extent of tumor precludes conservation surgery, and total laryngectomy is the only feasible surgical option, the alternative of enrolling the patient in larynx-sparing treatment protocols, including neoadjuvant chemotherapy and altered fractionation radiation therapy, is discussed with the patient and family.

RADIATION THERAPY

Most T_1 and many T_2 lesions are effectively treated by radiation therapy; this is the treatment of choice for early supraglottic cancer. Initial local control of approximately 90% is achieved with definitive radiotherapy for these lesions, with ultimate tumor control after surgery for recurrences of 95 to 98%.[20]

The treatment of the intermediate staged, T_2 and T_3 lesions, remains controversial.[21] Conventional radiotherapy delivering 180 to 200 cGy once per day to doses of 6500 to 7700 cGy has been reported to achieve control rates of 60 to 77% for T_2 lesions. At MDACC, we believe that most T_2 and many T_3 lesions can be treated effectively with primary radiotherapy provided appropriate selection criteria are applied.[20] The main contraindications to radiotherapy are bulky and/or infiltrative tumors with cord fixation, marked edema, or extensive preepiglottic space invasion. Tumors with these features are best treated by conservation laryngeal surgery when feasible or total laryngectomy when other considerations dictate.[1,20–22]

If total laryngectomy is the only option, the patient is offered the opportunity to enter a research protocol to evaluate the utility of neoadjuvant chemotherapy.

Since January 1984, all patients with stage T_2 or T_3 supraglottic larynx lesions who have been selected for definitive radiotherapy at the MDACC have been treated with a program of hyperfractionated therapy using 120 or 110 cGy twice daily. Hyperfractionated therapy exploits the differences in fraction size sensitivity between rapidly proliferating tissues such as tumor cells and mucosal cells, and slowly proliferating tissues such as cartilage.[23] The rapidly proliferating tissues are less sensitive to changes in fraction size. By reducing the fractional dose from 180 to 200 cGy to 110 to 120 cGy, it is possible to increase total tumor dose; increasing the probability of tumor control.

From January 1984 through December 1987, 38 patients with stages T_2 and T_3 supraglottic primary tumors were treated with hyperfractionated radiotherapy. This group included 23 T_2 lesions and 15 T_3 lesions. Three patients with fixed vocal cords had induction chemotherapy prior to radiotherapy, and three patients underwent planned preradiotherapy or postradiotherapy neck dissections.

Basic wide field therapy was delivered through lateral portals encompassing the larynx and upper neck nodes[20,23] For the first 30 patients, these fields were treated with 120 cGy fractions twice per day, with at least 4 hours between fractions. The remaining eight patients received 110 cGy fractions at a minimum interfraction interval of 6 hours. A field reduction, to spare the spinal cord, was made at 4400 to 4500 cGy; the tumor dose was carried to 5500 to 5760 cGy. If the neck was clinically positive, the posterior strips were supplemented with electron beam therapy to 550 cGy and the lower neck and supraclavicular areas were treated with a single anterior oppositional field to a dose of 5000 cGy using 200 cGy fractions once per day. Originally, patients with clinically negative nodes did not receive elective treatment to the posterior cervical or supraclavicular areas. Because two such patients, however, subsequently developed disease outside the radiated fields (one in a supraclavicular node and the other in a posterior cervical node) and because the additional morbidity of treating these areas is minimal, we recently adopted a policy of treating the entire neck in all patients.

Preliminary results of this treatment regimen with follow-up through June 1988 were reported by Wendt et al.[24] These results have now been updated through September 1989, providing a median follow-up of 31 months with a minimum of 20 months. Of the entire group of 38 patients, six have had local-regional failures: three at the primary site, one in both the primary and neck, and two in the neck only (outside the treatment fields). The actuarial 2-year local control rate is 90%, and the 2-year actuarial control rate above the clavicles is 84%. Five of the six

Table 17–1. Treatment of 404 Patients with Squamous Carcinoma of the Supraglottic Larynx, January 1974 through December 1987

1. Definitive therapy with intent of laryngeal preservation		
Radiotherapy only	199	
Requiring salvage surgery (2 partial, 10 total laryngectomy)	12	
Total treated by radiotherapy		211
Partial laryngectomy		
With postoperative radiotherapy	54*	
Without postoperative radiotherapy	11	
Total conservation surgery		65†
Neoadjuvant chemotherapy plus radiotherapy		3
2. Total laryngectomy		
With postoperative radiotherapy*	96	
Without postoperative radiotherapy	29	
Total		125

*Indications for postoperative radiotherapy: (1) significant extralaryngeal extension (base of tongue, pharyngeal wall, subglottis, neck tissues); (2) cancer in multiple lymph nodes; (3) extracapsular and connective tissue invasion; (4) perineural spread.

†Sixty supraglottic laryngectomies; one vertical hemilaryngectomy; four other conservation surgeries.

failures were successfully salvaged with surgery, yielding a total 2-year local-regional control rate of 96%.

When compared with a group of 100 matched stage T_2 and T_3 patients treated at the MDACC from 1970 through 1979 with conventional fractionation, these figures represent a 14% improvement in local control ($p = 0.027$), and an 11% improvement in overall local-regional control ($p = 0.056$) (Figs. 17–2, 17–3). As expected, acute reactions were more severe with twice-a-day treatment than with conventional fractionation. Severe acute reactions—defined as loss of more than 10% of pretreatment body weight, mucositis requiring a nasogastric tube, or persistent mucositis lasting more than 2 months after completion of radiotherapy—occurred in 12 of 38 (32%) patients treated with the hyperfractionated regimen. In an effort to reduce the severity of acute effects while maintaining the benefits of hyperfractionation, we reduced the fractional dose to 110 cGy to the large fields and increased the interfraction interval to at least 6 hours. For the smaller volume boost field, the dose per fraction has been maintained at 120 cGy. Only two patients treated with hyperfractionated therapy have developed severe late complications. One developed laryngeal necrosis, which was successfully managed with hyperbaric oxygen treatment; the other required a laryngectomy for necrosis without evidence of recurrent tumor. The incidence of severe complications is not greater than that of the historical series treated with conventional fractionation. Overall, 33 of 38 (87%) stage T_2 and T_3 patients have retained healthy, functioning larynges.

Follow-up Examinations After Definitive Radiotherapy

Patients are examined at 6 and 12 weeks after completing radiotherapy and then every 3 months for 2 years. As already noted, acute reactions may be protracted with superficial ulceration and edema persisting for several months after completion of treatment. These findings are *not* indications for biopsy to rule out recurrence. In the absence of frank recurrent disease, we believe the only indication for biopsy in the postradiation period is increasing pain that lasts longer than 6 weeks and/or worsening of ulceration or edema. Unwarranted biopsies may precipitate laryngeal necrosis and should be avoided. After 2 years, the follow-up intervals are increased to 6 to 12 months, depending on circumstances.

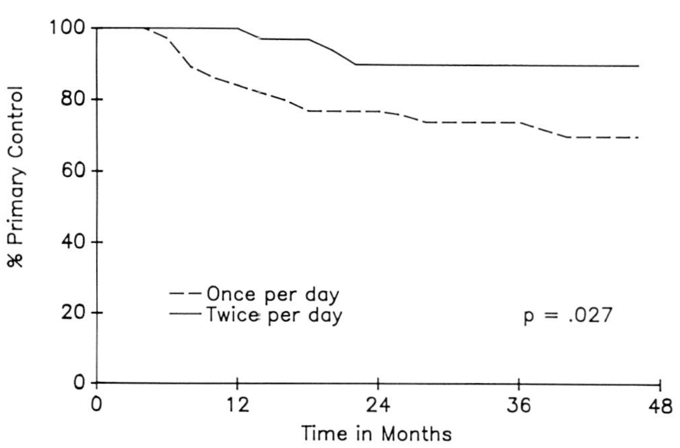

Figure 17–2. Primary control: Patients treated with radiotherapy.

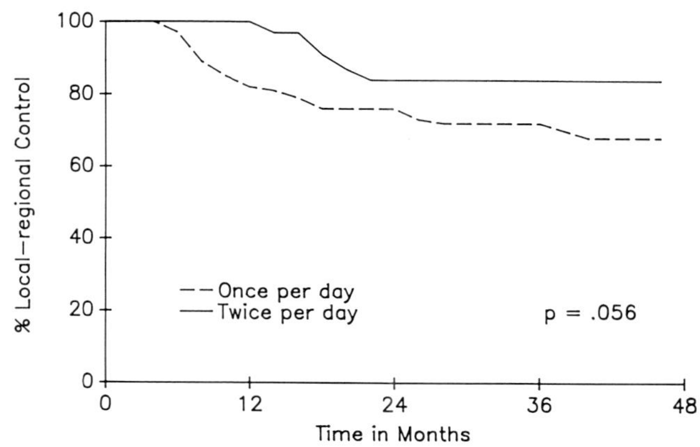

Figure 17–3. Local-regional control: Patients treated with radiotherapy.

SURGICAL THERAPY

The surgical techniques available for cancer of the supraglottic larynx are well established.[2,21,25] Treatment of the primary tumor is integrated with management of the neck disease. If surgery is chosen for the treatment of supraglottic larynx cancer and there is no clinically obvious metastatic disease in the neck, bilateral jugular node dissection is performed, with preservation of the spinal accessory nerve, the jugular vein, sternocleidomastoid muscles, and the contents of the submandibular triangles.[14] If obvious cancer is present in the lymph nodes, an appropriate neck dissection is performed; if necessary, a standard radical dissection is performed. Invasion of lymph nodes in the posterior triangle and in the submandibular area is extremely rare and occurs only when there is substantial invasion of lymph nodes along the jugular chain. These nodal areas, if involved, are included en bloc in the dissection.[10,11,14]

COMBINED SURGERY AND RADIOTHERAPY

Combination surgery and irradiation approaches use each to complement the other. Irradiation can eradicate microscopic diseases, whereas surgery is most effective with larger volumes of bulky tumors.[12,20,22] Partial removal of a tumor achieves little, since this does not reduce residual disease to the microscopic level required for effective radiation therapy. If the concept of combined treatment is to be successful, all gross tumor must be removed. Unnecessary dissection in areas unlikely to be affected by disease is avoided. The term "debulking" should be used cautiously because it usually implies incomplete removal of gross tumor. We do not recommend the use of laser procedures for supraglottic larynx cancer, since they distort the local anatomy and leave an indeterminable amount of cancer in the tissues injured by the procedure and further modified by subsequent healing. Evaluation of the histologic specimen at both the primary site and the cervical lymph nodes determines who will benefit from postoperative radiotherapy. Cancer growth outside the confines of the larynx in the preglottic and paraglottic spaces or close to the margins of resection requires postoperative radiation therapy to the primary tumors.[22] Because of our concern about aggravation of aspiration by arytenoid edema, the postoperative protocol applied following supraglottic laryngectomy is somewhat modified from our standard for other sites. The postoperative dose has been set at 5500 cGy in 30 fractions over 6 weeks, with the dose specified at the midplane of the larynx. If cancer is present in more than one node or in the lymph nodes outside of the primary echelon of drainage, or if there is evidence of extranodal extension, postoperative radiotherapy is indicated for the neck. In such cases a booster dose of electrons of appropriate energy to a dose of 6300 cGy is delivered to the neck.

Our policy is to use supraglottic laryngectomy in patients with disease considered unsuitable for definitive radiotherapy.[21,22] For this reason, most of the patients undergoing supraglottic laryngectomy have had bulky lesions for which postoperative radiotherapy had been recommended. Under most circumstances, postoperative irradiation after partial laryngectomy is started 3 to 4 weeks following surgery and, almost always, within 6 weeks.

Between 1974 and 1987, 60 patients underwent supraglottic laryngectomy as definitive initial therapy. Another two patients underwent the procedure for salvage after radiation therapy and one after failure to respond to chemotherapy. This group of 60 selected patients was derived from a total population of 404 treated at the MDACC for cancer of the supraglottic larynx. In Table 17–2 the distribution of tumors in these patients is listed according to AJCC staging criteria. Fifty-four patients (83%) received postoperative radiation therapy (Table 17–1). Radiation for one patient was discontinued during the third week of treatment due to a severe local reaction, with intense swelling of the mucosa over the arytenoids. All other patients finished the radiation therapy within 12 weeks of surgery. This regimen has been well tolerated, and the morbidity encountered in patients receiving postoperative radiotherapy has been only slightly greater than in those treated by surgery alone.

The histologic evaluation of the neck specimens revealed that the clinical nodal staging had been inappropriate in 36% of cases. In a majority of instances, the neck had been understaged: 25 of 104 (24%) were upstaged from N_0 to N_+, and 10 of 104 (10%) were upstaged from N_1 to a higher N stage. Only 3% were downstaged from N_+ to N_0 because histopathologic examination revealed no evidence of metastatic disease in the removed lymph nodes. Table 17–3 compares the clinical and pathologic staging of cervical lymph nodes.

All patients were followed for at least 2 years. Survival rates calculated by the Kaplan-Meier method were 96% disease-specific at 2 years, and 91% disease-specific at 5 years (Fig. 17–4). In this group, none of the stagings, that is, the primary, the neck, or the pathologic tumor grade, had statistical prognostic significance. Ten patients died of secondary primary cancers. Eight patients developed lung cancers. Two patients died of postoperative complications. All patients who died of undetermined causes 2 to 7 years after treatment had been free of cancer at the last follow-up visit and it is considered unlikely that they died of the index cancer. Five patients died of their laryngeal cancer: two from regional disease, two from distant metastasis, and one with both regional disease and distant metastasis. One patient alive 2½ years after treatment is receiving chemotherapy for a local recurrence (Table 17–4).

Patients who undergo partial laryngeal surgery with postoperative radiation therapy retain their plastic tracheostomy tubes until radiation therapy is completed. Most patients are able to breathe with the tube occluded; only a few require the tracheotomy for adequate respiration during the latter phase of radiotherapy.

Table 17–5 lists the complications of patients treated by conservation surgery.

Successful rehabilitation of deglutition is an important feature after conservation surgery for supraglottic carcinoma, particularly when postoperative irradiation is employed. We have

Table 17-2. Patients with Supraglottic Carcinoma Treated by Supraglottic Laryngectomy: Clinical Staging*

NODAL STATUS	TUMOR STATUS T1	T2	T3	T4	TOTAL NO. PATIENTS
N_0	3	21	15	1	40
N_1	0	5	4	1	10
$>N_1$	0	6	2	2	10
Total no. patients	3	32	21	4	60

*Adapted with permission from Lee et al.[26]

Table 17-3. Dissected Neck Specimens: Correlation between Clinical and Pathologic Staging

CLINICAL STAGE*	HISTOPATHOLOGIC STAGE	NO. SPECIMENS
N_0	Same	56
N_0	N+	25
N+	N_0	3
N+	Same	10
N+	Upstaged	10

*+: positive.

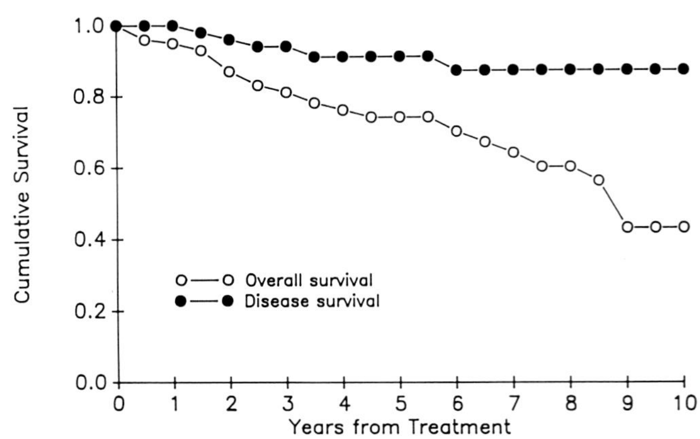

Figure 17–4. Survival after conservation surgery and radiation therapy for cancer of the supraglottic larynx. (From Lee et al.[26] Reprinted with permission.)

Table 17-4. Conservation Surgery for Six Supraglottic Cancers: Patients with Treatment Failures*

SITE†	TIME (MIN)	TREATMENT	OUTCOME†
Reg	39	None	DOD
Reg	10	Surgery	DOD
Reg	30	Chemotherapy	AWD
Reg/DM	16	Chemotherapy	DOD
DM	4	Chemotherapy	DOD
DM	18	Radiotherapy	DOD

*Adapted with permission from Lee et al.[26]

†Reg: regional recurrence; DM: distant metastasis; DOD: died of disease (cancer); AWD: alive with disease (cancer).

found fluoroscopic evaluation, beginning at about the 10th postoperative day, to be the most helpful means of identifying aspiration. Most patients are able to manage a complete diet of solid food by the 14th postoperative day, although they may need a longer period of rehabilitation before they can swallow liquids. We do not hesitate to maintain patients with tube feedings during the entire extent of postoperative radiation therapy if there is any indication that nutrition is inadequate prior to beginning the postoperative treatment. The patient's weight and sense of well-being are carefully monitored to avoid unnecessary morbidity and metabolic depletion. Replacement of the nasogastric tube is mandatory in assisting the patient through the periods of intense mucositis and dysphagia that often accompany postoperative radiation therapy. Figure 17–5 shows the curve plotting deglutition and successful oral nutrition. By the end of 3 months, 72% of the patients were swallowing well enough that their feeding tubes could be removed.

Three of 60 patients (5%) had intractable aspiration, necessitating conversion to a total laryngectomy. Residual tumor was

Table 17-5. Supraglottic Larynx Cancer, Conservation Surgery*

COMPLICATIONS	NO. PATIENTS
Minor	
Hematoma	1
Wound infection	1
Fistula	2
Dysphagia:	
Stricture	1
Esophageal dysmotility	1
Vocal cord paralysis	3
Significant	
Intravenous hyperalimentation	1
Gastrostomy tube	7
Tracheostomy	1
Major	
Pneumonia	2
Completion laryngectomy	3
Death	
Saddle embolus	1
Massive cerebrovascular accident	1

*Adapted with permission from Lee et al.[26]

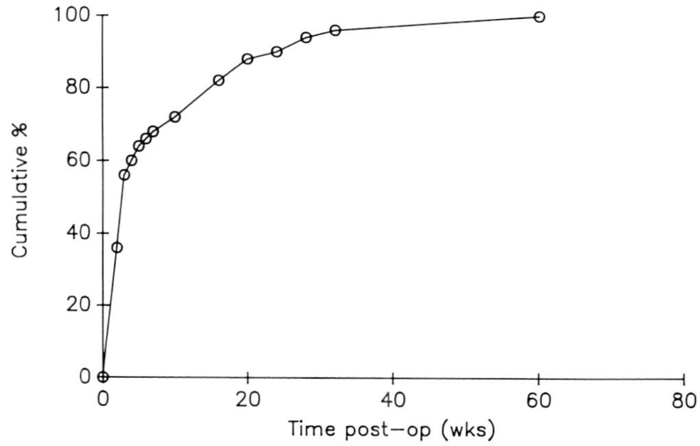

Figure 17–5. Supraglottic laryngeal carcinomas: Conservation surgery with postoperative radiation therapy—resumption of oral intake. (From Lee et al.[26] Reprinted with permission.)

not present in the larynx of any of these patients. Tracheal decannulation was accomplished in 65% of our patients by 12 weeks postoperatively (Fig. 17–6). Four of the 12 patients whose decannulation required longer than 3 months had undergone extended supraglottic laryngectomy. Fatal aspiration pneumonia occurred in one patient. The complication rate was greatest in patients who underwent extended laryngectomy with sacrifice of an arytenoid, particularly when postoperative radiation therapy had been administered (Table 17–6).

Total laryngectomy, with or without postoperative radiation therapy, is frequently required (Table 17–1). Under these circumstances, when feasible and depending on the wishes and motivations of the patient, a voice restoration procedure (tracheoesophageal fistula) is performed at the time of surgery. Our experience has shown, however, that the primary fistula necessary for voice restoration tends to be a source of complications in those patients who receive postoperative radiation therapy, particularly when the tracheostoma has been in the field of radiation therapy. For this reason, we recommend delayed voice

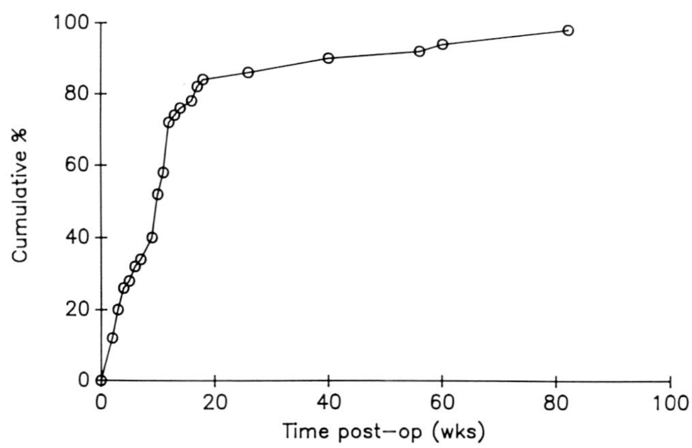

Figure 17–6. Supraglottic laryngeal carcinoma: Conservation surgery with postoperative radiation therapy—tracheostomy removal. (From Lee et al.[26] Reprinted with permission.)

Table 17-6. Extended Supraglottic Laryngectomy in Nine Patients*

ARYTENOIDECTOMY	OUTCOME
Partial	Decannulation, 10 weeks
Partial	Decannulation, 13 weeks
Partial	Decannulation, 10 months
Partial	Decannulation, 20 months
Partial	Permanent tracheostomy
Partial	Completion laryngectomy
Total	Decannulation, 6 weeks
Total	Decannulation, 13 months
Total	Decannulation, 6 weeks Occasional aspiration; died of aspiration, 7 years

*Adapted with permission from Lee et al.[26]

rehabilitation surgery in most patients after total laryngectomy. The use of combined treatment for advanced cancer of the supraglottic larynx has reduced the failure rate above the clavicles and, in our opinion, improves the 5-year survival rate of these patients.

Recurrent carcinoma of the supraglottic larynx secondary to radiation therapy is seldom amenable to conservation surgery, and total laryngectomy and appropriate neck dissection are usually necessary. All requisite precautions should be taken when operating in radiated tissue.

A consistent, careful evaluation to identify the sites of failure of local control demands the collaborative effort of all members of the treatment team for the best possible functional and oncologic results of any treatment chosen for the individual patient. Both conservation surgery and hyperfractionation radiotherapy have particular acute and delayed morbidity. It is the responsibility of the members of the treatment team to monitor carefully these patients throughout the post-treatment period, at least once a year, to recognize side effects of treatment and to prevent further complications. Whenever radiation therapy is used, the oropharyngeal mucositis may need supportive care for proper nutrition and alimentation. By the same token, patients submitted to supraglottic laryngectomy need the support of a trained speech pathologist for rehabilitation of deglutition and prevention of aspiration.

REFERENCES

1. Fletcher GH, Goepfert H. The role of irradiation in the treatment of cancer of the larynx. In: Ferlito A, ed. *Cancer of the larynx,* vol. 3. Boca Raton, FL: CRC Press. 1985:69–114.
2. Million RR, Cassissi NJ, eds. *Management of head and neck cancer: a multidisciplinary approach*. Philadelphia: JB Lippincott, 1984.
3. Cohen J, Guillamondegui OM, Batsakis JG, Medina JE. Cancer of the minor salivary glands of the larynx. Am J Surg 1985;150:513–8.
4. Batsakis JG, Fox JE. Supporting tissue neoplasms of the larynx. Surg Gynecol Obstet 1970;131:989–97.
5. Till J, Bruise WR, Elwan A, et al. A preliminary analysis of end results for cancer of the larynx. Laryngoscope 1975;85:259–75.
6. Pressman JJ, Simon MB, Monell C. Anatomic studies related to the dissemination of cancer of the larynx. Trans Am Acad Opthalmol Otolaryngol 1960;64:628–38.
7. Olofsson J, Van Nostrand AWP. Growth and spread of laryngeal and hypopharyngeal carcinoma with reflections on the effect of preoperative irradiation. Acta Otolaryngol Suppl (Stockh) 1973;308:1–84.
8. Coates HL, DeSanto LW, Devine KD, Elveback LR. Carcinoma of the supraglottic larynx. A review of 221 cases. Arch Otolaryngol 1976;102:686–9.
9. Lindberg RD. Distribution of cervical lymph node metastasis from squamous cell carcinoma of the upper respiratory and digestive tracts. Cancer 1972;29:1446–8.
10. Byers RM. Modified neck dissection. Am J Surg 1985;150:414–21.
11. Shah JP, Tollefson HR. Epidermal carcinoma of the supraglottic larynx: role of neck dissection in initial surgical treatment. Am J Surg 1974;128:494–9.
12. Fletcher GH. Elective irradiation of subclinical disease in cancers of the head and neck. Cancer 1972;29:1450–4.
13. Ogura JH, Biller HF, Wett ER. Elective neck dissection for pharyngeal and laryngeal cancers and evaluation. Ann Otol Rhinol Laryngol 1971;80:646–51.
14. Byers RM, Wolf PF, Ballantyne AJ. Rationale for elective modified neck dissection. Head Neck Surg 1988;10:160–7.
15. Kirchner JA, Som ML. Clinical and histological observations of supraglottic cancer. Ann Otol Rhinol Laryngol 1971;80:638–45.
16. Mancuso AA, Hanafee WN. *Computed tomography of the head and neck*. Baltimore: Williams & Wilkins, 1982:1–65.
17. Lehmann QH, Fletcher GH. Contribution of the laryngogram to the management of malignant laryngeal tumors. Radiology 1964;83:486–500.
18. Fletcher GH, Jing BS. *Head and neck, an atlas of tumor radiology*. Chicago: Yearbook Medical Publishers, 1968.
19. American Joint Committee *Manual for Staging of Cancer,* 3rd ed. Philadelphia: JB Lippincott, 1988:39.
20. Goepfert H, Jesse RH, Fletcher GH, et al. Optimal treatment for the technically resectable squamous cell carcinoma of the supraglottic larynx. Laryngoscope 1975;85:14–32.
21. Robbins KT, Davidson W, Peters LJ, et al. Conservation surgery for T_2 and T_3 carcinomas of the supraglottic larynx. Arch Otolaryngol Head Neck Surg 1988;114:421–6.
22. Goepfert H, Lindberg RD, Jesse RH. Combined laryngeal conservation surgery and irradiation: Can we expand the indications for conservation therapy? Otolaryngol Head Neck Surg 1981;89:974–8.
23. Peters LJ, Ang KK. Unconventional fractionation schemes in radiotherapy. In: DeVita VT, Hellman S, Rosenberg SA, eds. *Important advances in oncology 1986*. Philadelphia: JB Lippincott, 1987:269–86.
24. Wendt CD, Peters LJ, Ang KK, et al. Hyperfractionated radiotherapy in the treatment of squamous cell carcinomas of the supraglottic larynx. Int J Radiat Oncol Biol Phys, 1989; (in press).
25. Sisson GA, Goldstein JC, Becker GD. Surgery of limited lesions of the larynx. Otolaryngol Clin North Am 1970;3:529–41.
26. Lee NK, Goepfert H, Wendt CD. Supraglottic laryngectomy for intermediate stage cancer: UTMD Anderson Cancer Center experience with combined therapy. Laryngoscope 1990;100:831–6.

18

Subtotal Laryngectomy With Contralateral Laryngoplasty

William H. Friedman, George P. Katsantonis

Horizontal subtotal partial laryngectomy has been the preferred treatment for supraglottic cancers of the larynx for more than three decades. Alonso, Ogura, Som, Biller, Dedo, Sessions, and many other workers have established the anatomic, functional, and oncologic advantages of supraglottic laryngectomy over all other methods for the treatment of supraglottic cancers in selected patients.[1–7] Patient selection has been the most critical determinant of success in the performance of supraglottic laryngectomy, as it is in most cancer operations. The extent of supraglottic cancer requiring excision is critical to the preoperative determination of the indications for conservation surgery of the larynx, the limitations of supraglottic laryngectomy, and extensions of the supraglottic resection that may be feasible or necessary in attempting to encompass a specific lesion.

The supraglottic laryngectomy was initially limited conceptually to strictly epiglottic lesions or epiglottic lesions extending to a false vocal cord. The realization by laryngeal surgeons that supraglottic resection could encompass larger tumors led to expansion of the indications of the procedure to include tumors beyond the confines of the supraglottic larynx (medial wall of pyriform sinus, arytenoid, vallecula, and base of tongue).[8,9] The history of conservation laryngeal surgery in general has been one of increased indications, fewer contraindications, and extensions of partial laryngectomy to include anatomic regions outside the original anatomic compartments for which these procedures were designed. Pressman et al's[10] classic studies of laryngeal lymphatic compartmentalization led to the pioneering work of the first partial laryngectomies. Extensions of these efforts have proven to be oncologically and physiologically sound despite their relative lack of anatomic rationale. Indications for supraglottic laryngectomy now include extensions into the tongue base or vertical extensions to include an arytenoid, a true vocal cord, or even subglottic extension. The so-called horizontal subtotal partial laryngectomy with vertical extension or three-quarter laryngectomy was first described by Ogura and Dedo[11] in 1965 for T_2 supraglottic cancers involving the arytenoids and glottis with minimal subglottic extent.

Evaluation of patients with extensive lesions for possible laryngeal conservation surgery poses two questions to the surgeon: is the procedure oncologically sound and can the laryngeal remnant be successfully reconstructed while preserving phonatory, respiratory, and sphincteric functions of the larynx. Significant contributions have been made in the literature to answer these questions and support the belief that selected T_3 supraglottic or transglottic cancers are amenable to laryngeal conservation surgery.[12] Kirchner and Som[13] in 1971 reported 60% local control and an overall 60% survival rate for selected T_3 glottic cancers that were not transglottic, did not extend subglottically more than 8 mm anteriorly or 4 mm posteriorly, and did not involve the petiole region. In 1975, Ogura et al[14] reported 94.5% 3-year survival after hemilaryngectomy for T_3 lesions. However, the definition of T_3 carcinoma in their study included any tumor extending 10 mm or more subglottically regardless of vocal cord mobility. In 1986, Biller and Lawson[15] reported a 72% 2-year disease-free rate for similar lesions treated with conservation surgery.

Studies of serial whole-organ histopathologic sections of the larynx have demonstrated that a significant portion of T_3 laryngeal supraglottic or transglottic cancers do not invade the cartilaginous framework.[16] Kirchner,[17] in his classic 1977 study, reported that approximately 40% of large laryngeal lesions (those exceeding 2.0 cm) do not invade the cartilaginous laryngeal framework and therefore may be amenable to conservation surgery. Kessler et al[18] retrospectively examined 27 patients with selected T_3 lesions undergoing hemilaryngectomy and reported an 85% absolute 2-year disease-free survival rate. Assessment of disease extent was based on data obtained from physical examination, magnetic resonance imaging, or computed tomographic (CT) scanning, and direct laryngectomy. The investigators concluded that under the present staging system, T_3 cancers of the larynx are a heterogenous mixture of different tumor-spreading patterns and sizes and that carefully selected T_3 lesions can be cured with laryngeal conservation surgery.

PREOPERATIVE ASSESSMENT AND SELECTION OF PATIENTS

Accurate topognostic assessment of laryngeal tumors based on data obtained from CT scanning is of paramount importance in the preoperative evaluation and selection of patients with supraglottic cancers. Fourth generation CT scanners have proven to be extremely helpful in assessing laryngeal patterns of cancer spread preoperatively. The authors as well as others have previously reported the feasibility of determining cartilaginous invasion by utilizing CT of the larynx (Figs. 18–1 to 18–4).[19,20] Certain limitations exist; false-positive and false-negative CT results are common. Calcified cartilaginous portions of the larynx may contrast with adjacent uncalcified cartilage, producing a false impression of cartilaginous erosion. In addition, tumor infiltration of calcified cartilage with well-formed and enlarged intratrabecular spaces may not disrupt trabeculae enough to produce radiographic evidence of destruction.[21]

Nevertheless, certain histopathologic characteristics and known spread patterns of laryngeal tumors enhance the ability of the CT scan to determine accurately cartilaginous framework invasion preoperatively. Archer et al[22,23] have shown that maximal dimensions of laryngeal cancer exceeding 16 mm and involvement of the area below the apex of the arytenoid are associated with an increased probability of laryngeal cartilage invasion. In addition, these tumors are more likely to invade particular areas; the anterior commissure, the junction between the anterior one fourth and posterior three fourths of thyroid lamina, the cricothyroid membrane, the cricoarytenoid joint, and the cricotracheal membrane.*

INDICATIONS

The horizontal subtotal partial laryngectomy with vertical extension is indicated for supraglottic carcinomas extending onto the arytenoid or the vocal cord, or both. The procedure may also be used for transglottic cancers with minimal subglottic extension and minimal cephalic extension onto the ventricle and the false cord. Contraindications to the operation are similar to those for conventional supraglottic laryngectomy noted elsewhere in this text. Cartilage invasion, major supraglottic extension, pyriform fossa obliteration, and poor pulmonary function are the primary deterrents. Vocal cord fixation or previous radiotherapy are not considered absolute contraindications.[24,25]

RECONSTRUCTIVE OPTIONS

The resection of glottic structures to encompass extensive supraglottic lesions is likely to result in postoperative functional problems and requires reconstruction of the resected cord and/or arytenoid. Three features of laryngeal reconstruction after partial laryngectomy emerge as constant requirements for the preservation of the sphincteric, respiratory, and phonatory functions of the laryngeal remnant. These are: (1) preservation of at least one mobile arytenoid, (2) restoration of posterior glottic bulk to prevent aspiration, and (3) maintenance of sufficient anteroposterior diameter of the glottic remnant to preserve an adequate airway and phonation.[26–28]

A variety of techniques for reconstruction have been described in vertical, anterior, frontolateral, and bilateral hemilaryngectomies.[29–36] Only a few contributions have been made to reconstruction following extended supraglottic procedures.[37–40] According to one technique, the resected vocal cord is reconstructed by a large, inferiorly based sternohyoid pedicle muscle flap. This is sutured posteriorly to the cricoid cartilage as

*Editor's note: The pattern and mechanisms of laryngeal framework invasion are discussed in further detail by Gregor in Chapter 3.

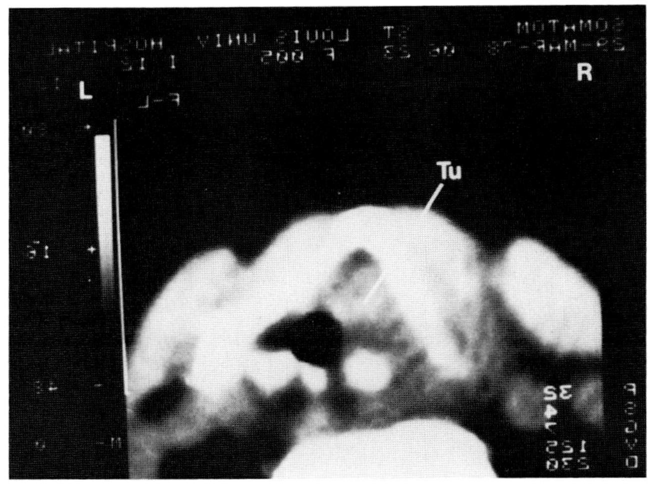

Figure 18–1. Preoperative computed tomographic scan of the larynx at the level of the arytenoid cartilages. Note tumor (Tu) filling the ventricle and involving the superior paraglottic space. The thyroid cartilage appears to be intact.

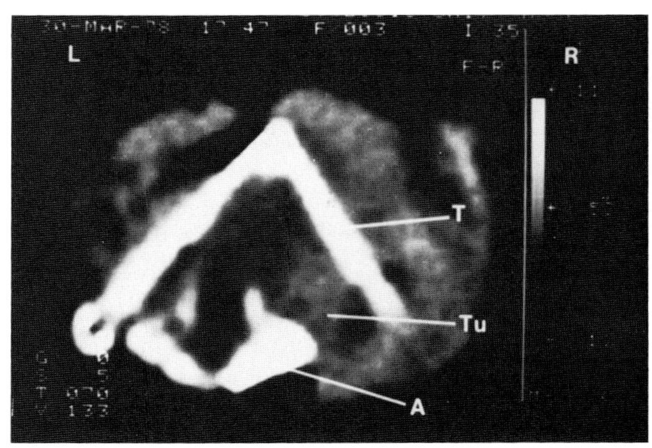

Figure 18–2. Preoperative computed tomographic scan at the level of the arytenoid cartilages demonstrating a right transglottic tumor (Tu) invading the paraglottic space. Thyroid cartilage (T) is intact.

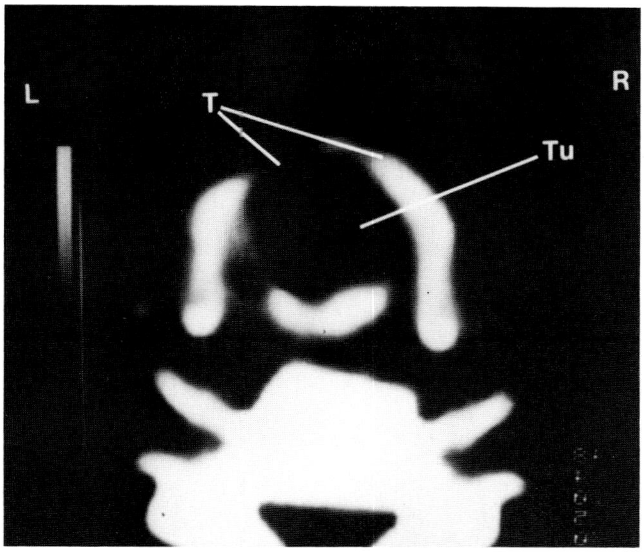

Figure 18–3. Preoperative computed tomographic scan showing thyroid cartilage invasion (T) by right transglottic tumor (Tu).

closely as possible to the remaining contralateral arytenoid. A flap of pyriform sinus mucosa is utilized to cover the muscle flap.[37] Although this method provides a vascularized bulky graft, there are certain drawbacks because the flap is subject to atrophy, distortion, and subsequent failure. The same tendency is encountered with free cartilage grafts, which occasionally are used for laryngeal reconstruction.

In 1976, Ogura and Dedo[38] reported the use of ipsilateral thyroid cartilage for reconstruction of the resected vocal cord. A triangular segment of the thyroid cartilage adjacent to resected vocal cord and pedicled on the internal perichondrium is "infractured," anchored into place and covered with pyriform sinus mucosa to create a pseudocord. Biller and Lawson[39] described reconstruction of the vocal cord using posterior thyroid cartilage pedicled on the inferior pharyngeal constrictor muscle. The posterior portion of the thyroid lamina adjacent to the resected vocal cord site, with attached muscle, is preserved. The cartilage-muscle graft is wired into position on the anterior commissure and the midcricoid posteriorly. Pyriform sinus mucosa is advanced to cover the graft. Both methods are compromised if preservation of a sufficient portion of thyroid cartilage is not feasible because of tumor bulk or subglottic extension.

In 1981 we described the contralateral laryngoplasty for laryngeal reconstruction in patients who had undergone supraglottic laryngectomy with vertical extension for transglottic cancers.[25,40] In this technique, the thyroid cornu of the uninvolved side of the larynx is mobilized and extended across the posterior commissure, greenstick fractured* anteriorly, and anchored into place to form a pseudocord (Fig. 18–5). This muscle-cartilage pedicled graft provides bulk for the posterior glottis, preserves the anteroposterior diameter, and provides a good vocal baffle.

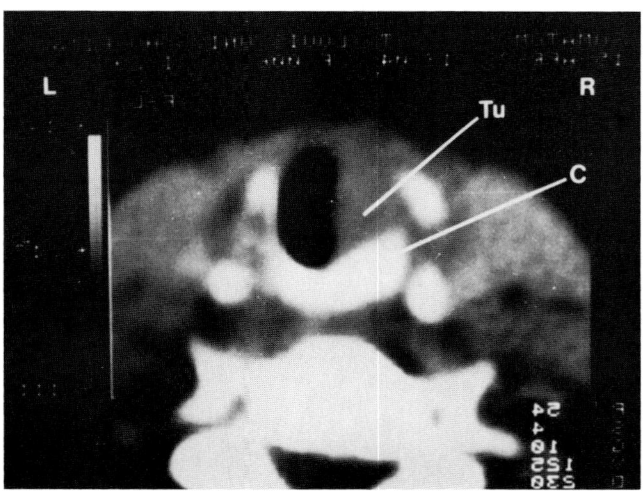

Figure 18–4. Preoperative computed tomographic scan showing cricoid cartilage invasion (C) by a right transglottic tumor (Tu).

TECHNIQUE OF CONTRALATERAL LARYNGOPLASTY

A preliminary tracheostomy, with wire-embedded endotracheal tube, is performed under local anesthesia. A horizontal midcervical incision is used, as in the approach for supraglottic laryngectomy (with posterior and superior extension for ipsilateral radical neck dissection when indicated). Thyroid perichondrium is elevated at the outset and left attached, when possible, to the inferior border of the thyroid cartilage. In each case, the specimen is resected; the ipsilateral arytenoid is removed along with a portion or all of the adjacent true vocal cord and thyroid cartilage (Figs. 18–6, 18–7).

The contralateral cartilage cuts spare the posterolateral border of the contralateral thyroid cartilage to preserve continuity with the superior cornu. The resection may be extended anteriorly on the anterior commissure or beyond, including a small amount of the opposite true vocal cord if indicated. In cases of minimal subglottic extension of tumor the largest portion of the ipsilateral thyroid lamina is resected, preserving only the inferior rim of the lamina on the involved side (Figs. 18–8, 18–9).

The reconstruction utilizes the contralateral superior thyroid cornu covered by its perichondrium and preserves its attachments with the inferior and middle pharyngeal constrictor muscles. A medial and vertical incision in the overlying mucosa exposes the cornu. The superior cornu is a long, narrow, conical extension of thyroid cartilage, directed upward, backward, and inward, and larger and bulkier in male patients. It terminates at its attachment to the lateral thyrohyoid ligament. A scissors is used to create a fracture point along the posterior thyroid ala so that the thyroid cornu can be mobilized and fractured medially, bringing with it fibers from the inferior constrictor muscle, the stylopharyngeus muscle, and the lower border of the middle constrictor muscle (Fig. 18–10). This cartilage-muscle pedicle

---

*Editor's note: A "greenstick" fracture of bone or cartilage is one in which the cortex of only one side is broken; the other is bent.

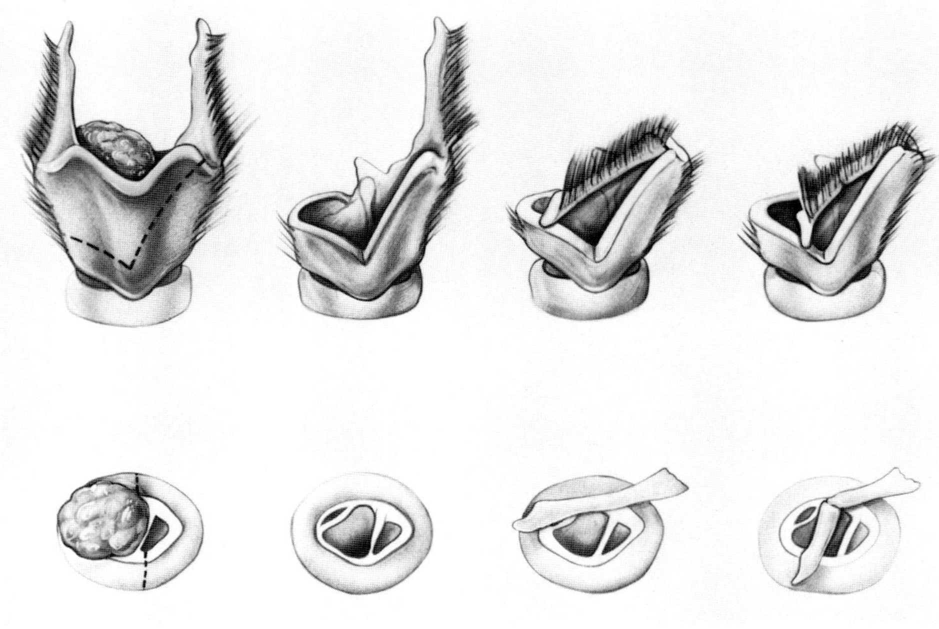

Figure 18–5. Schematic representation of the contralateral laryngoplasty technique. The superior thyroid cornu on the side contralateral to the resection site is preserved with the inferior pharyngeal constrictor attached to it. The cornu is mobilized, extended across the posterior commissure, and greenstick fractured anteriorly to form a pseudocord.

can exceed 3 cm in length and is easily displaced to the resection site across the posterior commissure of the laryngeal remnant. An additional greenstick fracture of the distal (formerly superior) tip of cornu is created so the cartilage can be sutured to the anterior midline. The cornu is anchored to the thyroid cartilage remnant anteriorly and posteriorly with 00 nylon sutures. Pyriform sinus and hypopharyngeal muscosa is then advanced superiorly to cover the cartilage-muscle pedicle, securing the mucosal flap to the cut edges of thyroid cartilage (Figs. 18–11, 18–12). Inferior constrictor and cricopharyngeal myotomies are performed.

In most patients, particularly males, the superior cornu is usually a substantial structure, long enough to accommodate the two greenstick fractures with sufficient extension to reach to the anterior commissure while replacing the resected cord. In about 10% of individuals, the cornu may be nonexistent or of insufficient length to employ for contralateral laryngoplasty. If the cornu is too short, an alternative to the described technique is to detach the posterior border of the thyroid cartilage, leaving it attached to the inferior thyroid constrictor. This cartilage-muscle pedicle flap can then be transferred to the area of the resected vocal cord (Fig. 18–13).

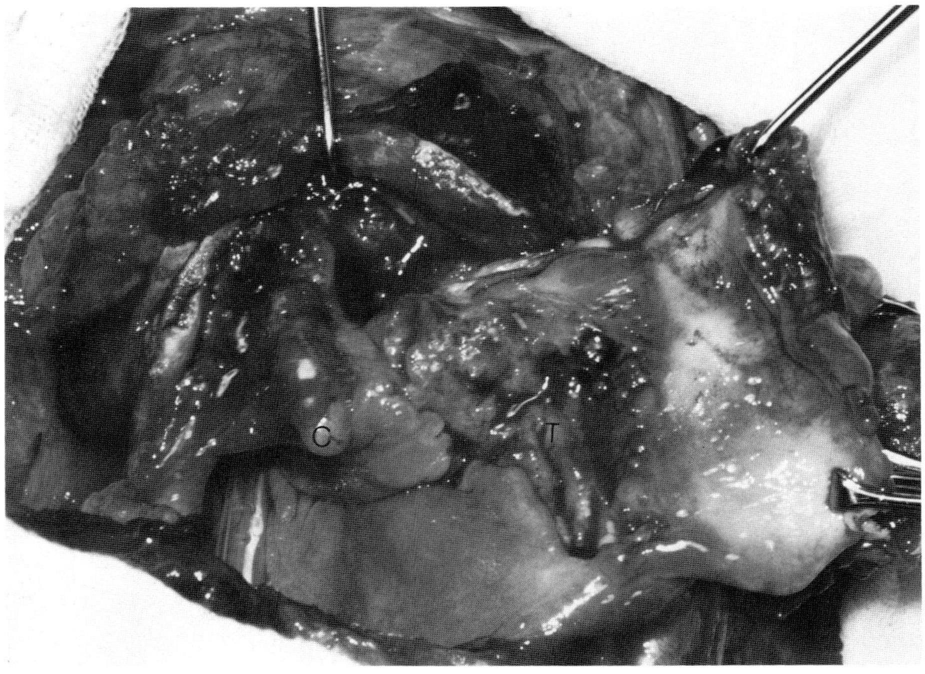

Figure 18–6. Operative photograph of a three-quarter laryngectomy for a large supraglottic tumor (T) extending onto the right arytenoid, posterior portion of the true vocal cord and subglottis. Note superior thyroid cornu (C) on the contralateral side.

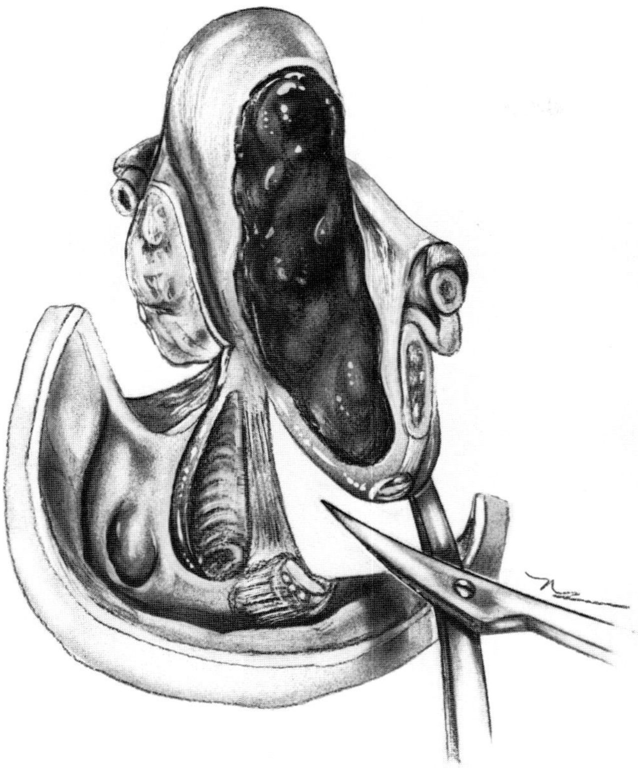

Figure 18–7. Schematic representation of a three-quarter laryngectomy. Note bulky supraglottic tumor extending onto the arytenoid and true vocal cord.

RESULTS

The postoperative course of patients who have undergone contralateral laryngoplasty is virtually identical to that of those who have undergone supraglottic laryngectomy without vertical extension. All patients aspirate in various degrees after oral feedings have been reinstituted, but the aspiration subsides in the majority of patients as rehabilitation occurs. The rate of conversion to total laryngectomy or need for long-term gastrostomy feedings because of persistent aspiration is no greater than that following supraglottic laryngectomy. Tracheostomy decannulation occurs at approximately the same time (17 days) as that of patients who have undergone routine supraglottic laryngectomy. In most cases pharyngeal and cricopharyngeal myotomy have been performed on patients undergoing supraglottic laryngectomy with or without vertical extension. In isolated instances, when there appears to be a troughlike entry into the esophagus, cricopharyngeal and pharyngeal myotomies are not considered necessary.

Since 1979, the authors have performed 24 contralateral laryngoplasties following supraglottic laryngectomy with vertical extension. The patient's age and sex, tumor maps, staging, and follow-up information can be seen in Table 18–1. Fifteen of 24 patients had palpable cervical lymphadenopathy at the time of surgery and underwent unilateral radical neck dissection in conjunction with their laryngectomy. Two of the patients had preoperative radiotherapy to 5500 cGy with cobalt-60. The remainder of the patients underwent postoperative radiotherapy to the tumor bed and necks to 6000 cGy. Three patients had N_2 cervical adenopathy and 12 had N_1. There were seven T_3 and 17 T_2 supraglottic tumors staged according to the 1983 American Joint Committee classification for supraglottic cancer.[41]

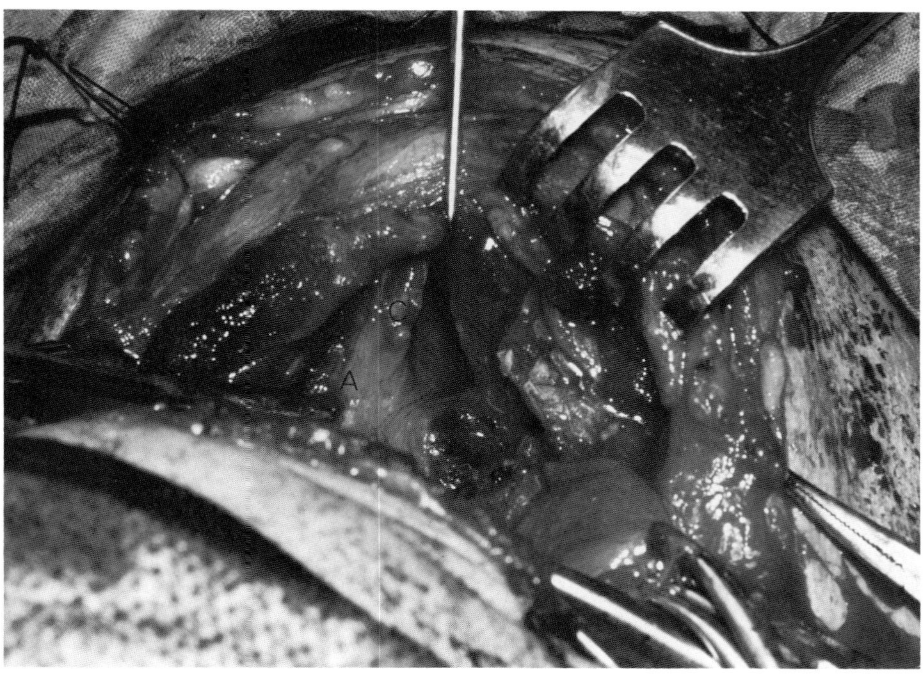

Figure 18–8. Intraoperative photograph following completion of the three-quarter laryngectomy. The contralateral arytenoid (A) and true vocal cord are seen on the left.

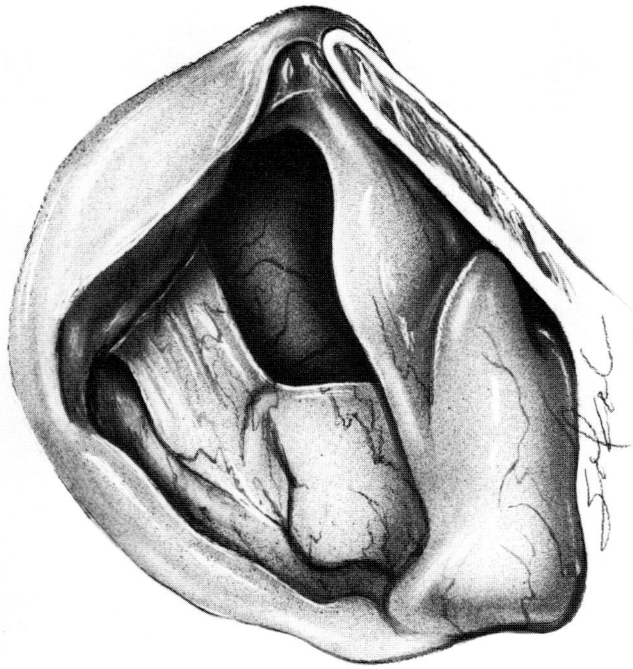

Figure 18–9. Schematic representation of the laryngeal remnant following three-quarter laryngectomy on the left.

The 3-year absolute survival rate was 70%. This rate is comparable to survival rates reported by others.[38,39,42] Fourteen of the 24 patients were alive 12 months to 10 years following surgery (Table 18–2). Six patients died of metastatic disease from 11 to 28 months following surgery; two of these patients also had local recurrences. One patient had thyroid cartilage invasion that was not determined until local recurrence required conversion laryngectomy. One patient died of local and regional nodal recurrence without evidence of widespread metastases.

Four patients developed widespread metastatic disease without local or neck recurrence. There were no neck recurrences other than in the three patients already described. Palpable lymphadenopathy had been present prior to surgery in each patient who died of cancer; three of these six patients had N_2 disease. The three patients with stage IV disease are dead of disease. Nine of 13 patients with stage III and eight of eight with stage II disease have survived from 12 months to 10 years (Tables 18–3, 18–4). Two patients required conversion to total laryngectomy because of persistent aspiration. Two other patients underwent conversion to total laryngectomy because of local recurrence. The length of time to decannulation approximated that of our patients who had undergone supraglottic laryngectomy without vertical extension. Aspiration has been a problem in one patient in the survival group (patient 11). This patient has intermittent swallowing difficulty and a feeding jejunostomy was recently inserted.

These results suggest that although tumor size and presence of cartilage invasion determine the feasibility of a three-quarter laryngectomy and may affect local recurrence rates, the presence of neck disease is the most important determinant of survival; there were no deaths due to cancer among patients who did not have palpable cervical adenopathy prior to surgery (Table 18–5).

The use of fourth generation CT has enabled us to determine preoperatively cartilage invasion with accuracy, when the size and location of the tumor was also taken into consideration. In this series, there has been no local recurrence in any patient since the availability of fourth generation CT scanners for preoperative assessment.

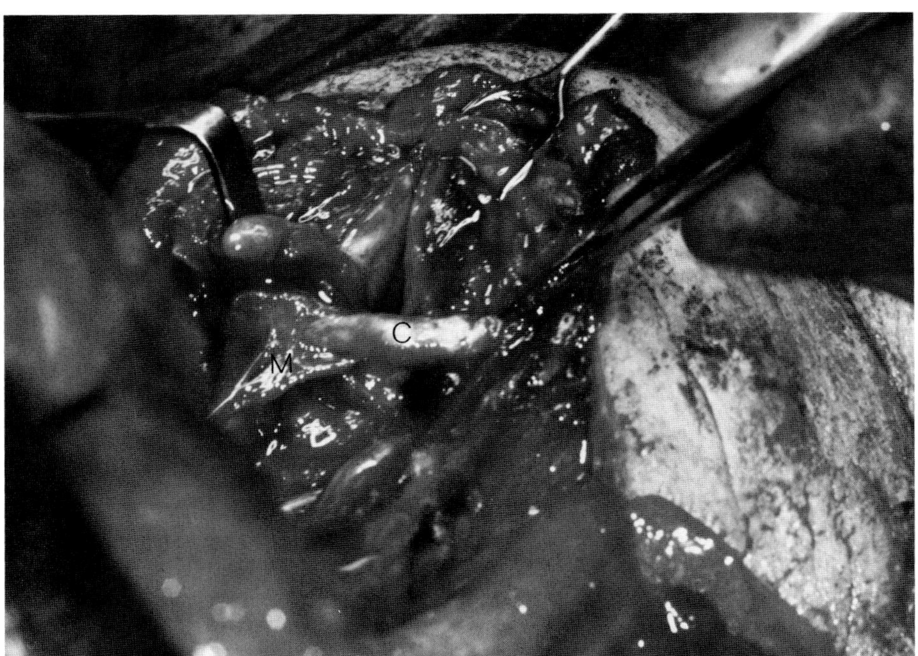

Figure 18–10. Intraoperative photograph of the contralateral laryngoplasty. The left superior thyroid cornu (C) with the inferior pharyngeal constrictor attached to it (M) is greenstick fractured across the posterior commissure.

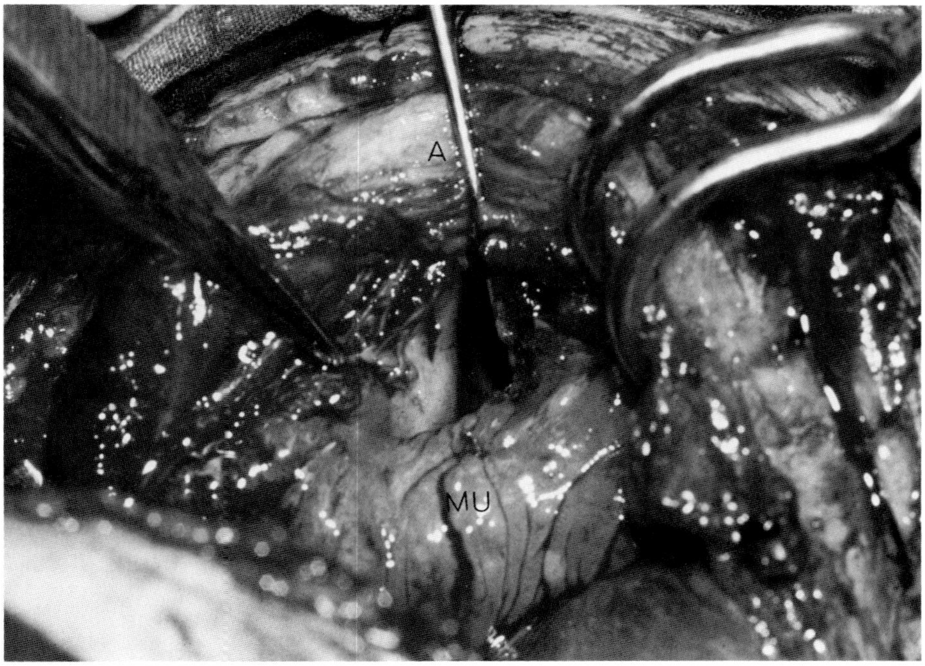

Figure 18–11. Following a second greenstick fracture, the thyroid cornu is attached to the anterior commissure (A) and covered with pyriform sinus mucosa (MU).

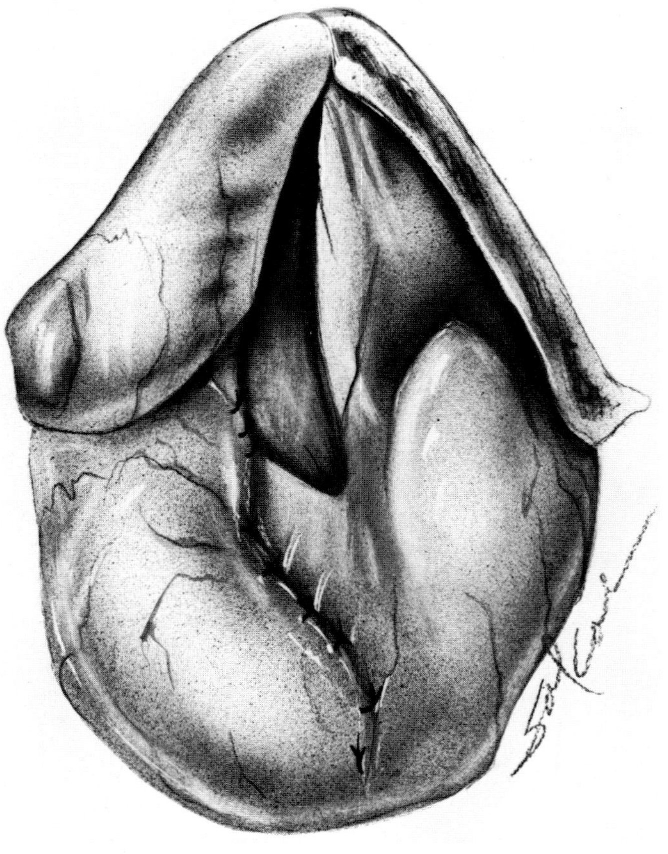

Figure 18–12. Schematic representation following completion of contralateral laryngoplasty on the left.

COMMENT

Biller and Lawson[39] in 1984 concluded that proper case selection, to include only patients with tumors of 2 cm or less, enhanced survival in patients who had undergone partial laryngectomy for transglottic cancers. In our opinion the criteria may be extended to include patients with tumors larger than 2 cm, when preoperative CT unequivocally demonstrates absence of cartilage invasion. The result of this series indicates that horizontal subtotal laryngectomy with vertical extension is an oncologically sound procedure for T_2 and selected T_3 lesions. Although resection and reconstruction may be feasible in patients with larger lesions and in patients with neck metastasis, treatment of T_4 lesions by supraglottic laryngectomy with vertical extension is not oncologically sound.

The described technique has been found to be effective for reconstruction of the larynx following horizontal subtotal supraglottic laryngectomy with vertical extension. Preservation of laryngeal function following this operation is not different from that in patients who had routine supraglottic laryngectomy. A particular advantage of the contralateral laryngoplasty compared with reconstruction of the larynx with ipsilateral thyroid cartilage graft is the fact that it utilizes cartilage at some distance from the lesion and therefore does not compromise tumor resection in cases with bulky tumors adjacent to thyroid cartilage. For this reason the contralateral laryngoplasty has proven to be both a functional and oncologically sound reconstruction of the larynx following horizontal subtotal laryngectomy with vertical extension for supraglottic and selected transglottic cancers.

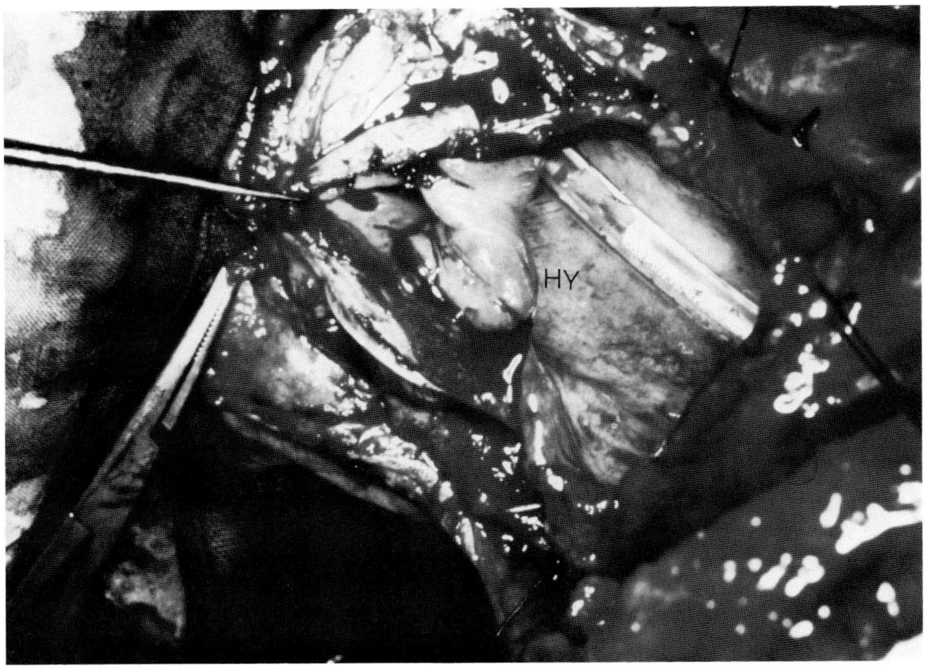

Figure 18–13. Intraoperative photograph at the completion of the contralateral laryngoplasty. Note that this procedure does not affect the patency of the hypopharyngeal lumen (HY). The nasogastric tube is clearly visible.

Table 18–1. Data on 24 Patients Treated by Contralateral Laryngoplasties Following Supraglottic Laryngectomy with Vertical Extension

PATIENT NO./ AGE/SEX	TUMOR MAP	TUMOR CLASSIFICATION	STAGE	STATUS
1/48/M	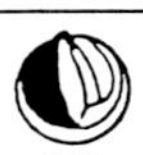	T_2N_1	III	Dead at 10 years, lung cancer
2/64/M	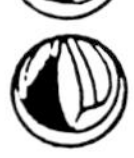	T_2N_0	II	Alive at 10 years, no evidence of disease
3/45/F	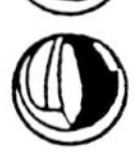	T_2N_1	III	Alive at 10 years, no evidence of disease
4/52/F	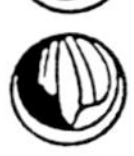	T_2N_1	III	Alive at 9 years, no evidence of disease
5/66/F	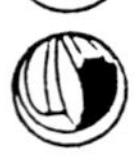	T_2N_1	III	Dead at 4 years, heart disease
6/49/F	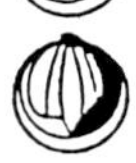	T_3N_2	IV	Dead at 11 months, local recurrence, metastatic disease
7/48/M	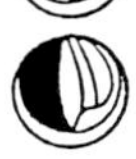	T_3N_0	III	Alive at 8 years, no evidence of disease
8/58/M	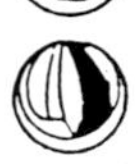	T_2N_1	III	Dead at 16 months, local recurrence, metastatic disease
9/57/M	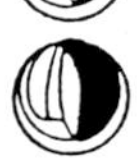	T_3N_0	III	Alive at 7 years, no evidence of disease
10/63/F	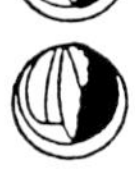	T_3N_1	III	Dead at 18 months, metastatic disease
11/77/F	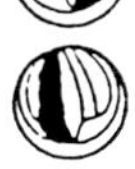	T_3N_0	III	Alive at 7 years, no evidence of disease, intermittent swallowing difficulty responds to dilation
12/59/F	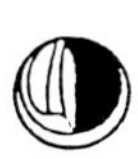	T_3N_2	IV	Dead at 16 months, metastatic disease, no local recurrence

Table 18-1. Data on 24 Patients Treated by Contralateral Laryngoplasties Following Supraglottic Laryngectomy with Vertical Extension (Continued)

PATIENT NO./ AGE/SEX	TUMOR MAP	TUMOR CLASSIFICATION	STAGE	STATUS
13/40/F	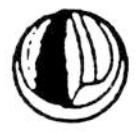	T_2N_2	IV	Dead at 28 months, distant metastasis, no local recurrence
14/51/M	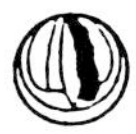	T_2N_0	II	Alive at 5 years, converted to total laryngectomy because of aspiration, no evidence of disease
15/63/M	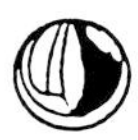	T_2N_0	II	Alive at 5 years, no evidence of disease
16/69/F	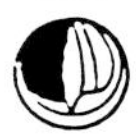	T_2N_1	III	Dead at 2 years, regional and local recurrences
17/67/M		T_2N_0	II	Alive at 4 years, no evidence of disease
18/39/M	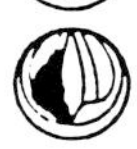	T_2N_1	III	Alive at 3 years, no evidence of disease
19/70/M	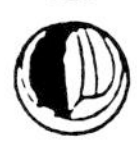	T_2N_1	III	Alive at 2½ years, no evidence of disease
20/61/M	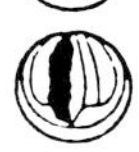	T_2N_1	III	Alive at 3 years, no evidence of disease
21/58/F	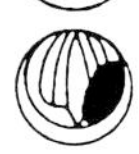	T_3N_1	III	Dead at 2½ years, metastatic disease, converted to total laryngectomy because of aspiration
22/61/M	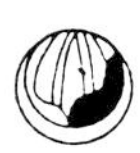	T_2N_0	II	Alive at 1½ years, no evidence of disease, converted to total laryngectomy because of aspiration
23/60/M	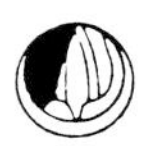	T_2N_0	II	Alive at 1 year, no evidence of disease
24/54/M	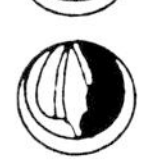	T_3N_1	III	Alive at 1 year, no evidence of disease

Table 18-2. Survival of Patients in Series

	TIME		
STAGE	*1-3 Years*	*3 Years*	*5 Years*
T_2N_0	2	1	3
T_2N_1	3	3	3
T_2N_2	1		
T_3N_0			3
T_3N_1	3		
T_3N_2	2		
Total	11	4	9

Table 18-4. Survival According to T Classification

	T_2	T_3
Alive	13	4
Dead	3*	4
Total no. patients	16	8

*All three patients had positive cervical lymph nodes.

Table 18-3. Survival According to Stage

	STAGE		
	II	*III*	*IV*
Alive	8	9	0
Dead	0	4	3
Total no. patients	8	13	3

Table 18-5. Survival According to Lymph Node Involvement

	N_0	N_1	N_2
Alive	9	6	0
Dead	0	6	3
Total no. patients	9	12	3

REFERENCES

1. Alonso JM. Conservative surgery of cancer of the larynx. Trans Am Acad Opthalmol Otolaryngol 1947;51:633.
2. Ogura JH. Supraglottic subtotal laryngectomy and radical neck dissection for carcinoma of the epiglottis. Laryngoscope 1958;68:983.
3. Som ML. Conservation surgery for carcinoma of the epiglottis by lateral pharyngotomy. Trans Am Acad Opthalmol Otolaryngol 1959;63:28.
4. Ogura JH, Sessions DJ, Spector GJ. Conservation surgery for epidermoid carcinoma of the supraglottic larynx. Laryngoscope 1976; 85:1808.
5. Ogura JH, Biller HF, Calcaterra TC, et al. Surgical treatment of carcinoma of the larynx, pharynx, base of tongue and cervical esophagus. Int Surg 1969;52:29–40.
6. Ogura JH, Spector GJ, Sessions DG. Conservation surgery for epidermoid carcinoma of the marginal area (aryepiglottic fold extension). Laryngoscope 1975;85:1801–7.
7. Goepfert H, Jesse RH, Fletcher GH, et al. Optimal treatment for the technically resectable squamous cell carcinoma of the supraglottic larynx. Laryngoscope 1975;85:14–32.
8. Ogura JH, Sessions DG, Ciralsky RH. Supraglottic carcinoma with extension to the arytenoid. Laryngoscope 1975;85:1327–31.
9. Ogura JH, Mallen RW. Partial laryngopharyngectomy for supraglottic and pharyngeal carcinoma. Trans Am Acad Opthalmol Otolaryngol 1965;69:832.
10. Pressman J, Simon M, Monell C. Anatomical studies related to the dissemination of cancer of the larynx. Trans Am Acad Opthalmol Otolaryngol 1960;64:628–38.
11. Ogura JH, Dedo HH. Glottic reconstruction following subtotal glottic-supraglottic laryngectomy. Laryngoscope 1965;75:865–78.
12. Biller HF, Blaugrund SM, Som ML. Decreasing limitation of partial laryngectomy for vocal cord cancer. Can J Otolaryngol 1975;4:432–3.
13. Kirchner JA, Som ML. Clinical and histological observations on supraglottic cancer. Ann Otol Rhinol Laryngol 1971;80:638.
14. Ogura JH, Sessions DG, Spector GJ. Analysis of surgical therapy for epidermoid carcinoma of the laryngeal glottis. Laryngoscope 1975;85:1521–30.
15. Biller HF, Lawson W. Partial laryngectomy for vocal cord cancer with marked limitation or fixation of the vocal cord. Laryngoscope 1986;96:61–4.
16. Harrison DFN. Significance and means by which laryngeal cancer invades thyroid cartilage. Ann Otol Rhinol Laryngol 1984;93:293–6.
17. Kirchner JA. 200 laryngeal cancers: patterns of growth and spread as seen in serial section. Laryngoscope 1977;87:474–82.
18. Kessler DJ, Trapp TK, Calcaterra TC. The treatment of T_3 glottic carcinoma with vertical partial laryngectomy. Arch Otolaryngol Head Neck Surg 1987;113:1196–9.
19. Archer CR, Friedman WH, Yeager VL, et al. Evaluation of laryngeal cancer by computed tomography. J Comput Assist Tomogr 1978;2:618–24.
20. Friedman WH, Archer CA, Yeager CL. Computed tomography of the larynx: choices and characteristics in CT. Proceedings of the Eighth Congress of the European Society of Neuroradiology; Strasbourg, France, September, 1979. Kugler Publications, 1980:215–20.
21. Katsantonis GP, Archer CR, Rosenblum BN, et al. The degree to which accuracy of preoperative staging of laryngeal carcinoma has been enhanced by computed tomography. Otolaryngol Head Neck Surg 1986;95:52–62.
22. Archer CR, Yeager VL. Computed tomography of laryngeal cancer with histopathological correlation. Laryngoscope 1982;92:1173–80.
23. Archer CR, Yeager VL, Herbold DR. Computed tomography vs histology of laryngeal cancer: their value in predicting laryngeal cartilage invasion. Laryngoscope 1983;93:140–7.
24. Thawley SE, Sessions DJ. Surgical therapy of supraglottic tumors. In: Thawley SE, Panje WR, eds. *Comprehensive management of head and neck tumors*. Philadelphia: WB Saunders, 1987.
25. Friedman WH, Katsantonis GP, Siddoway JR, et al. Contralateral laryngoplasty after supraglottic laryngectomy with vertical extension. Arch Otolaryngol 1989;107:742–5.
26. Flores TC, Wood BG, Levine HL. Factors in successful deglutition following supraglottic laryngeal surgery. Ann Otol Rhinol Laryngol 1987;91:579–83.
27. Adram GM, Kemp FH. The protection of the laryngeal airway during swallowing. Br J Radiol 1952;25:406–16.
28. Sessions DG, Zill R. Deglutition after conservation surgery for cancer of the larynx and hypopharynx. Otolaryngol Head Neck Surg 1979;87:779–96.
29. Blaugrund SM, Kurland SR. Replacement of the arytenoid following vertical hemilaryngectomy. Laryngoscope 1975;85:935–41.
30. Biller HF, Som ML. Vertical partial laryngectomy for glottic carcinoma with posterior subglottic extension. Ann Otol Rhinol Laryngol 1977;86:715–8.
31. Ogura JH, Biller HF. Glottic reconstruction following extended frontal lateral hemilaryngectomy. Laryngoscope 1969;79:2181–4.
32. Som ML. Cordal cancer with extension to vocal process. Laryngoscope 1975;85:1298–307.
33. Bailey BJ. Glottic reconstruction after hemilaryngectomy: bipedicle muscle flap laryngoplasty. Laryngoscope 1975;85:960–77.
34. Biller HF, Lawson W. Bilateral vertical partial laryngectomy for bilateral vocal cord carcinoma. Ann Otol Rhinol Laryngol 1981; 90:489.
35. Quinn HJ. Free muscle transplant method of glottic reconstruction after hemilaryngectomy. Laryngoscope 1975;85:985–6.
36. Pearson BW, Donald PJ. Larynx. In: PJ Donald, ed. Head and neck cancer: management of the difficult case. Philadelphia: WB Saunders, 1984.
37. Sylva N, Lore JM. Partial horizontal supraglottic laryngectomy: a method of reconstruction. Laryngoscope 1977;87:1164–8.
38. Ogura JH, Dedo HH. Glottic reconstruction following subtotal glottic-subglottic laryngectomy. Laryngoscope 1976;75:865–78.
39. Biller HF, Lawson W. Partial laryngectomy for transglottic cancers. Ann Otol Rhinol Laryngology 1984;93:297–300.
40. Friedman WH, Rosenblum BN, Katsantonis GP. Contralateral laryngoplasty: an update on reconstruction of the larynx following supraglottic laryngectomy with vertical extension. Arch Otolaryngol 1985;111: 742–6.
41. Beahrs OH, Meyers MA. *Manual for staging cancer,* 2nd ed. Philadelphia: JB Lippincott, 1983.
42. Shu CZ. The results of 31 patients of supraglottic vertical hemilaryngectomy. Ann NZJ Surg 1988;58:213–5.

19

Subtotal Laryngectomy With Epiglottic Reconstruction

Gary L. Schechter

Vocal cord stripping, radiotherapy, and laser cordectomy, have taken significant positions in the treatment armamentarium for early glottic cancer. The vertical hemilaryngectomy continues to be a treatment modality offered to patients for carcinoma of the true vocal cord. In recent years, however, it is being used more selectively for radiotherapy failures and in patients who are unable or unwilling to have radiotherapy. In most of these cases, an extended hemilaryngectomy, or subtotal laryngectomy, is required, in which more than half of the larynx is removed and reconstruction is required.

The objective of reconstruction after subtotal laryngectomy is to restore the functional competence of the larynx. These funtions include maintenance of the airway, protection of the airway during swallowing, and voice production. Achieving these goals with a single reconstructive procedure in all patients is difficult. In order to choose the reconstructive technique that is most applicable to a patient's problem, the structural components required for these functions must be understood.

There are competing forces in the physiology of the larynx. The demands of the airway require a variable lumen at the glottic level. This same lumen must be reduced markedly for airway protection during swallowing. The glottic configuration is modified in a variety of ways for efficient voice production, a function that is equally dependent on the mobility and fluidity of the mucosal covering of the vocal cords. These characteristics are significantly compromised when 50 to 75% of the vocal cord structure has been excised and reconstructed.

The history of reconstruction after partial laryngectomy dates back to the beginning of the 20th century. Most efforts have been directed at the defect created by cordectomy or by the standard hemilaryngectomy, in which there is a need to prevent anterior commissure web formation and to fill in the tissue loss at the cord level. In the subtotal laryngectomy, however, additional structures are removed that result in more extensive functional defects. These are detailed later. Although various combinations of reconstructive techniques may correct these defects, the only approach described that offers an immediate mucosal lining, cartilaginous support, and flexibility, in a single-stage procedure, is epiglottic reconstruction.

The use of the epiglottis for reconstruction of glottic defects was reported in the European literature by Bouche et al in 1965,[1] Sedlacek in 1965,[2] and Kambic in 1977.[3] Tucker and colleagues,[4] at the Cleveland Clinic, introduced epiglottic reconstruction in the United States in 1979. Since then, there have been numerous reports,[5,6] including my initial series of 12 patients in 1983,[7] describing the use of the epiglottis for reconstruction of a variety of laryngeal, tracheal, and pharyngeal defects.

SURGICAL ANATOMY

The epiglottis primarily consists of elastic cartilage and is divided into upper, or suprahyoid, and lower, or infrahyoid, portions according to their relationship to the hyoid bone. The suprahyoid portion is thin, and its anterior perichondrium is loosely attached. The infrahyoid portion is thick, contains numerous perforations, and its inferior border, or petiole, is approximately 1 cm above the anterior commissure. The perichondrium of the anterior surface of the infrahyoid portion of the epiglottis is more intimately attached due to the perforations.

The epiglottis is suspended in its retrolingual and supraglottic position by a combination of anterior ligaments. In the midline, at the junction of the suprahyoid and infrahyoid portions, is the loosely attached hyoepiglottic ligament. The paired pharyngoepiglottic ligaments are positioned laterally and are more firmly attached. The epiglottis is anchored inferiorly by the thyroepiglottic ligament, which extends from the petiole to the anterior commissure and Broyle's ligament. The infrahyoid epiglottis and the thyroepiglottic ligament serve as the posterior wall of the preepiglottic space.

The mucosal histologic features of the epiglottis vary. The suprahyoid portion is usually covered with squamous epithelium, whereas the infrahyoid mucosa consists of pseudostratified ciliated columnar epithelium. The latter is more characteristic of the respiratory system and may assist in mucous transport when the epiglottis is used in reconstruction at the glottic level.

The epiglottis provides the following advantages when used as a reconstructive material:

1. An immediate mucosal lining consistent with the intrinsic larynx.
2. Structural replacement for maintenance of the anteroposterior diameter of the larynx.
3. Flexibility that allows movement of the remaining arytenoid cartilage and redevelopment of sphincter action.
4. Development of varying pseudocord configurations.
5. No requirement for stent placement.
6. A one-stage reconstructive procedure.

INDICATIONS FOR EPIGLOTTIC RECONSTRUCTION

Patients undergoing subtotal laryngectomy must be chosen very carefully, since this surgery requires difficult rehabilitation that is associated with decannulation and aspiration problems to be outlined later in this chapter. The epiglottic reconstruction technique, in particular, produces more stress than other reconstructive techniques because of the loss of food bolus diversion and decreased superior laryngeal nerve sensory function when the epiglottis is mobilized and moved inferiorly. Good pulmonary function and a strong desire to achieve function are absolute requirements. The latter depends on motivational factors that go beyond the scope of this chapter, and the former requires considerable judgment beyond the confines of the pulmonary function laboratory.

Epiglottic reconstruction should be used only in patients who require the unique attributes of the epiglottis that cannot be obtained in a less complicated manner. It is most useful when at least 60 to 70% of the larynx at the glottic level must be replaced. Defects smaller than this can be reconstructed using muscle laryngoplasty techniques. The maximum defect is one in which only one arytenoid remains, with enough of the cricoid ring to maintain its integrity as a circular structure. This subtotal, or three-quarter, laryngectomy leaves a defect that requires reconstitution of the anteroposterior diameter of the airway, bilateral tissue bulk for glottic competence, flexibility for pseudocord movement, and mucosal lining for voice enhancement and mucous transport.

I use a combination of findings from the history, physical examination, and laboratory to assist in the decision-making process relative to a patient's ability to adapt to this procedure. In the history, I look for work ethic and the motivation of a family environment. Hard-working patients with strong family support groups do not always do well after conservation surgery of the larynx, but my worst results have occurred in patients who have been jobless and have had no family support systems.

I have often been puzzled by certain patients with laryngeal cancer who have evidence of moderately severe pulmonary disease on physical examination and pulmonary function testing, but have a history of aggressive physical activity in their daily work. The latter, of course, must be confirmed by a spouse or fellow worker. If this dichotomy exists, it can be tested by the "Ogura Stair Test," personally conducted by the examining surgeon. The patient is walked briskly down the hallway to the nearest stairway while carrying on a conversation. Without stopping, the examiner walks the patient up a flight of stairs at a slow but steady pace. If the patient is able to follow this procedure through to completion and is able to continue the conversation without severe shortness of breath, he or she is a candidate for most conservation surgery procedures of the larynx. Since a general internal medical examination is imperative in all of the patients who are to undergo subtotal laryngectomy with epiglottic reconstruction, these judgments can be made with the help of a medical colleague.

Radiographic imaging is essential in the evaluation of these patients. The computed tomography (CT) scan and magnetic resonance imaging (MRI) are used for tumor evaluation. The barium swallow is equally important, since it provides an opportunity to evaluate the esophagus for second primary tumors and also to determine if there is esophageal reflux. Esophageal reflux is a factor that contributes to serious aspiration problems after conservation surgery of the larynx and must be treated aggressively to avoid complications. The esophagus is evaluated further at the preoperative staging endoscopy.

OPERATIVE TECHNIQUE

This chapter will not deal with the intricacies of performing the extended hemilaryngectomy. It is assumed that the anterior halves of each thyroid cartilage have been resected with the anterior commissure. In order to mobilize the epiglottis, it must be freed from all of its anterior soft tissue and ligamentous attachments. This is accomplished by grasping the petiole with a thyroid tenaculum, exerting traction in an inferior direction, and using sharp dissection technique, with scissors, against the cartilage (Fig. 19–1). After a few millimeters of cartilage have been exposed, the subperichondrial plane can be identified using a sharp Freer or Cottle elevator. A knife, or scissors, is required for sharp dissection where the perichondrium dips into cartilage perforations. The latter are only present in the infrahyoid portion of the epiglottis. Once the sharp dissection is completed, it is helpful to replace the thyroid tenaculum with a 000 silk suture through each side of the petiole for further retraction. All dissection above this level, except where the lateral pharyngoepiglottic ligaments are attached, is easy and similar to the mucoperichondrial elevation in a nasal septoplasty.

The epiglottis must be freed up to the tip, which is easily identified. During the latter stages of the dissection, the retraction sutures are used to pull the epiglottis inferiorly to determine if the petiole reaches the cricoid without significant tension (Fig. 19–2).

At this point in the operation, the hypopharynx is still accessible, and my preference is to create a cervical esophagostomy for feeding. First, a no. 18 sump feeding tube is placed into the cervical esophagus via the laryngotomy and hypopharynx. Then, the muscular wall of the cervical esophagus is identified by dissecting to its posterolateral aspect at the level of the middle thyroid vein. Here, the esophagus and contained feeding tube are grasped with a Babcock clamp, and a 7 mm vertical

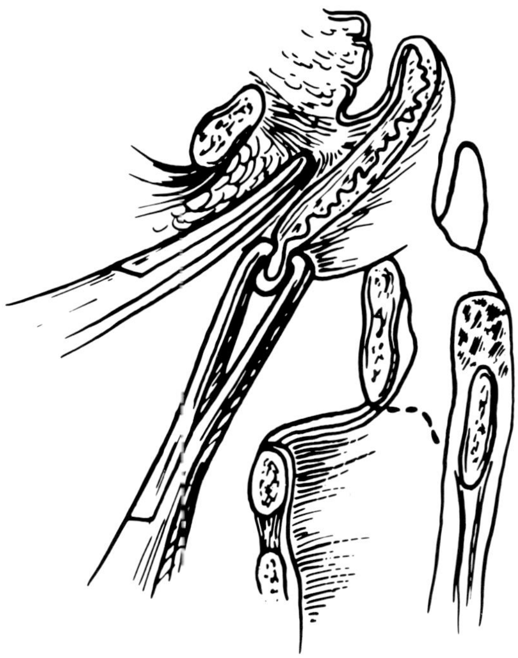

Figure 19–1. With the tenaculum applied to the base of the epiglottis, sharp dissection is begun with scissors to define the subperichondrial p ane.

esophagotomy is performed with a no. 15 knife blade. Once the mucosal edges of the esophagotomy are grasped with fine hemostats, the Babcock clamp is released, the feeding tube is withdrawn from the pharynx, and it is reinserted through the esophagotomy down into the stomach. A pursestring suture of 000 long-acting absorbable suture is placed around the tube at the esophagotomy site, and the tube is led out through a stab incision in the sternomastoid muscle and the skin of the lower neck. It is secured with a 00 silk skin suture and an umbilical tape.

Prior to suturing the epiglottis into position, it is essential to remove the shoulder roll that is placed during initial phases of the operation and to flex the patient's head slightly (Fig. 19–3). This relieves suture line tension in most patients. It is preferable to use individually placed long-acting absorbable sutures, such as nondyed 000 Vicryl (Fig. 19–4).

The suture technique for securing the epiglottis may influence the quality of the voice. I have found that a coarse and more masculine quality occurs when few sutures are used and are placed into the epiglottic cartilage but not through the intraluminal mucosa. This appears to encourage the development of a prominent pseudochord and more low-frequency sounds. The use of many sutures passed through the intraluminal mucosa apparently encourages a smoother surface at the suture line and results in a breathy and high-pitched voice more suitable for a female patient.

Once the epiglottis has been sutured in place, the strap muscles are sutured together in the midline, and the wound is

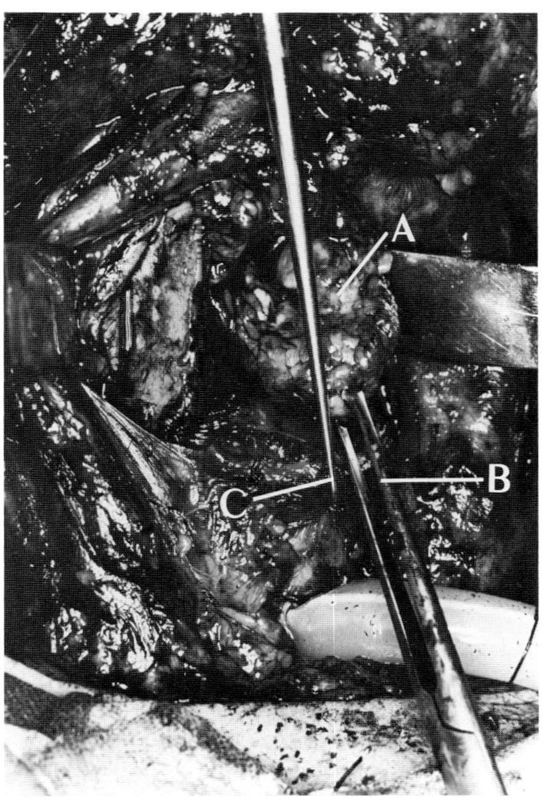

Figure 19–2. As dissection proceeds, the epiglottis (A) is drawn down with the tenaculum (B) toward the cricoid (C).

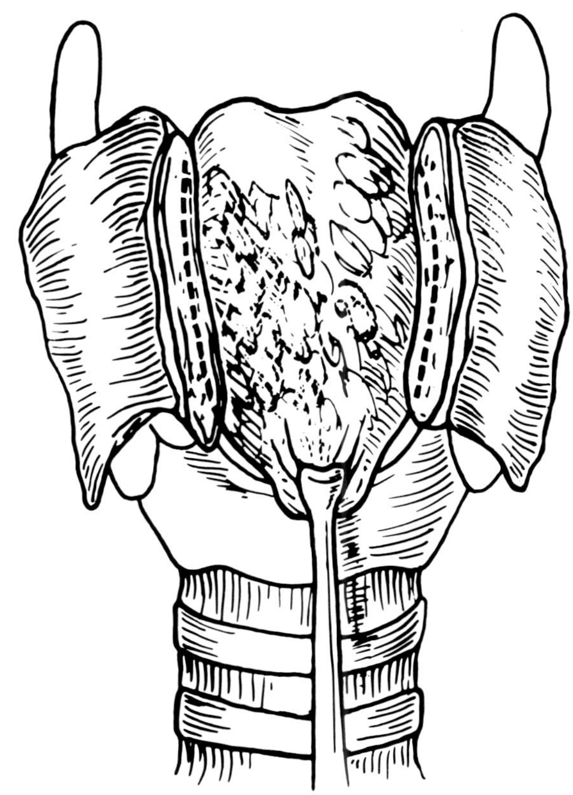

Figure 19–3. When dissection is completed, the petiole of the epiglottis easily reaches the cricoid cartilage and may overlap it.

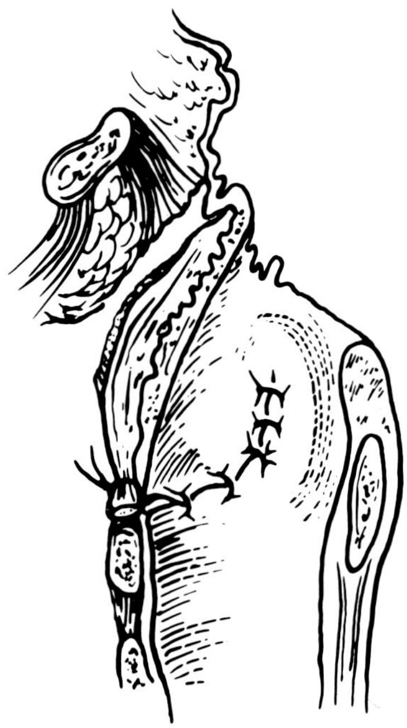

Figure 19–4. The epiglottis is sutured in place. Note: Sutures are passed through the mucosa in this illustration. This may decrease pseudocord formation and enhance a higher pitched voice.

drained using constant suction. The wound is closed in the standard fashion. A cuffed tracheotomy tube is placed at the end of the procedure.

POSTOPERATIVE CARE

Care during the immediate postoperative period is no different from that of any head and neck surgery patient. Early ambulation is important, and tube feedings are begun on the second or third postoperative day. The cuffed tracheotomy tube is replaced with a noncuffed tube, one size smaller, on the fifth postoperative day, and the laryngeal lumen may be tested by occluding the tracheotomy tube.

In patients who have not had previous radiotherapy, the postoperative edema subsides quickly, and the tracheotomy may be decannulated as early as the fifth or sixth postoperative day. In previously irradiated patients, however, the edema may last for 2 or 3 weeks. Patients should be warned about this possible delay in order to prevent depression and to help their families prepare for tracheotomy care at home.

I feel strongly that patients do better if oral rehabilitation is delayed until the third postoperative week. This allows pain and edema to diminish and the muscles of the pharynx to become more flexible. Most patients have achieved tracheotomy decannulation by this time, a factor that greatly aids the oral rehabilitation process.

ORAL REHABILITATION

The epiglottic reconstruction procedure results in major disruptions to the deglutition process. Dissection in the preepiglottic space restricts the posterior movement of the tongue base and the upward movement of the larynx. It also results in trauma to branches of the superior laryngeal nerves with resultant diminished sensation in the laryngeal introitus. The epiglottis is also lost as a diverting force to the food bolus. Finally, the spincteric action of the larynx is diminished. The net result is extremely conducive to aspiration.

The rehabilitation process must work around the defects produced by the operative procedure. Laryngeal and tongue base movement will increase with time if the tracheotomy tube is removed and the patient is encouraged to swallow saliva as quickly as possible. Diminished sensation is countered by having the patient swallow foods and liquids with harsh textures and extremes of temperature, that is, carbonated beverages, hot or iced liquids, coarse rather than pure textures. Lateral or supine positioning will help develop neosphincteric action in the reconstructed larynx.

RESULTS

Subtotal laryngectomy with epiglottic reconstruction is a good oncologic and reconstructive procedure. The overall 3-year survival rate in our present series is 71% (27 of 38 patients). Four of these survivors required total laryngectomy for salvage. All of the deaths occurred in previously irradiated patients; 11 of the 27 survivors had not received prior irradiation.

In this group of 38 patients there were no patients who required the tracheotomy tube beyond the sixth postoperative week. All of the patients had some degree of aspiration that prevented total oral intake for the first 3 to 6 weeks. Only four patients required feeding tube supplements beyond 3 months. All patients were independent of the feeding tubes within 6 months of surgery.

In general, the patients' voices were good. Some of the female patients in the early part of the series were unhappy with the harsh low-pitched character of their voices. The higher pitched, breathy voice obtained with closer approximation of the mucosal edges has been more satisfactory.

CONCLUSION

Subtotal laryngectomy and epiglottic reconstruction is an oncologically sound procedure that offers the patient with extensive cancer at the glottic level an opportunity for laryngeal conservation, even after radiation failure.

REFERENCES

1. Bouche J, Frecje CH, Husson U. Ann d'Otolaryngole 1965;T82, No 6, 643.
2. Sedlaček K. Československá Otolaryngologie 1965;XIV,8,328.
3. Kambič V. Epiglottoplasy—New technique for Laryngeal Reconstruction. Radiologia Iugoslavica 1977; Suppl II:33–43.
4. Tucker H, Wood B, Levine H, et al. Glottic reconstruction after near-total laryngectomy. Laryngoscope 1979;89:609–17.
5. Sobol SM, Wood B, Levine H. Epiglottic laryngoplasty for laryngeal stenosis. Ann Otol Rhinol Laryngol 1981;90:409–11.
6. Olson R, Sullivan MJ. Epiglottis in reconstruction of the larynx and trachea. Ann Otol Rhinol Laryngol 1985;94:437–41.
7. Schechter GL. Epiglottic reconstruction and subtotal laryngectomy. Laryngoscope 1983;93:723–34.

20

Deglutition Following Partial Laryngectomy

Harvey M. Tucker

Partial or "conservation" laryngectomy has become a widely accepted treatment modality for carcinoma of the larynx. Whether it is employed in conjunction with planned radiotherapy, as salvage surgery after failed primary radiotherapy, or as a sole means of therapy, difficulties with deglutition can be a distressing aftermath. Understanding the mechanisms of deglutition and how they may be compromised by the various resections and reconstructions employed in the management of laryngeal cancer can help to minimize swallowing difficulties and permit more effective rehabilitation of such patients.

PHYSIOLOGY OF DEGLUTITION

Several critical activities must occur at precisely the right moment to permit the act of swallowing to go to completion without aspiration or regurgitation. These include: (1) closure of the glottic sphincter, (2) depression of the epiglottis over the laryngeal introitus by the downward movement of the base of the tongue, (3) anterosuperior excursion of the laryngotracheal complex under cover of the base of the tongue, and (4) timely relaxation of the cricopharyngeus muscle. This sequence of events results in a rise in subglottic pressure to counteract the concomitant rise in supraglottic pressure as the food bolus approaches the larynx, and in simultaneous opening of the hypopharynx to receive the bolus. All of these activities depend on normal sensation in the posterior oropharynx and hypopharynx to trigger them at appropriate times during deglutition.

If one or perhaps two of these functions are compromised by partial laryngectomy (as they often are), most otherwise healthy patients can tolerate them with relatively little interference with the swallowing mechanism. When three or more are interfered with, almost every patient will experience severe difficulty or even complete inability to swallow.

SURGICAL CONSIDERATIONS

Vertical Partial Laryngectomy (Hemilaryngectomy)

Hemilaryngectomy usually results in removal of one vocal fold, thus rendering the glottis incompetent. Since there is no interference with sensation in the hypopharynx or any other critical function, most patients do not experience much difficulty in relearning swallowing after this procedure. If the arytenoid cartilage must be removed (extended hemilaryngectomy), however, about 50% of patients will experience significant aspiration unless the buttress between the pyriform sinus and the glottic introitus is reconstructed.[1,2] The technique I prefer employs an inferiorly pedicled flap of sternothyroid muscle brought through the preserved perichondrium and sutured to the bed of the excised arytenoid cartilage (Fig. 20–1).[3]

Near-Total Laryngectomy with Epiglottic Reconstruction*

This procedure effectively removes both membranous vocal folds and may even include arytenoidectomy on one side, thus rendering the glottis totally incompetent (Fig. 20–2).[4] Patients who undergo this procedure relearn swallowing rather easily,

---

*Editor's note: The term employed here as "near-total laryngectomy" refers to a different procedure than the operation described in Chapter 24. The latter does not reconstruct a functional airway, but leaves the patient with a permanent tracheotomy. Many authors would term the procedure described here by Dr. Tucker as a bilateral anterofrontal or extended frontolateral laryngectomy.

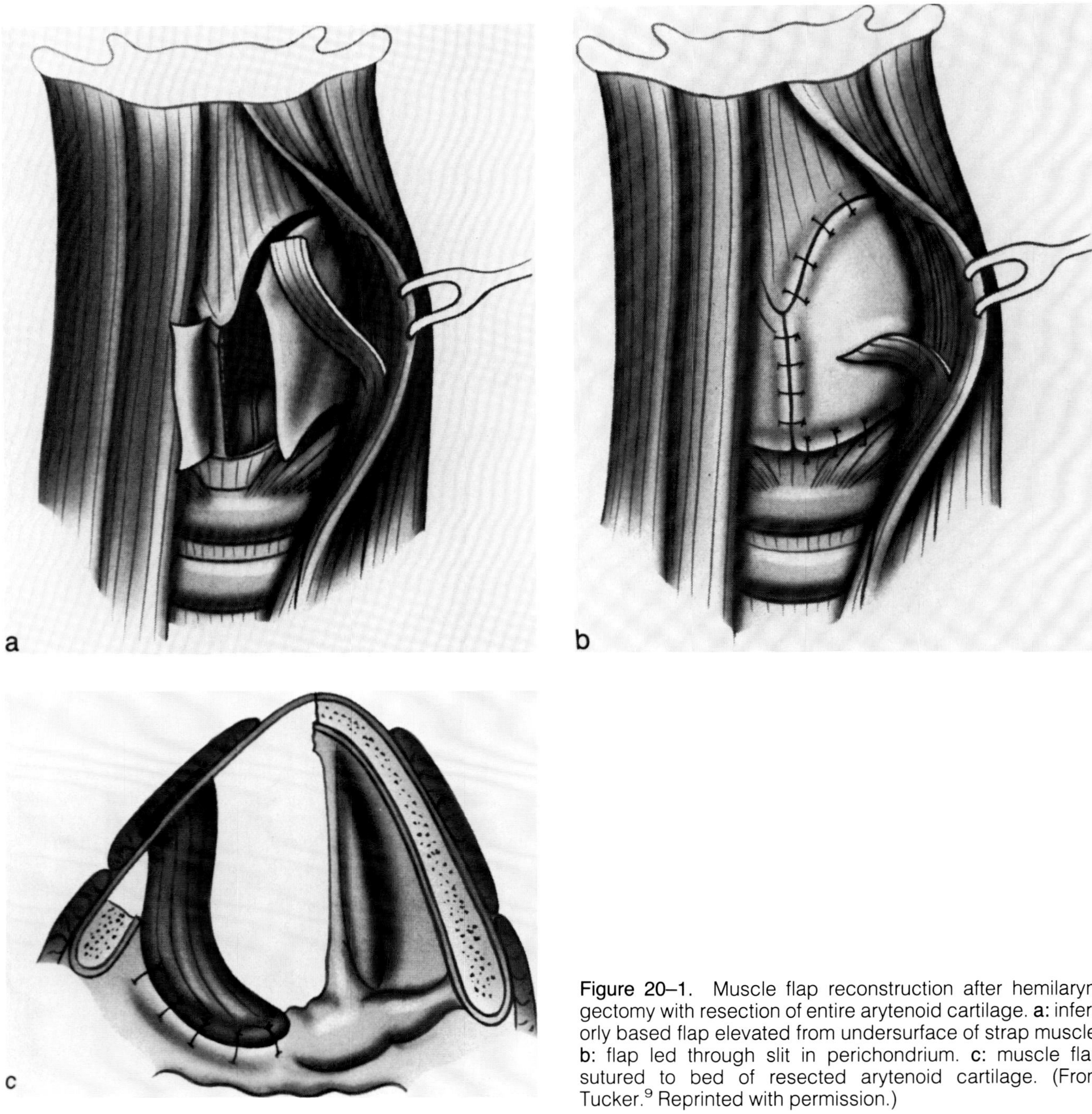

Figure 20–1. Muscle flap reconstruction after hemilaryngectomy with resection of entire arytenoid cartilage. a: inferiorly based flap elevated from undersurface of strap muscle. b: flap led through slit in perichondrium. c: muscle flap sutured to bed of resected arytenoid cartilage. (From Tucker.[9] Reprinted with permission.)

however, because there is no disruption of hypopharyngeal sensation or of the active upward mobility of the larynotracheal complex under cover of the base of the tongue. Thus, even though the epiglottis is greatly diminished in size, there is still protection for the glottic introitus. There is more often temporary aspiration following near-total laryngectomy than after simple vertical partial laryngectomy, as might be expected, but less than usually occurs after supraglottic laryngectomy (see later).

Horizontal Partial Laryngectomy

Supraglottic procedures can be divided into supraglottic laryngectomy, extended supraglottic laryngectomy, and partial laryngopharyngectomy. In addition to resection of the supraglottic larynx, the extended procedure includes removal of the base of the tongue, whereas partial laryngopharyngectomy usually refers to resection of the pyriform sinus with up to half the circumference of the hypopharynx as well.

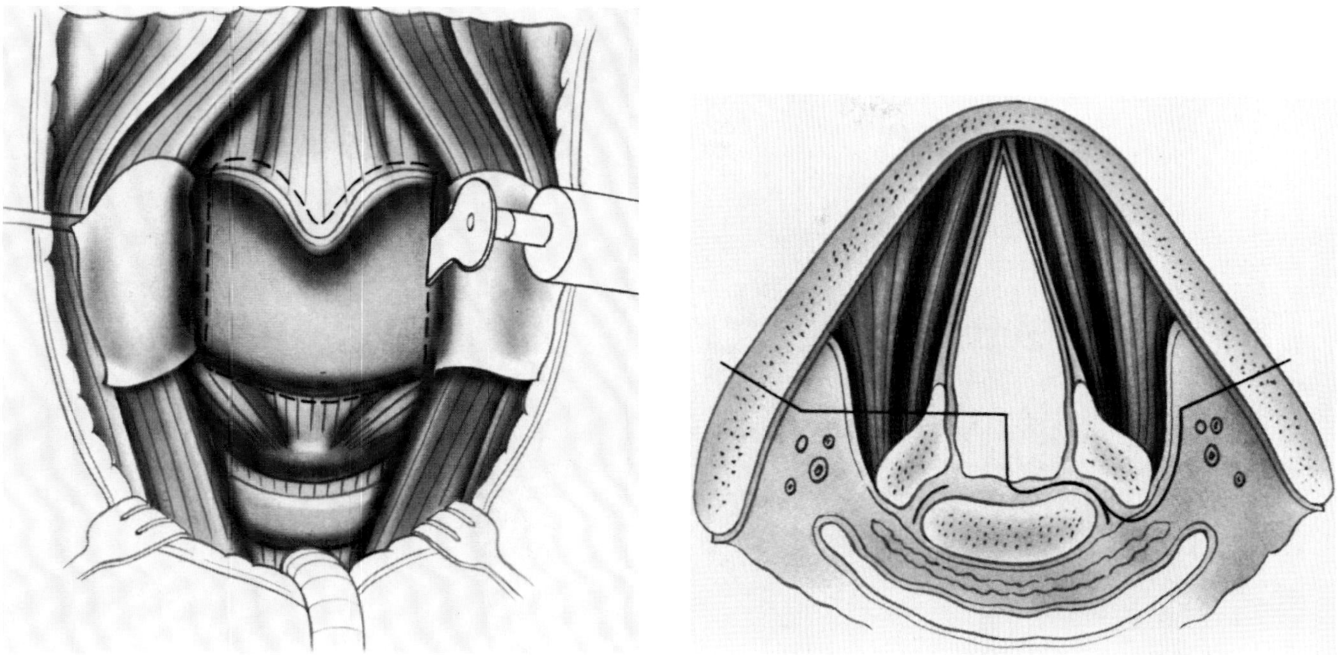

A B

Figure 20–2. Near-total laryngectomy. A: cartilage cuts. B: possible maximal extent of resection leaves posterior cartilage strut bilaterally and the body of at least one arytenoid cartilage. (From Tucker.[9] Reprinted with permission.)

All of these procedures result in significantly greater interference with the normal mechanisms of swallowing than does vertical partial laryngectomy. Not only does the patient incur loss of the supraglottic structures (that is, epiglottis and false vocal folds, base of tongue) that normally protect the laryngeal introitus, but he must, as a result of removal of the hypopharynx or base of tongue, or both, also adapt to ablation of significant portions of the sequential sensory input so important to timely relaxation of the cricopharyngeus muscle. It is this sensory derangement that seems to result in increased aspiration more than any other single anatomic or functional loss.

The problem is of such magnitude that return of swallowing function to near-normal levels can be expected in only 85 to 90% of patients after supraglottic laryngectomy.[5] Approximately half of the remaining 10 to 15% will swallow and cough well enough to protect the airway from their own secretions but will not be able to maintain adequate peroral nutrition without significant pulmonary soilage. These patients will have to choose between an alternate means of feeding (such as gastrostomy and cervical esophagostomy[6]) to retain speech and avoid a tracheostoma, and "completion" total laryngectomy in order to avoid life-threatening pneumonia. The remaining 5 to 7% of patients will have sufficient severe compromise of ability to protect the airway that they will be unable to tolerate even their normal secretions without development of aspiration pneumonia. Completion laryngectomy is the only alternative for this latter group of patients.

Flores et al[5] analyzed several parameters that can affect swallowing after supraglottic laryngectomy and various extended procedures. They found that:

1. Extended procedures resulted in significantly higher incidence of failure to swallow (supraglottic laryngectomy, 10%, extended supraglottic laryngectomy, 17%, partial laryngopharyngectomy with flap reconstruction, 66%).
2. Preservation of the hyoid bone facilitated closure, but affected deglutition only insofar as it permitted retention of both superior laryngeal nerves, thus preserving timely cricopharyngeus function.
3. Age, per se, was not a factor.
4. Cricopharyngeal myotomy could not be proven to influence ultimate swallowing success, but seemed to hasten return of deglutition.

Therefore the keys to successful deglutition after supraglottic laryngectomy include:

1. Reestablishment of the relationship between the remaining laryngotracheal complex and the base of the tongue. This maneuver permits the larynx to rise up and forward during swallowing and opens the hypopharynx.
2. Preservation of at least one and preferably, if possible within constraints of tumor removal, both superior laryngeal nerves to maintain sensory input and timely relaxation of the cricopharyngeus muscle.
3. Cricopharyngeal myotomy, particularly if there is suspicion that hypopharyngeal sensation has been lost.

NONSURGICAL CONSIDERATIONS

Other factors can play a major role in successful reestablishment of deglutition after partial laryngectomy. Although they are only indirectly related to the surgery itself, careful attention to these details of rehabilitation can "make or break" patient recovery.[7,8] They include:

1. Removal of the tracheotomy tube and taping of the wound at least 24 to 28 hours *before* swallowing is attempted. This sequence prevents air leakage that can interfere with reestablishment of appropriate rise in supraglottic pressure during swallowing to help prevent aspiration. It also removes any impediment to movement of the laryngotracheal complex and avoids even the slight delay in passage of the bolus of food because of the impression of the tracheotomy tube on the party wall between the trachea and esophagus.
2. The nasogastric tube should be removed at least 12 hours before attempted swallowing to allow cricopharyngeal irritation and edema to subside.
3. Speech and language pathologists trained in swallowing therapy are extremely helpful in initial reestablishment of deglutition. When such a professional is not available, the surgeon must do the necessary coaching. A three swallow sequence has been successful. The patient takes a deep breath and holds it. A small sip of semiliquid material is taken, swallowing is initiated, the patient immediately swallows a second time, then coughs and swallows a third time before taking a breath. In this manner, most of the swallowed material goes down with the first swallow, most of the rest with the second swallow, and the cough and third swallow serve to clear any material still resting on the glottis before a breath is taken.
4. Proper psychologic support cannot be emphasized too strongly. It is critical that the patient approach his first attempts at swallowing with as positive an attitude as possible. He must also understand that initially swallowing is likely to be difficult and frustrating. The three swallow technique is unnatural and very time consuming, but usually within a day or two the patient can expect to be taking sufficient nutrition by mouth, without significant aspiration, to be able to leave the hospital.

In time, swallowing will automatically become more spontaneous and closer to normal and the diet can usually be advanced to most table food and liquids. Nevertheless, all supraglottic laryngectomy patients aspirate to some degree, and most of them continue to aspirate from time to time, although not enough to threaten pulmonary function or nutrition.

CONCLUSIONS

Restoration of adequate deglutition is essential after partial laryngectomy, especially since the alternative of total laryngectomy is not only as effective in obtaining a cure, but allows alimentation with little or no difficulty. The one real advantage of subtotal laryngectomy is preservation of voice without the need for permanent tracheostomy, but this is of questionable value if ability to maintain nutrition by mouth is lost in the process. Understanding the critical elements in normal swallowing and how they can be compromised by the various subtotal laryngectomy procedures can help the surgeon to optimize the possibility of successful postoperative deglutition.

REFERENCES

1. Quinn JH. Free muscle transplant method of glottic reconstruction after hemilaryngectomy. Laryngoscope 1975;85:985–6.
2. Bailey BJ. Glottic reconstruction after hemilaryngectomy: bipedicled muscle flap laryngoplasty. Laryngoscope 1975;85:960–77.
3. Ogura JH, Biller H. Glottic reconstruction following extended frontolateral hemilaryngectomy. Laryngoscope 1969;79:2181–4.
4. Tucker HM, Wood BG, Levine HL, Katz R. Glottic reconstruction after near-total laryngectomy. Laryngoscope 1979;89:609–18.
5. Flores TC, Wood BG, Levine HL, et al. Factors in successful deglutition following supraglottic laryngeal surgery. Ann Otol Rhinol Laryngol 1982;91:579.
6. Tucker HM, Broniatowski M, Chase S. Tube esophagostomy. Arch Otolaryngol 1985;111:187.
7. Tucker HM. Management of the patient with an incompetent larynx. Am J Otolaryngol 1979;1:47.
8. Tucker HM. Rehabilitation of patients with postoperative deficits, cranial nerves VIII through XII. Otolaryngol Head Neck Surg 1980;88:576.
9. Tucker HM: *The Larynx*. New York: Thieme Medical Publishers, 1987.

21

Partial Laryngectomy: Trends in the United Kingdom

Henry J. Shaw

Conservative surgery for laryngeal cancer has been performed for almost 140 years, in fact preceding by 20 years the first recorded total laryngectomy for cancer, but inability to control infection, ignorance of surgical pathology and limited technical expertise discouraged progress.[1–3]

It is only in the last 40 years that real improvements in surgical technique and results have been achieved. Mainly, this is due to more widely available and effective antibiotics coupled with more precise knowledge of the compartmented lymphatics and of the histologic pathways of tumor spread within the larynx.[4–7]

As a result principally of the work of Alonso,[8] Ogura,[9] Som,[10] and Biller[11] in the Americas and of Leroux-Robert,[12] Bocca,[13] Guerrier,[14] and others in Europe, surgical techniques have been refined and extended to include "hemi-laryngectomy"[2] and "extended supraglottic laryngectomy,"[9] and even to the concepts of "partial laryngo-pharyngectomy"[15] and "near total laryngectomy."[16,17]

In the same period, with better sources and techniques of irradiation, the results of radiotherapy for cancer of the larynx have also steadily improved so that they can now match the excellent results for early tumors reported by primary surgical resection, usually with no functional damage.[18–20]

A further refinement in conservation during the past 15 years has been the introduction and development of carbon dioxide laser therapy for some premalignant lesions[21] and the earliest glottic tumors. It will be seen that a gradual consensus has now arisen that, with certain exceptions, most early laryngeal cancers are best treated by irradiation, using partial or total resection for salvage.

TUMOR VARIABLES IN RELATION TO CHOICE OF TREATMENT

In general, treatment for laryngeal cancer concerns the 98% histologically squamous or epidermoid carcinomas that will form the basis for discussion in this chapter. Rare tumors other than lymphoma, such as verrucous carcinoma, adenocarcinoma, sarcomas, and melanoma, are best treated primarily by conservation surgical techniques when circumstances permit and will not be considered in further detail.

Squamous carcinoma varies widely in histologic grading, with the majority of primary lesions being predominantly low-grade and well-differentiated, especially on the true vocal cords. High-grade or pleomorphic poorly differentiated tumors, more frequent in other regions of the larynx, have a lower cure rate and are usually less suitable for conservation surgery. A further biologic variable, more difficult to assess since it may not be directly related to histologic grade, is the growth rate and aggressive potential of each individual tumor.

The correct treatment decision requires accurate identification of the precise site and extent of disease with an approximate point of origin. An underestimate of these variables is frequent, especially with lack of experience or after failure of irradiation, and leads either to inappropriate reliance on partial laryngectomy for cure or to early recurrence of disease, or both. It follows that precise TN classification is essential for a proper choice of treatment. Furthermore, the chance of cure by surgery should not be compromised by a desire to preserve laryngeal function.

TREATMENT OPTIONS IN EARLY LARYNGEAL CANCER

Glottic Carcinoma

Epithelial dysplasia of the true vocal cords will lead progressively to the changes of carcinoma in situ in about 10% of cases if no effective measures are taken. This in turn may progress to microinvasive and later to true invasive cancer or the coexistence of these lesions.[22] If resolution does not take place with removal of etiologic factors such as smoking, vocal abuse, and local infection, it is usually agreed that treatment should be surgical rather than by radiotherapy;[18] stripping of the cord under microscopy or the use of a carbon dioxide laser is effective in many cases. If the lesion is single and recurrent, treatment by simple cordectomy or hemilaryngectomy may rarely be required. When the lesions are multiple and sometimes also in the supraglottic area, the same measures should be used initially, but greater vigilance and regular histologic review is required to detect invasive changes.

For the early invasive single T_1 glottic tumor, it is now generally accepted that initial treatment, whatever the histologic grade, should be by external teleradiation. Cure rates of 85 to 95% are obtainable, seldom bettered by surgery, and leave the patient with a normal voice in most cases.[20] Vertical partial laryngectomy can certainly produce equally good survival figures, although with vocal impairment. Initial surgery should be best reserved for young patients and those with established edematous laryngitis, due to an increased chance of long-term recurrence or second primary cancer within the larynx after irradiation.[23] It is also useful for patients who are unable or unwilling to attend regularly for outpatient radiotherapy.

It will be apparent that the above philosophy limits the application of vertical partial laryngectomy mainly to small glottic tumors recurrent after irradiation. Extension of disease beyond the confines of the true vocal cords and anterior commissure to be classified as T_2 (without fixation of the vocal cord, extension to the posterior arytenoid mucosa, invasion of thyroid cartilage, or appreciable subglottic extension) is still amenable to the same philosophy of external irradiation for cure with the possibility of extended partial or total laryngectomy for early recurrence in most cases. Exceptions to primary surgery by vertical partial laryngectomy, or sometimes extended hemilaryngectomy, have already been given. Again it must be emphasized that success will depend greatly on accurate clinical assessment before any choice of treatment.

Contrary to the opinion of some surgeons,[16] the consensus for treatment of T_3 glottic carcinoma is that conservation surgery, whether initial or secondary, is rarely indicated or feasible. This is due to the common difficulty of assessing these tumors with accuracy, especially after irradiation, usually resulting in an underestimate of their true extent.

Supraglottic Carcinoma

The development of the horizontal supraglottic partial laryngectomy procedure and its extensions has been an impressive contribution to conservation surgery of the larynx.[24] It is suitable for T_1 and on occasions T_2 tumors of the supraglottic area, especially when confined to the anterior part of the laryngeal vestibule. Supraglottic surgery can excise the lesion successfully even with a narrow margin of 2 mm and can give excellent curative results with good voice preservation, but it cannot be regarded as a simple procedure. Success again depends on precise preoperative assessment of disease extent and on a fit patient with good cardiopulmonary function. It is not for the occasional laryngeal surgeon. In addition, it carries an appreciable regular complication rate and hospital morbidity, especially for restoration of a normal swallow.

For these reasons and because precise irradiaiton of such tumors when neck metastases are clinically absent can give comparable survival results with minimal complications, primary treatment of such cases by teleradiation is again the preferred choice except in young patients.[20] However, the same authors offer good evidence that when neck nodes are clinically positive, better results are likely if partial laryngectomy is the primary treatment coupled with radical neck dissection. Depending on the degree of neck involvement, postoperative irradiation to both sides of the neck may also be advantageous.

Horizontal partial laryngectomy for recurrence following full-dosage irradiation is certainly hazardous but can be used successfully in a small number of cases if strict criteria are observed in selection, with meticulous surgery and after care.

Subglottic Carcinoma

In general, conservation surgery has no part to play in the treatment of cancer of true subglottic origin. However, when a cordal tumor extends downward up to 10 mm anteriorly below the cord of 5 mm posteriorly, an extended vertical partial laryngectomy (hemilaryngectomy) can properly be considered in the absence of other contraindications.

TREATMENT TRENDS FOR LARYNGEAL CANCER IN THE UNITED KINGDOM

The number of new cases in the United Kingdom appears to have been relatively stable over the past 20 years, although there is slight evidence of a recent relative increase in females.[25,26] It is also well-established in Britain that glottic primary lesions are more frequent than supraglottic lesions (32% supraglottic including epilaryngeal sites to 60% glottic).[18] In most of Northern Europe this pattern of regional frequency also holds good, but the exact reverse is apparent for people of Southern European origin and in Finland, who show a much greater relative incidence of supraglottic lesions (60% supraglottic to 30% glottic) and also a higher total incidence of laryngeal cancer.[26,27]

In the United Kingdom for the last 40 years laryngologists have enjoyed the facilities and support of skilled radiotherapists often isolated but working in regional departments readily accessible to the larger population groups. These facts together with excellent figures for cure obtained by irradiation in the more common cases of limited glottic cancer, coupled with the potent philosophies of "painless cure" and "saving the patient from surgical mutilation," have resulted in many years of radiotherapeutic domination in the treatment of laryngeal cancer. In recent years this attitude has been slowly changing with a realization of the greater effectiveness of combined treatment in advanced lesions and the more selective application of irradiation or surgery in other cases, deriving mainly from experience in combined head and neck clinics.

The economic and geographic factors of "free at the time" treatment and "free" transportation provided by a National Health Service have also tilted the balance in favor of the more prolonged but less traumatic outpatient treatment by irradiation. As a result of this predominance of radiotherapy, hospital centers are in a unique position to assess the application of surgical techniques after failed full-dosage irradiation.

Material Studied

To illustrate contemporary usage in the United Kingdom, two approximately parallel time periods have been chosen at two hospitals in London dealing frequently with laryngeal cancer. At the Royal Marsden Hospital, the period 1963–1988 is taken, and at The Royal National Throat, Nose and Ear (TNE) Hospital, partial laryngectomy for the period 1961–1988 is reviewed.

A total of 50 patients underwent forms of either vertical or horizontal partial laryngectomy at the former hospital. Only one malignant tumor of the vertical group was treated initially by surgery. During the same period all 11 patients with supraglottic tumors had initial supraglottic laryngectomy without prior irradiation; five were for benign lesions. Altogether 15 patients underwent horizontal partial laryngectomy after irradiation. For the same period a total of 410 total laryngectomies were carried out (Table 21–1).

A total of 60 partial laryngectomies were performed at the TNE hospital from 1961 through 1988. Vertical partial laryngectomy accounted for 57 of these, extended in 12 patients into a frontolateral operation. Surgery followed irradiation in 37 and 16 were nonirradiated. Five of 11 horizontal partial laryngectomies were performed after irradiation, and six were treated initially by surgery, two with postoperative irradiation. In the same period 650 total laryngectomies were carried out (Table 21–2).

In laryngeal cancer recurrent after irradiation, clinical classification and suitability for a conservation procedure cannot be finally determined, at least until the direct laryngoscopy that should precede any surgical intervention. In many doubtful cases it was also found on direct exploration of the larynx at operation that extensions of the tumor rendered partial resection unwise or impossible despite a favorable endoscopic assessment. This underlines the practical necessity to obtain prior permission for total laryngectomy in every case and to refrain from unqualified positive assurances to the patient regarding conservation before the event.

Table 21–1. Partial Laryngectomy: The Royal Marsden Hospital, 1963–1988*

TYPE OF OPERATION	NO.
Vertical	
After full irradiation	23
Nonirradiated	1
Subtotal	24
Horizontal	
After full irradiation	15
Nonirradiated	11
(5 benign lesions)	—
Subtotal	26
Total	50

*The age range of patients was 24 to 78 years (median, 59). Sex incidence was M/F: 37/11. Total laryngectomies in same period were 410.

Table 21–2. Partial Laryngectomy: Royal National Throat, Nose, and Ear Hospital, 1963–1988*

TYPE OF OPERATION	NO.
Vertical	
After full irradiation	37
Irradiated postoperatively	4
Nonirradiated	16
Subtotal	57
Horizontal	
After full irradiation	5
Irradiated postoperatively	2
Nonirradiated	4
(3 benign lesions)	—
Subtotal	11
Total	68

*The age range of the patients was 43 to 85 years (median, 62). Sex incidence was M/F: 61/6. Total laryngectomies in same period were 650.

Radiotherapy

Irradiation of patients from both hospitals was administered in the Radiotherapy Department of The Royal Marsden Hospital. The radiation source has been almost entirely the 5000 C cobalt telecurie therapy apparatus. In a few earlier cases, the older 12 gm radium "bomb" was used. Total tumor dose per patient has averaged 65 Gy to the larynx fractionated once daily 5 days per week over a period of 6 to 7 weeks.[18]

The two lateral fields used for glottic cancer (5×4 cm) were confined to the larynx itself. However, lateral fields for supraglottic cancer (10×8 cm) also included the upper neck lymphatics and thyrohyoid area where irradiation was concentrated during the latter part of the treatment. It is clear that the laryngeal vestibule and preepiglottic tissues probably received a maximal tumor dose that, of necessity, has influenced healing after surgical salvage.

Types of Operation

At both hospitals, the vertical operations were of a standard pattern using a midline vertical skin incision or a horizontal incision at the level of the lower third of the thyroid cartilage. After thyrotomy, the resection then extended from the anterior commissure posteriorly to include the whole vocal cord and intrinsic laryngeal musculature back to the arytenoid vocal process, and from the upper surface of the ventricular band to 5 mm below the edge of the true cord. In all cases a major portion of the thyroid cartilage on the affected side was excised (Figs. 21–1, 21–2).

In the period studied at the two hospitals, there were 16 extended vertical operations (hemilaryngectomies); five included the anterior commissure and the anterior third of the opposite vocal cord.

Most horizontal supraglottic operations were also standard, mainly following the technique of Som,[10] using a T-shaped skin

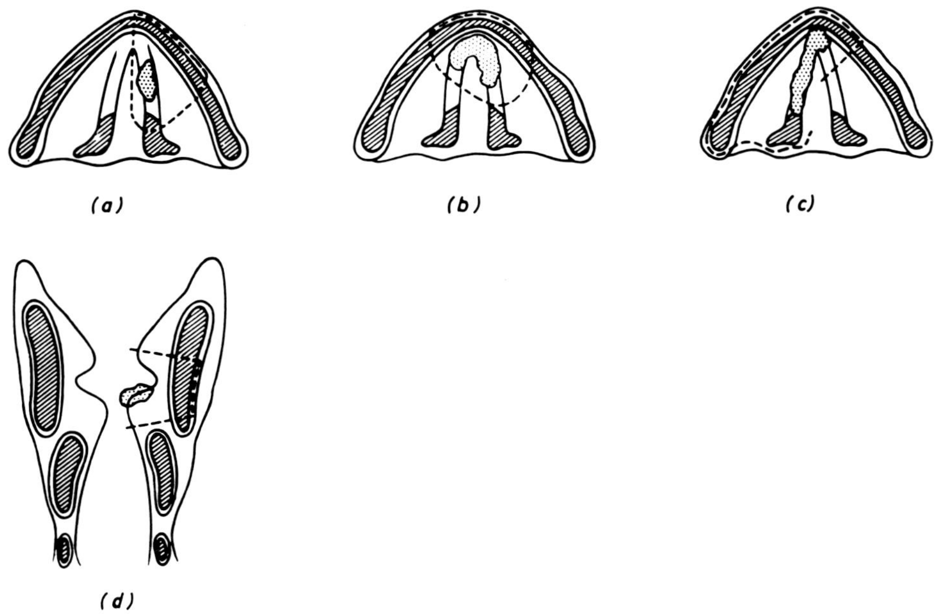

Figure 21–1. Types of resection for vertical partial laryngectomy. **a**: standard glottic resection; **b**: fronto-lateral resection; **c**: extended hemilaryngectomy; **d**: coronal view, standard resection.

incision with the horizontal component at the hyoid level and the vertical component offset about 5 cm from the midline to the side mainly involved. Resection then included the epiglottis, valleculae, preepiglottic space and hyoid bone, ventricular bands, and ventricles with parts of the aryepiglottic folds. However, in seven of 26 operations at The Royal Marsden Hospital, the resection was extended. Two operations included one arytenoid cartilage in each specimen, one of these also being extended to resect a vocal cord and adnexae on the same side, and one to include the top of the pyriform fossa on the same side. Five others were extended to resect part of the tongue base (Figs. 21–3, 21–4, 21–5).

The majority of patients had undergone one previous full course of telecobalt irradiation to a total dose of approximately 56 Gy at varying intervals prior to surgery. Of the 15 radical neck dissections carried out, all but one were for clinically positive nodes. One was simultaneous with a vertical partial laryngectomy and another performed in a separate stage after the

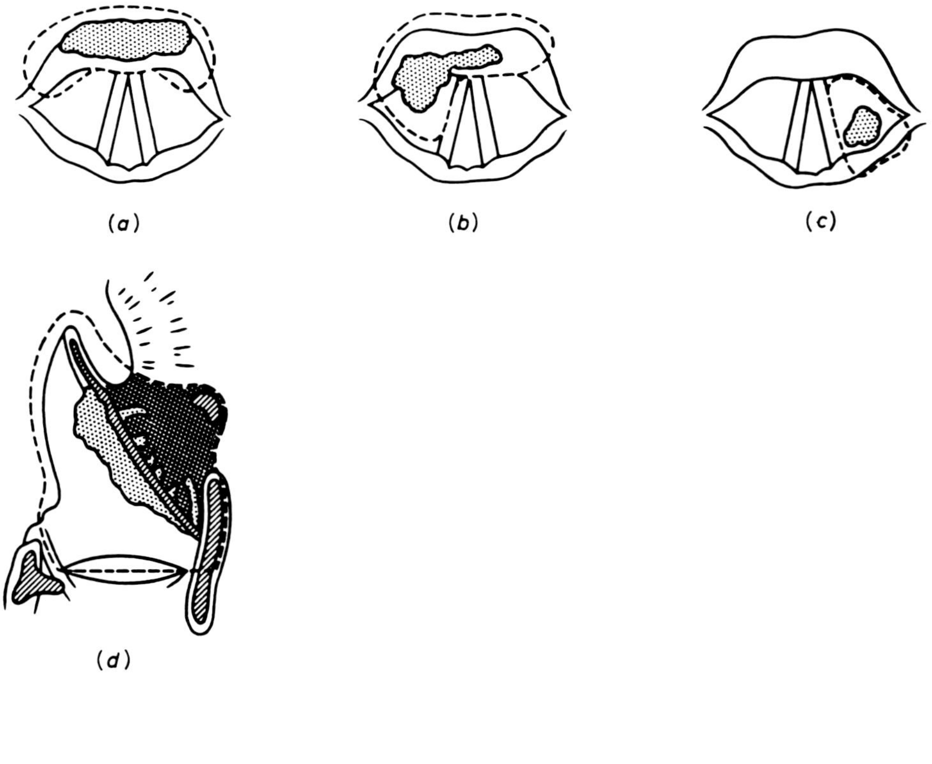

Figure 21–2. Types of resection for horizontal partial laryngectomy. **a,b,c**: standard supraglottic resection for three differing sites of lesion; **d**: sagittal view, standard resection with clearance of the preepiglottic space.

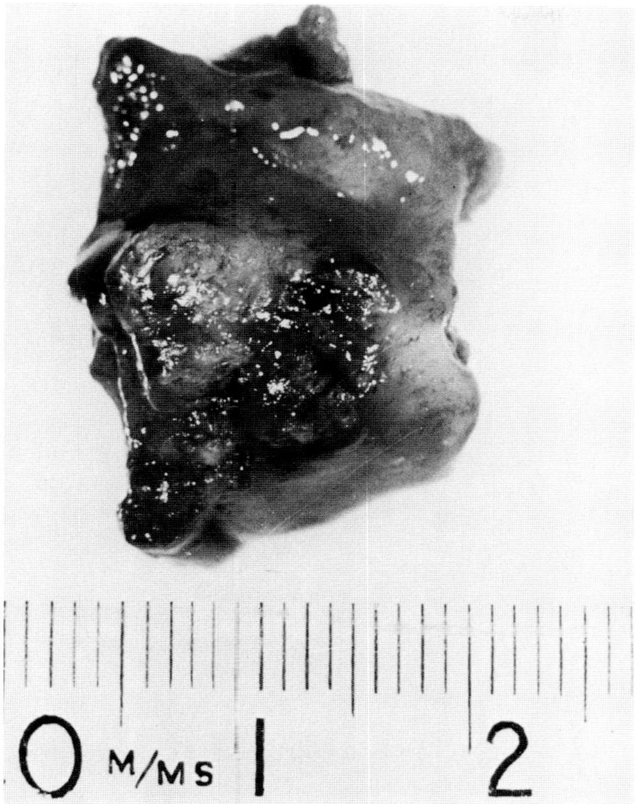

Figure 21–3. Specimen following postradiation vertical partial laryngectomy showing intact false cord with tumor involving true cord and ventricular floor, margins histologically clear.

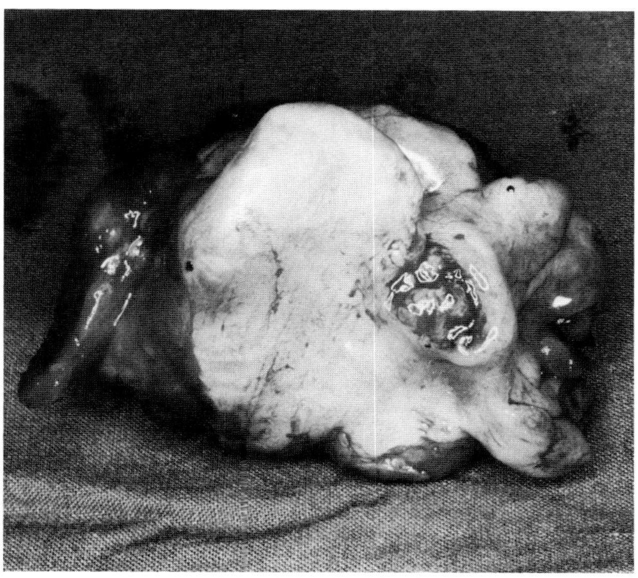

Figure 21–4. Specimen following postradiation horizontal partial laryngectomy showing tumor involving aryepiglottic fold and border of right pyriform fossa, margins histologically clear.

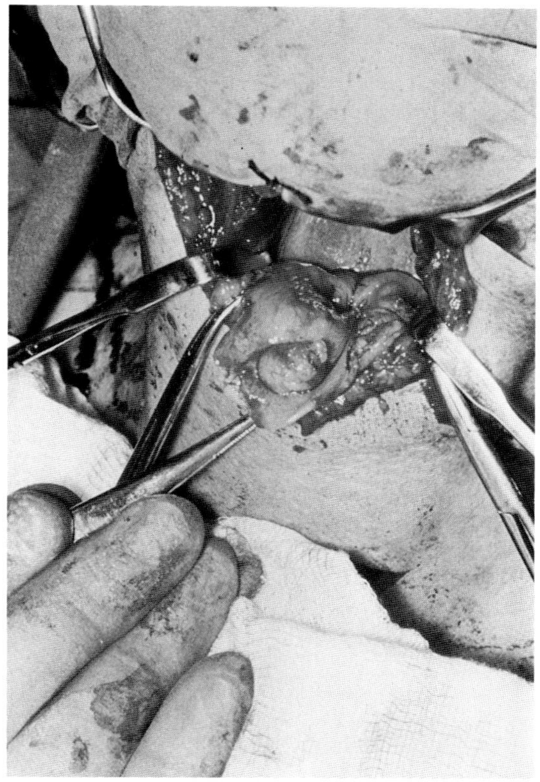

Figure 21–5. Exposure of postradiation recurrent tumor of epiglottis by transverse pharyngotomy for horizontal partial laryngectomy.

initial procedure. The other 13 were for supraglottic lesions and, when thought advisable, were also separately staged in order to minimize healing and swallowing difficulties.

Complications

Ward[28] draws necessary attention to at least a dozen major complications of laryngeal conservation surgery, which require careful management if they are to be avoided. In the series of 81 vertical operations carried out at the two hospitals most complications occurred in the 60 cases operated on after full irradiation. Even so, they were usually temporary and seldom serious. Perichondritis causing delayed decannulation, subcutaneous emphysema, and mild chest infections in a few cases were the main problems. One patient developed an intralaryngeal granuloma 6 months after surgery. In another, laryngeal edema following perichondritis lasted 16 months, and in a third, subglottic stenosis, requiring surgical correction, developed 7 years after operation.

The postoperative picture for the 37 horizontal partial laryngectomy cases gave more cause for concern, particularly in the 20 operated on after irradiation. Only eight of the latter healed per primum with no complications and none had undergone an extended procedure (Figs. 21–6, 21–7). At least half experienced delayed return of normal swallow up to 8 weeks. One patient required gastrostomy for 1 year and another for 6 years

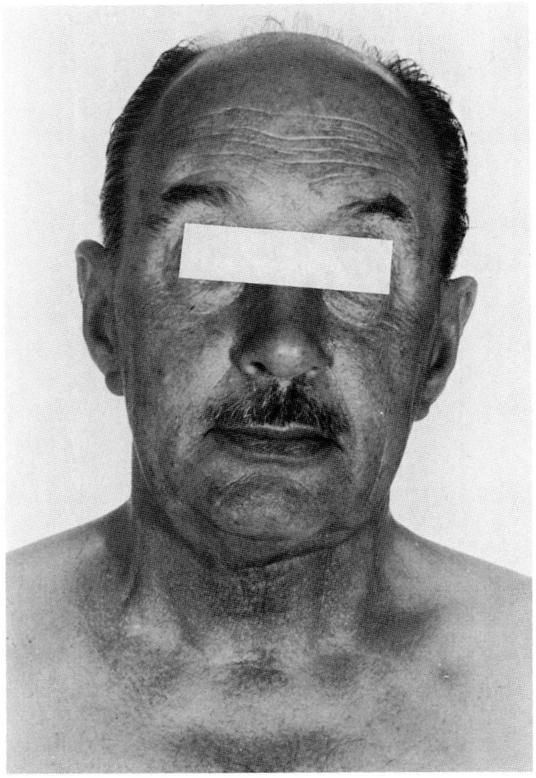

Figure 21–6. Patient after primary healing and functional rehabilitation following postradiation horizontal laryngectomy. Completed 5-year survival disease-free.

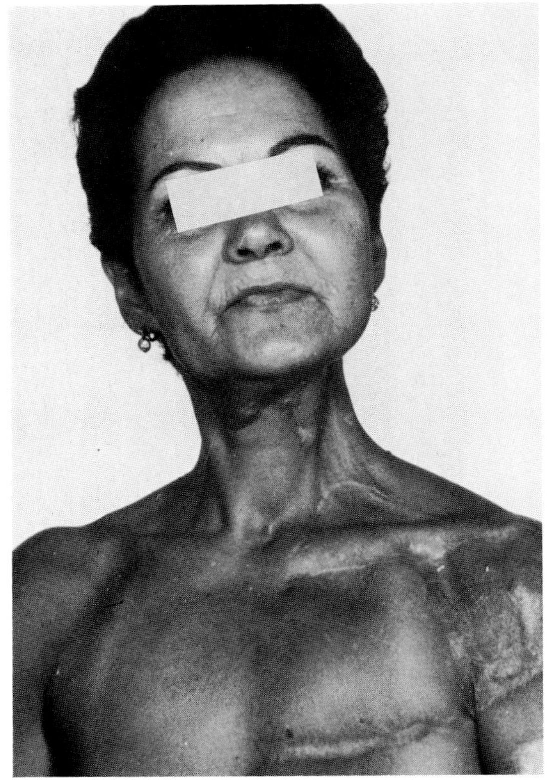

Figure 21–7. Patient after secondary fistula repair and functional rehabilitation following postradiation horizontal laryngectomy with radical neck dissection. Completed 5-year survival disease-free.

when total laryngectomy became necessary for recurrence. A variable degree of bronchitis and bronchopneumonia up to 6 weeks postoperatively was also common in many patients with delayed swallow; one required total laryngectomy for relief.

Another serious problem following the horizontal operation after irradiation was wound breakdown and fistula formation. This occurred in four patients, three who had extended procedures and required secondary repair by regional flap (Fig. 21–8).

Tracheal decannulation was usually possible within 7 days of operation after the vertical procedure and 14 to 21 days after the horizontal operation in patients with no complications. There were no postoperative deaths directly attributable to surgery.

Functional Rehabilitation

Healing is inevitably delayed in fully irradiated tissues to an unpredictable degree. It is believed that removal of three quarters of the ala of the thyroid cartilage in the vertical operation facilitates healing, which is probably not complete for at least 6 weeks. In the horizontal operation partial removal of the upper parts of the thyroid cartilage may also assist healing and is essential for access and closure. Care must be taken in these maneuvers to avoid unnecessary damage to the external and recurrent laryngeal nerves or their main branches.[28]

The assistance of the speech therapist is of great benefit to a patient's morale after operation and to the eventual quality of speech regained. During the immediate healing period, attempted use of the voice should be minimal with an absolute ban on smoking, vocal stress and alcohol.

Following the horizontal supraglottic operation, the greatest problem relates to regaining the natural swallow and the prevention of chest infection by spillover. Much has been written on this subject. The problem is intensified in irradiated patients by the increased local edema and delayed healing as well as by surgical trauma to the external laryngeal nerve. Experience so far would indicate that any extension of the standard supraglottic operation invites disaster in such patients, more especially since repair of the sphincter mechanism cannot be carried out with any assurance in the irradiated larynx. Furthermore, even when swallowing has recovered, with increasing age there is a likely increase in morbidity and even mortality from recurrent spillover due to dyskinesia of the swallow reflexes. Stell[29] reported recurrent chest infection in half of his nonirradiated supraglottic laryngectomy patients. This conclusion is well supported radiologically by Murray,[30] who assessed retrospectively the high incidence of postoperative pulmonary complications in these patients. Another report by Ellis[31] indicates that salvage by total laryngectomy was required for repeated aspiration and lower respiratory complications in two of three patients who had partial supraglottic operations for recurrence after irradiation (Table 21–3).

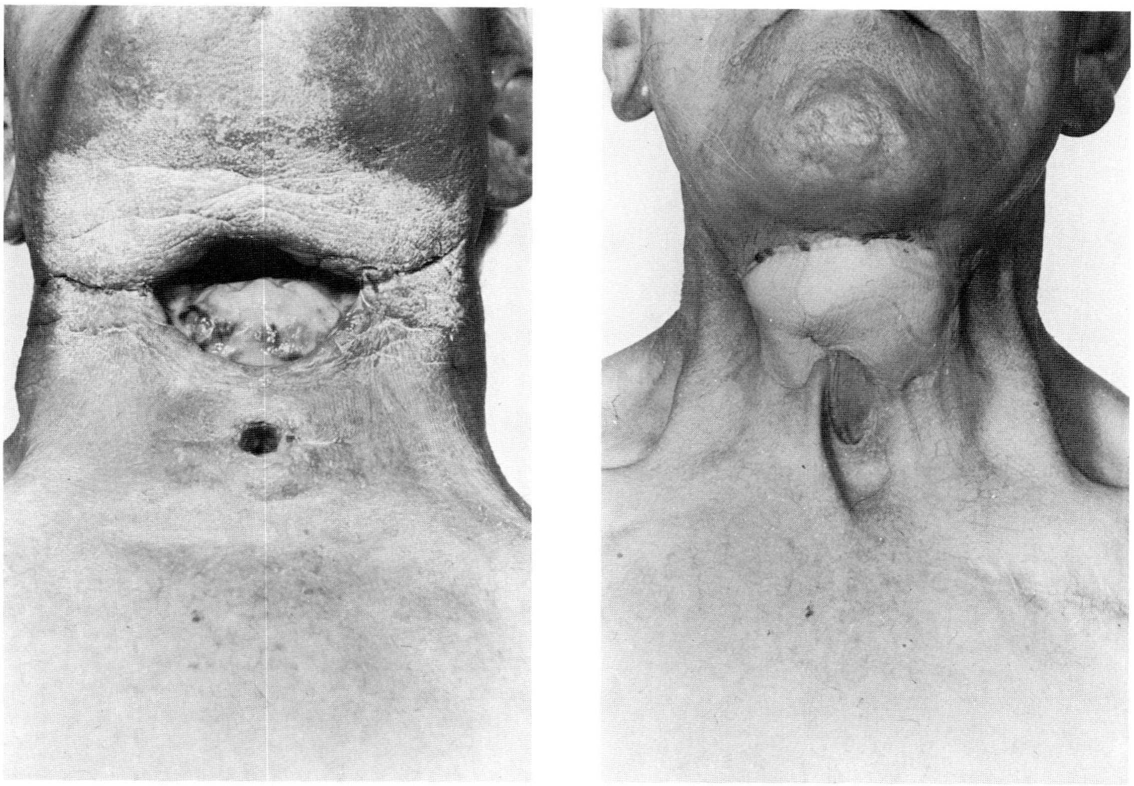

A B

Figure 21–8. Patient before (A) and after (B) repair of large fistula and tissue defect following postradiation horizontal laryngectomy with partial tongue base excision.

The value of cricopharyngeal myotomy seems equivocal. In all, it was carried out in only eight of the total 26 supraglottic operations at The Royal Marsden Hospital. Four of the eight, having had extended operations, were not adequately rehabilitated and two subsequently required gastrostomy. Myotomy, however, is a simple step that may assist swallowing and is easily performed at the time of supraglottic laryngectomy.

After full dosage irradiation, it is believed that there is no place for the more sophisticated reconstructive procedures such as cartilage transposition, muscle transplants, or fat and fascia

Table 21-3. Partial Laryngectomy: End Results After Full Irradiation

TYPE OF OPERATION	NO. PATIENTS	LOCAL RECURRENCE	CERVICAL METASTASIS	NECK DISSECTION	DIED OTHER CAUSES	DIED OF DISEASE	ALIVE AND WELL >3 YEARS
Royal Marsden Hospital 1963-1985							
Vertical	19	3	1	1	2	2	13 (68.4%)
Horizontal	13	2	7	7 (3 bilateral)	2	5	5 (38.4%)
Royal National Throat, Nose, Ear Hospital, 1961-1985							
Vertical	35	6	2	1	6	4	23 (65.7%)
Horizontal	4	1	4	3	1	2	1 (25.0%)
Total							
Vertical	54	9	3	2	8	6	36* (66.6%)
Horizontal	17	3	11	10 (3 bilateral)	3	7	6 (31.7%)

*Does not include seven patients salvaged by total laryngectomy.

grafts.[11] Repairs in this series comprised only the use of local mucosal rotation flaps and simple approximations, except for the use of twin deltopectoral skin flaps to close the large anterior cervical defect in the case of total breakdown previously mentioned, and the use of a single deltopectoral flap in other cases of partial breakdown.

Other Measures

No special attempt is made to spare the finer branches of the ipsilateral internal laryngeal nerve, since it is thought that they must inevitably be divided at some point during the resection. The external and recurrent laryngeal nerves and main branches, however, should be preserved. Radical neck dissection was needed for clinically positive nodes on 12 occasions in patients requiring horizontal partial laryngectomy. Three of these patients underwent bilateral dissections. These were all performed at separate stages in view of the increased risks to healing and swallow had they been done simultaneously. This was emphasized in one patient who developed quite severe dysphagia for a few weeks immediately after neck dissection, although swallow had recovered well after the initial laryngeal resection.

Normal blood cytology and hemoglobin levels were mandatory and all patients were placed on wide spectrum antibiotic cover for at least 3 weeks from the day before operation. Surgical technique was intentionally as atraumatic and meticulous as possible and omitted the routine use of coagulating diathermy. Any septic foci in the teeth or upper air passages were also eliminated before surgery.

Finally, criteria for selection should include good cardiopulmonary function and general health. A chronological upper age limit of about 65 is desirable[10] but approximately 20% of patients in the quoted series were over that age. Blood loss at surgery must be made good without delay by whole blood replacement and strict attention must be given to postoperative drainage, dressings, and intensive care.

End Results

The numbers of patients treated were insufficient to draw any absolute conclusions, but enough to indicate certain trends. There would seem little doubt that for the two hospitals combined, a minimum 3-year survival rate of 66.6% for patients undergoing vertical partial laryngectomy after failed irradiation is significant in spite of some healing delays and other minor complications. This does not include seven patients subsequently salvaged for a minimum of 3 years, after further local recurrence, by total laryngectomy (Table 21–3).

By contrast, a minimum 3-year survival of only six of 17 patients having horizontal operations, producing a survival rate of 31.7%, considered together with the serious complications and the high rate of local and regional recurrence (seven patients also died with metastatic disease), would indicate great caution in proposing these operations after full dosage irradiation (Table 21–3).

CONCLUSIONS

Given the availability of complete therapeutic facilities, the majority of limited glottic cancers with unimpaired cord mobility should initially be treated by full dosage external irradiation. Exceptions are likely to be in young patients, heavy smokers and drinkers, and those with diffuse keratosis or edematous chronic laryngitis for reasons previously given. The smaller number of treatment failures will have a good chance of salvage by vertical partial laryngectomy if recurrence or a new primary lesion can be detected early. These results are consistent with reports by various authors.[32–37]

It is believed that contraindications to the vertical partial operation or its extensions as applied to recurrence after irradiation can be given as follows:

1. Immobility of the affected vocal cord.
2. Arytenoid cartilage or mucosa directly involved by tumor.
3. More than one third of the opposite vocal cord involved by tumor.
4. Definite evidence of transglottic or subglottic spread of disease.
5. Evidence of perichondritis or thyroid cartilage invasion.

In supraglottic cancer the principle of primary irradiation (up to 65 Gy) for the majority of T_1 or T_2 cases followed by partial or total laryngectomy for salvage also seems acceptable. Initial treatment by supraglottic laryngectomy with neck dissection should generally be chosen for cases with clinically positive nodal metastases, perhaps followed by irradiation to the neck as combined therapy.[20]

It must also be said that for experienced surgeons initial treatment by horizontal partial laryngectomy and its extensions, with neck dissection on an elective basis, may give as good results for cure but with greater morbidity than using primary external irradiation.[13,14,17] A degree of flexibility in the choice and sequence of the two main treatment modalities will be rewarded with good results.[38]

There would appear to be no advantage in preoperative planned irradiation to a modified dosage of 20 to 40 Gy with the then possibility of increased postoperative morbidity.[10,14,28,37] It is believed that salvage by horizontal partial laryngectomy for supraglottic cancer recurrent after irradiation will be contraindicated unless:

1. The primary lesion is small and confined to the anterior laryngeal vestibule, free of the anterior commissure from the start of irradiation.
2. The lesion is histologically well differentiated.
3. The patient has good cardiopulmonary function, is under age 65 years, and has good general health.
4. Exceptional circumstances are present, such as refusal of total laryngectomy in a borderline situation or a similar situation in a professional voice user.

It is also desirable that these patients should have been closely followed throughout treatment by the surgeon and radiotherapist. In all other situations and when in doubt, the safest and best treatment for persistent supraglottic cancer after full course teleradiation therapy is total laryngectomy.

ACKNOWLEDGMENT

The author wishes to acknowledge the assistance of Dr. David Golding-Wood of the Royal National Throat, Nose and Ear Hospital and Dr. Paul Gluckman of the Royal Marsden Hospital for their valuable assistance in collection of statistical information required for this chapter.

REFERENCES

1. Buck G. On the surgical treatment of growths within the larynx. Trans Am Med Assoc 1853;6:509.
2. Gussenbauer C. Uber de erste durch T. Billroth am Menschen ausgefuhre Kehlkopf extirpation. Arch Klin Chirurg 1874;17:343–56.
3. Billroth T. (quoted) In: *Cancer of the larynx*. New York: Macmillan, 1930:136–42.
4. Pressman JJ. Submucosal compartmentation of the larynx. Ann Otol Rhinol Laryngol 1956;65:766–71.
5. Kirchner J, Som ML. Clinical and histological observation in supraglottic cancer. Ann Otol Rhinol Laryngol 1971;80:638–45.
6. Bryce DP, van Nostrand AWP, Broderec L. Growth and spread of laryngeal cancer. Adv Otolaryngol 1983;29:9–23.
7. Welsh LW, Welsh JJ, Rizzo TA. Internal anatomy of the larynx and the spread of cancer. Ann Otol Rhinol Laryngol 1989;98:228–34.
8. Alonso JM. Conservative surgery of cancer of the larynx. Trans Am Acad Ophthalmol Otolaryngol 1947;51:633–42.
9. Ogura JH. Supraglottic subtotal laryngectomy and radical neck dissection for carcinoma of the epiglottis. Laryngoscope 1958;68:983–1003.
10. Som ML. Conservative surgery for carcinoma of the supraglottis. J Laryngol Otol 1970;84:655–78.
11. Biller HF. Conservation surgery, past, present and future. Laryngoscope 1987;97:38–41.
12. Leroux-Robert J. Indications for radical surgery, partial surgery and combined surgery and radiotherapy for cancer of the larynx and hypopharynx. Ann Otol Rhinol Laryngol 1956;65:137–53.
13. Bocca E, Pignataro O, Mosciaro O. Supraglottic surgery of the larynx. Ann Otol Rhinol Laryngol 1968;77:1005–76.
14. Guerrier Y, Pinel J, Cachin Y. *La chirurgie conservatrice dans le traitement des cancers du vestibule, larynge et du sinus pyriforme*. Paris: Arnette, 1972.
15. Ogura JH, Jurema A, Watson R. Partial laryngo-pharyngectomy and neck dissection for pyriform sinus cancer. Laryngoscope 1981;91: 1904–12.
16. Pearson BW. Subtotal laryngectomy. Laryngoscope 1981;91:1904–12.
17. DeSanto LW, Pearson BW, Olsen KD. Utility of near total laryngectomy for supraglottic, pharyngeal, base of tongue and other cancer. Ann Otol Rhinol Laryngol 1989;98:2–7.
18. Lederman M. Radiotherapy of cancer of the larynx. J Laryngol Otol 1970;84:867–96.
19. Stewart JG, Brown JR, Palmer MR, Cooper A. The management of glottic cancer by primary irradiation with surgery in reserve. Laryngoscope 1975;85:1477–84.
20. Stell PM, Dalby JF. The treatment of early (T_1) glottic and supraglottic carcinoma. Does partial laryngectomy have a place? Eur J Surg Oncol 1974;3:533–5.
21. Strong MS. Laser management of pre-malignant lesions of the larynx. Can J Otolaryngol 1974;3:560–4.
22. Bauer WC. Concomitant carcinoma in situ and invasive carcinoma of the larynx. Can J Otolaryngol 1978;3:533–5.
23. Kaiser TN, Session DG, Harvey JE. Natural history of treated T_1N_0 squamous carcinoma of the glottis. Ann Otol Rhinol Laryngol 1989;98:217–9.
24. Silver CE. *Surgery for cancer of the larynx*. New York: Churchill Livingstone, 1981.
25. Thames Cancer Registry. Periodic Statistical Reports 1970–1986. Surrey: Sutton, 1988.
26. Robin PE, Powell J, Holme GM. Cancer of the larynx. In: Clinical *Cancer Monographs,* vol 2, New York: Stockton Press, 1989.
27. Cachin Y. Personal communication, 1976.
28. Ward PH. The Second JH Ogura Memorial Lecture: Complications of laryngeal surgery. Laryngoscope 1989;98:54–7.
29. Stell PM. Proc R Soc Med Lond 1977;70:780.
30. Murray GM. Pulmonary complications following supraglottic laryngectomy. Clin Otolaryngol 1976;1:241–7.
31. Ellis PDM. Conservative laryngectomy after radiotherapy. J Laryngol Otol 1982;91:209–15.
32. Norris CM, Peale AR. Partial laryngectomy for irradiation failure. Arch Otolaryngol 1966;84:558–62.
33. Kelly MD, Spaulding CA, Constable WC, et al. Definitive radiotherapy in the management of Stage I and II carcinoma of the glottis. Ann Otol Rhinol Laryngol 1989;98:235–9.
34. Shaw HJ. A view of partial laryngectomy in the treatment of laryngeal cancer. J Laryngol Otol 1987;101:143–54.
35. Biller HF, Blaugrund SM, Som ML. Decreasing limitation of partial laryngectomy for vocal cord cancer. In: Alberti PW, Bryce DP, eds. *Workshops From the Centennial Conference on Laryngeal Cancer*. New York: Appleton Century Crofts, 1976, pp 424–5.
36. Harwood AR. Cancer of the larynx—the Toronto experience. J Otolaryngol Suppl 1982;II:10–13.
37. Croll GA, Vandenbroek P, Tiwari RM, et al. Vertical partial laryngectomy for recurrent glottic carcinoma after irradiation. Head Neck Surg 1985;7:390–3.
38. Ogura JH, Biller HF. Pre-operative irradiation for laryngeal and laryngo-pharyngeal cancers. Laryngoscope 1970;80:802–10.

22

Total Laryngectomy

Philip M. Stell

The first total laryngectomy was carried out on 30th December 1873, by Billroth.[1] It is often stated[2] that a laryngectomy had been performed by Watson of Edinburgh for syphilis in 1866, but Watson's paper* shows that this is untrue.[3] Watson described the larynx and trachea obtained at postmortem of a patient who had syphilis: the only operation carried out during life was a tracheotomy.

Sporadic cases were reported for the next 30 years,[4] but the operation did not gain general acceptance until the pioneering work of Gluck in the early years of the present century.[5] Gluck's contributions were to separate the trachea from the larynx (either at a preliminary operation or early in the definitive operation) to form an end stoma and to close the pharynx primarily, thus protecting the patient from aspiration pneumonia.

About 1920, radiotherapy began to produce beneficial results[6] and for the next 30 years was the treatment of choice. Not until the 1950s did surgery again become a reputable form of treatment for advanced or recurrent carcinoma.[7]

INDICATIONS

Total laryngectomy may be indicated in the following circumstances:

1. For squamous carcinoma. Total laryngectomy may be required in the treatment of squamous carcinoma of the larynx or of the hypopharynx in the following circumstances:
   (1) as primary treatment,
   (2) for failed radiotherapy,
   (3) as a completion laryngectomy for failed conservative laryngectomy, either vertical or horizontal,[8]
   (4) as an emergency procedure if the patient's airway is obstructed by tumor, and
   (5) for chondroradionecrosis, often, incorrectly, called perichondritis.
2. For rare tumors (see Chapter 6 for discussion of unusual tumors of the larynx). In addition to squamous carcinoma, primary total laryngectomy is probably the treatment of choice for the following rare tumors: adenocarcinoma,[9] verrucous carcinoma (indeed, in this tumor, radiotherapy is absolutely contraindicated, since anaplastic transformation may occur),[10] the tumors of salivary type (adenoid-cystic and mucoepidermoid carcinoma,[11]) fibrosarcoma,[12] melanoma,[13] chondroma and chondrosarcoma,[14] and paraganglioma.[15]

Squamous Carcinoma of the Larynx

Total laryngectomy may be needed as a primary form of treatment for extensive multiregional carcinoma of the larynx, for salvage after failed radiotherapy, or for local recurrence that may follow about 10% of partial laryngectomies.[16] About half of the latter patients are saved by "completion laryngectomy," a term coined by Ogura and Bello.[7] Approximately 10% of their laryngectomies were carried out for the removal of the remaining part of the larynx following a preceding partial laryngectomy. In 60% of the cases the preceding operation was a vertical hemilaryngectomy, in 20% a supraglottic hemilaryngectomy, and in 20% a partial laryngopharyngectomy. In 10% of the patients the operation was required for the treatment of a fistula: nearly all patients in this group had undergone previous partial laryngopharyngectomy for a carcinoma of the pyriform fossa. The operation was carried out most commonly between the 6th and 12th months after the previous operation.

*The report to the Medico-Chirurgical Society of Edinburgh, published in the *Edinburgh Medical Journal*[3] was as follows: "III. Ulceration of Larynx, Tracheotomy, Haemoptysis. Dr. Watson showed the larynx and trachea of a patient on whom he had performed tracheotomy on account of ulceration of the glottis, with destruction of the left aretaenoid cartilage and part of the epiglottis. The disease was due to syphilis. No ulceration had been going on for some time, but with every change of weather, especially from dry to moist, symptoms of oedema glottidis set in. It was on this account tracheotomy was practised. There was no bleeding to speak of during the operation; but after the patient had been in bed for about half an hour, violent haemopytsis set in, which, although not directly fatal, induced such extreme feebleness that the patient sunk in the course of a few days. After death, although the wound, larynx, trachea, bronchi, and lungs were carefully examined, the source of the bleeding could not be detected."

Squamous Carcinoma of the Pyriform Fossa

The treatment of squamous carcinoma of the pyriform fossa is almost exclusively by surgery. The results of radiotherapy for this disease are poor, with 5-year survival rate below 5% when there are palpable lymph nodes in the neck, which indeed are present in at least 75% of cases.[17] For lesions of the pyriform fossa, a total laryngectomy is always essential, but partial pharyngectomy suffices for two thirds of patients[18]; the remaining third require total pharyngolaryngectomy.

Emergency Laryngectomy

A proportion of patients with laryngeal carcinoma present with stridor, particularly if the carcinoma is large and multiregional, or if it affects the subglottic space. The customary procedure is to carry out an emergency tracheostomy and then treat the tumor at leisure. This policy however, leads to a high incidence of recurrence in the tracheostoma.[19] In order to prevent this outcome some have suggested "emergency" laryngectomy.[20] Surprisingly, most patients accept this operation, since they realize that their larynx is not only useless, but a positive danger. The postoperative course is usually smooth. Whether this form of treatment does indeed reduce the incidence of stomal recurrence remains to be proven. In a personal series of 20 patients, the stomal rate was 5%, but the mortality rate from the operation was 15%.

Chondroradionecrosis

This complication is without doubt the worse disaster that can befall a patient undergoing radiotherapy for a laryngeal carcinoma. Although the incidence appears to be falling with improving techniques, approximately 5% of patients undergoing radiotherapy for a laryngeal carcinoma will have this complication. A more usual term for this disease is "perichondritis," but since it is the cartilage itself that undergoes necrosis, the term "chondroradionecrosis' is preferable. The epiglottic cartilage is the most frequently affected. Almost all these patients present within the first 6 months of radiotherapy.[21] Pathologic studies have shown that, in addition to cartilage necrosis, 70% of patients have recurrent tumor within the larynx. The important predipósing factors include peripheral vascular disease, chronic laryngitis, and large irradiation fields.[22]

The disease appears to have two phases: in the first there is pronounced edema of the laryngeal soft tissues, particularly over the arytenoids. This edema gradually becomes more pronounced, but may regress, particularly if the larynx is "rested" with a tracheostomy. Progression to chondronecrosis may follow, at which point the breath becomes foul, the mucosa begins to ulcerate, pieces of sequestrated cartilage may be expectorated, and the patient may have aspiration pneumonia.

A further potent cause of chondronecrosis is surgery to an irradiated larynx, particularly horizontal, partial, supraglottic laryngectomy, which is almost guaranteed to precipitate this event.

Treatment is dicated by the type of disease. If the larynx is merely edematous and there is no fetor or ulceration of the mucosa, the disease will probably resolve with steroids, possibly antibiotics (although it is doubtful if the antibiotics reach the intended site, since the basic problem is lack of blood supply), and putting the larynx at rest by a tracheostomy. If there is no clinical evidence of ulceration of the mucosa at this point, biopsy is absolutely contraindicated, particularly the so-called deep biopsy through the ventricle, which is sometimes advocated. Such a procedure seldom provides a histologic diagnosis, and there is a high risk of precipitating necrosis of cartilage.

If the disease progresses to the second stage with fetor and ulceration, the patient may die of aspiration pneumonia, sepsis, and cachexia. Furthermore, there is also a very high chance that tumor is recurrent within the larynx, although this may be difficult to prove by biopsy. A total laryngectomy should therefore be undertaken and the following precautions observed:[22]

1. The operation should be carried out through a vertical midline incision.
2. At the end of the operation, the carotid sheath must be protected by a sternomastoid or levator scapulae muscle graft.
3. The pharyngeal suture line should be closed in the usual way.
4. Since it is dangerous to close such a highly infected wound, it should be packed open, with an acriflavine pack changed every few days. When clean, the wound is closed by secondary suture. If a vertical incision has been used, the wound edges are easy to approximate at this time, whereas the edges of a horizontal wound tend to separate and cannot be brought together again.

NECK DISSECTION

If a patient to undergo total laryngectomy has a palpable lymph gland in the neck, all are now agreed that the correct policy is to carry out a radical neck dissection en-bloc at the same time. The main area of controversy is the place of prophylactic neck dissection, carried out when no nodes are palpable in the hope that nodes containing microscopic deposits ("occult nodes") will be removed early and that the patient's prognosis will thus be improved. Occult nodes occur in approximately 15% of patients undergoing surgery for laryngeal cancer.[23]

On the basis of the incidence of local recurrence in the neck in patients with negative nodes, occult nodes and palpable nodes, Ogura et al[23] have shown that the maximal increase in survival rate that can be achieved by prophylactic neck dissection is 4%. Whether this is true benefit can almost certainly never be decided by a clinical trial because the numbers required would be enormous (more than 7000) and because such a small difference is easily swamped by differences in surgical practice, nursing care, etc.

If the patient has bilateral neck nodes, bilateral neck dissection in either one[24] or two stages has been advocated but the results are disappointing: only about half the patients heal primarily, and the 5-year survival rate is of the order of 5%.[25]

Contralateral metastases may also occur in as many as 30% of patients with supraglottic tumors.[26] Late contralateral metastases can also occur, again being most frequent with supraglottic tumors. The prognosis in this case is quite good.

TECHNIQUE

Anesthesia

It is now generally accepted that total laryngectomy should be carried out under general endotracheal anesthesia. Previously, some authors believed that the operation should be carried out under local anesthesia[27] because of fear of implantation of malignant cells, but this has been shown not to be the case.[28]

Incision (Requirements)

1. Provide good exposure of the larynx and the contents of the neck if a radical neck dissection is to be carried out.
2. Allow a stable stoma to be created separate from the incision.
3. Allow reconstructive procedures to be carried out.
4. Avoid tension and subsequent necrosis of flaps.
5. Be capable of covering vital structures such as the carotid sheath.
6. Respect the vascular anatomy of the skin.
7. Have a good cosmetic result.

For a patient undergoing laryngectomy alone, these criteria are best achieved by a skin-crease incision, midway between the hyoid bone and the upper end of the sternum.

If the patient requires a radical neck dissection, this incision is easily extended as the "half H" incision[29] in which the vertical limb runs down the anterior border of the trapezius muscle (Fig. 22–1). The upper and lower flaps are thus nourished by the upper and lower vascular pedicles derived from the external carotid and subclavian arteries, respectively, and the horizontal limb lies in the watershed between these two territories.[30]

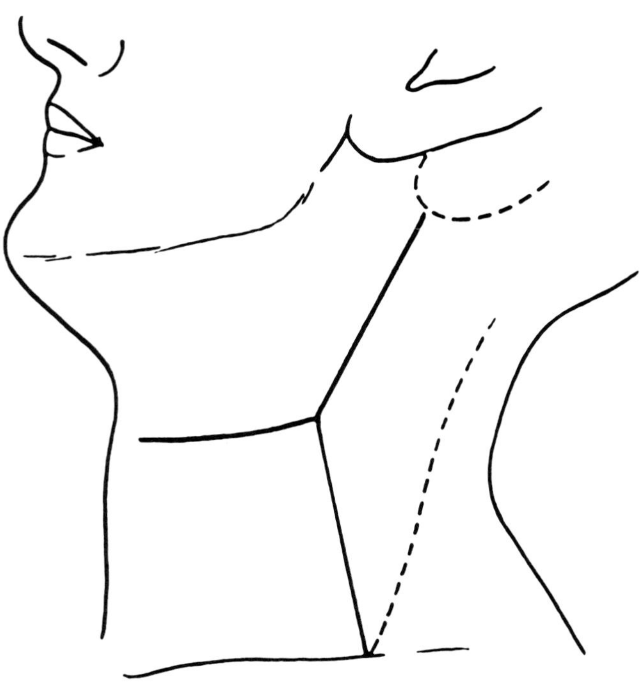

Figure 22–1. "Half H" neck incision. (From Stell and Maran.[59] Reprinted with permission.)

Excision

Since the operation is usually being carried out for a large multiregional tumor, all those structures that may be invaded by such a tumor must be resected. These include:[31]

- Preepiglottic space
- Strap muscles
- Lobe of the thyroid gland on the same side
- Mucosa overlying the cricoarytenoid joint
- Paratracheal lymph nodes

Mobilization of the Larynx

The skin flaps, including the platysma, are raised and stitched out of the way. If a radical neck dissection has been carried out, it is left attached to the larynx with as wide a pedicle as possible.

The medial border of the sternomastoid muscle is identified and mobilization of the larynx begun by dissection in the plane medial to the muscle (Fig. 22–2); the carotid sheath is retracted laterally. Dissection is carried down to the clavicle and up to the hyoid bone. The branches of the anterior jugular veins are tied, and the superior and inferior thyroid artery and vein and the middle thyroid vein are identified and transfixed on the side on which the thyroid lobe is to be removed. Dissection is continued through the fat lateral to the trachea until the tracheal wall is exposed. The paratracheal chain of nodes is dissected at this point, using blunt dissection with a finger in the superior

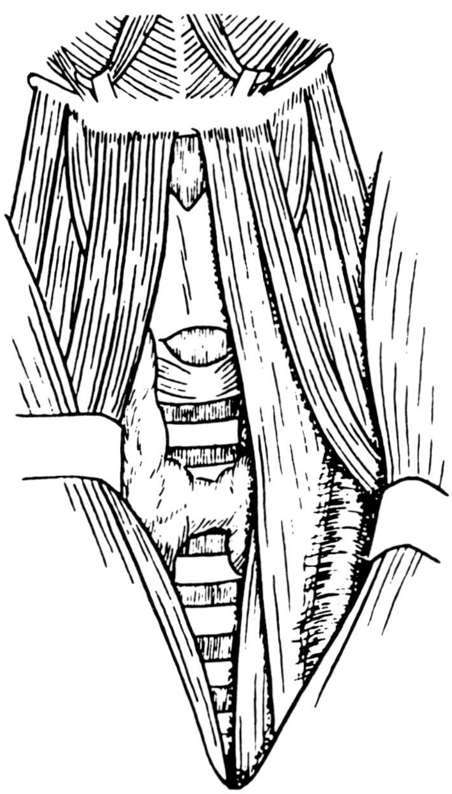

Figure 22–2. Beginning of dissection medial to carotid sheath. (From Stell and Maran.[59] Reprinted with permission.)

mediastinum. The recurrent laryngeal nerve lying in the tracheoesophageal groove is divided.

Next, the strap muscles are divided immediately above the sternum (Fig 22–3), and the muscles attached to the superior edge of the hyoid bone also are divided immediately above their attachment. The inferior thyroid veins are ligated and divided.

The larynx is now freed on the opposite side; the carotid sheath is first identified and retracted laterally. The lobe of the thyroid gland is preserved on this side so that the inferior thyroid artery is not divided. The larynx is now mobile up to the level of the hyoid bone (Fig. 22–4).

Division of the Trachea

The trachea can be divided at any stage in the operation from now onward, but the easiest method is to divide it now (Fig. 22–5). After estimating the position of the final tracheostomy in the skin flap, a hole is made at this site about an inch in diameter.

It is often said that the cut through the trachea should be beveled from below upward so that the end of the trachea will be vertical when it is swung forward. However, this technique cuts through cartilage that often then becomes necrotic and is expelled, leading to stomal stenosis. It is much better to divide cleanly through one of the spaces between the tracheal rings. Before proceeding further, a small swab is placed in the laryngeal remnant to prevent contaminated secretions running down into the wound. A cuffed tube is now placed in the trachea and anesthesia is continued through this. The tracheal stoma is now created in two layers.

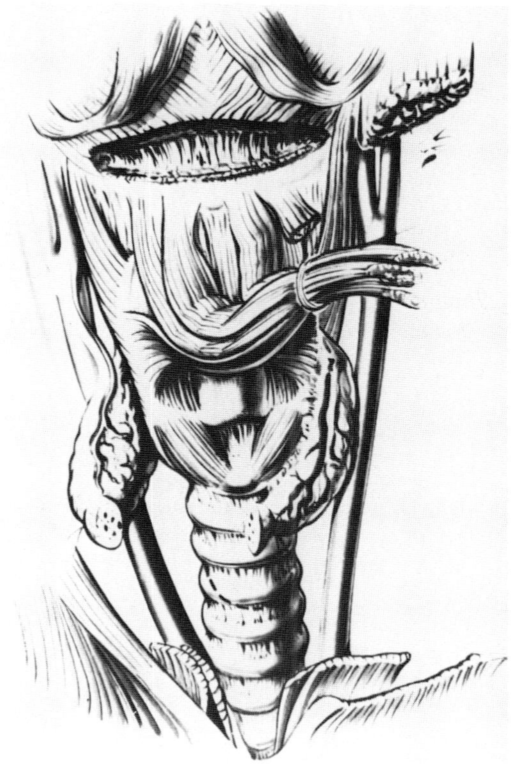

Figure 22–4. Completed mobilization of the larynx, prior to division of trachea. (From Silver.[60] Reprinted with permission.)

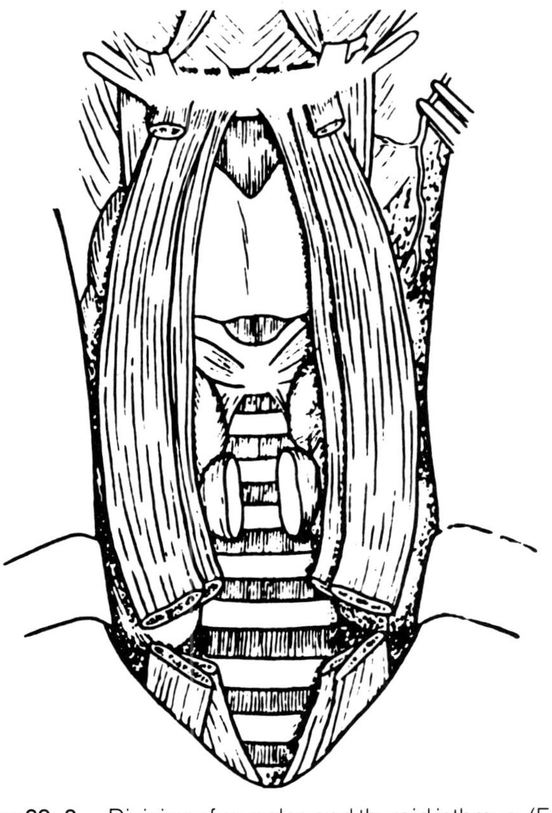

Figure 22–3. Division of muscles and thyroid isthmus. (From Stell and Maran.[59] Reprinted with permission.)

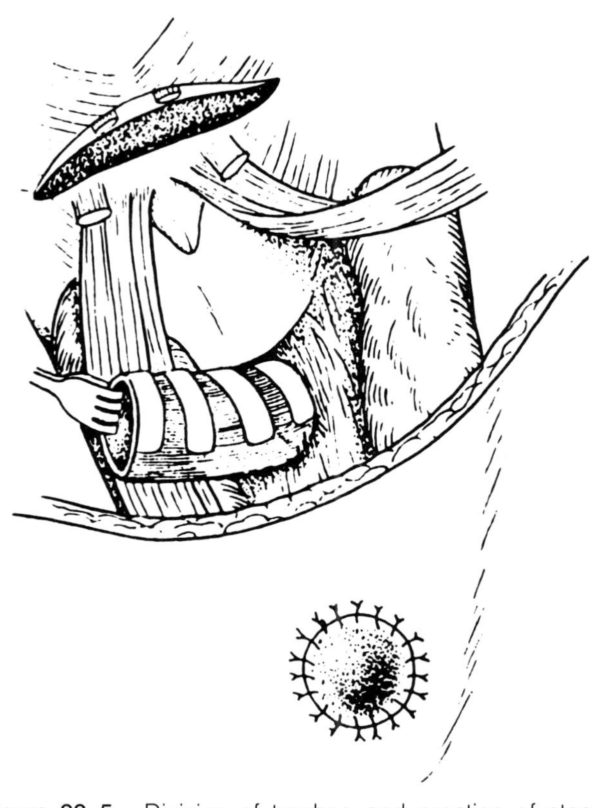

Figure 22–5. Division of trachea and creation of stoma. (From Stell and Maran.[59] Reprinted with permission.)

Removal of the Larynx

The larynx can be removed from below upward or above downward, but the latter is safer because the inside of the larynx can be seen, and there is no danger of cutting into tumor.

The body of the hyoid bone is grasped with a large forceps and pulled forward. The base of the tongue is divided and the pharynx opened, taking care not to open into the preepiglottic space. As soon as the pharynx is opened, the first assistant retracts the base of the tongue with a retractor placed through the opening into the larynx. Then the tip of the epiglottis is grasped with forceps and pulled anteriorly and inferiorly. The pharyngeal mucosa is cut with scissors on each side of the epiglottis aiming toward the superior cornu of the thyroid cartilage. The surgeon should now be standing at the head of the table, so that he can see into the larynx. The larynx is released by dividing the constrictor muscles along the posterior edge of the thyroid cartilage. The pharyngeal mucosa is divided on each side in the region of the superior cornu of the thyroid cartilage, aiming downward toward the posterior part of the arytenoid cartilage (Fig. 22–6).

These two cuts are joined posteriorly, below the cricoarytenoid joint, where there is a good plane of cleavage on the posterior cricoarytenoid joint. This is developed downward between the trachea and the esophagus. The larynx can now be removed.

If the operation is being carried out for a subglottic carcinoma, several rings of the trachea and the paratracheal chain of nodes must be removed. In addition, manubrial resection has also been advised.[32]

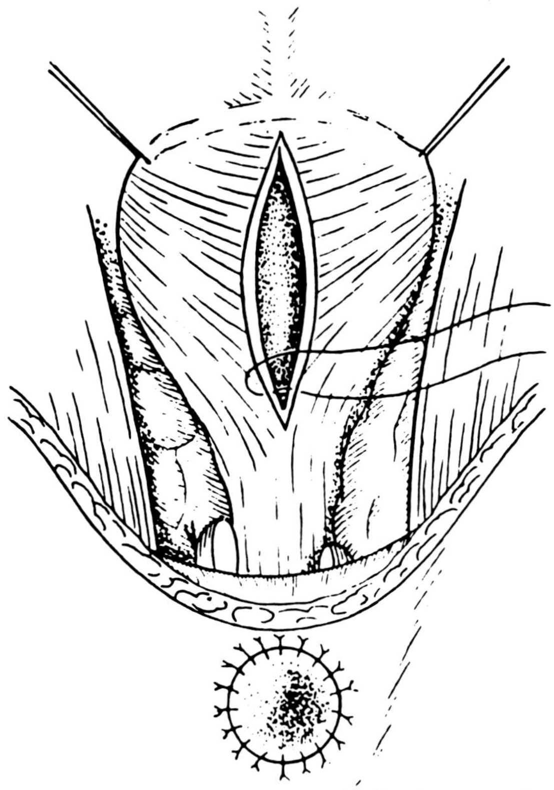

Figure 22–7. Pharyngeal repair. (From Stell and Maran.[59] Reprinted with permission.)

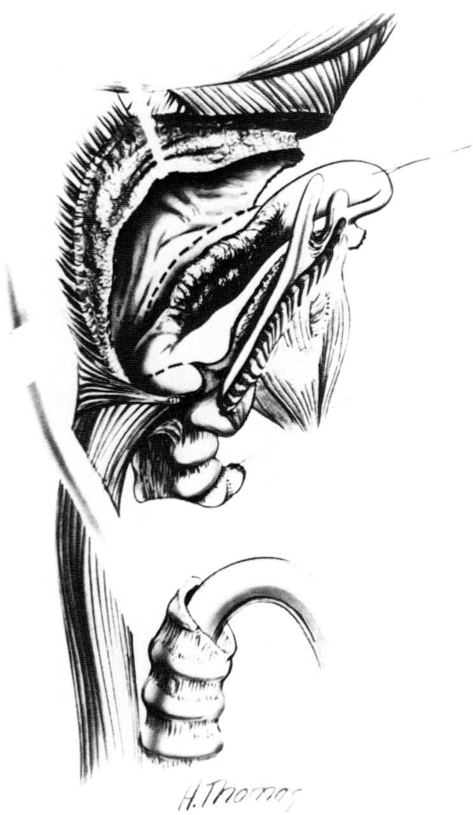

Figure 22–6. Final stage of excision. (From Silver.[60] Reprinted with permission.)

Repair of the Pharynx and Closure

The pharynx should be closed in three layers: mucosal, fascial, and muscular (Fig. 22–7*). A running Connell-type suture is often advised for the first mucosal layer. It is usual to invert the mucosal edge, but it has been shown experimentally that an everting closure is just as secure and preserves more mucosa, which is important if the procedure has been combined with partial pharyngectomy for a carcinoma of the pyriform fossa.[33]

Before closing the skin, if the patient has been irradiated, the carotid sheath is protected with a muscle flap of the levator scapulae[34] if a neck dissection has been performed, or the sternomastoid muscle if not. The skin is closed in two layers with suction drains.

AFTERCARE

Both the aftercare and complications of total laryngectomy may be considered under the following headings: (1) immediate

*Editor's note: The linear vertical closure depicted here is favored by many British surgeons. In the United States, a transverse or T-shaped closure is often employed.

(within 24 hours), (2) intermediate (before the patient leaves the hospital); and (3) long-term (after the patient leaves the hospital).

Immediate Care

This includes the general care of the patient undergoing a major operation, general care of a tracheostomy, and the specific care of a patient undergoing laryngectomy.

General care usually indicates monitoring of the various body systems, and may include some or all of the following:[35]

- Cardiovascular system: Pulse rate, electrocardiogram, arterial blood pressure, central venous pressure, cardiac output (or index), and total peripheral resistance
- Respiratory system: Respiration rate, respiratory volume, respiratory flow rate, respiratory pressure, respiratory compliance, respiratory gases (partial oxygen and carbon dioxide pressures), blood gases (pH, partial arterial oxygen and carbon dioxide pressures), and chest radiography
- Central nervous system: electroencephalogram and ventricular pressure
- Gastrointestinal system: fluid intake by mouth and nasogastric or intestinal tube drainage and electrolyte analysis of recovered fluid
- Hematopoietic system: complete blood count, hematocrit, coagulation studies, platelet count, and blood volume (red cell, plasma, total)
- Urinary system: urine output (hourly), urinalysis (routine and microscopic), blood urea nitrogen, serum creatinine, creatinine clearance, urine/plasma osmolarity ratio, and urinary electrolytes (sodium to potassium ratio)
- Metabolism: temperature, body weight, and intravenous fluid volume (electrolyte colloid, blood)
- Tracheostomy care

Intermediate Care

ANTIBIOTIC CHEMOPROPHYLAXIS

The incidence of infection after major head and neck surgery may be as high as 70% [36] Infection depends on many factors, including the dose and virulence of the organisms, hematoma, foreign materials, host resistance, and improper surgical technique.

The consequences of wound infection after major head and neck surgery include fistula, tissue necrosis, wound breakdown, and carotid artery "blowout." The risk of wound sepsis is much greater if the pharyngeal mucosa is breached, exposing the operative field to the oropharyngeal microbial flora. These may include several potential pathogens that may be enhanced by the tumor, poor dentition, or previous antibiotics.

Infected wounds usually harbor multiple bacterial species and genera, the main groups being intestinal aerobic gram-negative bacilli (IAGB), staphylococci, streptococci, and oral anaerobes. Preoperative cultures of the oral cavity do not correlate well with subsequent wound pathogens and, in particular IAGB are rarely present before the operation. However, they are often present in infected wounds: they have been shown to originate in the stomach and to ascend to the pharynx via the nasogastric feeding tube.[37] Thus, they are not present when the wound is open and at greatest risk of pathogenic contamination. This concept is important when considering the choice of antibiotics. The spectrum of cover need not be effective against IAGB, and prolonged use of unnecessarily broad-spectrum agents induces and encourages the selective growth of opportunistic pathogens. Erythromycin given over the perioperative period is effective. If a nasogastric tube has been inserted several days before major surgery, IAGB are likely to be present and a broad-spectrum antibiotic, such as Augmentin, is recommended. A prospective randomized trial has shown that intraoperative prophylactic antibiotics reduce the infection rate from 75 to 25%[38] in patients undergoing major head and neck surgery. The use of metronidazole has also been recommended to reduce infection by anaerobes.

Long-Term Care

STOMA BUTTON

At the end of the operation, the patient is usually left with either one of the silver laryngectomy tubes or one of the plastic varieties. The latter have the advantage of having a cuff that can be inflated to provide an airtight seal so that the patient can be ventilated if necessary. The suture line around the stoma can be protected by a dressing. In the longer term it may be necessary to provide some sort of permanent cannula to prevent stenosis of the stoma, and for this the stoma button described by Adams[39] can be used. If the patient expectorates a lot of mucus, Buchanan's protector can be worn to absorb this.

COMPLICATIONS

Immediate Complications

These include bleeding, airway obstruction, and pneumothorax and require no further description here.

Intermediate Complications

These may be general or local. The general complications are those of any major operation, mainly those affecting the chest. For reasons that are not entirely explained, the incidence of pulmonary embolism after major head and neck surgery is very low.

The major local complications include wound breakdown, pharyngeal fistula, and rupture of the carotid artery. Wound breakdown may be due to an ill-advised incision, particularly in a patient who has been irradiated, to a preoperative tracheostomy, and to sloppy surgical technique. Probably the most potent source of infection is the inevitable contamination of the wound by oral and pharyngeal organisms when the pharynx is opened.[40] Rupture of the carotid artery occurs in about 10% of patients undergoing laryngectomy.[41] Factors predisposing to rupture are fistula, wound breakdown, prior irradiation, and persistent tumor at the margins of resection: as many as 20% of the latter patients have carotid rupture.[41,42] Preventive measures include a correct incision, careful closure of the pharynx, and protection of the carotid sheath by the sternomastoid muscle (if it is still present), or the levator scapulae muscle.[34] The use of dermal graft[43] has now been largely abandoned.

Fistula

Probably the most common complication after total laryngectomy, and that which prolongs the patient's stay in hospital more than any other, is pharyngocutaneous fistula, due to dehiscence of the pharyngeal suture line or to actual necrosis of tissue. It is widely held that the most frequent cause of the latter is previous radiotherapy,[44] but, surprisingly, a careful review of a large series of cases by Lavelle and Maw[45] showed no difference in the incidence between patients who had and those who had not been irradiated previously. These authors showed that in patients who had been irradiated previously, fistulas were more common under certain circumstances: when the laryngectomy needed to be carried out between the 3rd and 6th month after radiotherapy; if the patient had a preoperative tracheostomy; if the postoperative hemoglobin was not maintained above 12.5 g/dl; and if a radical neck dissection was carried out, but only if this was combined with previous radiotherapy. Residual tumor is also a cause of fistula. Preoperative hemoglobin, the incision used, the material used for repair of the pharynx, the stage and site of the tumor, and the type of drainage employed did not appear to affect the incidence of fistulas. Furthermore, the occurrence of a fistula had no effect on the ultimate survival rate. The overall incidence of fistula in the series previously mentioned was 36.7%.

Fistulas may be treated conservatively or with surgery. Fistulas occurring in patients who have not been irradiated will generally heal spontaneously.[46] Most fistulas in irradiated patients will also heal spontaneously. A period of 40 days must be allowed for any necrotic tissue to demarcate and for local infection to be controlled. Surgery to close the fistula should therefore not be embarked on in the first 6 weeks after operation.

A fistula must be closed by two epithelial surfaces: one to line the pharynx and one to provide skin cover. Depending on the availability of local tissue, fistulas may be classified, according to the method required for repair, as follows:[47]

I. Both surfaces may be developed locally.
II. One surface may be developed locally and one from a distance.
III. Both surfaces must be provided by distant flaps.

CLOSURE OF TYPE I FISTULA

In this type, the inner layer is provided by two ellipses of skin turned inward. A crescentic flap is marked out on each side of the fistula, each being the same width, at its widest point, as the fistula (Fig. 22–8A,B). The ends of each ellipse are close to the margin of the fistula to avoid bunching of excess tissue.

The flaps are elevated and suturing begins at one end (Fig. 22–8C); the inner layer of sutures should be of the Connell inverting type. It is preferable to begin suturing from each end of the defect and to tie the knot in the middle to ensure that the skin at each end of the defect is inverted into the lumen. After suturing the flaps, the resultant pressure of the excess tissue forces the edges of the flaps down into the lumen, producing good apposition of their edges. A second, and preferably a third, layer of subcutaneous sutures is inserted to strengthen the closure.

The resulting raw surface must be covered with skin. A local flap, nearly always a rotation flap, fashioned in accordance with the basic principles of reconstructive surgery, may be used as follows. An isosceles triangle is drawn around the defect with pen and ink (Fig. 22–8D), the sides of the triangle on either side of the fistula being equal. To ensure viability of the flap, the angles at the base of the triangle must be more than 70°. The radius of the rotation flap is the same length as the side of the triangle, and the entire flap forms a semicircle with the triangle subtracted. The flap is raised, rotated into the defect, and sutured in place (Fig. 22–8E). If the donor site cannot be closed primarily, it may be resurfaced with a split-thickness skin graft.

CLOSURE OF TYPE II FISTULA

In this case there is enough local tissue to provide an inner lining but not enough for an outer lining. Since there is no actual mucosal loss, the inner layer can be resutured by turning in local flaps, as in a closure of a type I fistula, but the large skin defect must be resurfaced by tissue brought in from a distance because of lack of sufficient local tissue. At the present time, either freely transplanted or myocutaneous flaps are the preferred sources of this tissue. A free forearm flap has the advantage of providing a thin, pliant cover consisting only of skin; its disadvantage is the microsurgical expertise required. A pectoralis major myocutaneous flap, rotated 90° into the defect, has the advantage of speed, reliability, and simplicity. Its disadvantage is the superfluous muscle bulk that is carried with the skin paddle. A free omental flap (Fig. 22–9) provides a third option that may be particularly useful for the patient with heavy irradiation damage, particularly after "fast neutron" therapy. With this technique a piece of omentum of sufficient size is harvested with gastroepiploic artery and vein included. The omentum is transferred to the neck where its artery and vein are anastomosed by microsurgical techniques to vessels well away from the irradiated area; the acromiothoracic axis is usually an excellent choice. The revascularized omentum is then led through a subcutaneous tunnel to appear in the neck. The skin around the fistula is undermined widely and the omentum laid over the closed fistula and beneath the undermined skin edges. It is secured by nonabsorbable sutures, led through the overlying skin, and tied over buttons or rubber tubing. The external raw surface may be covered with a split-thickness skin graft a few days later or left to granulate if the fistula is small.

CLOSURE OF TYPE III FISTULA

In this case two surfaces must be supplied from a distance: much the best technique is the pectoralis major flap (Fig. 22–10). The flap is designed to include a skin island large enough to provide complete cover for the fistula once the flap has retracted by 10 to 15% in all dimensions. It is developed so that about 2 cm of muscle will protrude beyond the edge of the skin island in all directions. The pectoralis major flap is led through a cervical tunnel to emerge in the neck with its skin surface inward. The edges of the flap are then sutured to the inside edges of the fistula

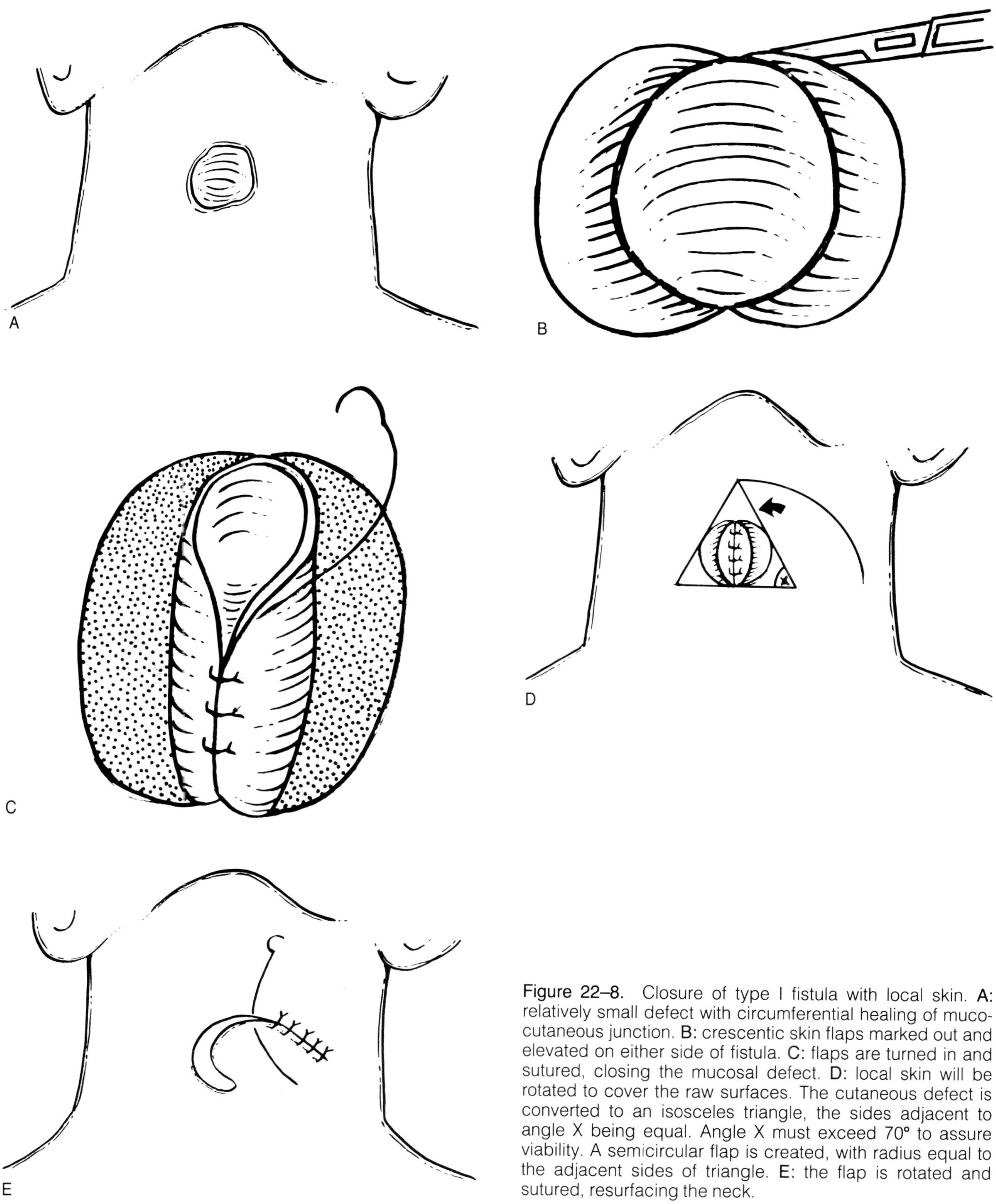

Figure 22–8. Closure of type I fistula with local skin. A: relatively small defect with circumferential healing of mucocutaneous junction. B: crescentic skin flaps marked out and elevated on either side of fistula. C: flaps are turned in and sutured, closing the mucosal defect. D: local skin will be rotated to cover the raw surfaces. The cutaneous defect is converted to an isosceles triangle, the sides adjacent to angle X being equal. Angle X must exceed 70° to assure viability. A semicircular flap is created, with radius equal to the adjacent sides of triangle. E: the flap is rotated and sutured, resurfacing the neck.

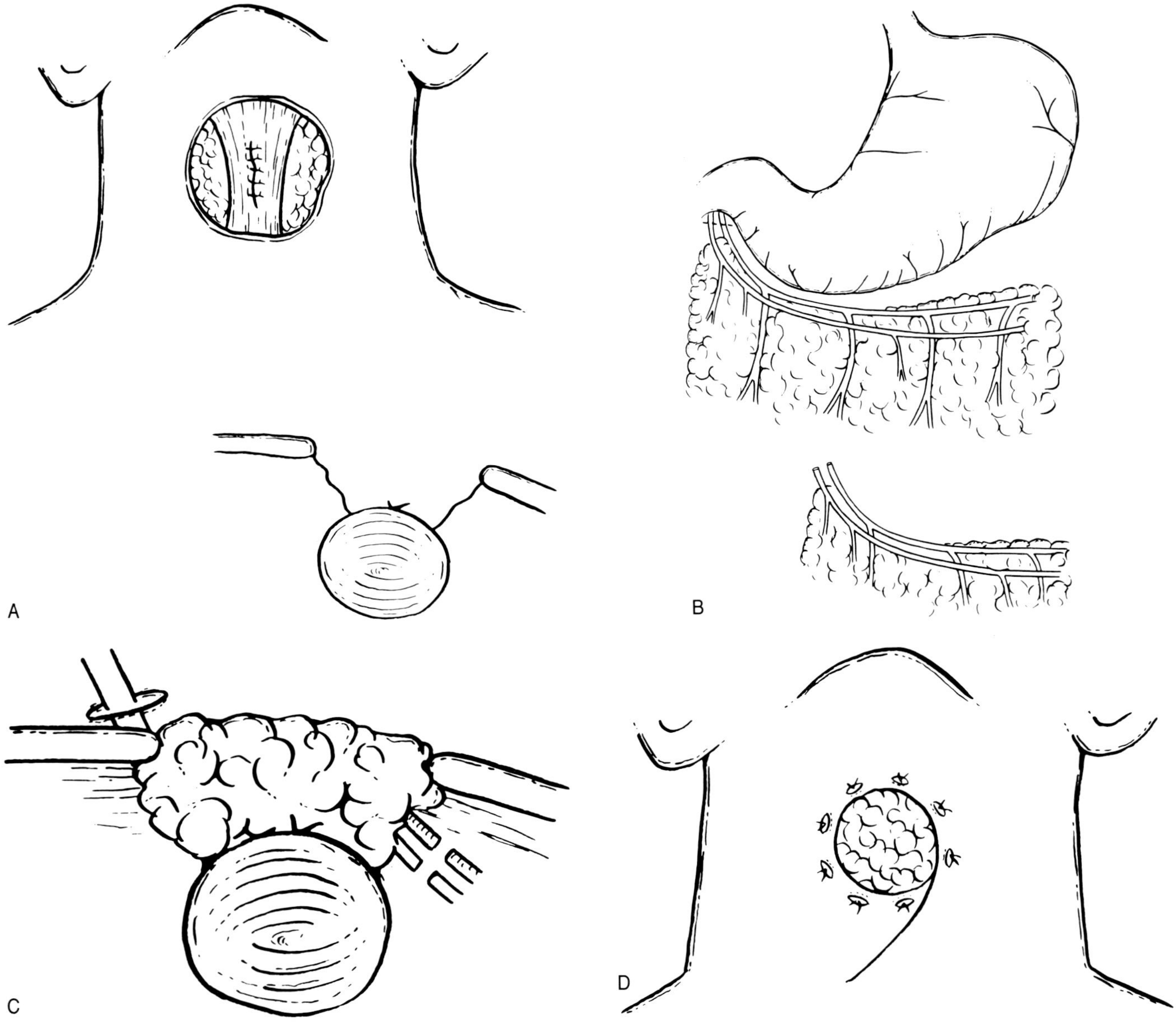

Figure 22–9. Closure of type II fistula with transplanted omentum. A: the mucosal defect is closed with local tissue, but the defect in skin and subcutaneous tissues is too large for closure. B: a portion of omentum is harvested, pedicled on the omental vessels. C: the omentum is transferred to the cervical defect, and revascularized by anastomosis of omental to local vessels, well away from the irradiated area. D: omentum is laid over the closed fistula and led under the undermined skin edges, where it is fixed by nonabsorbable sutures tied over buttons or rubber tubing. The external raw surface is grafted with split skin.

in two layers to create a watertight closure. To reinforce the closure, the redundant muscle surrounding the skin island is tucked beneath the undermined cervical skin surrounding the fistula and secured with nonabsorbable sutures tied over buttons or a catheter. In this way the flap is anchored and its weight is supported during the healing phase.

The outer surface of the flap may now be covered with another flap, but a very satisfactory result can be achieved by covering this area with split skin, preferably using the primary delayed technique.

An effective alternative is to rotate the pectoralis major muscle through 90° so that the skin surface is outward. A cavity 3 cm deep is developed all around the fistula and the muscle is then inset beneath the undermined cervical skin and fixed as before by nonabsorbable sutures anchored externally. The skin of the flap is stitched to the skin edge of the defect. The inner muscular layer lies over the fistula, but no attempt is made at formal closure. Surprisingly, the results are usually very good, leakage tends to be minor and temporary. The pharyngeal mucosa reepithelializes spontaneously.

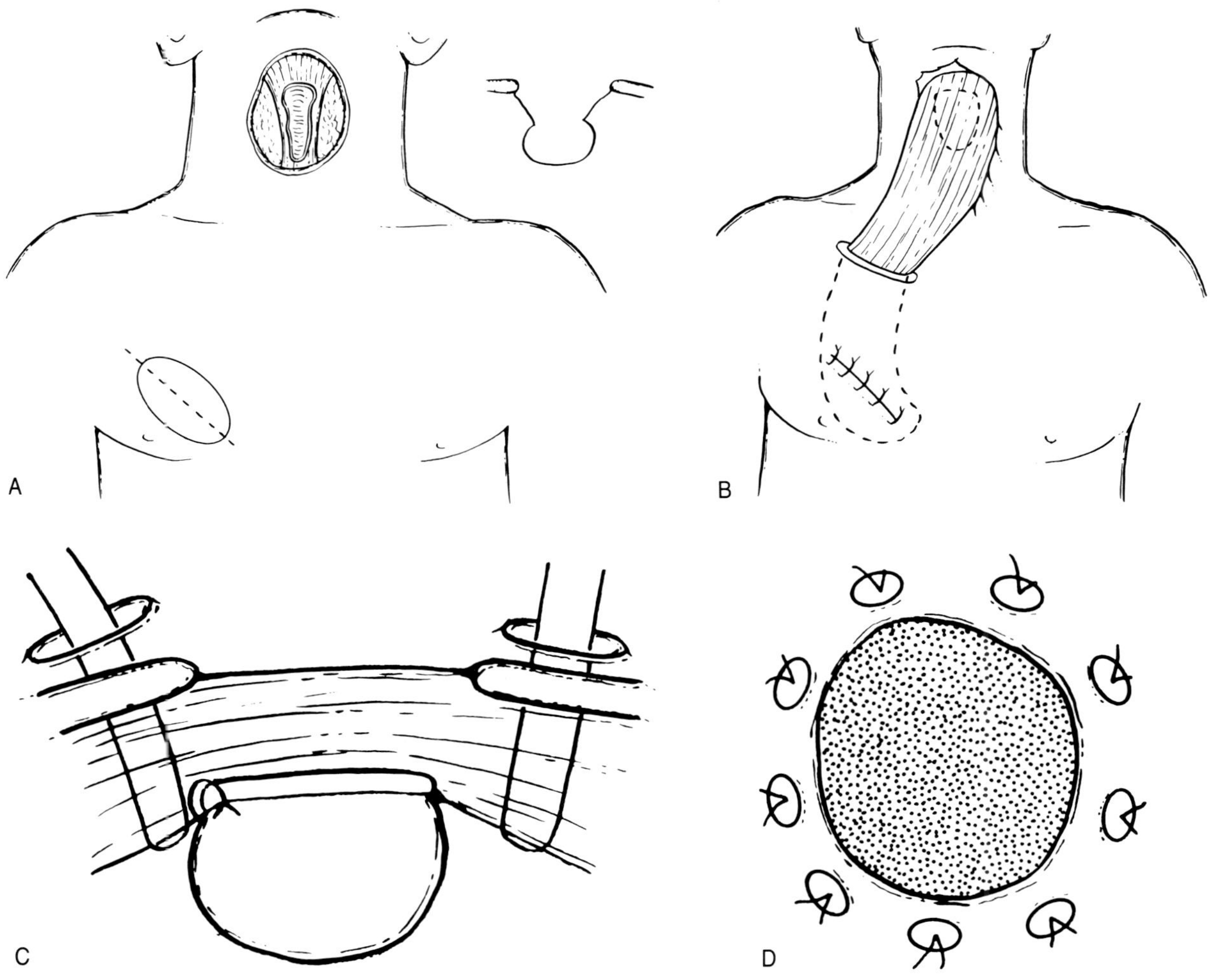

Figure 22–10. Closure of type III fistula with pectoralis major myocutaneous flap. A: large defect of mucosa and overlying cervical tissue. Both surfaces must be supplied by transfer of distant tissue. A pectoralis major myocutaneous flap is designed on the chest wall. B: the flap is raised and transferred, with about 2 cm of muscle extending beyond the skin island in all directions. C: edges of the skin island are sutured to inside edges of fistula. The surrounding cervical skin is undermined for about 2 cm, and the pectoralis muscle is tucked into this pocket all around the fistula. D: the muscle is secured with nonabsorbable sutures tied over buttons or catheters. The external surface may be covered with another flap, or skin graft.

LONG-TERM COMPLICATIONS

Stomal Recurrence

This is dealt with in Chapter 25.

Thyroid and Parathyroid Failure

After total laryngectomy and hemithyroidectomy for failed radiotherapy, the level of thyroid gland activity falls.[48] Since psychologic depression due to a minor degree of hypothyroidism may be thought to be due to the laryngectomy, the diagnosis is often not recognized. All patients with carcinoma of the larynx should undergo investigations of thyroid function prior to any treatment, so that a base line is determined for that individual patient. A patient who undergoes laryngectomy (which includes partial or total thyroidectomy) should have thyroid and parathyroid function assessed periodically: once a year is probably adequate, although some authors advise every 2 months. It is thought that the cause of the thyroid and parathyroid failure is damage to the blood supply of the remaining tissue.

Stomal Stenosis

This is dealt with in Chapter 26.

LONG-TERM EFFECTS OF LARYNGECTOMY

Lung Function Before and After Laryngectomy

After laryngectomy, pulmonary resistance increases to reach a maximum after 6 months when it is about ten times higher than before operation. The values fall thereafter, and 1 year after operation the resistance is only twice that of the original value. By that time, lung function is normal in respect to working capacity and arterial blood gas.[49]

Psychiatric Aspects

About 50% of patients undergo depression after laryngectomy. This appears to be related mostly to loss of the voice,[50] but also to the quality of domestic support. Since many patients requiring laryngectomy are thought to be alcoholics or heavy drinkers, it may be that this group is one that is prone to psychiatric disorder in any case.[51]

Hyposmia

Hyposmia ultimately occurs in all patients undergoing laryngectomy. This is type 1 hyposmia, that is, olfactory responsiveness is lost at the primary olfactory area but is retained at accessory olfactory areas. It is not known whether these changes are due to alterations in blood flow in the nasal mucosa or indirectly due to division of nerves, notably the recurrent laryngeal nerves.[52]

Alterations in Esophageal Motility, and Dysphagia

Marked derangements of the upper esophageal sphincter can be demonstrated by manometric studies in 50% of patients after laryngectomy.[53] This may be responsible for the dysphagia that occurs in some of these patients.

In an excellent review, McConnel et al[54] tell us that the reported incidence of dysphagia after total laryngectomy varies enormously, from 10 to 58%. The incidence may be underestimated, especially in retrospective analyses, since the patient may not complain actively of the dysphagia. All laryngectomees have an altered swallowing mechanism as a result of the removal of the larynx.

During normal swallowing, laryngeal elevation aids in opening the pharyngoesophageal (PE) segment. The PE segment develops a negative pressure that is important for bolus passage, but after removal of the larynx, negative pressure cannot develop in the PE segment. Without negative pressure in front of the bolus, the tongue must generate increased propulsive force.

Following total laryngectomy, the absence of prebolus negative pressure in the PE segment and lack of active opening of the pharynx secondary to laryngeal elevation diminish the pressure gradient to drive the bolus flow. This decreased pressure gradient is reflected in an increased pharyngeal transit time (1217 msec compared with 835 msec in normal subjects) and a decreased pharyngeal bolus velocity (6.6 cm/sec versus 8.7 cm/sec in normal subjects). The alteration in pressure gradient is greatest in the hypopharynx. Thus, the greatest increase occurs in the hypopharyngeal transit time: 1061 msec compared with 790 msec in normal subjects. The increase in oropharyngeal transit time is less marked; 658 msec compared with 570 msec in normal subjects.

The increased transit time is not due to decreased propulsive force when bolus-driving parameters are considered. In the oropharynx, the tongue-driving momentum is increased in total laryngectomees: 4.4 mmHg · sec compared with 1.5 mmHg · sec for normal subjects. Although normal tongue-driving pressure is 18 mmHg on the tail of the bolus, it is 32 mmHg in laryngectomees. Of greater significance is the increase in the oropharyngeal propulsive pump force in total laryngectomees: 9.0 mmHg · sec compared with 3.0 mmHg · sec in normal subjects. This reflects the relative obstruction in the PE segment. If the output of a pump is obstructed, then the pressure of the pump output increases until the obstruction is overcome.

Patients with tongue impairment in addition to laryngectomy cannot produce the necessary force for complete passage of the bolus in one swallow. They make multiple efforts that result in only weak pressure generation, greatly prolonged transit time, poor mucosal clearance, considerable clinical and radiologically visible swallowing impairment, and prolonged pharyngeal transit time of 3.0 seconds for the first swallow compared with 1.2 seconds for total laryngectomees and 0.8 seconds for normal subjects.[54]

Stenosis

Stenosis of the hypopharynx is a relatively frequent complication after total laryngectomy, reported in 73% of laryngectomies for pyriform sinus lesions.[55] Only 8% of patients acquired esophageal speech after surgery for pyriform sinus lesions in one series[56] probably because of the high incidence of hypopharyngeal stenosis.

The most important cause of hypopharyngeal stenosis appears to be the site of the lesion. Cancer of the larynx does not require a partial pharyngectomy, but pyriform sinus lesions do. Primary closure of the pharynx with less than 3 cm of hypopharyngeal mucosa remaining is to be avoided because of the high incidence of stenosis. The "tight closure" around the nasogastric tube has been discouraged by a number of surgeons. However, primary closure using flaps or free grafts is not without complication. The morbidity of postoperative stenosis is considerable: the diet must be restricted to soft or pureed foods, and there is a decreased acquisition of esophageal speech.

The most common form of therapy is dilation. Some patients will be able to dilate themselves and will have to perform it daily. If dilation is not successful, the surgical options include an extraluminal procedure, such as release of a band of scar tissue, myotomy, or a Z-plasty for narrow-band strictures. Repairs with a deltopectoral flap and myocutaneous flaps have been reported, but probably the best current option is a single-stage repair using free microvascular jejunal graft, either as a patch side graft or as a full luminal graft.[54]

SOCIAL AND ECONOMIC CONSEQUENCES

This is a vast field that would surely be fruitful for further research. Snow and colleagues have shown that only 40% of employed patients return to work; it must be remembered, however, that many of these patients are already of retiring age.[57] Furthermore, many of those returning to work do so at a lower level.[58] Half of all patients undergoing laryngectomy have family problems as a result of the operation, occasionally leading to divorce. Surprisingly, suicide is rare after this operation.

REFERENCES

1. Gussenbauer C. Uber die erst durch Th. Billroth am Menschen ausgefuhrte Kehlkopf Exterpation. Arch Clin Chir 1872;17:343.
2. MacComb WS, Fletcher GH. *Cancer of the Head and Neck*. Baltimore: Williams & Wilkins, 1967:245.
3. Watson PH. Ulceration of larynx, tracheotomy, haemoptysis. Edinburgh Med J 1866;11:78.
4. Holinger PH. A century of progress of laryngectomies in the northern hemisphere. Laryngoscope 1975;85:322–32.
5. Gluck T. Die chirurgische Therapie des Kehlkopfkarzinoms. Jahreskurse Artzt Fortbild 1912;2:20–41.
6. Coutard H. Roentgentherapy of epitheliomas of the tonsillar region, laryngopharynx and larynx from 1920 to 1926. Am J Roentgenol 1921;28:313–31.
7. Ogura JH, Bello JA. Laryngectomy and neck dissection for carcinoma of the larynx. Laryngoscope 1952;62:1–52.
8. Myers EM, Ogura JH. Completion laryngectomy. Ann Otol Rhinol Laryngol 1979;88:172–7.
9. Whicker JH, Neel BH, Weiland LH, Devine KD. Adenocarcinoma of the larynx. Ann Otol Rhinol Laryngol 1974;83:487–90.
10. Van Nostrand WP, Olofsson J. Verrucous carcinoma of the larynx. Cancer 1972;30:691–702.
11. Spiro RH, Lewis JS, Hajdu SI, Strong EW. Mucus gland tumors of the larynx and laryngopharynx. Ann Otol Rhinol Laryngol 1976;85:498–503.
12. Flanagan P, Cross RMP, Locke JH. Fibrosarcoma of the larynx. J Laryngol Otol 1965;79:1049–56.
13. Moore ES, Martin H. Melanoma of the upper respiratory tract and oral cavity. Cancer 1955;8:1167–76.
14. Swerdlow RS, Som ML, Biller HF. Cartilaginous tumors of the larynx. Arch Otolaryngol 1974;10:269–72.
15. Adlington P, Woodhouse MA. The ultrastructure of chemodectoma of the larynx. J Laryngol Otol 1972;86:1219–32.
16. Bauer WC, Lesinski SG, Ogura JH. The significance of positive margins in hemilaryngectomy specimens. Laryngoscope 1975;85:1–4.
17. Lederman M. Cancer of the pharynx. J Laryngol Otol 1967;81:151–72.
18. Stell PM. Cancer of the hypopharynx. J R Coll Surg Edin 1973;18:20–30.
19. Kiem WF, Shapiro MJ, Rosin HD. Study of post laryngectomy and stomal recurrence. Arch Otolaryngol 1965;81:183–6.
20. Baluyot ST, Shumrick DA, Faerts EC. Emergency laryngectomy. Arch Otolaryngol 1974;94:414–7.
21. Goodrich WA, Lenz M. Laryngeal chondronecrosis following roentgentherapy. Am J Roentgenol 1948;60:22–8.
22. Stell PM, Morrison A. Etiology and management of radiation necrosis of the larynx. Arch Otolaryngol 1973;80:111–3.
23. Ogura JH, Biller HF, Weth R. Elective neck dissection for pharyngeal and laryngeal cancers. Ann Otolaryngol 1971;80:646–51.
24. Moore OS, Frazell EL. Simultaneous bilateral neck dissection. Am J Surg 1964;107:565–8.
25. Stell PM, Green JR. Management of metastases to the lymph glands of the neck. Proc R Soc Med 1976;69:411–3.
26. Biller HF, Davis WH, Ogura JH. Delayed contralateral cervical metastases with laryngeal and laryngopharyngeal cancers. Laryngoscope 1971;81:1499–502.
27. Macbeth R. The treatment of cancer of the hypopharynx. The gutter graft operation. J Laryngol Otol 1969;83:119–32.
28. Condon HA. Postlaryngectomy stomal recurrence. Br J Anaesth 1969;41:531–4.
29. Hetter GP. Neck incisions relative to the cutaneous vasculature of the neck. Arch Otolaryngol 1972;95:84–7.
30. Rogers JH, Freeland AP. Arterial vasculature of cervical skin flaps. Clin Otolaryngol 1976;1:325–31.
31. Olofsson J, van Nostrand AWP. Growth and spread of laryngeal and hypopharyngeal carcinoma. Acta Otolaryngol Suppl (Stockh) 1973;308:1.
32. Harrison DFN. Laryngectomy for subglottic lesions. Laryngoscope 1975;85:1208–10.
33. Sobol S, Tucker W, Tucker HM. Everting closure of pharyngoesophageal defects. Arch Otolaryngol 1974;100:148–50.
34. Sealey GJ. A muscle cover for the carotid artery after radical neck dissection. Am J Surg 1961;102:815–7.
35. Wilson JI. Postoperative care. In: *Current surgical diagnosis and treatment*, 3rd ed. Los Altos, CA: Lange, 1977:14–36.
36. Robinson JMP. Wound infection following laryngectomy. J Laryngol Otol 1976;90:415–25.
37. Swift AC, et al. Wound sepsis, chemoprophylaxis and major head and neck surgery. Clin Otolaryngol 1988;13:81–3.
38. Raine CH, Bartyokas CA, Stell PM, et al. Chemoprophylaxis in major head and neck surgery. J R Soc Med 1984;77:1006–9.
39. Adams D. A newly developed permanent tracheostomy tube. J Laryngol Otol 1975;89:767–9.
40. Suarex Nieto C, Martin R, Mendez JD, Prendez P. Comparative studies of the two systems of prophylactic antibiotics in head and neck surgery. Clin Otolaryngol 1981;6:159–64.
41. Gall AM, Sessions DG, Ogura JH. Complications following surgery for cancer of the larynx and hypopharynx. Cancer 1977;39:624–31.
42. Stell PM. Catastrophic haemorrhage after major head and neck surgery. Br J Surg 1969;56:525–7.
43. Corso P, Gerold F. Use of autogenous dermis for protection of the carotid artery and pharyngeal suture lines in radical head and neck surgery. Surg Gyncol Obstet 1963;117:37–40.
44. Horgan EC, Dedo HH. Prevention of major and minor fistulae after laryngectomy. Laryngoscope 1979;89:250–60.
45. Lavelle RL, Maw AR. The aetiology of post-laryngectomy pharyngocutaneous fistulae. J Laryngol Otol 1972;86:785–93.
46. Maw AR, Lavelle RJ. The management of postoperative pharyngocutaneous pharyngeal fistulae. J Laryngol Otol 1972;86:795–805.
47. Stell PM, Cooney TC. Management of fistulae of the head and neck after radical surgery. J Laryngol Otol 1974;88:819–35.
48. Lavelle RJ. Thyroid function after radiotherapy and total laryngectomy in the treatment of carcinoma of the larynx. Ann Otol Rhinol Laryngol 1971;80:593–8.
49. Harris S, Johnson B. Lung function before and after laryngectomy. Acta Otolaryngol (Stockh) 1978;78;187–294.
50. Kiyzing P, Toremalm NG. The situation of the laryngectomised patient. Acta Otolaryngol Suppl (Stockh) 1970;263:119–23.
51. Davis H, Blaumont PJV. Psychiatric aspects of laryngectomy. S Afr Med J 1973;11:2192–4.
52. Davis RI, Larsen AL. On the mechanism of hyposmia following laryngectomy in man. Laryngoscope 1972;80:836–41.
53. Duranceau A, Jamieson G, Horowitz AL, et al. Alteration in esophageal motility after laryngectomy. Am J Surg 1976;131:30–5.
54. McConnel FMS, Cerenko D, Mendelsohn MS. Dysphagia after total laryngectomy. Otolaryngol Clin North Am 1988;21:721–6.
55. Kaplan JN. The incidence of hypopharyngeal stenosis after surgery for laryngeal cancer. Otolaryngol Head Neck Surg 1981;89:656–95.
56. Gates GA. Predicting esophageal speech. Ann Rhinol Laryngol 1982;91:454–7.
57. Brouwer B, Snow GB, Van Dam FSAM. Experiences of patients who undergo laryngectomy. Clin Otolaryngol 1979;4:109–18.
58. Savary P. Vocal and social situation of laryngectomees. Laryngoscope 1977;87:1516–22.
59. Stell PM, Maran AGD. *Head and neck surgery*, Philadelphia: JB Lippincott, 1972.
60. Silver CE. Surgical management of neoplasms of the larynx, hypopharynx and cervical esophagus. Curr Prob Surg 1977;14:1–69.

23

Pyriform Sinus Carcinoma

John S. Rubin

Cancers of the pyriform sinus constitute the majority of hypopharyngeal tumors seen in the United States, comprising 65 to 75% of reported tumors.[1] Predisposing factors, as in other areas of the head and neck, include tobacco and alcohol abuse. In Carpenter et al's[2,3] series 96% of patients were smokers and 93% had abused alcohol.

The incidence of pyriform sinus carcinoma in females has increased, undoubtedly related to an increase in smoking by women.[4] Nonetheless, in most series the male to female ratio is at least 4 to 1, in some as high as 9 to 1. In certain areas of Northern Europe, however, the disease predominates in women.[5]

The average age of patients at presentation is 60 years and the duration of symptoms prior to diagnosis varies from 6 to 12 months. Since the primary tumor is not evident on simple physical examination, patients are often treated initially with antibiotics or undergo cervical lymph node biopsy before the diagnosis of pyriform sinus carcinoma is determined.[4,6]

Palpable lymph node metastases are found in 65 to 75% of patients at the time of presentation.[1–3] Occult positive nodes occur in 38% of cases with clinically negative necks.[7] Late contralateral metastases have been reported in 36% of patients.[8] The presence of lymph node metastases has been found to be unrelated to the size of the tumor at presentation.[9]

Although some investigators have reported improvement in survival of stages III and IV pyriform sinus carcinomas with combined therapy,[10,11] others have failed to demonstrate this benefit.[2,3,12] Some reports have even documented lower survival rates following combined therapy.[13–15] Recently, an increase in distant metastases has been reported in some series of combined therapy.

One center has reported improvement in survival following induction, or neoadjuvant, chemotherapy.[16,17] The majority of centers do not corroborate these findings, however. The few articles describing immunotherapy have not to date demonstrated any significant survival improvement.

ANATOMY

The term "pyriform" is derived from the Latin "pirum" or "pear."[18] It is used to describe the two pear-shaped grooves of the hypopharynx which are created by the intrusion of the larynx into the anterior aspect of the pharynx.[18,19] The pyriform sinus has also been described as "horn-shaped"[20] and "comma-shaped."[21]

A century ago, Mackenzie described the pyriform as follows: "the posterior wall of this portion of the pharynx is channelled out, and not flat as in the upper regions. Its anterior wall is wanting centrally, owing to the opening of the larynx. Laterally, the anterior wall of this part of the pharynx presents a fossa on each side, the pharyngo-laryngeal sinus, which is about half an inch in its antero-posterior diameter and somewhat broader laterally."[22]

The pyriform sinus is made up of three walls: the anterior, lateral, and medial. The medial wall is the laryngopharyngeal wall, the free edge of the aryepiglottic fold separating the pyriform sinus from the intrinsic larynx. The lateral wall is bordered by the thyroid cartilage. The upper limit of the pyriform is the pharyngoepiglottic fold. The lower limit is the apex of the pyriform sinus, which lies in a plane related to the border of the cricoid cartilage. The apex lies slightly below the ventricle of the larynx and extends anteriorly close to the anterior commisure, where it comes in contact with the loose areolar tissues of the paraglottic space. This tissue allows the sinus to balloon out with deglutition, and thus to subserve its basic function, that of a passive gutter for transportation of the food bolus from the oropharynx to the cervical esophagus.[1,10,18,20–23]

A mucosal fold is visible in the lateral wall at the junction of the middle and lower third of the pyriform sinus, covering the internal branch of the superior laryngeal nerve; this proximity accounts for the frequent complaints of otalgia in cases of tumors in this region.

Lymphatics

Lymphatic drainage is profuse, primarily accompanying the superior laryngeal neurovascular bundle to the superior and middle deep jugular chain.[10] The subdigastric node is most commonly involved by metastatic disease, followed by midjugular node involvement. Spinal accessory chain involvement occurs but is relatively uncommon.[1,19,24] Extension of the tumor to the posterior hypopharynx places the retropharyngeal node of Rouviere at risk. Involvement of the postcricoid region may jeopardize the paratracheal nodes.[10]

PATTERNS OF SPREAD

Tumors of the pyriform sinus can arise from any of the walls and rapidly become infiltrating and ulcerative.[1] Furthermore, submucosal extension is the rule, frequently with as much as 10 mm of spread.[1,25] Pyriform sinus carcinoma tends to spread centrifugally in a stepwise fashion.[26]

Kirchner's studies[9,27,28] demonstrated frequent medial spread into the paraglottic space with displacement or fixation of the lateral laryngeal wall. Other causes of laryngeal fixation included invasion of the cricoarytenoid joint or, less commonly, invasion of the recurrent laryngeal nerve. Even small medial wall tumors tended to invade soft tissues around the homolateral arytenoid. Larger growths extended to the posterior wall of the hypopharynx or across the postcricoid region to the opposite pyriform sinus. Spread superiorly into the base of the tongue was also seen, whereas spread into the cervical esophagus rarely occurred.

Lateral wall lesions frequently invade thyroid cartilage and do so early in the disease.[19] Kirchner found a 40% incidence of thyroid cartilage invasion in his series; all of these cases demonstrated lateral wall involvement as well as apical invasion. Larsson et al[21] speculate that ossification of cartilage actually provides the vascular channels and medullary spaces through which tumor cells can invade and destroy thyroid cartilage.[21] The thyroid gland can be involved through direct invasion of the thyroid cartilage. The gland can also be involved even without thyroid cartilage invasion via lymphatic tumor emboli or through intraglandular vascular channels.[29]

Extralaryngeal spread of disease can occur directly through the cricothyroid membrane, or out behind the posterior margin of the posterolateral thyroid cartilage. It can then follow the superior thyroid vessels in an antigrade fashion.[9,27,28,30]

PATIENT EVALUATION

The pyriform sinus is a clinically "silent" area. Early lesions have no associated symptoms. Advanced lesions produce a characteristic triad of odynophagia, referred otalgia, and dysphagia.[1,10] Tumor ulceration may produce bloody sputum.[1] Approximately 20 to 25% of patients with pyriform sinus tumors present initially with an asymptomatic neck mass.[1-3,10]

Signs

Absence of normal postlaryngeal crepitation indicates an abnormality between the cervical spine and laryngeal cartilages.[1] Fullness may also be noted at the thyrohyoid or cricothyroid membranes as a result of extralaryngeal spread.[10]

Edema and erythema of the postcricoid and arytenoids with pooling of saliva in the pyriform sinus are frequently the only findings noted on office examination of the larynx. Vocal cord mobility and laryngeal function may be impaired.

Radiographic Studies

Esophagram should be performed prior to endoscopy. It serves two purposes: it helps to rule out a second aerodigestive primary, and to establish, preoperatively, the likelihood of extension of the tumor into the cervical esophagus. Computed tomography (CT) may be helpful in demonstrating cartilage invasion as well as soft tissue extension. It can also be helpful in identifying nonpalpable lymphadenopathy. CT has predominantly replaced laryngography, tomography, and soft tissue lateral films for evaluation of laryngeal and pyriform sinus tumors. Nevertheless, some centers still utilize contrast laryngograms to aid in localization of tumor with respect to the pyriform apex. This information can be useful in decision-making regarding conservation surgery.[1,3,20] The role of magnetic resonance imaging in this region is still somewhat undefined. (Radiographic imaging of the larynx is discussed in detail in Chapter 7.)

Endoscopy

Traditionally, direct endoscopy, including laryngoscopy esophagoscopy, and bronchoscopy, has been performed in all patients.[10] Cervical esophagoscopy is certainly important in order to evaluate the lower extent of the lesion. Rigid bronchoscopy, however, does not appear to be of value in the presence of a normal chest radiograph.

STAGING

The current staging system of the American Joint Committee on Cancer[31] for tumors of the hypopharynx is presented in Appendix B. The hypopharynx is divided into three sites: pyriform sinus, postcricoid, and posterior hypopharyngeal wall.

A classification for tumors restricted to the pyriform sinus does not exist at present. Previously, Lederman[32] and Leroux-Robert[33] each devised staging systems dividing the pyriform sinus into regions. Neither system, however, came into general use. The current classification of "T" status of the pyriform sinus is somewhat misleading. A T_1 lesion that involves the medial, anterior, and lateral walls is more worrisome than a T_2 lesion involving the medial wall and extending to the postcricoid region.[8] Similarly, medial wall tumors appear to have better prognosis than lateral wall tumors.[9,27,28]

SELECTION OF TREATMENT

History

In the early decades of this century, Trotter[34] established the need for surgical excision of cancers of the hypopharynx. He treated lateral wall lesions with partial pharyngectomy via a lateral transthyroid pharyngotomy. The procedure never achieved widespread popularity, primarily due to the high morbidity and mortality from blood loss and sepsis. Once supervoltage radiation therapy was introduced, it became the accepted treatment for these lesions. Surgery was withheld for salvage. In the United States, prior to 1950, carcinoma of the pyriform sinus was generally regarded as inoperable.[35] Unfortunately, cure rates with radiotherapy were low and attempts at surgical salvage often unsuccessful.[2,3,32–36]

Combined treatment with surgery and radiation was first introduced by Schinz and Zuppinger.[2,3] In 1956 it was advocated by LeRoux-Robert[33] as initial treatment for pyriform sinus carcinoma. By 1962, Andre and Pinel had reported on their 5-year follow-up of patients treated with combined therapy of radiation followed by surgery, with a 17% survival.[36]

Conservation surgery of the pyriform sinus was also undergoing reconsideration in the mid-1950s. In 1956 Jesburg noted "until we possess better preoperative and diagnostic aids . . . it will be impossible to select cases for (conservation procedures)."[35] Ogura believed that laryngograms gave him this preoperative diagnostic advantage and reintroduced partial laryngopharyngectomy. In 1964 his group reported a series of partial laryngopharyngectomies with a 43% 5-year survival rate.[37]

Current Selection of Treatment

Treatment is determined by a series of factors, including extent of local-regional disease, evidence of distant metastases, and underlying medical condition. A summary of results of treatment of pyriform sinus carcinoma by various modalities, reported in the contemporary literature, is presented in Table 23–1.

Early T_1 lesions of pyriform sinus, with normal mobility, can be well controlled with single modality therapy: surgery or irradiation. In some institutions surgical intervention is preferred. Partial pharyngectomy, without any resection of the larynx, can be performed for lateral wall lesions. Partial laryngopharyngectomy is appropriate for medial wall lesions.[2,3,38] (Technical aspects of these procedures are discussed in detail by the editor in Chapter 13.)

Satisfactory control of early pyriform sinus lesions has been reported with radiation therapy. In one series of nine patients local control was achieved in eight with radiation therapy.[39] These early lesions are uncommon, however, and few authors have compiled significantly large series of cases.

Management of lesions that extend beyond the confines of the pyriform sinus, but still have normal mobility, is more complex. Selection of treatment depends on the presence or absence of disease in the apex. T_2 lesions without apical invasion can be

Table 23–1. End Results—Treatment of Pyriform Sinus Carcinoma

STUDY (YR)	NO. PATIENTS*	MODALITY*	SURVIVAL (%)	YEARS*
Mendenhall et al[39] (1987)	54(P.S.)	X(X/salv)	39	5(A)
			56	5(D)
Routh and Hickman[24] (1987)	25(P.S.)			
	12	X	8	3(U)
	4	X + S	25	3(U)
	5	S + X	20	3(U)
	4	Palliation	0	3(U)
Sasaki et al[52] (1986)	50(P.S.)		26	2(U)
	13	S		
	5	X + S		
	32	S + X		
Vandenbrouck et al[41] (1987)	351(P.S.)			
	152	X	25/14	3/5(U)
	18	S(PLP) + X	67/39	3/5(U)
	181	S(TLP) + X	48/33	3/5(U)
Brasnu et al[16] (1986)	285(P.S.)			
	43	S+X	30/13	3/5(U)
	95	S + X + Bl	31/29	3/5(U)
	98	S + X + Vn/MTX		
		Bl or En	47/39	3/5(U)
	40	S + X + CDDP/Bl		
		5-FU or MTX	61	3(U)
Ahmad and Fayos[50] (1984)	61(P.S.)	X(X/salv)	26	5(A)
Flores[49] (1984)	97(P.S.)			
	64	X(X/salv)	40	5(U)
	4	S	50	5(U)
	7	X + S + X	43	5(U)
	11	X + Bl/Vn/MTX/5-FU	0	5(U)
	11	No Rx	33	5(U)

Table 23-1. End Results—Treatment of Pyriform Sinus Carcinoma (*continued*)

STUDY (YR)	NO. PATIENTS*	MODALITY*	SURVIVAL (%)	YEARS*
Yates and Crumley[15] (1984)	60(P.S.)			
	21	S	65/56	3/5(D)
	28	X + X	50/36	3/5(D)
	11	S + X	50/25	3/5(D)
Driscoll et al[11] (1983)	75(P.S.)			
	26	X	19	3(D)
	18	S	39	3(D)
	26	X + S	50	3(D)
	5	S + X	60	3(D)
El Badawi et al[20] (1982)	418(P.S.)			
	57	X(cure)	47	2(U)
	203	S	40	2(U)
	125	S + X	50	2(U)
	17	X + S	47	2(U)
	16	X(Palliative)	0	2(U)
Bataini et al[51] (1982)	434(P.S.)	X(X/salv)	26/19	3/5(A)
			47/41	3/5(D)
Persky and Daly[10] (1981)	51(P.S.)			
	18	X(X/salv)	6	5(A)
	4	S		
	18	X + S	33	5(A)
	4	X + chemotherapy		
	7	Palliation		
Ogura et al[42] (1980)	175(P.S.)			
	33	X	11	3(A)
	85	X + S(PLP)	59	3(A)
	57	X + S(TLP)	36	3(A)
Puhakka and Nordman[5] (1980)	20(P.S.)	X	21/20	3/5(U)
Baruah[48] (1980)	92(P.S.)	X	32.6/20.6	3/5(U)
Donald et al[6] (1980)	33(P.S.)			
	6	X	0	2(U)
	7	X + S	29	2(U)
	14	S + X	64	2(U)
Razack et al[79] (1978)	97(P.S.)			
	22	X	0	5(U)
	8	X/salv	37	5(U)
	67	S	25	5(U)
Eisbach and Krause[14] (1977)	84(P.S.)			
	33	X	9/8	3/5(A)
			10/9	3/5(D)
	19	S	47/47	3/5(A)
			56/56	3/5(D)
	32	X + S	31/20	3/5(A)
			40/31	3/5(D)
Harwick[8] (1975)	91(P.S.)	S	25.4	5(A)
Kirchner[9] (1975)	116(P.S.)			
	55	X	4	3(U)
	28	S	29	3(U)
	33	X + S	36	3(U)
Jesse and Lindberg[54] (1975)	116(P.S.)			
	67	S	22	5(U)
	49	S + X	33	5(U)
Marchetta et al[46] (1967)	119(P.S.)			
	93	X	2	5(U)
	26	S	20	5(U)

*P.S.: Patients studied; X: radiation therapy; S: surgery; X/salv: radiation followed by salvage surgery; X + S: radiation followed by surgery; S + X: surgery followed by radiation; PLP: partial Laryngopharyngectomy; TLP: total Laryngectomy Partial Pharyngectomy; Bl: bleomycin; Vn: vincristine; MTX: methotrexate; Em: CDDP: cisplatin; 5-FU: 5-fluorouracil; Rx: treatment; A: absolute; D: determinate; U: unspecified.

treated much like T_1 lesions. Million et al[19] reported approximately 60% control of such lesions with radiation therapy.

Good results have been reported with treatment of carefully selected early lesions by conservation surgery (partial laryngopharyngectomy) followed by postoperative radiation.[10,40,41]

Once tumor involves the apex of the pyriform, there is less disagreement regarding treatment. Total laryngectomy with partial pharyngectomy followed by postoperative radiation therapy is generally accepted.[10,19,38] Similarly, lesions with fixation of the hemilarynx or with extensive infiltration should be treated with combined therapy.[2,3,9,14,23,27,28,39–41] There are exceptions, however. One group suggests that exophytic lesions should receive a trial of preoperative radiotherapy and at 50 Gy decide whether to extirpate the larynx or complete a course of radical radiation therapy.[19]

With large infiltrating tumors, the question changes from how much laryngopharynx to remove to how much, if any, laryngopharynx to leave behind. In our institution we will perform total laryngopharyngectomy for lesions involving more than two thirds of the circumference of the hypopharynx. Smaller lesions are evaluated on a case-by-case basis. In general, any resection of more than half of the circumference of the hypopharynx will require reconstruction with distant tissue.[23]

Palliative treatment is offered to patients with extensive inoperable local-regional disease, patients with distant metastases, patients with extensive medical problems, and patients who are unwilling to undergo surgery.[6,19]

CONTROVERSIAL ISSUES IN TREATMENT PLANNING

Controversy regarding treatment has revolved around certain issues: indications for conservation surgery; single modality versus combined modality therapy; preoperative versus postoperative radiotherapy; and adjunctive immunotherapy and chemotherapy. These issues will be reviewed.

Indications for Conservation Surgery

Conservation surgery is not generally considered to be suitable in pyriform sinus carcinoma due to the extensive infiltration and submucosal spread. Ogura has developed a series of criteria to be fulfilled in order for patients to be candidates for partial laryngopharyngectomy. These include: (1) the vocal cords and the arytenoids must be free of gross disease and mobile; (2) there must be no invasion of the thyroid cartilage; and (3) there must be no involvement of the pyriform apex.[12,42] By following these criteria, Ogura was able to perform conservation surgery on 48% of his patients, many with indeterminate T stages. Fifty-two percent of these patients retained a useful voice after surgery. Three-year survival rate was 59%.[12,42]

Kirchner[9] generally agreed with Ogura's criteria, but believed that conservation surgery should not be attempted in cases with involvement of the lateral wall, due to the high incidence of cartilaginous invasion. In retrospect he considered only one of 51 specimens to be suitable for conservation surgery. Shah et al[43] also found very few pyriform sinus tumors (46 of 301) suitable for conservation surgery.

Florant et al[44] reported on 48 cases of conservation surgery for pyriform carcinomas, 92% T_1 or T_2. He extended Ogura's criteria to include gross disease of the homolateral arytenoid, providing that there is no diminution in mobility of the vocal cords. In Florant et al's series, arytenoid involvement was fairly common; its presence was not deleterious to the survival rate (46%).

Pearson et al approached the problem of conservation from the standpoint of near-total laryngectomy.[45] In their review of 20 whole-mount specimens, only one of 20 fulfilled Ogura's requirements; yet 13 could have been excised with a near-total laryngectomy procedure. Contraindications, which they devised for performance of near-total laryngectomy on pyriform sinus carcinoma, include bilateral cord fixation, postcricoid involvement, and extension to the posterior commissure. (See Chapter 24 for detailed discussion of near-total laryngectomy.)

Silver[23] found a greater percentage of lesions suitable for conservation surgery as he became more willing to accept conservation surgery as adequate oncologic treatment for certain hypopharyngeal carcinomas.

Radical Radiation Versus Combined Modality Therapy

A wide diversity exists in survival statistics reported for radical radiation therapy for pyriform sinus carcinomas. These range from 3 to 41%.[5,14,26,46–51] In one series, survival as high as 56.5% was reported for patients with stage III disease.[50]

Reports that compare radiation therapy with combined therapy generally note an improvement in survival with the latter. In three series, survival with combined therapy was reported to be at least four times better than with radiation alone (one reported statistical significance of $p = 0.001$).[4,26,47] There is a problem inherent to these studies, however. The combined treatment groups tend to treat only curable patients, whereas the radiation groups tend to include inoperable patients and patients who are medically unstable, along with curable patients. Nevertheless, it is generally accepted that, except in T_1 and early T_2 lesions, surgery combined with preoperative or postoperative radiotherapy is preferred over radiotherapy as single modality treatment.

Surgery Alone Versus Combined Modality Therapy

The literature again contains somewhat discordant results. Certain studies[13–15] have found that patients treated with single modality surgery actually do better than those treated with surgery combined with radiotherapy. Eisbach and Krause[14] pinpointed one problem as being that of inadequate local control with surgery combined with preoperative radiation therapy, presumably because the margins were obfuscated by the radiation. They conclude that these patients should receive postoperative rather than preoperative radiotherapy.

On the other hand, several large studies have come out in favor of combined therapy. Studies performed at the M.D. Anderson Cancer Center and at Yale University found combined treatment to produce slightly improved survival.[9,20,27,28] Other studies demonstrated more impressive survival statistics with combined therapy, one with almost twofold improvement in survival.[52]

Preoperative Versus Postoperative Radiation Therapy

For large tumors, the sentiment of major centers is now for combined therapy, specifically, for surgery followed by radiation therapy. Donald et al[6] found over twofold improvement in survival (64 versus 28%) when comparing postoperative to preoperative radiotherapy. In a randomized prospective study comparing postoperative and preoperative radiotherapy (in tumors of the hypopharynx), Vandenbrouck et al[40] found statistically better survival in the group treated with postoperative radiotherapy (56 versus 14%, $p = 0.01$). El Badawi et al[20] found a somewhat lower failure rate above the clavicles (11 versus 28%) in patients treated with postoperative radiotherapy.

Postoperative radiation therapy is generally believed to give fewer complications than preoperative radiotherapy, and better quality of life, as well as to be necessary for the control of subclinical residual disease.[40,41]

Distant Metastases with Combined Therapy

Whereas there is little question that combined therapy has decreased the incidence of local-regional recurrence, certain centers have noted a disturbing increase in distant metastases in patients so treated. This increase may be due to increased longevity in the combined group, to the extent that subclinical distant metastases become evident. On the other hand, it may be due to the more dubious possibility that combined treatment increases the likelihood of distant metastases.

Byers et al[53] reported a 47% incidence of distant metastases at 2 years following combined treatment in T_3 and T_4 carcinomas, with only a 19% incidence of local-regional disease. Yates and Crumley[15] noted a 50% incidence of distant metastases in patients treated with combined therapy versus 28% in patients treated with surgery alone. Schuller et al[13] reported a threefold increase in distant metastases in patients with cancer of the hypopharynx treated with combined therapy over those treated with surgery only (61.5 versus 20%, $p = 0.063$). Some reports[11,54] do not corroborate these findings; nevertheless, the trend exists and is disturbing.

IMMUNOLOGY

Immunologic Parameters in Patients Undergoing Radiation Therapy

It is well known that patients with squamous cell carcinoma of the head and neck demonstrate numerous impairments in cell-mediated immunity. These include decreased skin reactivity to dinitroclorobenzine, diminished lymphocyte reactivity to phytohemaglutinin and concanavalin A, alterations in macrophage function and accumulation, functional defects in T lymphocytes as well as natural killer cell alterations in tumor-draining lymph nodes.[55–64]

When patients in this population are treated with radiation therapy, further defects in immune responsiveness have been observed. This depression of cell-mediated immunity has been found to be persistent and prolonged.[65–67] It may well be that the addition of radiation therapy to surgery, while improving local-regional cure, may predispose the patient to distant metastatic disease by further diminishing his immunologic reserve.

Adjuvant Immunologic Therapy

In an attempt to overcome this problem, immunologic and chemotherapeutic trials have been attempted. Bacille Calmette-Guérin (BCG) has been administered to head and neck patients treated with radiation therapy. In a randomized trial no significant changes in survival were found, nor were there any differences in immunologic responsiveness between the groups post-treatment.[68] BCG has also been tested in a large group of randomized patients with carcinoma of the larynx and hypopharynx treated with combined therapy. Again, no effect was demonstrated.[69]

Currently, preliminary data suggest the possibility of therapeutic benefit from local injection of interleukin-2.[70] An Eastern Cooperative Oncology Group Phase I protocol is underway in an attempt to further investigate this phenomenon.

In summary, to date, there has been no consistent evidence that immunologic manipulation affects survival in patients with squamous cell carcinoma of the laryngopharynx.

ADJUVANT CHEMOTHERAPY

Systemic chemotherapy with single or multiple agents has been utilized for well over a decade. At least three agents, methotrexate, cisplatin, and bleomycin, have been shown to demonstrate consistent antitumor effects.[19] Several groups have demonstrated a response rate of 60 to 90% with multiple agent chemotherapy.[71–74] One group has recently reported results of treatment of a large series of patients with pyriform sinus carcinoma with combined therapy and then randomized to single agent bleomycin or multiple agent therapy. A statistically significant increase in survival was found with the multiagent group ($p = 0.01$), although a 35% incidence of distant metastases was noted in the group treated with cisplatin.[17]

Antitumor effects must be carefully weighed against toxicity. Cisplatin and methotrexate are potentially nephrotoxic. Cisplatin, methotrexate, bleomycin, 5-fluorouracil, doxorubicin, and vinblastine can cause myelosuppression, mucositis, or both. For drugs used in combination, cisplatin and bleomycin appear best in that their toxicities do not overlap.[19]

Several groups have been unable to document any improvement in survival using chemotherapy.[40,41,75] One study demonstrated significant decrease in survival in patients with tumors of the "buccopharynx" (including pyriform sinus) treated with radiation therapy and multiagent chemotherapy compared with those treated with radiation therapy only (0 versus 60%).[76]

In summary, there is, at present, no conclusive evidence that single or multidrug chemotherapy regimens either improve survival or solve the problem of distant metastases. To the contrary, the hypopharynx has been considered to be an area that responds poorly to chemotherapy.[7]

WHY WE FAIL

Generally speaking, the high failure rate in treatment of pyriform sinus carcinoma has been ascribed to the insidious onset of the disease coupled with the relative inaccessability to scrutiny, the early paraglottic invasion and frequent regional and systemic metastases, the high incidence of synchronous and metachronous disease, and the continued exposure to environmental carcinogenic agents.[26]

Tumor histologic grade has been correlated with survival. In hypopharyngeal tumors, Shah et al[43] correlated survival to histologic grade of the primary, with survival falling from 33% in grade I tumors to 16% in grade IV tumors. Martin et al[77] correlated keratinization of tumor to metastatic potential. Nonkeratinizing tumors (which correlated at $p = 0.005$ with poorly differentiated histologic features) had a greater likelihood of developing distant metastases ($p = 0.02$). Interestingly, keratinizing tumors were slightly more likely ($p = 0.11$) to be associated with local-regional recurrence.

Treatment plan has been noted to affect location of failure. As an example, in Ogura's series, radiation therapy often led to local recurrence, whereas partial laryngopharyngectomy preceded by radiation therapy would fail by recurrence in regional lymph nodes.[7,29,35,42]

Positive surgical margins have been implicated as an important cause of failure. Kirchner and Harrison have emphasized the extent of submucosal spread within the primary tumor.[9,25,27,28,78] One third of Vandenbrouck et al's[40,41] resected specimens had borderline or involved margins. Martin et al[77] and Marks et al[12] noted that positive margins are associated with a high incidence of local-regional recurrence and poor prognosis.

The presence of regional metastases is clearly related to poor survival. Several authors note a two- to threefold decrease in survival in patients with positive nodes.[43,79,80] Sasaki et al[52] found that survival decreased in direct correlation to the number of positive nodes: a 50% survival with none or one node, 31% survival with two to three nodes, and 16% survival with four or more nodes. The presence of positive lymph nodes in the posterior triangle portends a particularly poor prognosis.[10]

Subclinical cervical node disease is related to prognosis, but can be effectively sterilized with radiation therapy. Eisbach and Krause[14] reported a decrease in contralateral neck disease from 26 to 3% with the addition of radiation therapy to surgery. Similarly, in the series reported by Jesse and Lindberg,[54] regional failure fell from 15 to 4% in necks with positive lymph nodes in which radiation therapy was added to surgery.

Extracapsular spread of nodal disease and involvement of connective tissue have both been identified as important causes of failure.[15,20,40,41,77] The high incidence of distant metastases at a time when local-regional control is improving has been discussed. Similarly, immunodeficiencies in patients with head and neck cancer, compounded by radiation therapy, may be an important cause of failure.

REFERENCES

1. Suen JY, Myers EN, eds. *Cancer of the head and neck.* New York, Churchill Livingstone, 1981.
2. Carpenter RJ, De Santo LW, Devine KD, Taylor WF. Cancer of the hypopharynx: analysis of treatment and results in 162 patients. Arch Otolaryngol 1976;102:716–21.
3. Carpenter RJ, De Santo LW. Cancer of the hypopharynx. Surg Clin North Am 1977;57:723–35.
4. Plante DA, Piccirillo JF, Sofferman RA. Decision analysis of treatment options in pyriform sinus carcinoma. Med Decis Making 1987;7:74–83.
5. Puhakka H, Nordman EM. Radiotherapy of carcinoma of hypopharynx. Strahlentherapie 1980;156:315–7.
6. Donald PJ, Hayes HR, Dhalival R. Combined therapy for pyriform sinus cancer using postoperative irradiation. Otolaryngol Head Neck Surg 1980;88:738–44.
7. Ogura JH, Biller HF, Wette R. Elective neck dissection for pharyngeal and laryngeal cancers: an evaluation. Ann Otol Rhinol Laryngol 1971;80:646–51.
8. Harwick RD. Carcinoma of the pyriform sinus. Am J Surg 1975;130:493–5.
9. Kirchner JA. Pyriform sinus cancer: a clinical and laboratory study. Ann Otolaryngol 1975;84:793–803.
10. Persky MS, Daly JF. Combined therapy vs curative radiation in the treatment of pyriform sinus carcinoma. Otolaryngol Head Neck Surg 1981;89:87–91.
11. Driscoll WG, Nagorsky MJ, Cantrell RW, Johns ME. Carcinoma of the pyriform sinus: analysis of 102 cases. Laryngoscope 1983;93:556–60.
12. Marks JE, Kurnik B, Powers WE, Ogura JH. Carcinoma of the pyriform sinus: an analysis of treatment results and patterns of failure. Cancer 1978;41:1008–15.
13. Schuller DE, McGuirt WF, Krause CJ, et al. Symposium: Adjuvant cancer therapy of head and neck tumors. Laryngoscope 1979;89:582–94.
14. Eisbach KJ, Krause CJ. Carcinoma of the pyriform sinus: a comparison of treatment modalities. Laryngoscope 1977;87:1904–10.
15. Yates A, Crumley RL. Surgical treatment of pyriform sinus cancer: a retrospective study. Laryngoscope 1984;94:1586–90.
16. Brasnu D, Lacau-St-Guily, Fabre A, et al. La survie dans les cancers du sinus piriforme apres chimiotherapie d'induction. Ann Otolaryngol Chir Cervicofac 1986;103:83–9.
17. Brasnu D, Bassot V, Fabre A, et al. Induction chemotherapy in pyriform sinus carcinoma analysis of survival. Proc Am Soc Clin Oncol Annual Meeting, 1987, vol. 6, Abstr 551.
18. Barton RT. Surgical treatment of carcinoma of the pyriform sinus. Arch Otolaryngol 1973;97:337–9.
19. Million RR, Cassisi NJ, Wittes RE. Cancer of the head and neck. In: DeVita VT, Hellman S, Rosenberg SA, eds. *Cancer: principles and practice of oncology,* ed 2. Philadelphia: JB Lippincott, 1985.
20. El Badawi SA, Goepfert H, Fletcher GH, et al. Squamous cell carcinoma of the pyriform sinus. Laryngoscope 1982;92:357–64.
21. Larsson S, Mancuso A, Hoover L, Hanafee W. Differentiation of pyriform cancer from supraglottic laryngeal cancer by computed tomography. Radiology 1981;141:427–32.
22. Mackenzie M. *Diseases of the pharynx, larynx and trachea.* New York: William C. Wood, 1880.
23. Silver CE. *Surgery for Cancer of the Larynx and Related Structures.* New York: Churchill Livingstone, 1981.
24. Routh A, Hickman BT. Carcinoma of the pyriform sinus. South Med J 1987;80:177–81.
25. Harrison DFN. Pathology of hypopharyngeal cancer in relation to surgical management. J Laryngol Otol 1970;84:349–67.
26. Son YH, Habermalz HJ. Prognostic factors in pyriform sinus carcinoma. Acta Radiol Oncol 1979;18:561–71.
27. Kirchner JA. Two hundred laryngeal cancers: patterns of growth and spread as seen in serial sections. Laryngoscope 1977;87:474–82.
28. Kirchner JA, Owen JR. Five hundred cancers of the larynx and pyriform sinus: results of treatment by radiation and surgery. Laryngoscope 1977;87:1288–1303.
29. Ogura JH. Surgical pathology of cancer of the larynx. Laryngoscope 1955;65:867–926.
30. Lam KH. Extralaryngeal spread of cancer of the larynx: a study with whole-organ sections. Head Neck Surg 1983;5:410–24.
31. Beahrs OH, Henson DE, Hutter RVP, Myers MH, eds. *Manual for staging of cancer,* 3rd ed. Philadelphia: JB Lippincott, 1988.
32. Lederman M. Cancer of the laryngopharynx: classification, staging and results of radiotherapy. J Laryngol Otol 1956;68:333–69.
33. Leroux-Robert J. Indications for radical surgery, partial surgery, radiotherapy and combined surgery and radiotherapy for cancer of the larynx and hypopharynx. Ann Otol Rhinol Laryngol 1956;65:137–53.

34. Trotter W. Operations for malignant disease of the pharynx. Br J Surg 1929;16:485–95.
35. Ogura JH, Jurema AA, Watson RK. Partial laryngopharyngectomy and neck dissection for pyriform sinus cancer. Laryngoscope 1960; 70:1399–417.
36. McGavran MH, Bauer WC, Spjut JH, Ogura JH. Carcinoma of the pyriform sinus: the results of radical surgery. Arch Otolaryngol 1963;78:826–30.
37. Freeman RB, Marks JE, Ogura JH. Voice preservation in treatment of carcinoma of the pyriform sinus. Laryngoscope 1979;89:1855–63.
38. Pesavento G, Ferlito A. Management of squamous cell carcinoma of the pyriform sinus. Acta OtoRhinoLaryngol Belg 1984;28:156–63.
39. Mendenhall WM, Parsons JT, Cassisi NJ, Million RR. Squamous cell carcinoma of the pyriform sinus treated with radical radiation therapy. Radiother Oncol 1987;9:201–8.
40. Vandenbrouck C, Sancho H, LeFur R, et al. Results of a randomized clinical trial of preoperative irradiation versus postoperative in treatment of tumors of the hypopharynx. Cancer 1977;39:1445–9.
41. Vandenbrouck C, Eschwege F, De la Rochefordiere A, et al. Squamous cell carcinoma of the pyriform sinus: retrospective study of 351 cases treated at the Institut Gustave-Roussy. Head Neck Surg 1987;10:4–13.
42. Ogura JH, Marks JE, Freeman RB. Results of conservation surgery for cancers of the supraglottis and pyriform sinus. Laryngoscope 1980;90:591–600.
43. Shah JP, Shaha AR, Spiro RH, Strong EW. Carcinoma of the hypopharynx. Am J Surg 1976;132:439–43.
44. Florant A, Berreby S, Gilain L, et al. La chirurgie fonctionelle des cancers de l'hypopharynx: hemi-laryngopharyngectomies posterieures par abord cervical bilateral. Ann Otolaryngol Chir Cervicofac 1986;103:443–53.
45. Dumich PS, Pearson BW, Weiland LH. Suitability of near-total laryngopharyngectomy in pyriform carcinoma. Arch Otolaryngol 1984;110:664–9.
46. Marchetta FC, Sako K, Holyoke ED. Squamous cell carcinoma of the pyriform sinus. Am J Surg 1967;114:507–9.
47. Horwitz SD, Caldarelli DD, Henderickson FR. Treatment of carcinoma of the hypopharynx. Head Neck Surg 1979;2:107–11.
48. Baruah JD. Carcinoma of the pyriform sinus. Ind J Radiol 1980;34:207–10.
49. Flores AD. Carcinoma of the pyriform sinus: a review of treatment methods (meeting abstract). 3rd Annual Meeting of the European Society for Therapeutic Radiology and Oncology. Jerusalem, September 9–15, 1984:273.
50. Ahmad K, Fayos JV. High dose radiation therapy in carcinoma of the pyriform sinus. Cancer 1984;53:2091–4.
51. Bataini P, Brugere J, Bernier J, et al. Results of radical radiotherapeutic treatment of carcinoma of the pyriform sinus. Int J Radiat Oncol Biol Phys 1982;8:1277–86.
52. Sasaki TM, Baker HW, Yeager RA, et al. Aggressive surgical management of pyriform sinus carcinoma. Am J Surg 1986;151:590–592.
53. Byers RM, Krueger WWO, Saxton J. Use of surgery and postoperative radiation in the treatment of advanced squamous cell carcinoma of the pyriform sinus. Am J Surg 1979;138:597–9.
54. Jesse RH, Lindberg RD. The efficacy of combining radiation therapy with a surgical procedure in patients with cervical metastases from squamous cancer of the oropharynx and hypopharynx. Cancer 1975;35:1163–6.
55. Browder JP, Chretien PB. Immune reactivity in head and neck squamous carcinoma and relevance to the design of immunotherapy trials. Semin Oncol 1977;4:431–9.
56. Wanebo HJ, Jun MY, Strong EW, Oettgen H. T-cell deficiency in patients with squamous cell cancer of the head and neck. Am J Surg 1975;130:445–51.
57. Wolf GT, Lovett EJ, Peterson KA, et al. Lymphokine production and lymphocyte subpopulations in patients with head and neck squamous carcinoma. Arch Otolaryngol 1984;110:731–5.
58. Tan IB, Drehxage HA, Scheper RJ, et al. Immunosuppressive retroviral P15E-related factors in head and neck carcinomas. Arch Otolaryngol Head Neck Surg 1986;112:942–5.
59. Balm FJ, Von Blomberg-VanDeFlier BM, Drexhage HA, et al. Mononuclear phagocyte function in head and neck cancers: depression of murine macrophage accumulation by low molecular weight factors derived from head and neck carcinomas. Laryngoscope 1984;94:223–7.
60. Pierri I, Cordone G, Rogna S, et al. T-lymphocytes phenotype and functions in patients with head and neck cancer. Laryngoscope 1985;95:577–81.
61. Wolf GT, Schmaltz S, Hudson J, et al. Alterations in T-lymphocyte subpopulations in patients with head and neck cancer: correlations with prognosis. Arch Otolaryngol 1987;113:1200–6.
62. Herberman RB. Effects of biological response modifiers on effector cells with cytotoxic activity against tumors. Semin Oncol 1986;13: 195–9.
63. Wustrow TPU, Zenner HP. Natural killer cell activity in patients with carcinoma of the larynx and hypopharynx. Laryngoscope 1985;95:1391–1400.
64. Kessler D, Mickel R, Lichtenstein A. Depressed natural killer cell activity in cervical lymph nodes containing focal metastatic squamous cell carcinoma. Arch Otolaryngol Head Neck Surg 1988;114:313–8.
65. Stefani S, Kerman R, Abbate J. Serial studies of immunocompetence in head and neck cancer patients undergoing radiation therapy. Am J Roentgenol 1976;126:880–6.
66. Rafla S, Yang SJ, Melcka F. Changes in cell-mediated immunity in patients undergoing radiotherapy. Cancer 1978;41:1076–86.
67. Tarpley JL, Potvin C, Chretien PB. Prolonged depression of cellular immunity in cured laryngopharyngeal cancer patients treated with radiation therapy. Cancer 1975;35:638–44.
68. Stefani S. BCG and radiotherapy for head and neck carcinoma: a randomized controlled study—preliminary results. In Chretien PB, Wolf GT, eds. *International Head & Neck Oncology Research conference abstracts*. 9.13, 1980.
69. Cachin Y, Vandenbrouck C, Amiel JL, et al. Preliminary results of a randomized trial with BCG immunotherapy in laryngeal and hypopharyngeal carcinomas. In Chretien PB, Wolf GT, eds. *International Head & Neck Oncology Research conference abstracts*. 9.12, 1980.
70. Cortesina G, DeStefani A, Giovarelli M, et al. Treatment of recurrent squamous cell carcinoma of the head and neck with low doses of Interleukin-2 injected perilymphatically. Cancer 1988;62:2482–5.
71. Hong WK, Shapshay SM. Treatment of previously untreated stage III and IV squamous cell carcinoma of the head and neck. Otolaryngol Clin North Am 1980;13:521–8.
72. Spaulding C, Hahn SS, Constable WC. The effectiveness of treatment of lymph nodes in cancer of the pyriform sinus and supraglottis. Int J Radiat Oncol Biol Phys 1987;13:963–8.
73. Gordon RA, O'Brien E, Lipton A, Harvey HA, et al. Combined modality therapy of locally advanced stage IV squamous cell carcinoma of the head and neck. Proc Am Soc Clin Oncol 1985, vol. 4, Abstr C-527.
74. Phalguni M, Osman MR, Wajima T, et al. Combined modality therapy for previously untreated advanced squamous cell carcinoma of head and neck. Proc Am Soc Clin Oncol 1985, vol. 4, Abstract C-526.
75. Holoye PY, Grossman TW, Toohill RJ, et al. Randomized study of adjuvant chemotherapy for head and neck cancer. Otolaryngol Head Neck Surg 1985;93:712–7.
76. Stell PM, Dalby JE, Strickland P, et al. Sequential chemotherapy and radiotherapy in advanced head and neck cancer. In: Wigand ME, Steiner W, Stell PM, eds. *Functional partial laryngectomy: conservation surgery for carcinoma of the larynx*. Berlin: Springer-Verlag, 1984.
77. Martin SA, Marks JE, Lee JY, et al. Carcinoma of the pyriform sinus: predictors of TNM relapse and survival. Cancer 1980;4:1974–81.
78. Harrison DFN. Surgical management of hypopharyngeal cancer. Arch Otolaryngol 1979;105:149–52.
79. Razack MS, Sako K, Kalnins I. Squamous cell carcinoma of the pyriform sinus. Head Neck Surg 1978;1:31–4.
80. Wang CC, Schultz MD, Miller D. Combined radiation therapy and surgery for carcinoma of the supraglottis and pyriform sinus. Am J Surg 1972;124:551–4.

24

Near-Total Laryngectomy

Carl E. Silver, Idel I. Moisa

Near-total laryngectomy is a voice-preserving operation designed for the oncologic resection of selected, advanced, unilateral carcinomas involving the larynx.[1,2] Such tumors are usually treated with total laryngectomy, but when sufficiently localized to one side, an oncologically sound resection may be feasible with "true" hemilaryngectomy, including cricoid cartilage and superior tracheal rings, while preserving a portion of the uninvolved contralateral larynx. Cancers for which this procedure is generally indicated are too large for conventional conservation surgery, often being transglottic with invasion of the paraglottic space and fixation of the vocal cord. Such cancers may originate in the vocal cord or may fix the cord by extension from the ipsilateral subglottis, supraglottis, or pyriform fossa.

Near-total laryngectomy ablates one entire hemilarynx. The anterior portion of the contralateral vocal cord may be resected with the specimen when the primary tumor originates in the larynx while the entire contralateral vocal cord may be preserved for pyriform sinus carcinoma with minimal endolaryngeal involvement. Posteriorly, the operation extends beyond the arytenoid to the posterior commissure. Inferiorly, the resection includes the ipsilateral cricoid cartilage, thyroid lobe, and portions of the upper tracheal rings. Superiorly, the entire preepiglottic space, epiglottis, hyoid bone, and, if necessary, the valleculae are excised. On the uninvolved contralateral side, a segment of larynx is preserved, including the recurrent laryngeal nerve, posterior thyroid cartilage, arytenoid, and the contained section of thyroarytenoideus muscle.

Although the remaining laryngeal tissue is insufficient for reconstruction of an adequate airway, preservation of a myomucosal segment of intrinsic larynx along with its recurrent laryngeal nerve and arytenoid cartilage allows the creation of a "dynamic" tracheoesophageal shunt for preservation of voice. This mucosa-lined tube connects the trachea with the pharynx and can function as a neoglottis during expiration, allowing lung-powered voice production. Because the shunt is composed of endolaryngeal muscle innervated by the vagus nerve, sphincteric action during swallowing closes the shunt, thus preventing aspiration. Breathing is maintained by a permanent tracheotomy. The tracheotomy must be manually occluded to produce voice.

TERMINOLOGY

Although originally called an "extended hemilaryngectomy"[1] and subsequently termed a "subtotal laryngectomy,"[2] because of confusion with other surgical procedures bearing the same names, this procedure is now commonly referred to as "near-total laryngectomy (NTL)."[3–5] When applied to resection of hypopharyngeal (pyriform sinus) lesions, the term "near-total laryngopharyngectomy (NTLP)" is more specific.[6,7] In larger resections necessitating flap reconstruction of the pharynx, the name "extended near-total laryngopharyngectomy" has been suggested.[7]

INDICATIONS AND CONTRAINDICATIONS

Cancers that are oncologically encompassed by NTL include unilateral T_3 and T_4 laryngeal carcinomas, transglottic and pyriform sinus cancers (Table 24–1). On physiologic grounds, this procedure has been suggested instead of total laryngectomy for resection of tongue base and pharyngeal cancers requiring sacrifice of the larynx.[7,8]

Supraglottic carcinoma poses unique oncologic as well as physiologic dilemmas. Supraglottic laryngectomy may be oncologically feasible, but it may be physiologically contraindicated in some patients because of age, chronic lung disease, or the necessity of extending the resection into the tongue or pharynx. Although total laryngectomy is often recommended, NTL may have the advantage of preserving voice while diminishing the chance of developing uncontrollable aspiration.[7,8] In such patients, NTL may represent an alternative to supraglottic laryngectomy for smaller (T_1 and T_2) lesions as well.[8]

Extensive pyriform sinus carcinoma involving the aryepiglottic fold, tongue base, or tonsil, requiring pharyngectomy and

Table 24-1. Indications for NTL, NTLP, and Extended NTLP*

SITE	PEARSON AND KEITH[7]	DESANTO ET AL[8]	CHANDRACHUD ET AL[10]	SINGH AND HARDCASTLE[11]	TOTAL
Glottic	24		3	1	28
Transglottic	14		5	2	21
Supraglottic	32	28	3		63
Aryepiglottic fold	6				6
Subglottic	1				1
Pyriform fossa	24			1	25
Tongue base	5	1			6
Pharynx		8			8
Oral tongue	1				1
Thyroid with laryngotracheal invasion		1			1
Total	107	38	11	4	160

*NTL: near-total laryngectomy; NTLP: near-total laryngopharyngectomy.

flap reconstruction of the pharynx, does not represent a contraindication for NTL provided that the lesion is sufficiently localized to one side and one normal pyriform fossa can be preserved.[7]

Because one arytenoid and at least two thirds of the uninvolved cord must be preserved in order to create the vocal shunt, tumor involvement of the postcricoid area or interarytenoid region becomes the principal contraindications to this operation. The anterior portion of the opposite cord may be involved, but it must move normally and its arytenoid must be free of tumor.

Dumich et al[6] employed whole-organ sections to study the suitability of NTLP in carcinoma of the pyriform sinus. Although pyriform sinus carcinomas may involve the pyriform apex and paraglottic space, immobilize or involve the ipsilateral vocal cord, and invade the cricoid and thyroid cartilages, such findings do not necessarily represent oncologic reasons for removing uninvolved laryngeal tissues on the contralateral side. On the other hand, bilateral vocal cord fixation, postcricoid involvement, or extension across the interarytenoid area represent clear contraindications to NTLP. The value of preoperative assessment and frozen section monitoring in properly selecting patients for this procedure was emphasized. Robbins and Michaels[9] conducted a similar study of laryngeal cancers and noted comparable results. These authors concluded that NTL is a technically viable alternative for many patients who would otherwise undergo total laryngectomy.

The place of NTL for treatment of recurrent disease following radiation therapy is questionable. Total laryngectomy may be preferable in these cases because tumor margins may be obscure and the safety of preserving the contralateral arytenoid is uncertain.[5,7] NTL may be considered following radiation failure in cases treated when they were T_1 lesions but have become T_3 cancers when recurrence is recognized.[7] Although some authors are of the opinion that patients who have failed radiation therapy for supraglottic carcinoma are not considered candidates for NTL,[7] others have treated such patients successfully using this operation.[1,4]

Extralaryngeal spread does not represent a contraindication to NTL. When cervical metastases are present or suspected, a neck dissection may be performed before the laryngeal surgery begins.

Postoperative radiation therapy following NTL does not seem to have a deleterious effect on subsequent development of speech or deglutition.[8]

TECHNIQUE

The complex operative procedure has been described in detail by Pearson in previous publications.[1–3,7] The following description will outline the essential features of the operation. In the accompanying illustrations, resection of a right-sided transglottic carcinoma is demonstrated.

The ipsilateral (right) larynx is mobilized in the same manner as for total laryngectomy, with the thyroid lobe, prelaryngeal muscles, and adjacent lymphoareolar structures included in the resected specimen. On the contralateral (left) side, the larynx is skeletonized as for vertical hemilaryngectomy. The central portion of thyroid cartilage is outlined and will be removed (Fig. 24–1). This exposes the ventricular mucosal defect through which the larynx will be entered, at about the midportion of the contralateral vocal cord (Fig. 24–2) In resection of hypopharyngeal tumors that do not involve the endolarynx, the laryngotomy may be performed in the midline to preserve the entire contralateral mucosa. The mucosal incision is extended superiorly (Fig. 24–3) and inferiorly (Fig. 24–4) until the endolarynx is exposed and an adequate resection margin outlined (Fig. 24–5). The deep structures in the posterior midline, the interarytenoideus muscle and cricoid lamina are incised, with care not to injure the anterior hypopharyngeal mucosa (Fig. 24–6). Fracture of the cricoid lamina is facilitated by scoring the anterior perichondrium and by placing a finger in the hypopharynx, as shown. The specimen, consisting of the entire right hemilarynx, with the tumor and adequate mucosal margins is now excised (Fig. 24–7). Since the entire paraglottic space has been included, adequate extirpation of transglottic carcinoma is achieved.

The reconstructive phase of the procedure commences with submucosal dissection and piecemeal removal of a sufficient

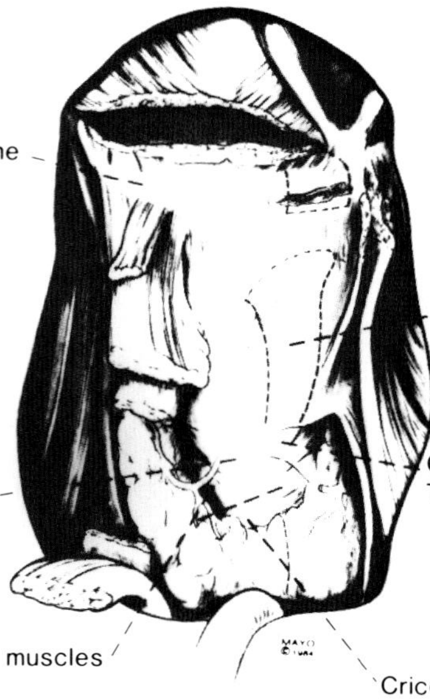

Figure 24–1. Near-total laryngectomy: Right hemilarynx mobilized as for total laryngectomy with laryngeal adnexae, including prelaryngeal muscles and thyroid lobe. The left side has been skeletonized, with prelaryngeal muscles divided near their insertion on the hyoid bone, in order to preserve them. The (central) portion of left thyroid cartilage, to be removed, is outlined. (From Pearson.[3] Reprinted with permission.)

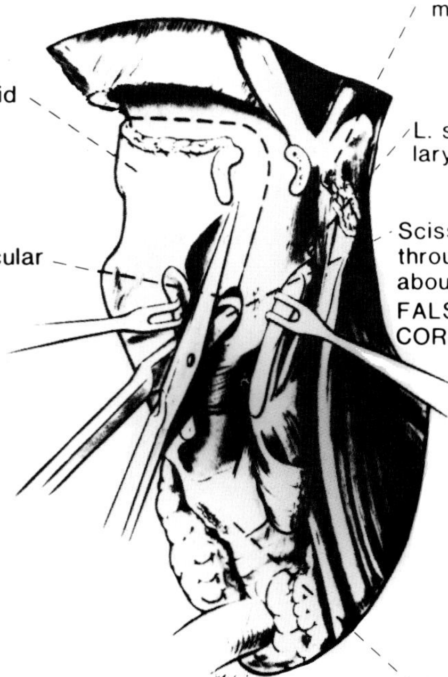

Figure 24–2. After division of the thyroid isthmus, a tracheostomy is placed through the third tracheal ring. The thyroid lobe is separated from the laryngotracheal complex with preservation of the recurrent laryngeal nerve. Removal of the central portion of thyroid cartilage exposes the ventricle, where laryngeal entry is made. (From Pearson.[3] Reprinted with permission.)

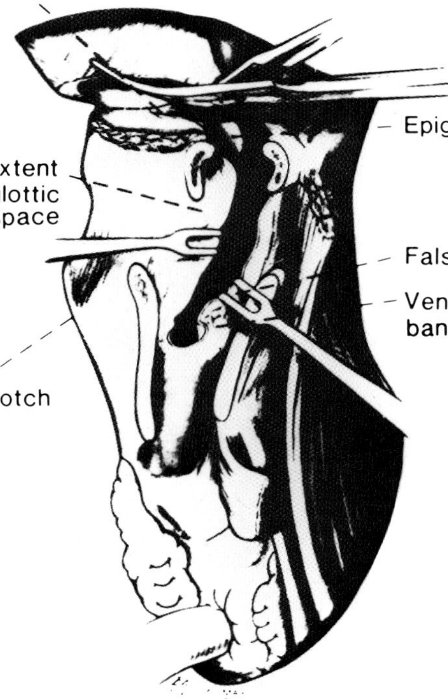

Figure 24–3. Laryngotomy is extended superiorly through the false vocal cord and medially through the valleculae. (From Pearson.[3] Reprinted with permission.)

amount of residual (left) cricoid cartilage to permit tubing of the subglottic mucosa (Fig. 24–8). The defect in the right pyriform sinus is sutured as far as the reflection of postcricoid mucosa (Fig. 24–9). In most cases of endolaryngeal tumor, there will be insufficient laryngeal mucosa remaining to form a shunt of adequate diameter (the mucosal tube should accommodate a 14 F–5 mm diameter–catheter). The mucosa available for tubing may be augmented by rotating a flap of pyriform sinus mucosa inferiorly, where it is sutured to the remaining laryngeal mucosa (Fig. 24–10). This newly constructed mucosal structure, with its overlying muscle, is rolled into a tube and sutured, using the 14 F catheter as a temporary template (Fig. 24–11). After closure of the remaining pharyngeal defect, a second layer is provided by suture of the preserved left infrahyoid to suprahyoid musculature. An anterior wall tracheotomy, placed through the third tracheal ring, is "matured" by suture to the skin. The resulting configuration is shown in sagittal section in Figure 24–12.

ADVANTAGES AND DISADVANTAGES

This operation has several advantages over total laryngectomy and subsequent voice rehabilitation procedures. Pearson noted that the ease and quality of speech through the biologic shunt created by NTL surpass those forms of fistula voice in which the upper esophageal sphincter is the vibrating source.[2] This observation, although subjective, has recently received some sub-

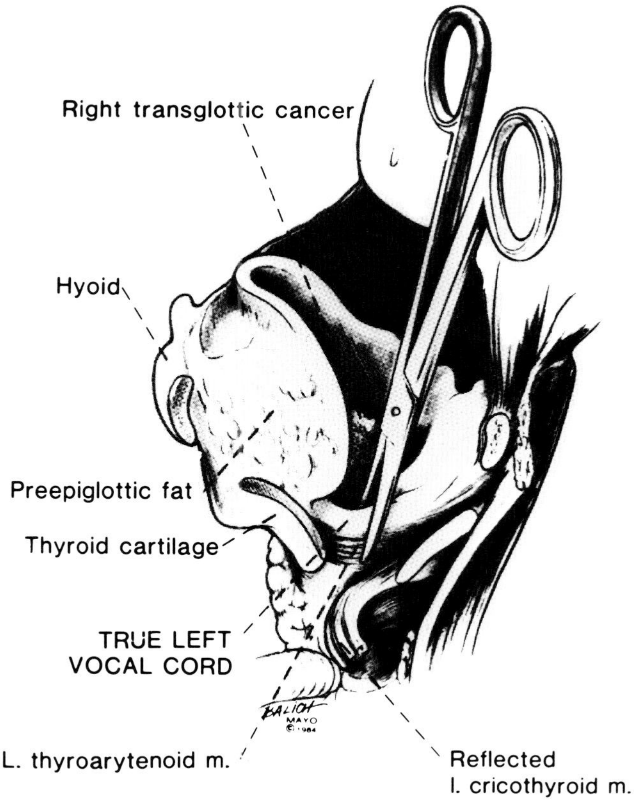

Figure 24–4. Inferiorly, the laryngotomy extends through the true vocal cord and subglottic region. (From Pearson.[3] Reprinted with permission.)

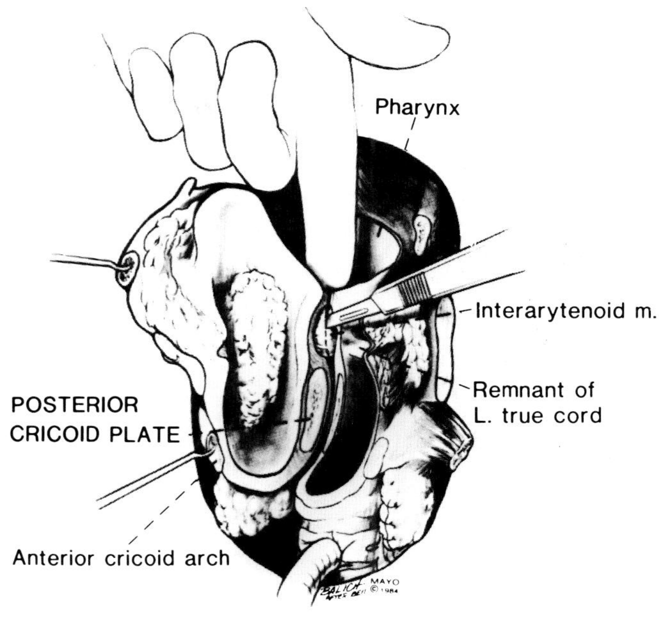

Figure 24–6. The deep structures in the posterior midline are bisected. Fracture of the cricoid lamina contributes greatly to liberation of the specimen from the portions of larynx to be preserved. (From Pearson.[3] Reprinted with permission.)

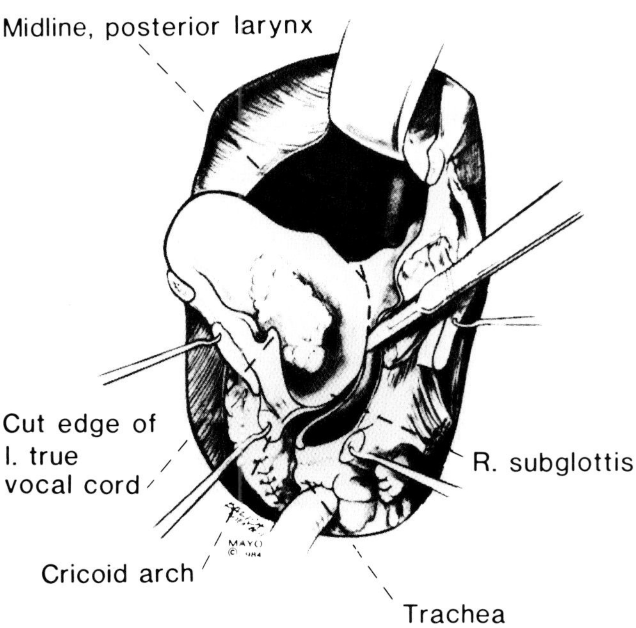

Figure 24–5. Subglottic mucosal incision is carried to the posterior midline, providing an adequate resection margin. (From Pearson.[3] Reprinted with permission.)

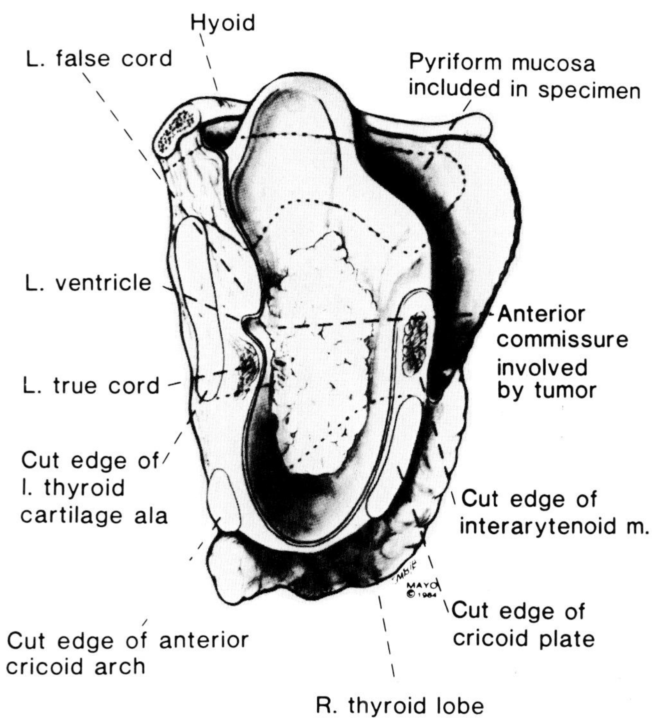

Figure 24–7. The surgical specimen has adequate mucosal margins and includes the entire paraglottic space. (From Pearson.[3] Reprinted with permission.)

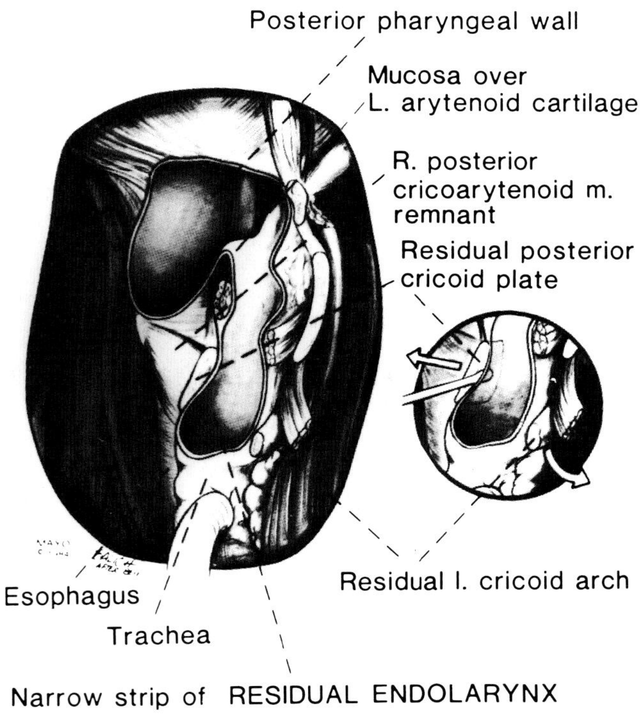

Figure 24–8. The residual cricoid plate is dissected submucosally and removed sufficiently to permit tubing of the segment. The intrinsic laryngeal musculature, cricothyroid muscle, and recurrent nerve of the laryngeal remnant are preserved. (From Pearson.[3] Reprinted with permission.)

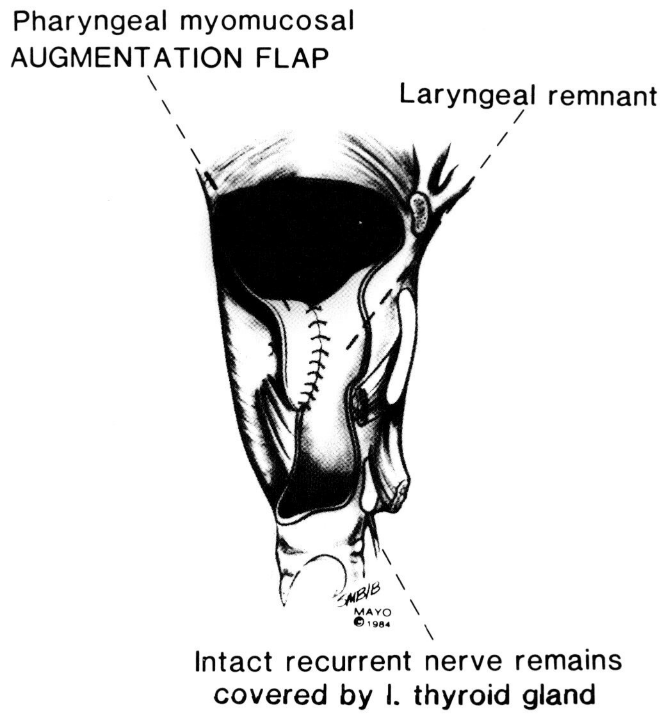

Figure 24–10. The pharyngeal augmentation flap is sutured to the mucosa of laryngeal remnant. (From Pearson.[3] Reprinted with permission.)

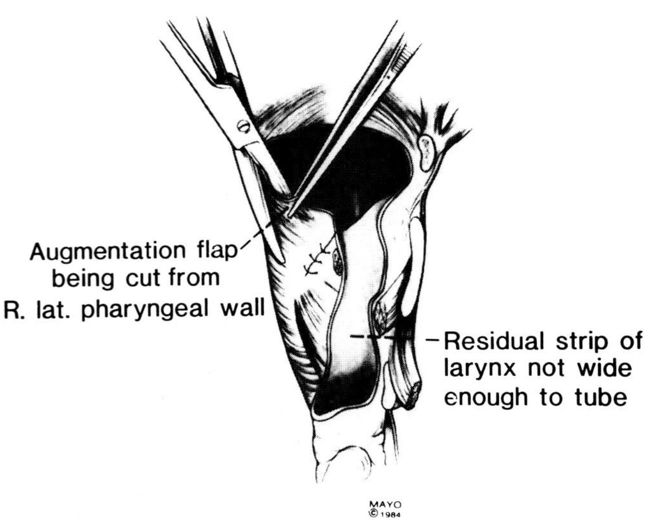

Figure 24–9. The pyriform sinus mucosa has been closed as far as the mucosal reflection of laryngeal remnant. An incision in the right lateral pharyngeal wall will create a flap of pyriform sinus mucosa that may be rotated inferiorly to augment the diameter of the tube that will be formed. (From Pearson.[3] Reprinted with permission.)

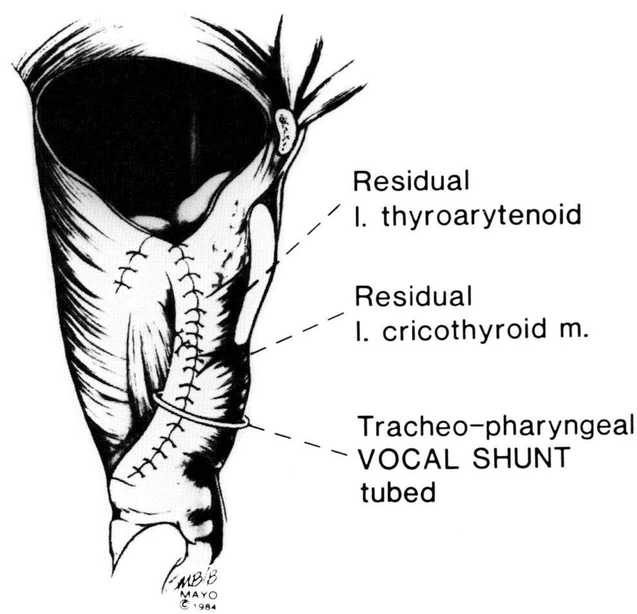

Figure 24–11. The myomucosal segment is now tubed by suture over a 14 F catheter. The catheter is not left in situ as a stent; it is removed after the tube has been fashioned. The tubed segment contains a mucosal lining as well as innervated portions of intrinsic laryngeal and cricothryoid muscle in its wall. (From Pearson.[3] Reprinted with permission.)

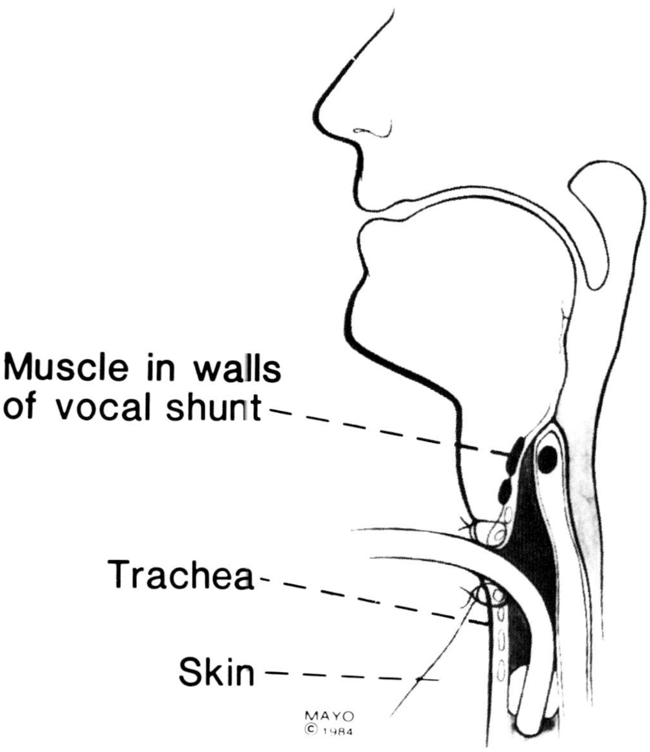

Figure 24–12. The sagittal section demonstrates tracheostomy and shunt in relation to pharyngeal mucosa. Occlusion of the tracheostomy with a finger will force exhaled air into the pharynx, producing voice. During swallowing, the innervated muscular wall of the shunt contracts, occluding the tube and thus preventing aspiration of food and liquids. The retained arytenoid cartilage helps in achieving watertight closure during deglutition. (From Pearson.[3] Reprinted with permission.)

stantiation and will be discussed later in this chapter. Another advantage of NTL is that since the shunt is epithelialized, it is stable and cannot quickly close.[2] In addition, since there is no prosthesis to care for, the NTL shunt is reliable and maintenance free.

This somewhat greater complexity of this procedure as well as the longer operative time (usually 30 to 60 minutes), compared to total laryngectomy, have been the chief disadvantages of NTL.[7]

RESULTS OF NEAR-TOTAL LARYNGECTOMY

Cure Rates

The local control rate of NTL appears to match that of total laryngectomy.[7] In a review from the Mayo Clinic, representing the largest experience with NTL to date, Pearson and Keith[7] reported an overall 3-year cure rate in 35 (53%) of 66 patients. If nine patients who died of causes unrelated to their laryngeal cancer are excluded, an overall cure rate of 61% was achieved.

Cure and recurrence rates for individual sites reported in this and other studies cited here are summarized in Tables 24–2 and 24–3. It is noteworthy that local recurrence was the cause of death in only two of the patients reported by Pearson and Keith; both had failed radiation therapy for supraglottic carcinoma. Distant metastases accounted for the highest number of deaths (8 of 20) in the patients with hypopharyngeal tumors.

Another report from the same institution involved 39 patients operated on between 1980 and 1985. Twenty-five (64%) demonstrated no recurrences and 13 (33%) died of their disease (Table 24–2).[8]

Chandrachud et al[10] reported no deaths and no local recurrences among 11 patients who underwent NTL between 1983 and 1987, although one patient developed cervical metastasis requiring neck dissection. Four patients in this series (two T_3N_0 supraglottic and two T_3N_0 transglottic) were radiation failures. Singh and Hardcastle[11] reported good short-term oncologic results in their series of four patients.

Voice Production

Voice production following NTL requires that the shunt walls be sufficiently healed so that air is not prevented, by postoperative edema, from entering the pharynx when the stoma is occluded.[7] Although an occasional patient may attain speech as early as the second postoperative week, the establishment of good fistula speech usually requires a longer period of healing and education. A dedicated speech pathologist is invaluable during this

Table 24-2. Cure Rates

STUDY	NO. PATIENTS	FOLLOW-UP OR STUDY PERIOD	CURE RATE BY SITE		CURE RATE OVERALL
Pearson and Keith[7]	66	3 years	Transglottic, glottic, and subglottic	20/29	53% (35/66)
			Supraglottic	8/17	
			Hypopharynx	7/20	
DeSanto et al[8]	39	1980-1985	Supraglottic		67% (26/39)
Chandrachud et al[10]	11	1983-1987	Transglottic	5/5	100% (11/11)
			Glottic	3/3	
			Supraglottic	3/3	
Singh and Hardcastle[11]	4	0.3-1.3 years	Transglottic	2/2	100% (4/4)
			Pyriform fossa	1/1	
			T_3 glottic	1/1	

Table 24-3. Recurrence Following NTL

STUDY	NO.	SITE	NONE	LOCAL	NECK	DISTANT	UNRELATED CANCER
Pearson and Keith[7]	29	Glottic, transglottic, subglottic	20	0	4	2	3
	17	Supraglottic	8	2	3	1	3
	20	Hypopharynx	7	0	2	8	3
DeSanto et al[8]	28	Supraglottic	19	3	3	3	
	8	Pharynx	5	1	0	2	
	2	Tongue	0	0	0	2	
	1	Thyroid	1	0	0	0	
Chandrachud et al[10]	11		10	0	1	0	
Singh and Hardcastle[11]	4		4	0	0	0	

phase and often an interim means of communication, such as an electrolarynx, may be required. As previously mentioned, voice production usually requires finger occlusion of the stoma. Alternatively, patients may be fitted with adhesive expiratory stomal valves, designed originally for tracheoesophageal puncture protheses.

Results of NTL have been most encouraging, with regard to the quality of voice as well the number of patients who have been able to achieve fistula speech (Table 24–4). Shunt dilation may sometimes be required to achieve or enhance voice.[7] Postoperative radiation therapy following NTL does not seem to have a deleterious effect on subsequent speech or deglutition.[8]

Several authors have described the laryngoscopic appearance following NTL.[7,10] The upper end of the shunt flutters and vibrates during phonation; it closes on swallowing, thereby preventing aspiration.

Singh[12] used electrolaryngography to study the site and mechanism of phonatory function of the neoglottis in eight patients who had undergone NTL. Substantial similarities were demonstrated in the functional nature of the neoglottis compared with the normal glottis. The resultant wave patterns revealed that the neoglottis not only controls airflow through it, but also acts as a source of vibration, similar to the normal vocal cords. In a subsequent report, Singh[13] discussed the utility of this modality for speech rehabilitation in patients following NTL.

Trudeau[14] studied the acoustical characteristics in a single patient who had undergone a NTL 4 years previously. Marked similarities were noted in the frequency, intensity, and timing of this patient's speech when compared with that of a patient judged to have acquired excellent tracheoesophageal speech using a Blom-Singer prosthesis for the same period of time. The study also suggested that the reconstructed valve offered little resistance to expiratory air and still prevented aspiration.

Videofluoroscopic studies by Chandrachud et al[10] demonstrated a distinct narrowing of the pharyngoesophageal segment above the myomucosal shunt. Based on this observation, these authors regard the pharyngoesophageal segment, rather than the neoglottis, to be the site of voice production following NTL.

Stomal pressures measured in NTL patients who have achieved successful speech average 25 ± 6 cm H_2O at threshold, and 32 ± 20 cm H_2O during phonation. In comparison, normal subjects with an intact larynx generate subglottic pressures of approximately 10 ± 5 cm H_2O. For speech to occur at physiologic airway pressures, the shunt diameter must be greater than 6 mm.[15]

COMPLICATIONS OF NTL

Aspiration and shunt stenosis are the major complications of NTL (Table 24–5). Although infrequent, aspiration is the more common. Pearson and Keith[7] reported serious aspiration in 8 of 66 patients, most of whom were subsequently corrected without sacrificing speech. Singh and Hardcastle[11] encountered no aspiration in four patients. Chandrachud et al[10] described one instance of aspiration and one of stenosis among a series of 11 patients.

In addition to the evidence previously cited there is some indirect information based on dye studies suggesting that the NTL shunt is dynamic and functions to prevent aspiration.[7]

THE AUTHORS' EXPERIENCE

During the period from 1986 through 1989, seven patients at the Montefiore Medical Center were believed, on the basis of preoperative imaging and endoscopy, to be suitable candidates for NTL and were explored with the intention of performing that

Table 24-4. Voice Production Following NTL

STUDY	SATISFACTORY FISTULA VOICE
Pearson et al,[7] 1989	82% (54/66)
DeSanto et al,[8] 1989	74% (29/39)
Chandrachud et al,[10] 1989	91% (10/11)
Singh,[12] 1987	100% (8/8)*

*Starting on postoperative day 8 to 10.

Table 24-5. Complications Following NTL

STUDY	ASPIRATION (SEVERE OR TRANSIENT)	STENOSIS
Pearson and Keith[7]	8/66	6/66
DeSanto et al[8]	6/39	
Chandrachud et al[10]	1/11	1/11
Singh and Hardcastle[11]	0/4	0/4

procedure. After laryngotomy through the contralateral ventricle, as already described, the procedure was converted to a total laryngectomy in three instances. These included one supraglottic and two transglottic carcinomas. In these cases the narrow resection margins attainable in order to preserve sufficient tissue for the dynamic shunt, while suitable for a true "conservation" type operation, were thought to be insufficient in proportion to the amount of laryngeal tissue that had to be sacrificed for resection of these large tumors.

NTL was completed in four patients; two had transglottic carcinomas, and two had hypopharyngeal tumors that could be resected with preservation of the entire contralateral hemilarynx. One patient required a pectoralis major myocutaneous flap for replacement of lateral hypo- and oropharyngeal wall. Two patients are alive and free of disease 6 months and 4 years after surgery. One, with transglottic carcinoma, developed recurrence 1 year after the operation; the contralateral resection margin had been reported as "close," and the patient had been treated with postoperative irradiation. The patient with the large hypopharyngeal tumor that required myocutaneous flap reconstruction died with both local-regional and distant metastatic disease. NTL had been chosen for that patient because of minimal laryngeal involvement with an otherwise extensive tumor; resection (and the outcome) had not been compromised by preservation of a portion of the larynx.

Two patients developed satisfactory shunt voice that was considered superior to esophageal voice, or to that obtainable with a prosthesis. One patient required dilation of his shunt, following which aspiration became a problem. This was solved by insertion of a "Shapiro" type periscope prosthesis into the fistula; this type of prosthesis fits almost perfectly into the tracheopharyngeal shunt created by the NTL operation. Following this, the patient had satisfactory voice and deglutition until his death from cancer. The fourth patient was never able to generate voice with his shunt, but developed excellent esophageal speech in the early postoperative period. As a result, no effort was made to dilate the shunt.

In commenting on this personal experience, we note that it is minute compared with that of the Mayo Clinic group, but may be significant in comparison with that of other institutions, where the procedure is never performed. Differing philosophies with regard to selection of patients are an obvious factor. Surgeons who strongly favor conservation surgery may prefer the latter for some lesions that might be eminently suitable for NTL. The same may apply in institutions where radiation therapy is employed as initial treatment for all but the most advanced laryngeal tumors.

Our experience of proceeding with total laryngectomy rather than NTL in almost half the operations attempted, as well as the indifferent oncologic results obtained, are perhaps reflective of our selection of patients with relatively advanced tumors for this operation, which, in turn, probably accounts for the small number of cases in our series.

CONCLUSIONS

NTL is a useful procedure for resection of large unilateral laryngeal and hypopharyngeal tumors, with preservation of a natural phonatory neoglottis. Results reported by groups with the largest experience are comparable to those achieved by total laryngectomy for the same disease, and voice achieved is easier to produce and superior in quality to esophageal voice or that generated with a prosthesis. Despite these facts, the operation has not gained widespread popularity, as is evident from the relatively small experience reported in the literature. This may partly be due to the technical difficulty of the procedure, as well as preference for either extended conservation surgery, irradiation, or, perhaps most often, the proven benefits of total laryngectomy performed with simultaneous or subsequent tracheoesophageal puncture and prosthesis if desired. The authors' small personal experience is reflective of these trends.

REFERENCES

1. Pearson BW, Woods RD, Hartman DE. Extended hemilaryngectomy for T_3 glottic carcinoma with preservation of speech and swallowing. Laryngoscope 1980;90:1950–61.
2. Pearson BW. Subtotal laryngectomy. Laryngoscope 1981;91:1904–12.
3. Pearson BW. Near-total laryngectomy. In: Silver CE, ed. *Atlas of head and neck surgery,* New York: Churchill Livingstone, 1986:235–51.
4. Pearson BW. The theory and techniques of near-total laryngectomy. In: Bailey BJ, Biller, HF, eds. *Surgery of the larynx.* New York: WB Saunders, 1985:336–46.
5. Donald PJ, Pearson BW. The larynx. In: Donald PJ, ed. *Head and neck cancer—management of the difficult case.* New York: WB Saunders, 1984.
6. Dumich PS, Pearson BW, Weiland LH. Suitability of near-total laryngopharyngectomy in pyriform carinoma. Arch Otolaryngol 1984;110:664–9.
7. Pearson BW, Keith RL. Near-Total Laryngectomy. In: Johnson JJ, Blitzer A, Ossoff RH, Thomas JR, eds. *American Academy of Otolaryngology-Head and Neck Surgery, Instructional courses,* vol. 2. St. Louis: CV Mosby, 1989:309–30.
8. DeSanto LW, Pearson BP, Olsen KD. Utility of near-total laryngectomy for supraglottic, pharyngeal, base-of-tongue, and other cancers. Ann Otol Rhinol Laryngol 1989;98:2–7.
9. Robbins KT, Michaels L. Feasibility of subtotal laryngectomy based on whole-organ examination. Arch Otolaryngol 1985;111:356–60.
10. Chandrachud HR, Chaurasia MK, Sinha KP. Subtotal laryngectomy with myomucosal shunt. J Laryngol Otol 1989;103:504–7.
11. Singh W, Hardcastle P. Near-total laryngectomy with myomucosal valved neoglottis. J Laryngol Otol 1985;99:581–8.
12. Singh W. Electrolaryngography in near-total laryngectomy with myomucosal valved neoglottis. J Laryngol Otol 1987;101:815–8.
13. Singh W. Clinical application of electrolaryngograph for speech rehabilitation in near-total laryngectomy with myomucosal valved neoglottis. J Laryngol Otol 1988;102:335–6.
14. Trudeau MD. Acoustical characteristics of speech following Pearson's subtotal laryngectomy: a case study. Folia Phoniatr 1987;39:178–82.
15. Woods RW, Pearson BW. Alaryngeal speech and the development of an internal tracheopharyngeal fistula. Otolaryngol Head Neck Surg 1980;88:64–73.

25

Management of Stomal Recurrence

Jordan S. Josephson, Yosef P. Krespi

Stomal recurrence is a dreaded complication in the management of laryngeal carcinoma and continues to result in poor survival rates. Radical en bloc dissection of the stoma, with a wide, deep border, including mediastinal dissection, yields the most promising chance of cure.[1] Death may be related to the recurrent disease, but in a significant number of patients it is related to surgical complications, including sepsis and great vessel rupture. Ultimate survival rates may be enhanced by diminution of these complications, thus decreasing morbidity and mortality.

The incidence of stomal recurrence ranges from 5 to 15% in most series.[2–6] Etiologic factors of stomal recurrence that have been implicated include the location of the primary tumor, the size of the primary tumor, and whether a preliminary tracheotomy was performed before the definitive resection. Inadequate resection of the tumor with positive margins, residual disease in the paratracheal nodes, and subglottic extension also may predispose to this potentially devastating recurrence.

Since the results of treatment have been poor, efforts at prevention have been discussed by many authors and seem to be promising. Hoover and King[7] reported the use of "emergency laryngectomy" for obstructing laryngeal carcinoma in an attempt to decrease the risk of implantation of viable tumor cells into the raw and granulating bed of a recent tracheostomy. Harris and Butler[8] advocated complete resection of the paratracheal and mediastinal lymph nodes for patients with subglottic or pyriform apex tumors. Schneider et al[9] employed postoperative irradiation, including the tracheal stomas, with favorable results.

Results of treatment of stomal recurrence have been poor. Sisson et al[5] in 1977 reported a 17% 5-year survival rate. Gluckman et al[10] 10 years later reported the overall 2-year survival rate for operated patients to be 16% with a 24% determinate survival. On further analysis of this study, however, surgery for early disease (types I and II) resulted in a 45% 5-year survival rate, with relatively low morbidity and mortality. Excellent palliation was achieved in those who failed to survive 2 years. In more advanced cases (types III and IV) surgery failed to produce acceptable survival, and perioperative morbidity was extremely high.

Nevertheless, radical surgery provides the best chance of cure. Various other modalities, including radiotherapy, chemotherapy, and a combination of both have been employed as palliative measures, but without predictable results.[11]

The concept of radical resection of stomal recurrence was stimulated by Sisson's work.[1,12] He stressed the importance of great vessel protection by employing the pectoralis muscle flap to obliterate the operative defect in the mediastinum and to act as a barrier between the trachea and the innominate artery. He later described staged techniques and emphasized the importance of proper flap selection. However, these staged techniques required elaborate planning and precise execution. The morbidity associated with these multiple staged procedures and the resultant increased hospital stay and associated mortality is well documented in the literature.

The pectoralis major myocutaneous flap has been advocated by Biller et al.[13,14] It is a one-stage procedure that provides good coverage of the great vessels with well-vascularized muscle tissue. The muscle mass also obliterates the mediastinal dead space. The donor site is closed primarily and skin and dermal grafts are not required.

CLASSIFICATION

Stomal recurrences are classified into four types (Fig. 25–1). Type I lesions are localized and usually present as a discrete nodule in the superior aspect of the stoma. These lesions do not involve the esophagus. Type II lesions are localized to the superior aspect of the stoma, but involve the esophagus. Type III lesions originate from the inferior aspect of the stoma and involve the superior mediastinum. Type IV lesions have lateral extension beneath both clavicles and into the superior mediastinum.

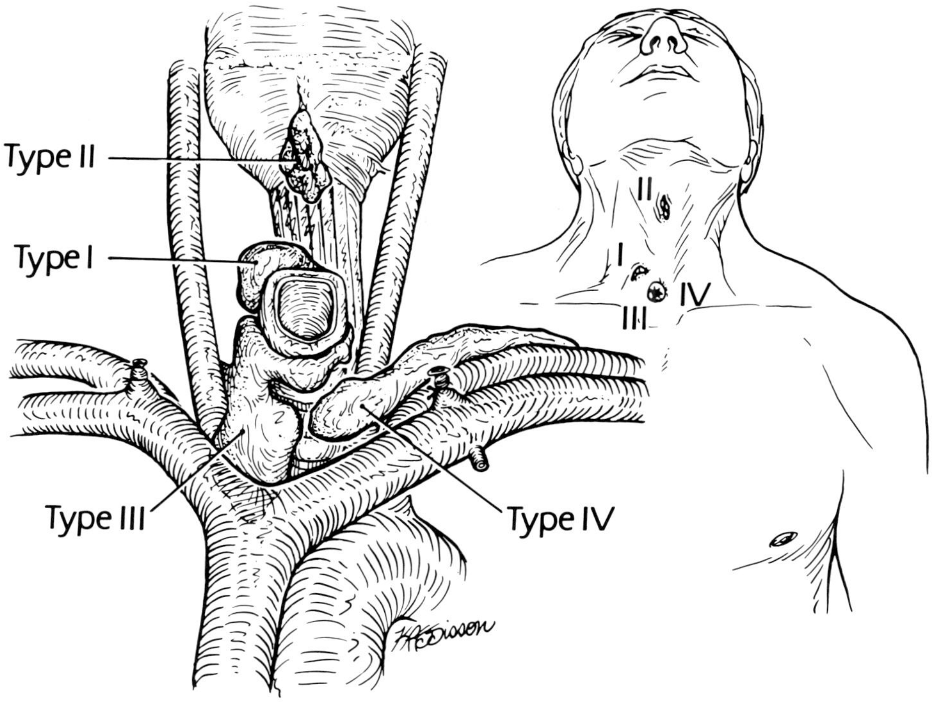

Figure 25–1. Classification of stomal recurrence.

SURGICAL TECHNIQUES

The operation is performed with the patient in the supine position. Figure 25–2 shows a type II lesion involving the esophagus. The tracheal stoma with the area of tumor involvement and a minimum of a 3 cm skin margin is excised. The cuts in the manubrium are made with an oscillating saw. The underlying structures are protected from the saw by a periosteal elevator that is placed between the posterior periosteum of the manubrium and the bone (Fig. 25–3). The dissection may be as far lateral as to include the sternal ends of the clavicles and the upper portion of the manubrium, which is then removed to permit en bloc resection of the involved tracheal stoma and to provide access for the superior mediastinal dissection and lymphadenectomy.

After removal of the manubrium, the posterior periosteum of the manubrium is carefully incised. The innominate artery and vein are identified. The node-bearing fat pad of the upper mediastinum is dissected, exposing all the great vessels. These vessels represent the greatest potential hazard for intraoperative catastrophe; on the left, the aorta and common carotid, and on the right, the innominate and carotid arteries. The surgical field should be inspected to determine that the tumor does not involve the great vessels. If they are uninvolved, the tumor is resectable. Ligation and transection of the innominate vein may be necessary for better visualization and also makes a lower tracheostoma possible. Other authors recommend resecting the clavicle, the first three ribs, and the upper third of the sternum, but the final resection must be dictated by the size of the lesion. The contents of the superior mediastinum are swept superiorly to connect with the neck dissection specimen. On the left side,

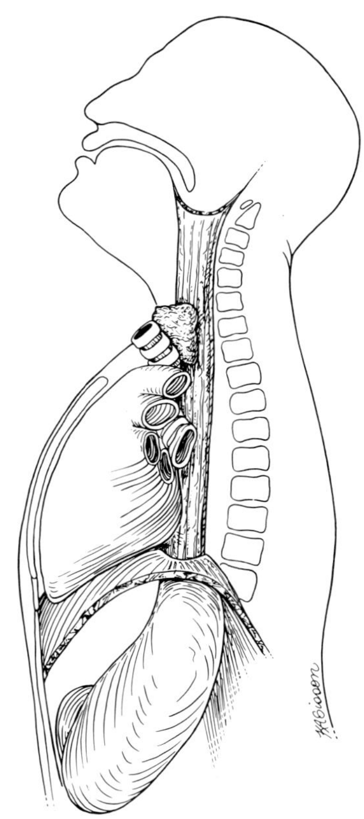

Figure 25–2. Type II lesion showing involvement of esophagus.

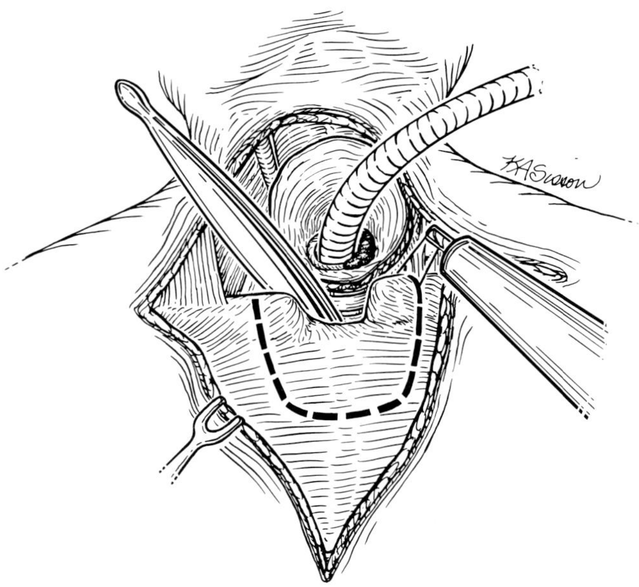

Figure 25–3. The cuts are made by oscillating saw in the manubrium. A periosteal elevator is placed between the posterior periosteum and the manubrium to protect the underlying structures.

the thoracic duct must be identified and preserved when possible. If damaged, it must be carefully ligated. Low paratracheal and tracheoesophageal nodes are also included with the specimen. The remainder of the thyroid gland should be removed. Since this may result in hypoparathyroidism, it is important to check calcium levels postoperatively.

The defect created after resection of a type I lesion (no pharyngeal involvement) is depicted in Figure 25–4. In the past, deltopectoral and pectoralis muscle flaps were utilized for reconstruction of this defect. More recently, use of the pectoralis major myocutaneous flap has decreased considerably the morbidity and mortality associated with this surgery.[11–13]

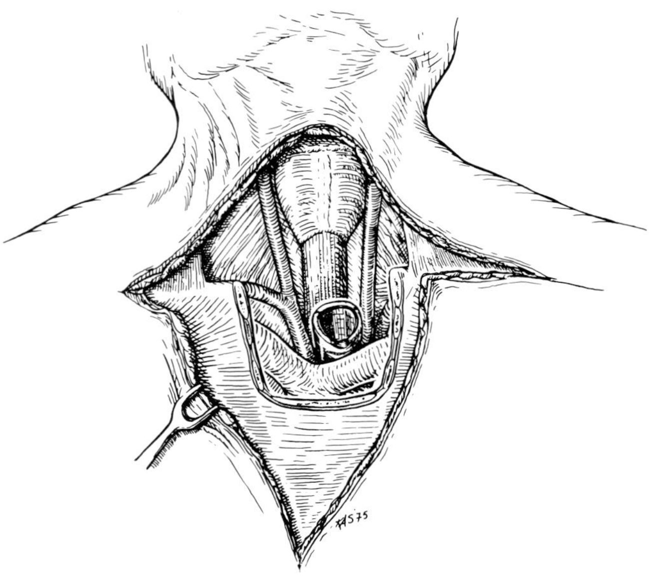

Figure 25–4. The defect created after a type I lesion has been removed.

The pectoralis major myocutaneous flap is usually developed from the right side because this facilitates its placement between the trachea and innominate artery. The flap must be designed to both protect the great vessels and obliterate the mediastinal dead space. The skin island is devised to conform to the surgical defect (Fig. 25–5). A circumferential incision is made and continued through the subcutaneous tissue to the pectoralis major muscle. The entire muscle is exposed by elevating medial and lateral chest flaps. Next, the skin is sutured to the underlying pectoralis major muscle to protect it from separating from the underlying muscle.

The lateral edge of the muscle is identified and separated from the chest wall. The myocutaneous flap is elevated superiorly and the lateral thoracic artery and pectoral branch of the thoracoacromial artery are easily identified. On the deep surface of the muscle, the tendinous insertion to the humerus is severed. The lateral thoracic artery is saved when possible but may be ligated if it limits the rotation arc. A large subcutaneous tunnel is made under the skin bridge between the neck and chest incisions. The flap is passed beneath the skin bridge and placed appropriately into the cervicomediastinal defect, where the skin is sutured to the cutaneous margins of the cervical defect and to the trachea.

The island skin can be designed in two ways. When the cutaneous defect following stomal resection is primarily superior to the stoma, as is often the case with types I or II lesions, the

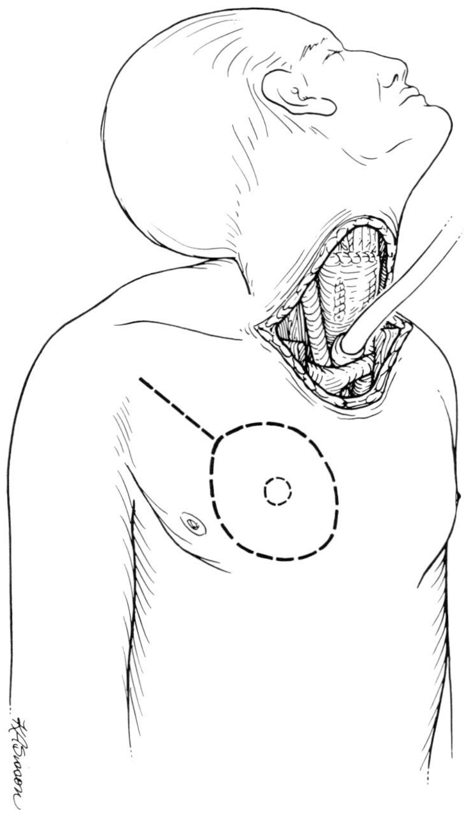

Figure 25–5. The skin island flap is designed.

skin island is designed in a semilunar shape. The myocutaneous flap covers the surgical defect above and at both sides of the stoma. The inferior margin of the new stoma is sutured to the upper chest skin. Resection of a type III stomal recurrence will often result in an extensive circumferential defect around the tracheal stump. The new stoma is placed in the center of the skin island, resulting in the "donut" shaped paddle demonstrated in Figure 25–6. A 1.5 to 2 cm skin ellipse is excised from the center of the skin island, and the subcutaneous tissue and muscle are bluntly spread to permit insertion and suturing of the trachea. In both methods, most of the pectoralis muscle is placed between the trachea and the great vessels. The chest donor defect is closed primarily (Fig. 25–7).

Lesions involving the cervical esophagus require esophagectomy with immediate reconstruction. The technique of blunt extrathoracic total esophagectomy with replacement by transposition of the stomach through the posterior mediastinum is most suitable for this (This technique, its applications and results, are discussed in detail by Professor Harrison in Chapter 28). Following resection of the proximal trachea, the common tracheoesophageal wall is exposed. The posterior tracheal wall is bluntly dissected from the esophagus. Tears at the posterior tracheal wall must be avoided by careful dissection. Once the tumor and upper esophagus are mobilized and a tumor-free tracheal stump is obtained, the lesion is determined to be fully resectable and suitable for gastric "pull-up" reconstruction (Fig. 25–8).

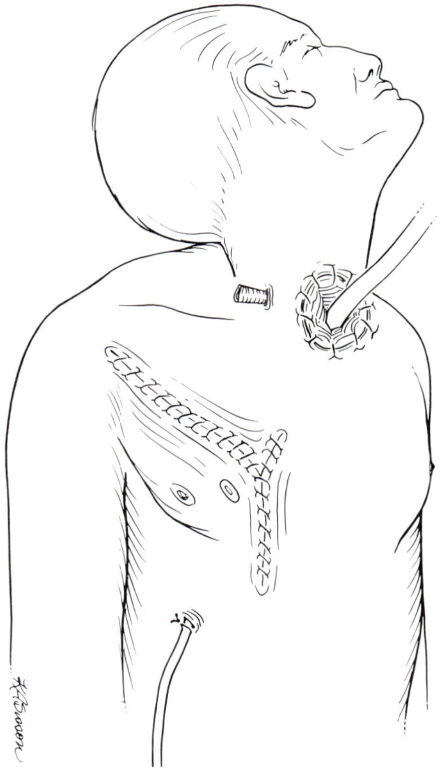

Figure 25–7. The skin island is sutured in place with the center of the "donut" forming the new tracheal stoma. The defect at the chest donor site is closed primarily.

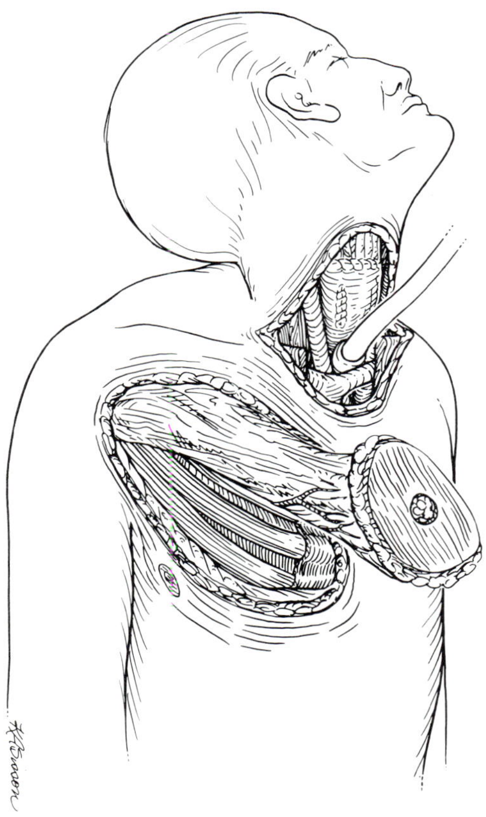

Figure 25–6. The new stoma is placed in the center of the skin island after the myocutaneous flap is raised.

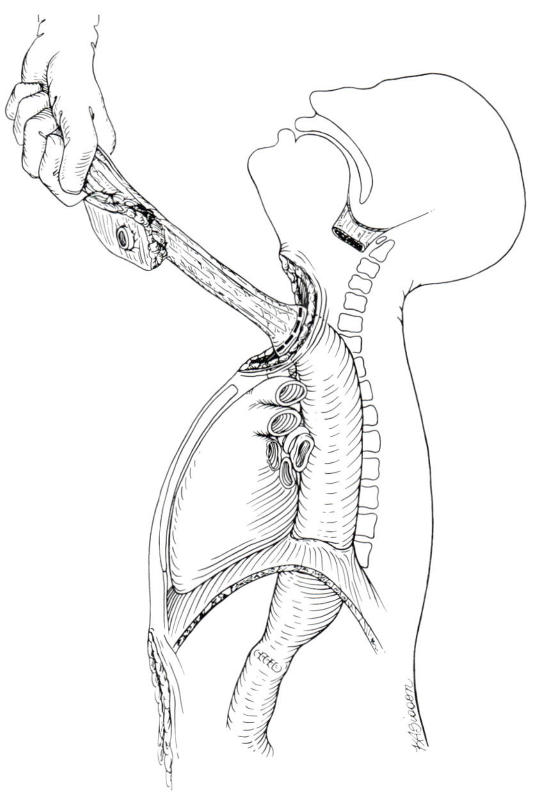

Figure 25–8. After the tumor and upper esophagus are mobilized, gastric pull-up reconstruction is performed.

The abdominal surgical teams enter the abdomen via a long midline incision. The stomach is mobilized, preserving the right gastric and gastroepiploic vessels. The left gastric and gastroepiploic vessels are ligated. The short gastric arteries are ligated. The surgeon must carefully protect the spleen with abdominal pads during this part of the procedure. A wide Kocher maneuver is performed to mobilize the duodenum. The esophageal hiatus is enlarged and both vagus nerves are clipped and transected. Pyloroplasty is mandatory in order to avoid gastric outlet obstruction.

Using sharp and blunt dissection, the esophagus is mobilized circumferentially in the posterior mediastinum. After complete mobilization of the esophagus, superiorly from the neck and inferiorly from the abdomen, the specimen is pulled up through the neck. The esophagus is then divided at the cardioesophageal junction with a stapler and the fundus of the stomach is positioned to create a gastropharyngeal anastomosis. Single layer, nonabsorbable sutures are used. A needle jejunostomy is created. The abdominal cavity is closed in layers in the usual fashion.

After completion of the gastropharyngeal anastomosis, the skin defect is measured and an appropriate sized pectoralis major myocutaneous flap is elevated as already described (Fig. 25–9).

Other options of reconstruction are available, although the described procedure is preferred by us. Esophageal involvement may require partial or total esophagectomy. A proximal pharyngostome (or blind pharyngeal pouch) and distal esophagostome may be formed. This is not ideal, but may be considered, if the patient's medical condition is not optimal for a long procedure. Later, second-stage esophageal reconstruction may be performed. Primary reconstruction with a previously prepared contralateral "Janus" pectoralis myocutaneous flap is another alternative.[15] A jejunal and rectus abdominal free-flap are other alternatives. These require surgical expertise with microvascular free flap techniques. The option chosen will depend on the extent of the lesion, the patient's medical condition, and the surgeon's skill and preference.

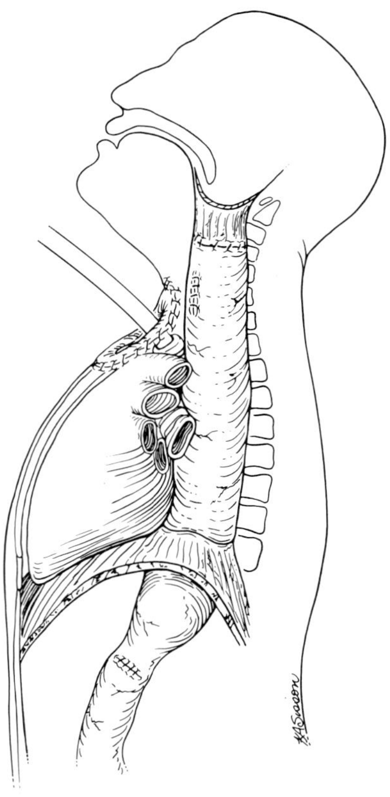

Figure 25–9. Completion of the gastric pull-up. Gastropharyngeal anastomosis and closure of the defect with an appropriately sized pectoralis major myocutaneous flap is performed.

Postoperative radiation therapy is indicated if the patient has not previously received adjunctive radiation therapy for the original lesion.

COMPLICATIONS IN SURGERY

The potential occurrence of every major complication of head and neck surgery exists in stomal recurrence surgery. A strong knowledge of the anatomy and dissection techniques is imperative. Improper identification or technical imprecision may lead to disastrous complications. These may be divided into three categories: immediate intraoperative, immediate postoperative, and late complications.

Intraoperative Complications

The immediate intraoperative complications are acutely life-threatening. Injury to the great vessels results in profuse hemorrhage, difficult to control, and often leading to fatality.

Air embolism is a second acute complication. A sudden rise in pulse and respiratory rate associated with venous bleeding should alert the surgeon to this life-threatening complication. The patient should be immediately placed in the left lateral decubitus position, tilting the table with the head down. This will protect the cerebral vessels from air embolism. If unrecognized, cardiorespiratory arrest and cerebral infarction may quickly result.

Pneumothorax is a complication that requires acute diagnosis and immediate action. Any change in respiration associated with a change in compliance or resistance should alert the surgeon. Immediate closed tube thoracotomy must be performed.

Chyle leaks may be obscured by scar or blood. Clear or milky liquid is the most common presentation. Most commonly, this occurs on the left side, occasionally on the right. It can be accentuated by increasing intravascular pressure. If found, the chyle leak should be suture ligated with nonabsorbable material at the time of surgery.

Immediate Postoperative Complications

The immediate postsurgical complications may occur during the first five postoperative days. Mediastinitis may be fatal. It may be secondary to an infected hematoma, seroma, or leaky suture line. A local wound infection can evolve into septicemia or septic shock. These complications may be diminished by the use of closed tube drainage, particularly important during the first 72 hours. If mediastinitis is diagnosed, immediate thoracotomy and drainage is important. Care must be taken not to compromise the myocutaneous flap vasculature. Proper intravenous antibiotic therapy and wound care are mandatory.

Late Postoperative Complications

Complications that appear after the fifth postoperative day may result in fatalities equal in number to those occurring earlier. Vascular accident is the most life-threatening of this group. With the tracheostoma in a lower position, the potential for arterial erosion into the trachea exists because of the intimate association of the trachea and the innominate artery and aortic arch. Prolonged mechanical ventilation increases the possibility of this catastrophe because it causes constant trauma to these structures.

Flap necrosis is first manifested by darkening of the wound edges and dehiscence of suture lines. Necrosis of skin is confirmed by absence of evidence of capillary filling in response to pressure. Minor flap necrosis occurs in 10% of cases, but major flap loss is rare.[16]

Hypothyroidism and hypoparathyroidism may occur. Mental status changes, bowel habit changes, or patient irritability should alert the surgeon of this possibility. Calcium and phosphorus levels and thyroid function should be monitored. Hypothyroidism may lead to depression and poor wound healing. Late hypoparathyroidism may result in psychosis.

Wound infection, or poor respiratory reserve, may lead to aspiration pneumonia. This can be devastating if not treated early. It is well known that previous radiation and poor nutritional status result in poor healing. This, as well as other complications, may result in fistula formation. Management of a fistula greatly prolongs hospitalization and is often frustrating to both patient and surgeon.

CONCLUSIONS

A significant number of patients with stomal recurrence have attained favorable palliative and curative outcomes as a result of the application and increased experience with mediastinal dissection. Radiotherapy and chemotherapy have offered little chance of cure and virtually no potential for palliation; surgery has produced the most promising results.

The basic techniques of transsternal mediastinal dissection for stomal recurrence, developed by Sisson[1] in 1962, form the basis for anatomic removal of disease. Employment of the single stage reconstructive procedures adapted by Biller and his group[14] in 1981 have reduced previously unacceptable morbidity and mortality to satisfactory levels. These methods have been employed by the authors to achieve successful disease control and to afford an improved quality of life for their patients.

REFERENCES

1. Sisson GA, Strachley CJ Jr, Johnson NE. Mediastinal dissection for recurrent cancer after laryngectomy. Laryngoscope 1962;72:1064–77.
2. Bauer WC, Edwards DL, McGavran MH. A critical analysis of laryngectomy in the treatment of epidermal carcinoma of the larynx. Cancer 1962;15:263–70.
3. Keim WF, Shapiro MJ, Rosen HO. Study of post laryngectomy stomal recurrences. Arch Otolaryngol 1965;81:183–6.
4. Modlin B, Ogura JH. Post-laryngectomy tracheal stomal recurrences. Laryngoscope 1969;79:239–50.
5. Sisson GA, Bytell DE, Becker SP. Mediastinal dissection 1976: indications and newer techniques. Laryngoscope 1977;87:751–9.
6. Myers E. Complications in surgery for stomal recurrences. Laryngoscope 1983;93:285–8.
7. Hoover WB, King BD. Emergency laryngectomy. Arch Otolaryngol 1954;59:431–3.
8. Harris HH, Butler E. Surgical limits in cancer. Arch Otolaryngol 1968;87:490–3.
9. Schneider JJ, Lindberg RD, Jesse RH. Prevention of tracheal stoma recurrences after total laryngectomy by postoperative irradiation. J Surg Oncol 1975;7:187–90.
10. Gluckman L, Hamaker RC, Weissler MC, et al. Surgical salvage for stomal recurrence: a multi institutional experience. Laryngoscope 1987;97:1025–9.
11. Kies MS, Gordon LI, Hauck WW, et al. Analysis of complete responders after initial treatment with chemotherapy in head and neck cancer. Otolaryngol Head Neck Surg 1985;93:199–205.
12. Sisson GA, Edison BP, Bytell DE. Transsternal neck dissection. Arch Otolaryngol 1979;101:46–9.
13. Biller HF, Krespi YP, Lawson W, Baek S. A one-stage flap reconstruction following resection for stomal recurrence. Otolaryngol Head Neck Surg 1980;88:357–60.
14. Biller HF, Baek S, Lawson WL, et al. Pectoralis major myocutaneous island flap and head and neck surgery. Arch Otolaryngol 1981;107:23–7.
15. Dennis D, Kashima H. Introduction of the Janus flap. Arch Otolaryngol 1981;107:431–5.
16. Withers EH, Davis L, Lynch JB. Anterior mediastinal tracheostomy with a pectoralis major musculocutaneous flap. Plast Reconstr Surg 1981;67:381–4.

26

Tracheal Stomal Stenosis Following Total Laryngectomy

Hector P. Rodriguez, Carl E. Silver

The tracheal stoma is an artifically created opening formed after laryngectomy by suturing the transected trachea to the skin of the anterior inferior neck. Ideally, the stoma should not require a cannula for stenting and should permit normal laminar flow of air with minimal turbulence during the ventillatory cycle. It should allow for normal clearing of tracheobronchial secretions and be wide enough to facilitate the insertion of a tracheoesophageal speech prosthesis. When the stoma is narrowed sufficiently to prevent these functions, tracheostomal stenosis, of some degree, may be considered to exist.

Although there is not a universally accepted definition for this complication, many surgeons consider it to be present in any patient who requires the use of a postoperative laryngeal cannula to maintain an adequate airway.[1,2] In order to avoid stenosis, it is helpful to identify preoperative risk factors. Meticulous surgical stomal construction and postoperative care are also required.

This chapter will examine the incidence, etiologic factors, and pathophysiology of tracheal stomal stenosis and describe the accepted principles of proper initial stomal construction as well as a variety of methods employed in dealing with secondary tracheal stomal stenosis.

INCIDENCE AND CLASSIFICATION

The reported incidence of tracheal stomal stenosis varies (Table 26–1). Loewy and Larker[3] found six occurrences (4%) in 138 patients. All had been performed by a single surgeon. Yonkers and Mercurio,[4] in a retrospective analysis of laryngectomies performed by various surgeons at nine different hospitals, reported a much higher incidence of 46 in 107 patients (43%).

Lam et al[5] was able to decrease the complication rate by varying the surgical technique. In the initial phase of *his* series of 141 total laryngectomies, a 31% incidence of stenosis occurred. After modifying the technique of stoma construction, the incidence was reduced to 4%.

There is no generally accepted classification for tracheal stomal stenosis. Montgomery[6,7] categorized stenosis into three different types, according to possible etiology and external stomal configuration. Concentric stenosis, caused by circumferential scar contracture or keloid formation, was most common, representing more than 60% of instances in his series. "Vertical shelf stenosis," caused by lateral encroachment from the sternomastoid muscle or remaining thyroid lobe, constituted the next most frequent type. "Inferior shelf stenosis," caused by redundant skin folds, accounted for fewer than 10% of the cases. Montgomery's classification is a practical guide for formulation of strategy for effective correction of stenosis.

EPIDEMIOLOGY AND RISK FACTORS

A number of etiologic factors may contribute to formation of tracheal stomal stenosis. For analysis, these factors can be grouped into three categories: those present prior to the procedure, developed during the operation, and resulting from the surgery.

Table 26–1. Incidence of Tracheal Stomal Stenosis

REFERENCE	NO. LARYNGECTOMIES	STENOSIS No.	STENOSIS %
Yonkers and Mercurio[4]	107	46	42
Langebrunner and Chandler[2]	124	43	34
Lam et al[5]	116*	36	31
	25†	1	4
Griffith and Luce[8]	89	19	22
Lowey and Larker[3]	138	6	4

*Early experience.
†Later experience.

Preoperative Factors

Factors inherent to the host can range from race and sex to body habitus. Black individuals have a higher incidence of keloid and hypertrophic scar formation. Females have up to a 30% smaller tracheal circumference and thinner, less rigid, tracheal cartilages than do male patients. The smaller, softer trachea is more easily affected by extrinsic pressure. Patients with short, stubby necks are at a higher risk due to excess skin laxity and thick subcutaneous tissue, that tends to bulge into the stoma, resulting in a pseudostenosis. Prominent thyroid glands and hypertrophic muscles may cause encroachment upon the tracheal walls. A rare occurrence is the congenital absence of tracheal rings.

Radiation therapy damages vascular tissue and may contribute to a higher incidence of infection and scar formation. Griffith and Luce[8] noted a 14% incidence of stomal stenosis in patients receiving postoperative radiation therapy, although other authors have not found this to be the case.[1,2,5]

Operative Risk Factors

Faulty construction of the tracheal stoma can produce several complications. Tensions at the tracheocutaneous junction can result from overstretching the tracheal stump. This is most likely to occur with laryngectomy following previous tracheotomy, or for resection of subglottic tumors. A predisposition to stenosis may be caused by failure to displace tissues that may encroach upon the stoma, to obliterate dead space, or to approximate precisely the mucocutaneous junction.

Postoperative Risk Factors

These include infection, which may be secondary to salivary fistulas causing healing by secondary intention with increased scarring. Balle and Bretlau[9] reported a 61% incidence of stomal stenosis in association with postoperative fistula formation. Other authors[4,5] differentiate between pharyngocutaneous and pharyngostomal fistulas. They believe the latter seem to play a more contributory role, due to the scar tissue and deposits adjacent, rather than lateral, to the stoma. Tracheitis at the mucocutaneous junction caused by irritation from the prolonged use of postoperative respirators, vigorous suctioning with rigid catheters, and ill-fitting cannulas are also considered contributing factors.

Several authors[1,3,9–12] concur that benign scar contracture, in the absence of other factors, plays a major role in the etiology of tracheal stomal stenosis. The natural tendency of cutaneous wounds to contract and shorten is the basic problem. Contraction of circular scars will reduce the luminal diameter. The area most vulnerable to contraction is the posterior membranous tracheal wall, due to absence of cartilaginous support in this area.

Tracheocutaneous separation is prone to occur in those patients whose closure is under tension, are hypoproteinemic, on steroid therapy, or have received preoperative radiation therapy. The gap created will promote increased deposition of scar tissue with reduction in luminal size.

Recurrent tumor is responsible for fewer than 5% of cases but constitutes an important cause of late stenosis.

PATHOPHYSIOLOGY

Once stenosis has occurred, signs and symptoms are variable. Dyspnea of varying degrees may ensue, depending on the size of the opening relative to the respiratory reserve. Bain[13] determined that a 50% stenosis in all diameters produces a 75% reduction in surface luminal area. Individuals with normal lung function can tolerate this degree of stenosis but the same deficit may produce considerable respiratory disability in patients with pulmonary disease.

Spirometric analysis of patients with stomal stenosis will demonstrate a reduction in forced expiratory volume ($A2_1$) in 1 second and in maximal voluntary ventilation in 1 minute.

Another aspect of the pathophysiology of tracheal stomal stenosis is the increase in air turbulence at the cutaneous opening, which causes desiccation and crusting. This in turn impedes the proper clearing of tracheal secretions, which may contribute to pulmonary infections. Use of a tracheal cannula to bypass the stenotic area may solve the immediate problem, but may lead to persistent irritation and crusting due to compression of the tracheal wall. A vicious cycle is begun which, if untreated, may deteriorate progressively.

TRACHEAL STOMA CONSTRUCTION

Although there are various accepted methods of stomal construction, most authors agree on three major steps to prevent tracheal stomal stenosis. These include tension-free anastomosis, displacement of encroaching tissues, and elongation and interruption of the tracheal perimeter.

Tension-Free Anastomosis

The trachea must be exteriorized at the proper level of the neck to avoid anastomotic tension. This is easily accomplished in patients with adequate tracheal stump length. The surgeon can either incorporate the tracheal stump into the transverse incision joining superior and inferior skin flaps or place it in the inferior flap, either through a separate incision or a vertical extension from the junction of flaps.

When the tracheal stump is excessively short, exteriorization at the level of the inferior flap, as already described, and placement of tension-releasing sutures through at least two cartilaginous rings and skin with heavy suture material (0 or 00 silk or nylon) will reduce anastomotic tension.[14]

In extreme cases in which the remaining trachea cannot reach the level of the suprasternal notch without excessive tension, a manubriectomy with creation of a mediastinal tracheostomy may be necessary.[15] Alternatives to this last situation may include funneling skin to the trachea by means of cutaneous advancement, pedicled or mycocutaneous flaps.[10,16]

Displacement of Encroaching Tissues

Lateral displacement or partial resection of bulky thyroid lobes and transection of the sternal attachments of the sternomastoid muscle, particularly in those patients with stomas located at the level of the suprasternal notch, will prevent the formation of superior and vertical shelf stenosis, respectively. The identification and resection of excessive cutaneous laxity and subcutaneous fat-laden tissue, particularly in obese individuals, will avoid formation of concentric stenosis. Proper trimming of protruding tracheal cartilaginous rings in order to obtain exact mucocutaneous approximation will allow primary healing and avoid concentric stomal stenosis.

Elongation and Interruption of the Tracheal Stomal Perimeter

These maneuvers are aimed at avoiding circumferential stomal stenosis secondary to benign scar contracture. The numerous ways to achieve this are listed in Table 26–2. Tracheal beveling increases the circumference of the stoma and changes the configuration of the opening from circular to elliptical. (An opposite opinion regarding tracheal beveling is expressed by Professor Stell in Chapter 22.) A 45° angle cut in an anteroposterior direction by transecting across at least two cartilaginous rings will create a satisfactorily large opening (Fig. 26–1).

Relaxing incisions in the trachea in combination with "Z" plasties and/or cutaneous flaps will alter the configuration of the stoma, creating an irregular perimeter and redistributing the forces of scar contraction, thus avoiding concentric stenosis. Both single and multiple Z-plasties have been described.[1,5] The single Z-plasties are usually placed in the posterior membranous tracheal wall allowing for transposition of both skin and mucosal triangles (Fig. 26–2). Trail[17] reported effective reduction of stenosis in 50 patients with single posteriorly located Z-plasties. Chandler[1,2] stressed the importance of making the posterior Z-plasties large enough by incising between 2 and 3 cm of posterior tracheal wall.

Dual Z-plasties, when employed, are usually created in the anterior and posterior portions of the stoma. Flaps created by incising through cartilaginous rings may be deficient in blood supply if angulated too sharply and may be cumbersome to transpose due to rigidity of the cartilage if the angulation is excessively broad.

Relaxing incisions in the trachea are created by simple perpendicular transection of the trachea or by wedge excisions. They usually extend through two cartilaginous rings, or 1.5 to 2.5 cm of tracheal wall. They may be placed at 12, 3, 6, and 9 o'clock of the tracheal perimeter and are reported as single (usually posterior), double (either anteroposterior or lateral), or multiple (all four quadrants). Skin may be interposed into the gaps created by the relaxing incisions by reapproximation of preserved skin wedges, or by advancement or rotation advancement flaps.

Table 26-2. Techniques for Tracheal Stomal Construction

TECHNIQUE	REFERENCE
1. Tantalum ring implantation	Mumma and Pressman[25]
2. Tracheal beveling	Catlin[26]
	Chandler[1]
	Clairmont[14]
3. Z plasties	Trail et al[17]
4. V-Y interdigitation flaps	
A. Anterior and posterior	Hartwell and Dykes[18]
	Myers and Gallia[20]
B. Lateral	Catlin[26]
	Panje and Kitt[12]
	Montgomery[6]
	Yonkers and Mercurio[4]
C. Multiple (4 flap)	Lam et al[5]
	Converse[27]
5. Combination Z-plasties and V-Y advancement	Ishiki and Tanabe[11]
	Murayama et al[22]

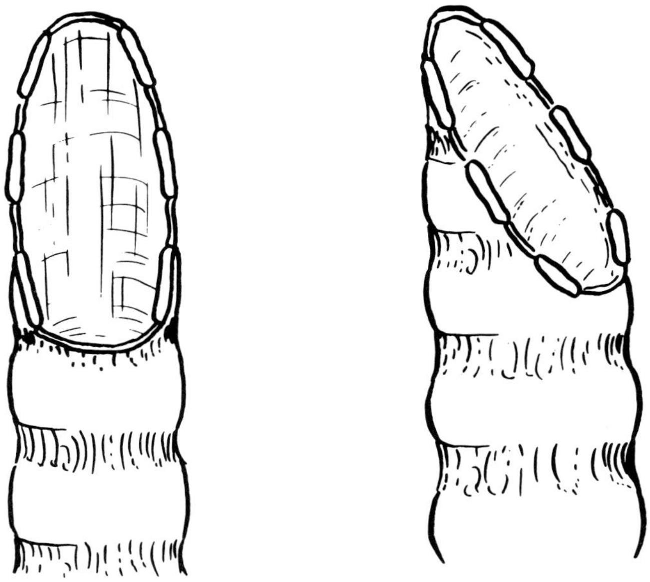

Figure 26–1. Beveling of cut end of trachea permits creation of tracheostoma with larger diameter than would simple transection.

Hartwell and Dykes[18] in 1967 and Carlton[19] in 1970 reported success with the use of a posterior tracheal relaxing incision, followed by the advancement of a superiorly based triangular flap. They employed this technique both for primary construction and secondary revision. The tracheal incision extends 2.5 cm in length, and two lateral cutaneous triangles are excised prior to the advancement of the flap (Fig. 26–3). Myers and Gallia[20] reported a similar technique but utilized a posterior tracheal wedge excision and a transposition cutaneous flap to fill the space. Montgomery[6,7] has utilized a single anterior wedge excision and a rotation interposition flap for revision of inferior shelf stenosis.

Double relaxing incisions have been reported by numerous authors.[8,14,18] When performed at the anterior and posterior tracheal walls, followed by interdigitation of triangular cutaneous advancement flaps, they create an external stomal configuration of a "bow tie" or "butterfly." The disadvantage of the posterior interdigitation flap is that it may interfere with the placement of a tracheoesophageal prosthetic device. The thickness of the newly interposed skin may not accept even the longest of the voice prosthetic devices and creation of the puncture at the posterior mucocutaneous junction may lead to undue widening of the tracheoesophageal fistula.

Double relaxing incisions placed on the lateral tracheal walls, with interdigitation of lateral cervical skin triangles, avoid the

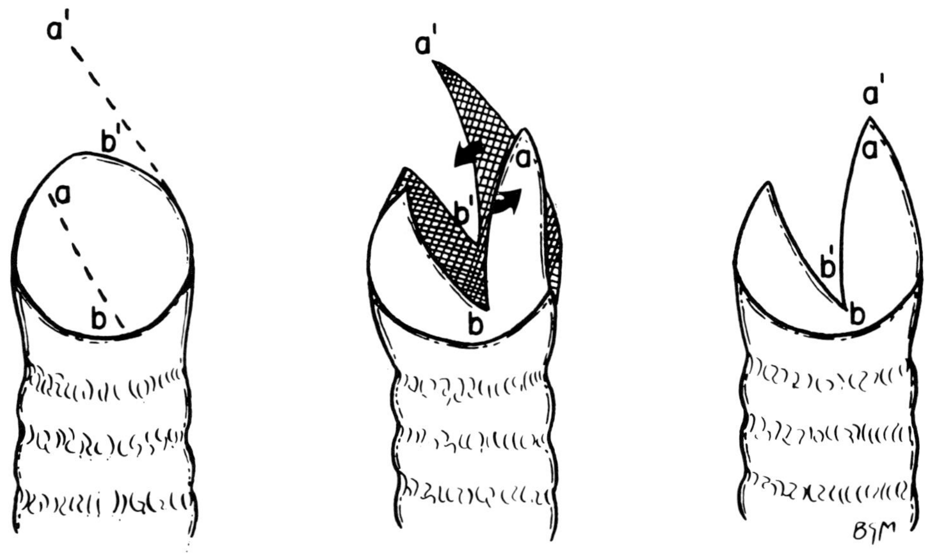

Figure 26–2. Single posterior Z-plasty. This technique may be employed for initial tracheostomal construction or for correction of stenosis.

inconveniences of the previously discussed technique (Fig. 26–4).[6,12]

Creation of multiple relaxing incisions at 12, 3, 6, and 9 o'clock on the trachea followed by interdigitation flaps will create a serrated or zig-zag configuration of the stoma. This has been reported by Lam et al[5] with 96% success rate.

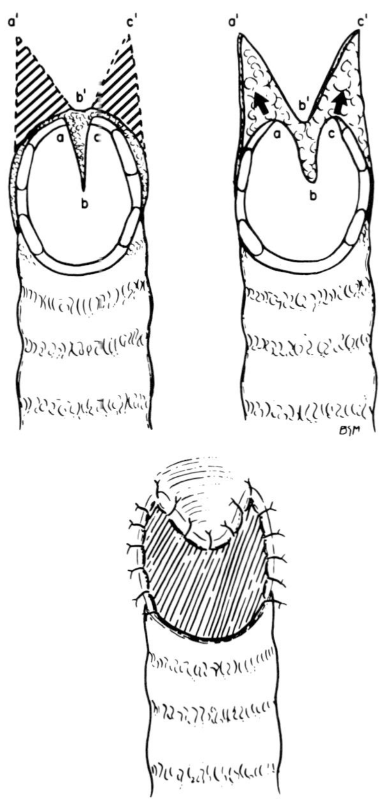

Figure 26–3. Posterior tracheal relaxing incision with advancement of superiorly based triangular skin flap.

SURGICAL REPAIR OF STOMAL STENOSIS

Many of the techniques that have been employed for correction of stomal stenosis are summarized in Table 26–3. A variety of nonsurgical techniques are often used initially, or in mild cases. These include the placement of progressively larger tracheostomy tubes or stomal buttons. Such measures may provide only a temporary solution, since removal of the stent will often result in recurrent stenosis.

Montgomery,[6,7] and later Callins and Applebaum[21] described the use of multiple radial incisions with an electrocautery carried through the mucous membrane, skin, soft tissues, and fibrous bands of the stenotic area. Care is taken not to extend the incisions more than 6 to 8 mm laterally to avoid injury to the major vessels. This is followed by the insertion of a no. 10 laryngeal cannula, which is left in place for 1 month. The results and long-term follow-up have not been reported.

More formal procedures carry a higher success rate and include excision of all cutaneous and cartilaginous scar tissue, and mobilization of "fresh" tissues with reconstruction following the principles enumerated in the section (see before) on stomal construction.

The use of Z-plasties and interdigitation flaps has been discussed. Other local alternatives include the five flap procedure described by Murayama et al,[22] which consists of a combination of two Z-plasties and a V-Y advancement flap interposed in the posterior suture line.

More extensive procedures, which include transposition of lateral cervical skin flaps sutured to the lateral tracheal walls and fenestrated deltopectoral flaps, have been advocated in patients who have severe skin compromise secondary to radiation therapy.[10,16]

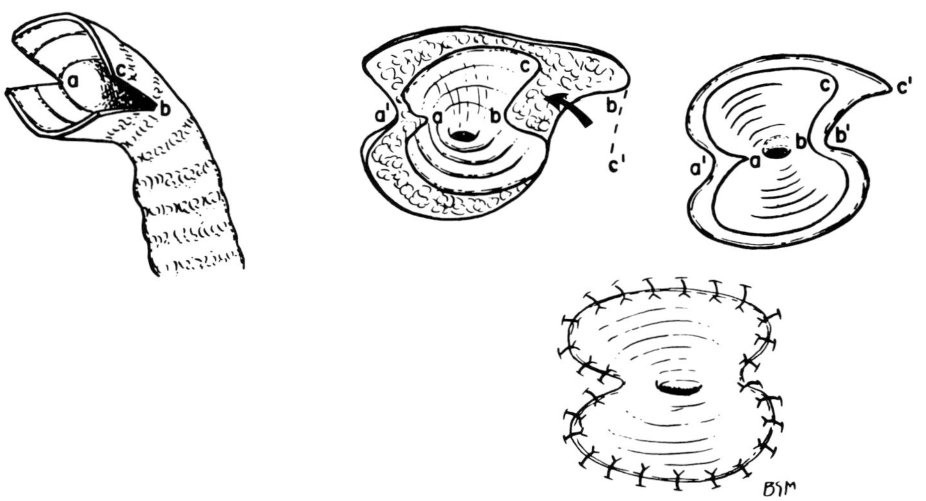

Figure 26–4. Laterally placed double relaxing incisions with interdigitation of triangular cutaneous advancement flaps. Note the typical "butterfly" appearance of the resulting stoma.

ANTERIOR MEDIASTINAL TRACHEOSTOMY (THORACOTRACHEOSTOMY)

Anterior mediastinal tracheostomy, created by resecting the manubrium of the sternum and transposing the trachea inferiorly into the chest skin, is utilized for patients who require excision of larger segments of tracheal stump for stomal recurrence. This has been described by Sisson et al,[23] Grillo,[15] and Oringer and Sloan[24] and is discussed in Chapter 25.

CONCLUSIONS

Tracheal stomal stenosis after laryngectomy is due to a variety of causes, including underlying anatomic, genetic or medical predisposition, excessive anastomotic tension caused by the extent of resection or faulty operative technique, or to postoperative events such as infection. Various surgical techniques may be employed to prevent stenosis by maximizing the tracheostomal perimeter and minimizing anastomotic tension. These range from simple beveling of the tracheal end to complex procedures involving transfer of local, or occasionally distant, skin flaps. Anterior mediastinal tracheostomy may be necessary in cases of extensive tracheal resection.

Table 26-3. Repair of Tracheal Stomal Stenosis

1. Radial incisions and dilation
2. "Donut" excision and reapproximation
3. Z-plasties
4. Local interdigitation flaps
   - Single V-Y
   - Double V-Y
   - Combination Z-plasty and V-Y advancement
5. Regional pedicled flaps
   - Lateral cervical advancement flaps
   - Fenestrated deltopectoral flap
   - Fenestrated pectoralis major flap

Procedures employed to correct stenosis after it has occurred usually include excision of the circumferential scar, advancement of sufficient skin to permit tension-free anastomosis, and use of the same techniques to interrupt and lengthen the tracheostomal perimeter that have been described for primary construction in order to prevent stenosis. Multiple radial incisions through the circumferential scar, combined with insertion of a tracheostomy tube of adequate diameter, may provide a simpler alternative in some cases.

The decision as to which measures should be taken, during initial laryngectomy, to prevent postoperative stenosis may depend on circumstances related to individual patients and may vary among surgeons. Some employ special techniques for perimeter interruption and lengthening in all laryngectomy cases; others, including us, are satisfied with the results obtained by simple construction, provided basic mechanical requirements, such as avoidance of tension and tissue redundancy, have been met.

REFERENCES

1. Chandler JR. Construction and reconstruction of the laryngeal stoma. Int Surg 1967;48:233–9.
2. Langebrunner DJ, Chandler JR. Tracheal stomal stenosis: causes and correction. South Med J 1968;61:838–42.
3. Loewy A, Larker HI. Tracheal stoma problems. Arch Otolaryngol 1968;87:477–81.
4. Yonkers AJ, Mercurio GA Jr. Tracheostomal stenosis following total laryngectomy. Otolaryngol Clin North Am 1983;16:391–405.
5. Lam KH, Wei WI, Wong J, Ong GB. Tracheostome construction during laryngectomy—a method to prevent stenosis. Laryngoscope 1983;93:212–5.
6. Montgomery W. Stenosis of tracheostoma. Arch Otolaryngol 1962;75:76–9.
7. Montgomery W. *Surgery of the upper respiratory system,* vol. 2, 2nd ed. Philadelphia: Lea & Febiger, 1979.
8. Griffith GR, Luce EA. Tracheal stomal stenosis after laryngectomy. Plast Reconstr Surg 1982;70:694–8.
9. Balle VH, Bretlau P. Tracheostomal stenosis following total laryngectomy. J Laryngol Otol 1985;99:577–80.
10. Doyle PJ, Dubeta KR. Post laryngectomy tracheostome stenosis—etiology and treatment. J Otolaryngol 1977;6:284–9.
11. Ishiki N, Tanabe M. A simple technique to prevent stenosis of the

tracheostoma after total laryngectomy. J Laryngol Otol 1980;94:637–42.
12. Panje WR, Kitt VV. Tracheal stoma reconstruction. Arch Otolaryngol 1985;111:190–2.
13. Bain J. Late complication of tracheostomy and prolonged endotracheal intubation. Int Anesthesiol Clin 1972;10:255–64.
14. Clairmont AA. Tracheostoma construction during laryngectomy: techniques to prevent stenosis. J Laryngol Otol 1978;92:75–8.
15. Grillo HC. Terminal or mural tracheostomy in the anterior mediastinum. J Thorac Cardiovasc Surg 1966;51:422–7.
16. East CA, Flemming AF, Brough MD. Tracheostomal reconstruction using a fenestrated deltopectoral skin flap. J Laryngol Otol 1988;102:282–3.
17. Trail ML, Chambers R, Leonard JR. Z-Plasty of tracheal stoma at laryngectomy. Arch Otolaryngol 1968;88:84–6.
18. Hartwell SW, Dykes ER. Construction and care of the end tracheostomy. Am J Surg 1967;113:498.
19. Carleton JS. Revision of the tracheal stoma. Laryngoscope 1970;80:260–6.
20. Myers EN, Gallia LJ. Tracheostomal stenosis following total laryngectomy. Ann Otol Rhinol Laryngol 1982;91:450–3.
21. Callins WP, Applebaum EL. Correction of laryngectomy stomal stenosis. Laryngoscope 1980;90:159–61.
22. Murayama Y, Kubota J, Nakasima H. A 5 flap procedure for repair of stenosed tracheostoma. Acta Chir Plast 1980;22:107–10.
23. Sisson GA, Straechley CJ Jr, Johnson NE. Mediastinal dissection for recurrent cancer after laryngectomy. Laryngoscope 1962;72:1064–77.
24. Orringer MB, Sloan H. Anterior mediastinal tracheostomy. J Thorac Cardiovasc Surg 1979;78:850–9.
25. Mumma C, Pressman J. A surgical technique to eliminate the tracheotomy tube after laryngectomy. Trans Am Acad Ophthalmol Otolaryngol 1951;55:418–23.
26. Catlin D. Making a large tracheal stoma during laryngectomy. Ear Nose Throat J 1966;45:87–90.
27. Converse JM. An operation for relief of stenosis of the stoma following total laryngectomy. Arch Otolaryngol 1950;52:950–1.

27

Surgical Approaches to Voice Restoration After Laryngectomy

Donald P. Shedd

Patients who have experienced long periods of voicelessness are able to report what a devastating disability is the complete inability to accomplish oral communication. Until recently, the usual approach to voice restoration after laryngectomy was training in esophageal speech (ES), and, if that failed, resort to an electrolarynx (EL). A significant number of individuals were not successful in developing adequate ES, and for some of these the EL was a less than satisfactory method of communication, for the monotonous vocal quality was often not acceptable. For these reasons, surgeons over the years have attempted to develop operative methods of voice restoration. The history of those attempts is a long and fascinating tale.

HISTORICAL BACKGROUND

If one were to consider all the possible methods of producing speech after laryngectomy, the possibilities could be summarized as shown in Table 27–1. Included are pneumatic, electronic, and electromechanical methods. The latter will not be covered in this review.

Electronic Methods

These can be divided into *surgical* and *nonsurgical* types. The latter includes the various transcervical devices, the peroral devices, and the intraoral approaches. All of these tend to produce a monotonous form of speech. Of the two surgical electronic methods, the transfistula approach of Goode[1] is not in current use. The idea of implantation of sound sources into the retropharyngeal area was explored by Griffith et al[2] and by Young et al[3] and is a fascinating concept.

Pneumatic Methods

These are techniques that use either pulmonary or nonpulmonary air. There are three of the latter, and two of them, buccal and pharyngeal speech, are not considered acceptable by speech pathologists. Buccal speech traps air in the cheek pouch and has low intelligibility. Pharyngeal speech, which traps air farther back at the faucial level, is also of poor quality.

ES, considered by some to be the best of all methods, was reported before the first laryngectomy. It is unfortunate that a significant portion of patients are unable to acquire proficiency in the use of this method. The pulmonary air nonsurgical method is the old stoma to mouth reed system, an approach that was popular before the advent of the electrolarynx.

Some of the surgical approaches utilize an appliance and some do not. In reviewing these, one can recognize historical

Table 27–1. Methods of Postlaryngectomy Speech Rehabilitation

- Pneumatic
  - Nonpulmonary air
    - Esophageal, buccal, and pharyngeal speech
  - Pulmonary air
    - Nonsurgical
      - Stoma-to-mouth appliances
    - Surgical
      - With appliance
        - Singer-Blom method
      - Without appliance
        - Staffieri method
- Electronic
  - Surgical
    - Transfistula
    - Implanted
  - Nonsurgical
    - Transcervical
    - Peroral
    - Intraoral
- Electromechanical
  - Dayal

channels named after individuals or after concepts. As in previous publications,[4] I have observed a conceptual rather than temporal sequence in describing the Asai channel, the Billroth channel, the Conley-Briani channel, and the "ice pick" channel.

ASAI CHANNEL

Some remarkably good results were achieved with the original Asai[5] operation, both in Japan and in the United States. The procedure required three operative stages and consequently a prolonged interval elapsed before speech was achieved. Various workers attempted to lessen the number of stages; Montgomery[6] reduced it to two, and McGrail and Oldfield[7] to one by using a deltopectoral flap. A direct fistula made from esophageal wall was utilized by Komorn[8] and by Calcaterra and Jafek.[9] The problem with many of these approaches was that of controlling salivary leakage from pharynx into trachea. Stallings[10] attempted to solve this by constructing a tendon sling around the fistula, with the idea that as the patient raised his chin to swallow, the sling would tighten and occlude the fistula.

The operation devised by Mario Staffieri[11] of Italy became quite popular in Europe. He constructed a phonatory neoglottis at the completion of laryngectomy by draping a flap of pharyngeal wall over the end of the trachea, and making a slit in this drape, through which air would flow when expiring against a finger-closed tracheostoma. This operation has not been widely accepted in the United States because of frequent problems with aspiration.[12] A similar but more ambitious effort was that of Arslan and Serafini,[13] who developed a procedure for voice restoration in which they elevated the first tracheal ring to the epiglottic level. In some of their patients they even carried out tracheal extubation after their voice rehabilitation operation, thus striving for total rehabilitation. Although occasional success was achieved, many patients experienced severe aspiration problems.

Amatsu[14] employed a portion of tracheal wall to construct an inclined fistula from trachea to esophagus. This procedure never became popular but served to lead Singer and Blom[15] into development of their practical technique (see later).

BILLROTH CHANNEL

Gussenbauer,[16] in 1874, described his efforts to fabricate a device for voice restoration in Billroth's first laryngectomy patient, utilizing a musical reed for sound production. Other workers utilized the reed concept, including Brown[17] of Australia, who employed an ear speculum and a standard musical pitch pipe with successful production of voice. The phenomenon of historical recurrence of ideas occurred when Taub and Spiro[18] in the 1970s again employed reeds for a speech appliance. The Roswell Park Memorial Institute group[19] also studied this approach with particular reference to those patients who had undergone pharyngolaryngectomy, patients who only rarely can develop ES.

CONLEY-BRIANI CHANNEL

The use of external appliances to route air from the trachea into the pharynx was developed in the 1950s by Briani[20] of Italy and John Conley[21] of New York. Briani's approach was to use a plastic appliance with valves, and Conley employed a side-arm on a tracheostomy tube. Years later, the same external appliance concept was employed by Taub and Spiro, and their device was marketed commercially under the name of Voicebak. This device had an ingenious respiratory valve, a feature that turned up years later in the work of Singer and Blom.

An external appliance approach was also utilized by the Roswell Park group in the 1970s, a system that they called the air-tunnel method. Their appliances were fabricated by the Department of Maxillofacial Prosthodontia. A similar approach was utilized by Sisson et al.[22] Sisson's device included a trimodal valve that stayed open for breathing, closed for speaking, and underwent prolapse when the patient coughed. Such a method was also described in a small series of British patients by Edwards.[23]

"ICE PICK" CHANNEL

The initiator of this concept, described by Guttman,[24] was an ingenious patient; a man who made his own fistula for speech purposes, using a red hot ice pick, which he passed through the posterior wall of his trachea into his esophagus. A good voice resulted, and the patient was able to maintain the fistula by using a goose quill.

It was in trying the method of Amatsu that Singer and Blom came up with their tracheoesophageal puncture method. To prevent leakage of saliva into the trachea, they first employed a homemade "duck-bill" valve. A commercial version was subsequently marketed.

Various modifications of the Singer-Blom method have appeared, one being that of Panje et al,[25] who used a different type of appliance and placed the fistula lower than their predecessors. Henly-Cohn et al's[26] modification was designed to be self-retaining, with the idea that frequent removal for cleaning would not be necessary. Shapiro and Ramanathan[27] conceived the idea that there would be advantages to combining the speech appliance with a tracheostomy tube, thereby simplifying retention of the appliance and at the same time maintaining stoma size. Workers in Holland[28] insert what is called the Groningen prosthesis designed to stay in place for approximately 3 months between changes. Strome et al[29] have described a procedure in which a tubular tracheoesophageal fistula is constructed, a method that eliminates the need for prosthesis in some of the patients.

The work of Singer and Blom is of further importance in respect to their later efforts. They found that not all patients having a tracheoesophageal puncture (TEP) developed good voices, and this led them to study the element of spasm. They employed myotomy and later neurectomy in dealing with the spastic element, efforts that increased the percentage of successful results. Their initial work dealt with patients who had the TEP done at some time subsequent to the laryngectomy, but at a later time they also studied the potential for doing the puncture at the time of the laryngectomy: the so-called "primary puncture."

Many ingenious approaches have been applied to the biologic problem of alaryngeal aphonia, and it is of interest to note the progression from complexity to simplicity, exemplified by a comparison between the Taub device and the later Singer-Blom appliance (Fig. 27–1). Over the years, one of the major problems has been how to connect the airway with the upper digestive tract in such a way that leakage will not occur. This has

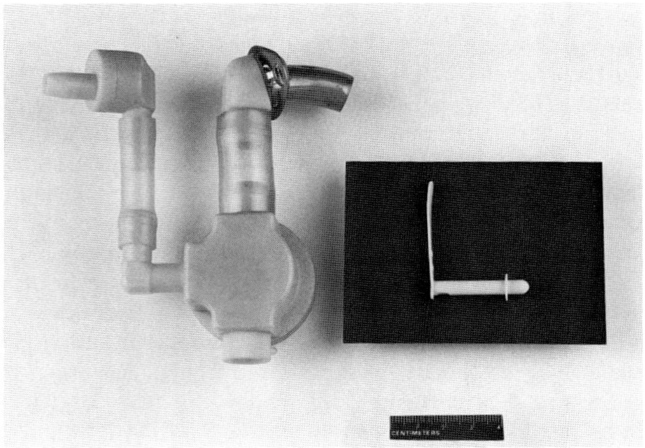

Figure 27–1. Comparison of the early Taub device with the Singer-Blom prosthesis. (From Shedd.[4] Reprinted with permission.)

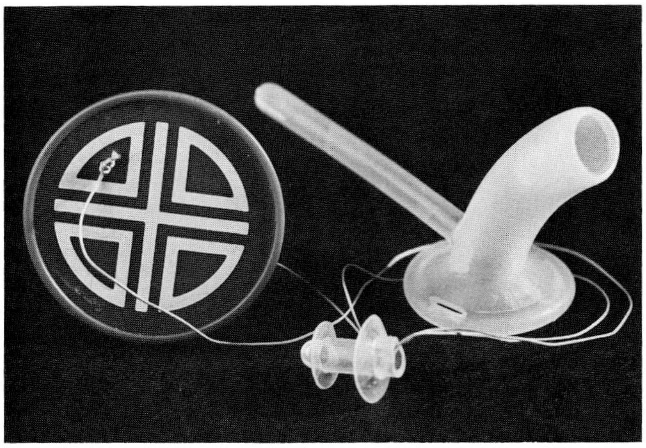

Figure 27–2. The Panje prosthesis (left) showing the two flanges, and the Shapiro appliance, (right) showing the periscope that fits into the speech fistula.

depended on creation of valves, made either of living tissues or from artificial materials. It is of interest to note how ideas recur in this field, an example being the revival in 1980 by Singer and Blom of the "ice pick" puncture first described in 1935.

PRESENT STATUS OF SURGICAL SPEECH REHABILITATION

Of the various options just presented, the one utilized by Singer and Blom has been associated with the most consistent success and relatively few problems. This prosthetic method, as well as the various modifications described, are those most widely employed at the present time. The remainder of this discussion will thus be devoted to the TEP type of procedure.

It is clear at this time that the laryngectomee who cannot achieve ES and who rejects the EL should be evaluated for a possible TEP. The success rate has been high enough that some speech pathologists would favor TEP for all laryngectomees, believing that the labor of teaching a patient ES is prohibitive. Many successful esophageal speakers would disagree with this position.[30] Certainly, good ES is an excellent method of communication that requires no secondary operation and no appliance.

Appliances Available

The first commercially marketed appliance for TEP was that of Singer and Blom, a simple "duck bill" valve having two external retention strips for taping in place. Panje's modification had internal and external flanges for retention, thus eliminating the need for adhesive tape. Shapiro's approach provided a valved fistula tube connected to a silicone rubber tracheostomy tube, which facilitated retention and helped to maintain stoma size (Fig. 27–2). The Bivona "Colorado" appliance is similar but has variation available in the length of the fistula tube. Singer and Blom later altered the valving mechanism to reduce the resistance to air flow, and they introduced prostheses not only of 16 F diameter but also of 20 F. Henley-Cohn designed an appliance that may be left in place for months at a time, whereas most of the others require daily removal and cleaning (Fig. 27–3). The existence of such a variety of devices implies that an ideal solution has not yet been found for the pertaining biomedical requirements. Familiarity of the surgeon with the various appliances available makes it possible to select the most suitable one for a given patient (Table 27–2).

COMPLICATIONS

Although the puncture is a simple procedure, complications occur. Ward et al[31] reported 26 complications in a series of 104 patients. Perioperative complications include peristomal cellulitis, mediastinitis, septicemia, and aspiration pneumonia. There was one fatality from the latter in the Ward series. Hypopharyngeal leakage can occur either perioperatively or

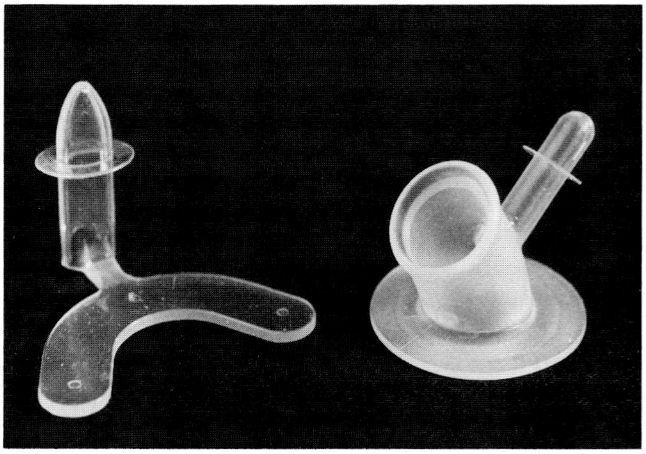

Figure 27–3. The Henley-Cohn prosthesis (left) showing flange for intraesophageal retention, and the Bivona Colorado appliance (right) showing the fistula tube, obtainable in various lengths.

Table 27-2. Commercially Available Appliances

COMPANY	PRODUCT
American V. Mueller	Voice prosthesis
Bivona	Voice prosthesis
	Low-resistance prosthesis
	Periscope prosthesis (Shapiro)
	Colorado prosthesis
Storz	Henley-Cohn prosthesis
Xomed	Panje button
Entermed (Holland)	Groningen voice prosthesis

chronically. Late postoperative complications include enlargement or migration of the fistula, tracheal stenosis, esophageal stenosis and colonization of the prosthesis by fungus.

In a few instances, spontaneous enlargement of the small speech fistula has resulted in a significant reconstructive problem. Aspiration of the prosthesis, a dangerous complication, occurred seven times in Ward's series. Curley and O'Donoghue[32] have indicated that complication rates can be reduced by adequate knowledge of the relevant anatomy, although a small but irreducible minimum of problems is to be expected with any surgical procedure.

Despite these liabilities, the opinion of most surgeons who utilize TEP is that the complication rate is acceptable, and the potential benefit of satisfactory speech provides adequate compensation for the difficulties.

SPECIFIC PROBLEMS IN SURGICAL SPEECH REHABILITATION

Selection of Patients for TEP

The various criteria for selection of candidates for surgical speech rehabilitation may be listed as follows:

1. Adequate stoma size
2. Absence of hypopharyngeal stenosis
3. Reasonable manual dexterity
4. Adequate visual acuity
5. Satisfactory pulmonary status
6. Sufficient intelligence
7. Good motivation
8. Mental stability
9. Good performance on insufflation test.

Assessment of the first five of these criteria should not prove difficult, but there are problems with respect to the remainder. It can be difficult to assess adequacy of intelligence in this context. Motivation and mental stability may also prove to be difficult to appraise. A patient with uncontrolled alcoholism is often unsuitable for such a procedure. The insufflation test, originally described by Taub and Bergner[33] is useful in predicting ability to produce sound. Blom et al[34] described a modification of the test and advocated myotomy at the time of puncture for patients whose phonation on insufflation is not good.

Selection of Appropriate Appliance

There is a considerable array of different appliances on the market. Choosing the proper one is not easy, for each may have specific advantages and disadvantages. These appliances fall into two broad categories: simple fistula tubes, and complex tubes in which the fistula portion is attached to a tracheostomy tube of some sort. In the latter type the attachment is at a fixed angle, which can prove detrimental to some patients. The advantages of this type of prosthesis are that the tracheal stent portion may augment a stoma of borderline size, and the self-retaining configuration of the device eliminates the need for application of adhesive to the skin.

The simple fistula tubes are held in place either by taping, by flanges, or by a combination of the two. Blom[35] has summarized the complex situation with respect to the various tracheoesophageal valves and their design in a recent article published as part of an overall summary of the results of a workshop on postlaryngectomy speech rehabilitation held in Baltimore in June of 1984.

Patients Who Present with a Narrow Stoma

The patient who presents for TEP with a significant narrowing of his stoma should have surgical revision before the puncture is done. Minimal narrowing may be managed by using one of the stented appliances. Judgment is required in choice of appropriate course of action.

Patients Who Do Not Get Good Voice from TEP

A small percentage of patients after puncture will not have a satisfactory voice. Various approaches to this problem have been recommended. Cheesman et al[36] have pointed out that studies can determine whether poor voice is due to hypotonicity, mild hypertonicity, spasm, or stricture. Stricture requires surgical correction, whereas spasm is an indication for a myotomy. Mild hypertonicity may respond to use of a low resistance prosthesis, and hypotonicity is helped by external compression.

Lack of Appropriate Speech Pathology Support

Achievement of success in TEP speech is dependent not only on the successful puncture, but also on the participation by a dedicated speech pathologist who is knowledgeable about the details of tracheoesophageal speech and who can handle some of the problems relating to selecting and fitting the optimal appliance. As time goes on, various problems may arise, many of which can be solved by the attention of the speech pathologist.

QUESTIONS AND ANSWERS

Although TEP has become widely accepted, some questions remain to be answered. They are as follows:

1. Should TEP be performed as a primary or secondary procedure?

After it became apparent that TEP done some time after laryngectomy would provide good voice for most patients, there began investigation of the possible value of performing primary

TEP at the time of resection of the larynx. A number of reports[37,38] have appeared on this subject, and some of them strongly advocate doing the puncture at the end of the laryngectomy. There are others who believe that the fistula may contribute excessive difficulty to the immediate postlaryngectomy period.[39] Some believe that experiencing a period of voicelessness will improve motivation for a patient to cope subsequently with the fistula and the prosthesis. Others think that the patient should be given the opportunity to acquire natural ES before opting for surgical rehabilitation. No clear-cut answer to the question of preliminary TEP is available at this time.

2. Is myotomy or neurectomy more effective in relieving aphonia due to cricopharyngeal spasm?

The work of Blom (see before) and others has shown that an element of spasm is often a factor in those patients who do not develop good speech after puncture. This problem has been approached by constrictor myotomy and by neurectomy of the pharyngeal plexus. These procedures have been used in respect to both primary and secondary TEP. Studies are underway to determine which is the operation of choice in respect to voice production, deglutition, and complications.

3. Will TEP provide voice in the patient who has undergone pharyngectomy in addition to laryngectomy?

Only a limited number of patients have had punctures done after total pharyngolaryngectomy, but present evidence suggests that such patients can develop satisfactory speech from TEP. A study by Medina et al[40] of ten such patients indicated that all were able to produce adequate voice. The series included five visceral transpositions.

4. What is the ideal appliance?

The ideal appliance would have the following properties:

- Ability to stay in place for many days without cleaning.
- Resistance to fungus.
- Changeable by patient without difficulty.
- Long survival of valving function.
- Low resistance to air flow.
- Compatibility with tracheal stoma valve.
- Compatibility with a small stoma.

None of the currently available prostheses meets all of these requirements, but work is continuing in order to meet the need.

One Option

Among the various options available, the writer favors not performing TEP at the time of a standard laryngectomy, but rather allowing the patient a few months to attempt development of ES. If he fails, he is given a trial with the EL to determine his level of acceptance of this method. Many patients will use the EL as an adjunct during their period of trial of ES. With failure of ES and rejection of the EL, the patient is evaluated for TEP by the methods described. For the patient who is to undergo pharyngolaryngectomy, present evidence would indicate that development of ES is quite rare, and early evaluation for TEP is appropriate.

CONCLUSIONS

The developments over recent years in restoration of voice by surgical means is an exciting chapter in the history of rehabilitation and oncology. Many lessons have been learned, and many patients have been helped to regain the priceless gift of oral communication. Reasonably good approaches to the problem of alaryngeal aphonia now exist, and there is reason to expect further progress in solution of the remaining problems in this fascinating area.

REFERENCES

1. Goode RL. The development of an improved artificial larynx. Trans Am Acad Opthalmol Otolaryngol 1969;73:279–87.
2. Griffith MV, Frederickson JM, Bryce DP. An implantable electronic sound source for speech production. Arch Otolaryngol 1976;102:676–82.
3. Young KA, Bailey BJ, Everett R, Griffiths CM. Electronic laryngeal prosthesis for implantation: a progress report in surgical and prosthetic approaches to speech rehabilitation. In: Shedd DP, Weinberg B, eds. *Surgical and prosthetic approaches to speech rehabilitation.* Boston: GK Hall, 1980:231–45.
4. Shedd D. A historical perspective on surgical speech rehabilitation. Probl Gen Surg 5:113, 1988.
5. Asai R. Laryngoplasty after total laryngectomy. Arch Otolaryngol 1965;95:114–9.
6. Montgomery WW. Postlaryngectomy vocal rehabilitation. Arch Otolaryngol 1972;95:76–83.
7. McGrail JS, Oldfield DL. One-stage operation for vocal rehabilitation at laryngectomy. Trans Am Acad Opthalmol Otolaryngol 1971;75: 510–2.
8. Komorn RM. Vocal rehabilitation after total laryngectomized patient with a tracheoesophageal shunt. Ann Otolaryngol 1974;83:445–51.
9. Calcaterra TC, Jafek B. Tracheoesophageal shunt for speech rehabilitation after total laryngectomy. Arch Otolaryngol 1971;94:124–8.
10. Stallings JO. Restoration of the voice after total laryngectomy: immediate and delayed neolaryngoplasty. In: Shedd DP, Weinberg B, eds. *Surgical and prosthetic approaches to speech rehabilitation.* Boston: GK Hall, 1980:191–7.
11. Staffieri M. Laryngectomie totale avec reconstruction De La Glotte Phonatoire. Rev Laryngol 1974;95:63–83.
12. Klima A, Ilberg CV. Laryngoplasty: results and problems after the creation of a neoglottis. J Laryngol Otol 1988;102:43–4.
13. Arslan M, Serafini I. Restoration of laryngeal functions after total laryngectomy, first 25 cases. Laryngoscope 1972;82:1349.
14. Amatsu MA. A new one-stage surgical technique for post-laryngectomy speech. Arch Otorhinolaryngol 1978;220:149–52.
15. Singer MI, Blom ED. Vocal rehabilitation after laryngectomy. Otolaryngol Clin North Am 1985;18:605–11.
16. Gussenbauer C. Uber die Erste durch Billroth am Menschen ausgefuhrte Kehlkopf-Extirpation and die Anwendung eines Kunstlichen Kehlkopfes. Arch Chir 1874;17:343–6.
17. Brown G. A simple but effective artificial larynx. J. Laryngol Otol 1925;40:793–7.
18. Taub S, Spiro R. Vocal rehabilitation of laryngectomees. Am J Surg 1972;124:87–90.
19. Shedd DP, Bakamjian V, Sako K, et al. Reed fistula method of speech rehabilitation after laryngectomy. Am J Surg 1972;124:510–4.
20. Briani AA. Riabilitazoine fonectica di laringectomazzati. Arch Ital Otorhinolaryngol 1952;63:469–75.
21. Conley J, DeAmesti F, Pierce JK. A new surgical technique for the vocal rehabilitation of the laryngectomized patient. Ann Otolaryngol 1958;67:655–64.
22. Sisson G, McConnel F, Logemann JA, Yeh S. Voice rehabilitation after laryngectomy. Arch Otolaryngol 1975;101:178–81.
23. Edwards N. Post-laryngectomy vocal rehabilitation using expired air and external fistula method. Laryngoscope 1975;85:690–9.
24. Guttman RG. Rehabilitation of the voice in laryngectomized patients. Arch Otolaryngol 1932;15:478–9.
25. Panje WR, VanDemark D, McCabe BF. Voice button prosthesis rehabilitation of the laryngectomee: additional notes. Ann Otorhinolaryngol 1981;90:503–5.
26. Henley-Cohn J, Hausfeld J, Jakubczak G. The artificial larynx prosthesis: comparative clinical evaluation. Larynscope 1984;94:43–5.

27. Shapiro MJ, Ramanathan V. Tracheal stoma vent voice prosthesis. Laryngoscope 1982;92:1126–9.
28. Manni JJ, van den Broek, de Groot MA, Berends E. Voice rehabilitation after laryngectomy with the Groningen prosthesis. J Otolaryngol 1984;13:333–6.
29. Strome M, Brasnu D, Laccoureye H. Current status of the myomucosal tracheoesophageal shunt. Head Neck Surg 1988; Suppl II:S151–5.
30. Ausherman WD. Immediate versus delayed surgical rehabilitation after laryngectomy: one patient's viewpoint. Head Neck Surg 1988; Suppl II:S139–40.
31. Ward PH, Andrews JC, Mickel RA, et al. Complications of medical and surgical approaches to voice restoration after total laryngectomy. Head Neck Surg 1988; Suppl II:S124–8.
32. Curley JW, O'Donoghue GM. Some complications of tracheoesophageal puncture for voice restoration. J Laryngol Otol 1988;102:558–9.
33. Taub S, Bergner LH. Air bypass voice prosthesis for voice rehabilitation. Am J Surg 1973;125:748–56.
34. Blom ED, Singer MI, Hamaker RC. An improved esophageal insufflation test. Arch Otolaryngol 1985;111:211–2.
35. Blom E. Tracheoesophageal valves: problems, solutions and directions for the future. Head Neck Surg 1988; Suppl II:S142–5.
36. Cheesman AD, Knight J, McIvor J, Perry A. Tracheoesophageal puncture speech—an assessment technique for failed esophageal speakers. J Laryngol Otol 1986;100:191–9.
37. Juarbe C, Shemen L, Eberle R, et al. Primary tracheoesophageal puncture for voice restoration. Am J Surg 1986;152:464–6.
38. Trudeau MD, Hirsch SM, Schuller DE. Vocal restorative surgery: Why wait? Laryngoscope 1986;96:975–7.
39. Ward PH, Andrews JC, Mickel RA, et al. Complications of medical and surgical approaches to voice restoration after total laryngectomy. Head Neck Surg 1988; Suppl II:S124–8.
40. Medina JE, Nance A, Burns L, Overton R. Voice restoration after total laryngopharyngectomy and cervical esophagectomy using the duckbill prosthesis. Am J Surg 1987;154:407–10.

PART SIX

Replacement of Cervical Esophagus

28

Replacement of Cervical Esophagus by Gastric Transposition

Donald F.N. Harrison

Failure to eradicate tumor at the primary site remains the largest single cause of patient mortality in head and neck carcinoma. Anatomic complexity or inaccessibility frequently results in positive margins after supposedly oncologic resections, and hope that postoperative radiotherapy or chemotherapy would compensate for inadequate surgery has proved overoptimistic.

Although primary carcinoma of the cervical esophagus is rare, extension from superiorly placed postcricoid neoplasms are common, necessitating removal of pharyngolarynx as well as involved esophagus. A decade or two ago, most tumors in this region were treated by primary pharyngolaryngectomy with removal of as much cervical esophagus as was readily available. Repair was both tedious and prolonged. Few patients regained ability to swallow prior to local recurrence of tumor. In 1970 Harrison[1] examined pharyngolaryngectomy specimens from 50 patients by whole-organ serial sectioning and found that submucosal extension was present for at least 10 mm superiorly and 5 mm inferiorly. The range of extension was considerable, however. The sections also showed that involvement of the thyroid gland, paratracheal lymph nodes and party wall between trachea and esophagus could result in inadequate resection with disease left in situ (Fig. 28–1).

Since these extensions were frequently undetectable clinically or radiologically (although they might have been suspected), it was clear that the operation of pharyngolaryngectomy was frequently inadequate, particularly when the cervical esophagus was involved. The problems of reconstruction following pharyngolaryngectomy that bedevilled the laryngologist in the 1960s resulted in many patients receiving radiotherapy, despite its limited value. Repair of surgical defects with cervical skin flaps, following failed radiation therapy, was performed in stages and required an average of approximately 6 months for completion. Even when this type of reconstruction was successful, swallowing was limited by stenosis at the skin-esophageal junction—a problem that still occurs with present-day repair utilizing the myocutaneous flap.

No matter how much esophagus is removed along with the pharyngolarynx, the problem remains of replacing a mucosa-lined cylinder sheathed in smooth muscle and covering it with viable skin. The new gullet will be a nonperistaltic conduit that functions with only tongue thrust and gravity to energize swallowing.

An excellent, comprehensive, historical review of the many varied and imaginative procedures used over the past two decades to deal with this problem has been given by DeSanto and Carpenter[2] and Surkin et al.[3] Most of the more esoteric or prolonged procedures have been abandoned and of the abdominal viscera, the gastric pull-up has emerged as probably the most effective means of combining radical resection with effective rehabilitation of swallowing.

GASTRIC TRANSPOSITION

At the early part of this century, a subcutaneous gastric tube was used in esophagoplasty. This was replaced by the reversed gastric tube of Heimlich, which occasionally could reach as high as the cricoid cartilage. However, blood supply to the superior margin was precarious and swallowing uniformly poor. Transposition of the whole stomach to the neck was pioneered by Ong and Lee in 1960[4] when they successfully anastomosed the gastric fundus to the pharynx in four patients following resection for advanced laryngeal cancer. All these patients had tumors extending through the posterior plate of the cricoid cartilage to involve the inferior hypopharynx, a common occurrence in the Chinese, who have small, often nonossified larynges. Their technique, with minor modifications has now been adapted

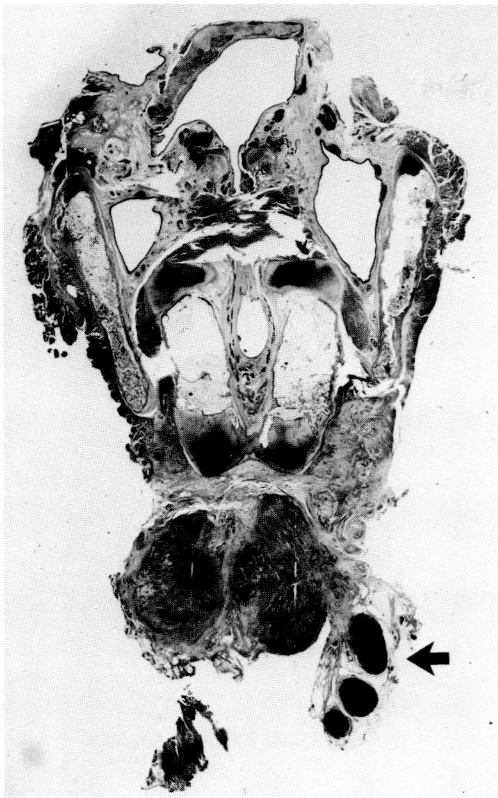

Figure 28–1. Whole-organ serial section cut at 20 μm of pharyngolaryngectomy specimen. Tumor present at lower end of excision. Paratracheal nodes indicated by arrow.

worldwide, although both morbidity and mortality rates reflect the expertise and experience of the surgical teams.

The advantages of the operation of pharyngolaryngoesophagectomy may be summarized as follows:

1. The procedure allows total removal of the esophagus, thus eliminating the possibility of inadequate inferior resection of multicentric lesions.
2. Removal of paratracheal lymph nodes is enhanced.
3. The operation is performed in one stage. An intra-abdominal anastomosis is not required.
4. Even after radical radiotherapy, the blood supply to the pharyngogastric anastomosis is excellent.
5. The cervically placed stomach readily accepts a skin graft, thus allowing resection of damaged or involved cervical skin without the need for local or distant skin flaps.
6. The postoperative stay is short and swallowing invariably trouble free.
7. Even when disease is left in situ within neck or superior mediastinum, swallowing remains good since penetration of the gastric wall by extrinsic tumor is unusual.

CHOICE OF PATIENT AND OPERATION

As the ultimate success of any oncologic operation lies in the ability to resect locally all neoplasm, preoperative assessment of both tumor and regional lymph metastasis is essential in both planning the operation and determining feasibility. These findings, or more frequently impressions, form the basis for preoperative classification and eventually comparisons of treatment modalities. Although computed tomography (CT) scanning and fiberoptic endoscopy has enhanced our ability to evaluate the mucosal extent of disease within the cervical esophagus, extension outside the muscle wall or involvement of paratracheal lymph nodes is rarely detectable. Manubrial resection as recommended by Harrison[5] in 1977 allows low resection of the trachea, minimizing risk of disease being left in the posterior wall of the tracheostome (Fig. 28–2) and also facilitates clearance of the paratracheal nodes. Even when disease is left on prevertebral fascia or at the root of the neck, effective palliation is obtained with pharyngogastric anastomosis and this is not an indication of inoperability. However, even though unilateral regional lymph node metastases indicate a need for combining neck dissection with primary resection, my personal experience of patients presenting with bilateral cervical metastasis is that their prognosis is so poor that in most cases they should be considered inoperable.

Every patient with hypopharyngeal or cervical esophageal cancer has dysphagia or at least discomfort on swallowing. Many have poor nutritional status. Although gastrostomy feeding does not preclude subsequent transposition of the stomach, delay in surgery may lead to extension of an initially resectable lesion and respiratory infection from overflow of saliva secondary to severe dysphagia. If the patient's nutritional condition cannot be improved within a brief period of time, gastric transposition may not be feasible.

Advanced age, extensive local disease, or systemic metastases are obvious contraindications to any form of surgery. Poor general condition is less easy to evaluate. My personal experience has been that diabetes, hypertension, or previous myocardial infarction magnify the danger of operative morbidity and mortality, but skilled anesthesia and nursing care may diminish such risk to a level appropriate to the otherwise lethal disease being treated. Such surgery, however, cannot be viewed as a "euthanasic" procedure. It is important to appreciate that trouble-free swallowing is a worthwhile alternative to dying with gastrostomy and tracheostomy.

Many patients will have been enthusiastic users of tobacco and alcohol. Although the latter will occasionally result in hepatic dysfunction, reduced vital capacity from emphysema or chronic bronchitis seriously increases operative morbidity and mortality. Although the degree of risk is difficult to quantify, patients considered as having serious respiratory dysfunction are in jeopardy of adult respiratory distress syndrome and, if elderly, may not survive such a major operation.

SURGICAL PROCEDURE

Although Ong and Lee had successfully shown that the stomach could be mobilized to reach the pharynx and remain viable, the anatomic basis for the operation was not demonstrated until nearly 20 years later. By injecting radiopaque media into the arterial supply of 22 postmortem human stomachs, it was shown that the right gastroepiploic artery alone will perfuse the fundus of the stomach, normally supplied by the left gastric artery.

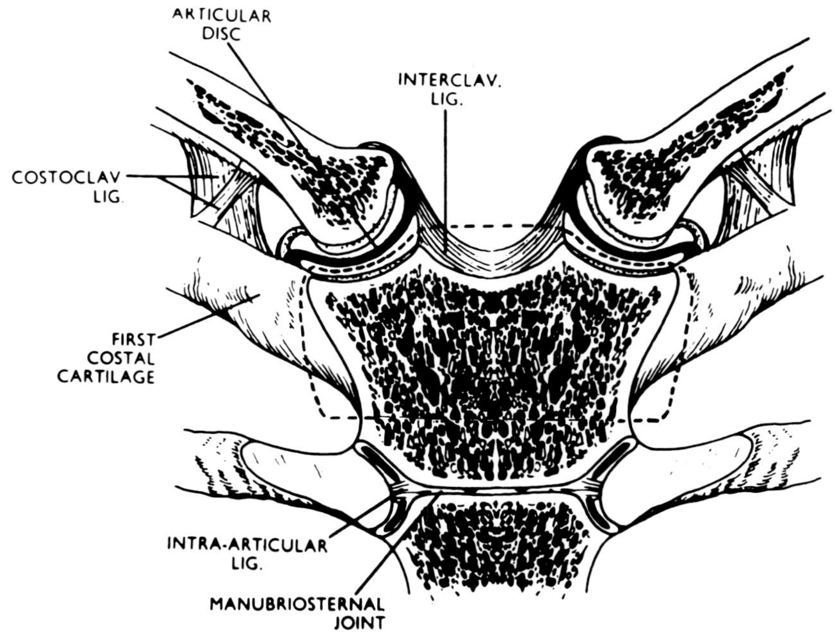

Figure 28–2. Schematic representation of line of excision of the upper part of the manubrium sterni.

Perfusion is independent of the left gastric arcade and occurs through the submucosal anastomotic plexus. Unless severe atherosclerosis is present, viability of the transposed stomach can be assured after preservation of the right gastroepiploic artery (Fig. 28–3). This has been the case in my personal series of 145 consecutive gastric pull-up operations in which fundus viability was consistently maintained. Initial accounts of the operation included thoracotomy, which has been found to be unnecessary and increases morbidity.

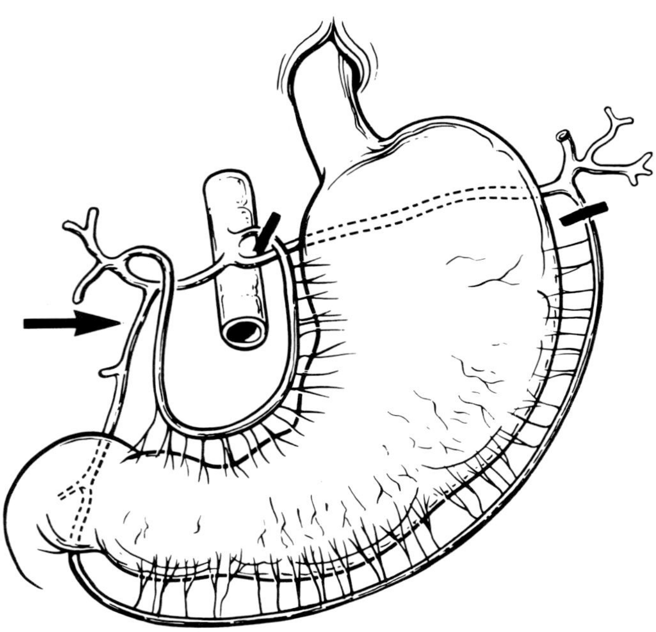

Figure 28–3. Gastric blood supply after ligation of left gastroepiploic and left gastric artery. (Right gastroepiploic artery indicated by arrow.)

Operative details have been described by Harrison and Thompson,[6] who recommend two surgical teams. The head and neck surgeon carries out a pharyngolaryngectomy with total thyroidectomy and manubrial resection if indicated. Radical neck dissection is included with preservation of accessory nerve, except in the rare instance in which metastasis in the upper cervical lymph nodes is suspected. The cervical and mediastinal esophagus is mobilized from above down to the level of the bifurcation of the trachea. This must be carried out with the endotracheal tube balloon deflated to prevent tearing of the posterior tracheal wall. Following mobilization of stomach, duodenum, and esophagus to the level of the carina, the stomach is drawn up through the empty posterior mediastinum by gentle traction on the pharyngolarynx and guidance from below (Fig. 28–4). Rotation of the fundus within the neck allows the highest part to reach the pharyngeal defect. After transecting the cardia, the esophagogastric opening is closed in traditional manner and an incision is made in the gastric fundus and tailored to fit the pharyngostoma. Anchoring the stomach to the prevertebral fascia assists in preventing gastric retraction while the pharyngogastric anastomosis is completed. If omentum is available, this can be used to cover suture lines or carotid artery following neck dissection. Drainage of both pleural cavities is essential for measurement of postoperative bleeding from the mediastinum. Average loss over 48 hours postoperatively is 1 liter. The drains are removed when dry.

Following pyloromyotomy, a feeding jejunostomy tube is placed 12 cm from the duodenojejunal flexure. A nasogastric tube is unnecessary.

Extramural Tumor Extension

Transposition of the stomach into the neck allows swallowing even when extramural disease is left in situ. Tumor invading the prevertebral fascia may be excised, providing the anterior longitudinal ligament is spared to preserve vertebral blood

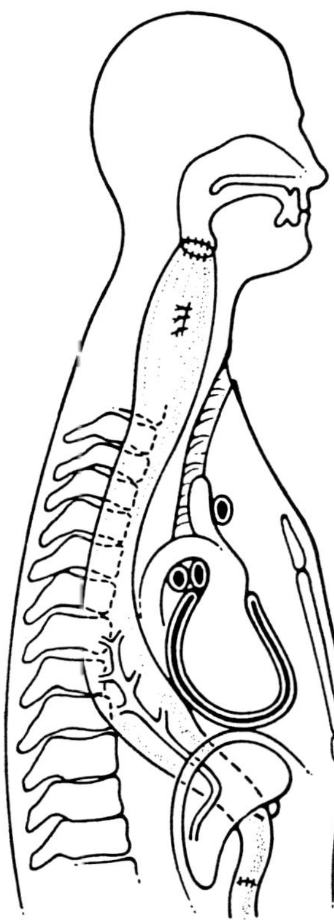

Figure 28–4. Schematic representation of pharyngogastric operation with stomach occupying the posterior mediastinum.

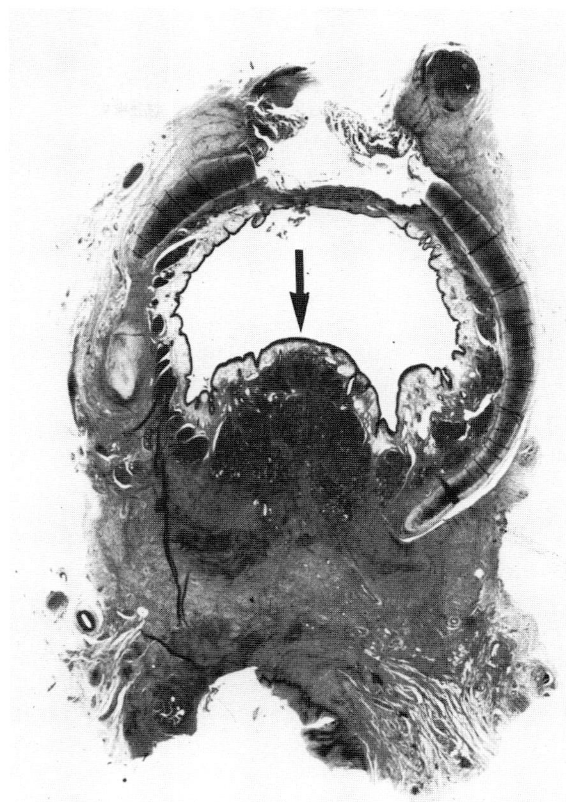

Figure 28–5. Section through tracheoesophageal junction showing involvement of posterior tracheal wall by esophageal cancer (arrow). Section cut at 5 μm.

supply. Neoplasm at the root of the neck invariably involves the carotid arteries, which are closely related to the tracheoesophageal groove. Excision of segments of these vessels with repair has proved unsuccessful in my hands and is not recommended.

Manubrial Resection

The clavicular heads and manubrium sterni often impede access to the trachea for transection below potentially involved tracheoesophageal party wall in large esophageal tumors. Removal of manubrium will provide adequate exposure of trachea as well as the oncologically significant paratracheal lymph nodes, as far inferiorly as the innominate (brachiocephalic) vein. The trachea inclines posteriorly as it descends; nevertheless, at least 3 cm more trachea can be resected via this approach than through the cervical incision (Fig. 28–5).

The surgical details of manubrial resection were reported by Harrison in 1977.[6] The only modification suggested after 72 operations (it is also recommended for subglottic extension in laryngeal neoplasms) is the use of the straight cutting Fisher burr, which reduces time in cutting through the clavicle and first rib (Fig. 28–6).

Tracheal Disruption

In many patients the esophagus is surrounded by fibrous bands and care is necessary when mobilizing the upper portion to avoid tearing muscle wall or, as previously stressed, posterior tracheal wall. The latter is avoidable providing the balloon of the endotracheal tube is completely deflated during mobilization. If this is not done, a tear may extend to the carina, posing considerable difficulty in repair.

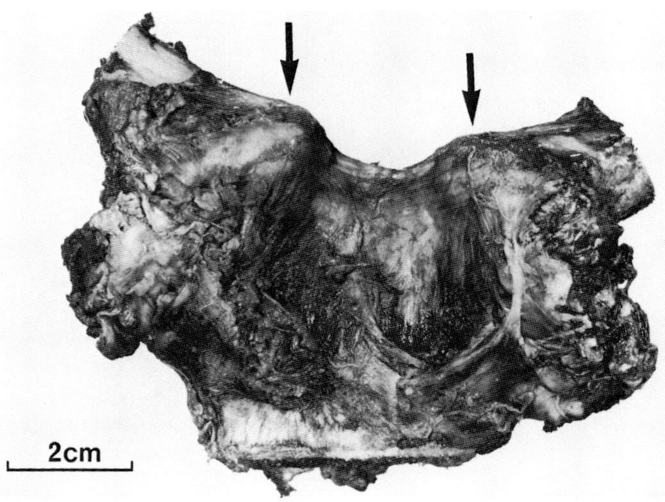

Figure 28–6. Excised manubrium sterni with both clavicular heads (arrows).

Skin Grafting

The transposed stomach is an excellent base for skin grafting. Used successfully in five of my own patients, this allows involved or radiation-damaged cervical skin to be resected along with the laryngopharynx (Fig. 28–7).

Anesthesia

Anesthesia presents no particular difficulty except avoidance of hypotension. During transabdominal mobilization of the stomach, cardiac irregularities and short-term hypotension are common—hypotension prior to this could be irreversible.

Thyroidectomy

In 1973 Harrison[7] discussed his rationale for advocating total thyroidectomy in "gastric pull-up" operations. The problems of postoperative maintenance of thyroid and parathyroid function are discussed later, but this philosophy has been maintained, although it is agreed that examination of the operative specimen confirms that fewer than 50% of patients could have safely had a less radical procedure. However, direct involvement of thyroid by extension from circumferential tumor or secondary involvement from metastatic disease in upper paratracheal lymph nodes is rarely discernible, particularly following radiotherapy. Disease left within a thyroid remnant following subtotal thyroidectomy is rarely detected before involvement of the closely related carotid artery and is inoperable. Since replacement of thyroid, and when necessary parathyroid, function has presented few problems in my 145 gastric pull-ups, I still consider this a worthwhile part of the operation.

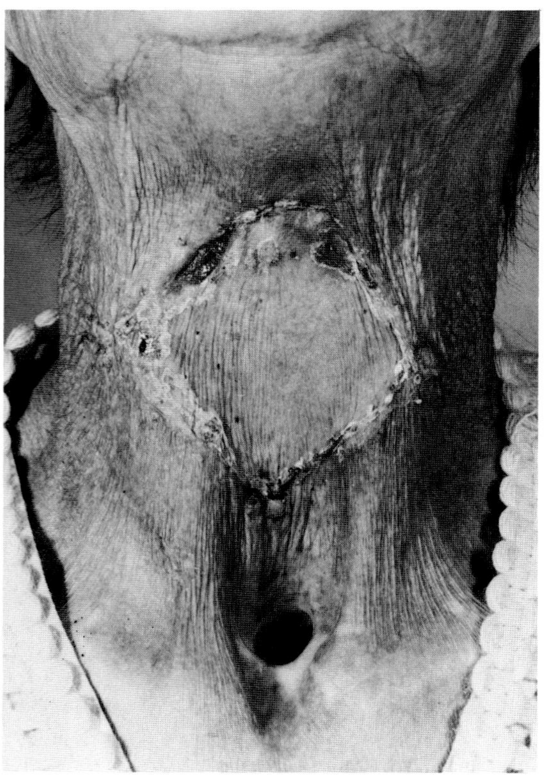

Figure 28–7. A split-skin graft has been applied to the transposed stomach following excision of involved cervical skin.

Hemorrhage

Despite the filling of the posterior mediastinum with transposed stomach, bleeding is inevitable and is best evacuated via drains inserted during the initial operation. This not only prevents hemothorax, but allows measurement and replacement of postoperative blood loss within the neck. Corrugated rubber drains have proved more satisfactory than traditional suction drainage, since the latter are soon blocked with omental fat. The dead space is minimal except after neck dissection, being filled with transposed stomach. Drains should reach as high as the pharyngogastric suture lines, although with careful suturing leakage should not occur.

OPERATIVE MORTALITY

Comparisons between operative mortality rates for any operation are hindered by lack of agreement on the time duration to be considered. Perhaps the most realistic definition is "the number of patients dying before they leave the hospital, irrespective of the cause." In patients with hypopharyngeal or esophageal cancer it is influenced by previous radiotherapy, poor general condition, and the method of repair.

Undeniably, gastric transposition is a potentially dangerous operation requiring considerable surgical and nursing expertise. Lam et al,[8] with the largest experience of 157 patients, reported a mortality rate of 31% over a 14-year period, although this had dropped to 18% during the last 2 years. Many of their patients were in poor general condition; over half had advanced primary laryngeal cancers. My own figures for 145 operations show a mortality of 9.3%. It is unlikely that further reduction can be expected without the most rigorous selection of patients.

Preoperative pulmonary infections, common in patients with obstructive lesions within hypopharynx and esophagus, are difficult to control, although surgery is carried out under an "umbrella" of metronidazole and cephalosporin. Emphysema and poor respiratory reserve in heavy smokers enhances the risk of operation, and pulmonary emboli or myocardial infarction remain hazards for all within the age group over 50 years. Hemorrhage and sepsis, although a major cause of death in the patients operated on by Lam et al,[8] have not been a problem in my own experience.

Table 28–1 is an analysis of the 13 patients who died postoperatively in the hospital. One patient with undetected aortic stenosis should not have been operated on and the two patients with irreversible hypotension alerted us to the need for drains to measure postoperative blood loss within the posterior mediastinum. One patient had severe stomach wall necrosis associated with loss of overlying skin. He had a radiation-induced cricoesophageal tumor, uncontrolled diabetes, and was in a poor general condition. Skin grafting on the transposed stomach was not then appreciated and skin loss led to fatal

Table 28-1. Hospital Deaths After Gastric Pull-Up

Operative death	
Aortic stenosis	1
Myocardial infarct	1
Pulmonary	
Embolism	1
Bronchopneumonia	2
Adult respiratory distress syndrome	2
Cardiovascular	
Myocardial infarction	2
Hypotension	2
Mesenteric thrombosis	1
Graft necrosis	1
Total	13/140 (9.3%)

secondary hemorrhage These deaths would now be considered avoidable.

The remaining operative deaths may be considered unavoidable, unless a policy of such rigorous selection were adopted as to deprive many patients of a lengthy period of worthwhile palliation or a chance of cure. At the present time, an operative mortality of approximately 10% would seem justifiable in view of the poor prognosis without surgical treatment; a higher mortality rate would appear to be ethically unacceptable.

POSTOPERATIVE COMPLICATIONS

Morbidity, defined as nonlethal complications, will be present to some degree after any operation. Table 28–2 quantifies those postoperative complications that occurred in my own series during hospitalization. They differ from those reported in other large series due to variations in surgical technique, nutritional status of patients, and selection criteria.

Despite previous radiotherapy (approximately 40% of our patients), healing was excellent and the few cases of small pharyngogastric fistulas were due to errors in surgical technique. Although potentially lethal chest infections were common, particularly in elderly debilitated patients, diligent postoperative physiotherapy was successful in preventing mortality. Pneumothorax was effectively prevented by mediastinal drainage, but some degree of clinically insignificant pleural effusion was often detected radiologically. The same drains obviated the risk of undetected mediastinal bleeding. Bile regurgitation invariably ceased with oral feeding although occasionally became a long-term problem. Diarrhea was common with jejunostomy feeding despite varying the preparations used.

Table 28-2. Morbidity After Gastric Pull-Up (Excluding Deaths)

Pleural effusion	All (routine drains)
Cardiac arrhythmia	All (during operation)
Pharyngogastric fistula	2 (2%)
Sloughing of skin—stomach	2 (2%)
Wound infection	0 —
Abdominal wound dehiscence	2 (2%)
Colon prolapse into chest	1 (1%)
Chest infection	15 (15%)
Bile regurgitation	22 (22%)
Diarrhea	All —

It is difficult to explain variations in both incidence and etiology of complications between my experience and that reported by Lam et al.[8] Our patients were possibly in better general condition, required neck dissection less often, and rarely had pharyngogastric fistulas. The latter is a prime initiator of infection and should be avoidable, since the repair is both easier and more substantial than after total laryngectomy. It is possible that the high incidence of this complication experienced by Lam with his population of ethnic Chinese patients may be due to discrepancy in relative size of the stomach with consequently precarious blood supply to the fundus. Prophylactic antibiotic coverage of all major head and neck operations with metronidazole and cephalosporin, as has been my practice for the past 8 years, has reduced the fistula rate after total laryngectomy to less than 5%, irrespective of previous irradiation.

Tension-free pharyngogastric anastomosis is essential and can be achieved without special modifications, simply by adequate mobilization of the stomach and low pharyngeal resection. Coverage of the suture line with omentum is helpful. This tissue, when available, may also be used to cover the carotid artery following neck dissection.

Most patients are able to swallow liquids by the fifth postoperative day, depending on the duration of postoperative ileus. Excellent deglutition may be expected by the tenth postoperative day, although this is in part related to patient motivation because the absence of pharyngeal constrictor muscles requires the sole use of the tongue to initiate deglutition. Hypoglossal nerve paralysis following neck dissection will seriously hamper subsequent swallowing.

Although influenced by factors such as neck dissection, concomitant chest infection, and the patient's ability to acquire adequate oral nutrition, the average period of hospitalization will be 2 weeks.

Control of Thyroid and Parathyroid Function

Histologic examination of the operative specimens of circumferential postcricoid and cervical esophageal cancers verifies that microscopic invasion of the thyroid gland, either by direct spread or metastatic disease in closely related paratracheal lymph nodes, occurs to varying degrees. Despite the potential value of thyroid scan and palpation, it is usually not possible to detect this invasion. As operative assessment by mobilization and close examination contravenes the dictum of minimizing tissue damage in proximity to malignant tumors, it is accepted that total thyroidectomy should accompany radical ablation of postcricoid and high cervical esophageal neoplasms. Not only does this enhance the opportunity for oncologic resection of the neoplasm but when combined with manubrial resection virtually guarantees avoidance of subsequent stomal recurrence. Although it is expected that following total thyroidectomy each patient would require replacement therapy with thyroxine, long-term thyroid function tests show that about 10% recover function spontaneously.

The problems of both short- and long-term calcium metabolism are more complex and serious and have been recently reviewed by Price and Ridley.[9] From their analysis of ten patients following gastric pull-up with various combinations of thyroparathyroidectomy and mediastinal dissection, they concluded that postoperative hypocalcemia should be controlled with intravenous calcium to maintain an adjusted serum calcium of 7.6 to 8.0 mg/dL. They also stress that exogenous thyroid hormone inhibits intestinal uptake of calcium and is unnecessary for several weeks, since significant hypothyroidism will not occur until that time.

With the beginning of jejunostomy feeding, calcium gluconate can be given together with vitamin D, although the dosage of the latter will vary from patient to patient. They also stress the need for continuous monitoring of serum calcium levels for signs of hypercalcemia. Their conclusions are similar to those reported by Buchanan et al[10] in 1975 and Harrison[6] in 1986. Some patients require large amounts of supplementary calcium, possibly because of dietary insufficiency or poor absorption. Hypercalcemia with metastatic calcification occurred in two patients because of inadequate monitoring.

In view of these difficulties, autotransplantation of parathyroid glands has been considered. Ideally, identification should be undertaken intraoperatively, but, because of the risk of disseminating tumor, this can be carried out, with some difficulty, on the freshly excised specimen. Although mediastinal dissection appears to result in complete ablation of parathyroid function, this is not so in total thyroidectomy alone. Measurements of parathyroid hormone levels have shown that return of normal levels can occur within 2 years postoperatively, suggesting that at least one parathyroid remains in situ, possibly because of variations in number or location.

LONG-TERM PROBLEMS

Most patients are able to eat a normal diet, although many elderly patients require small but frequent feedings. The sensation of discomfort or frank "dumping" syndrome is not common, although video studies on swallowing transit time does reveal delay at the gastroduodenal junction in some individuals (Fig. 28–8).

Regurgitation of both food and bile may occur, particularly when lying down after eating. This probably relates to slow emptying of the stomach and is avoided by reducing the quantity of food eaten, together with avoidance of a supine position for an hour or so after eating.

Although gastritis can be detected on gastric biopsy, few patients complain of relevant symptoms and ulceration is rare. Acid secretion is reduced following bilateral vagotomy and ulceration would be expected to respond to H_2-antagonists.

Despite the young age of many patients treated by pharyngolaryngoesophagectomy and the high degree of motivation, few acquire an acceptable "gastric voice." Elimination of tactile and kinesthetic sensation from the gastric reservoir affects the patient's awareness of air distension and release. A few highly motivated younger patients have received a tracheogastric shunt successfully, whereas others manually compress their cervical stomach to speak.

SURVIVAL

Many patients with cervical esophageal cancer present with locally advanced or disseminated disease and although they may possibly be palliated with gastric pull-up, they will not be cured. Extramural tumor or paraesophageal nodal metastases markedly reduce prognosis even when surgery is followed by radiation therapy. Total esophagectomy will ensure adequacy of distal margins and removal of subclinical multifocal neoplasm, although there was only one instance of second primary esophageal tumor in the 145 patients in our series (Fig. 28–9). Table 28–3 shows an analysis of cause of death in patients who died while free of local disease. Most of the pathologic conditions are to be expected within the age group treated and relate to the effects of continuing systemic disease and further primary

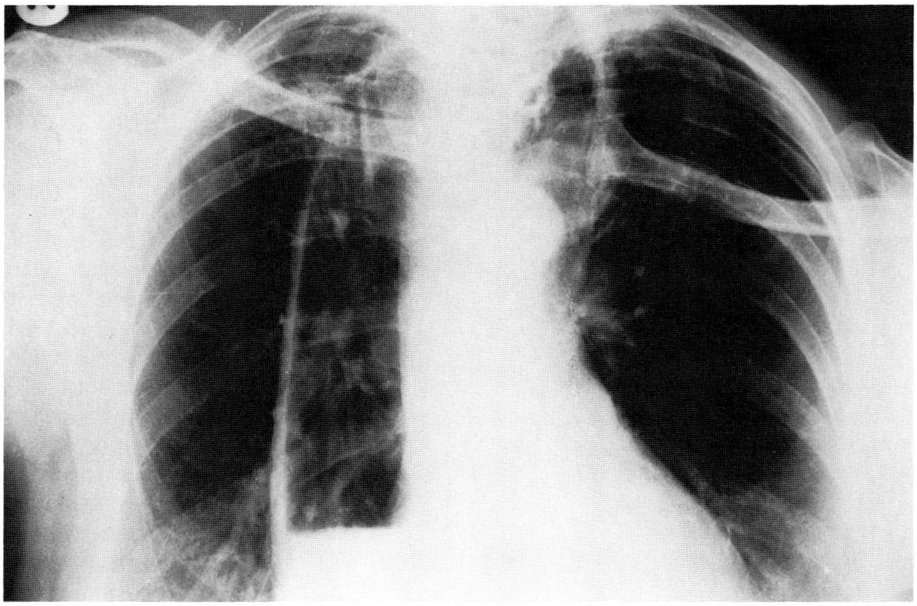

Figure 28–8. Barium swallow following gastric pull-up to show distended "thoracic" stomach.

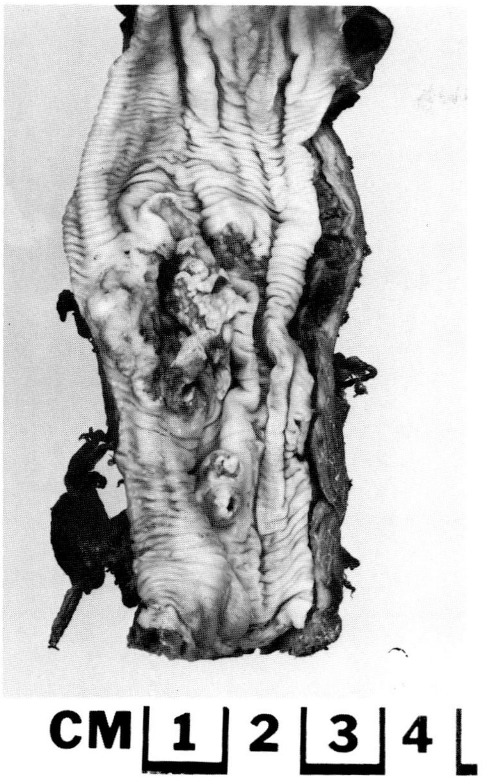

Figure 28–9. Section of excised esophagus cut at 5 μm showing a second malignant tumor. Primary was in the cricoesophageal region.

neoplasms, but no effects are directly attributable to the operation of gastric pull-up except possibly nephrocalcinosis, the risk of which is now recognizable and avoidable.

The greatest concern is the late development of systemic metastases in patients with apparently complete local control. Whereas survival within the first postoperative year is primarily related to extent of primary tumor and cervical lymph node metastases, long-term survival is less easy to predict. Although the operation described here produces excellent local control of potentially curable neoplasms of the cricoesophageal region, improvement in long-term survival may possibly require prolonged administration of systemic chemotherapy. The risk remains, however, that usage of immunosuppressent drugs might actually increase the risk of systemic metastases.

Table 28–3. Deaths Occurring More Than 1 Year After Discharge From the Hospital—92 Patients

Second primary neoplasm	
Lung	8
Breast	2
Uterus	1
Oral cavity	2
Systemic metastasis	15
Myocardial infarct	8
Cerebrovascular accident	6
Pulmonary embolism	3
Mephrocalcinosis	2
Hepatic failure (alcoholic cirrhosis)	3
Bleeding duodenal ulcer	1
Traffic accident	1
Senility	5

REFERENCES

1. Harrison DFN. Pathology of hypopharyngeal cancer in relation to surgical management. J Laryngol 1970;84:349–64.
2. DeSanto LW, Carpenter RS. Reconstruction of the pharynx and upper esophagus after resection for cancer. Head Neck Surg 1980;2:369–79.
3. Surkin MI, Lawson W, Biller HF. Analysis of the methods of pharyngoesophageal reconstruction. Head Neck Surg 1984;6:953–70.
4. Ong GB, Lee TC. Pharyngogastric anastomosis after oesophagopharyngectomy for carcinoma of the hypopharynx and cervical esophagus. Br J Surg 1960;48:193–200.
5. Harrison DFN. Resection of the manubrium. Br J Surg 1977;64:374–7.
6. Harrison DFN, Thompson AE. Pharyngolaryngoesophagectomy with pharyngogastric anastomosis for cancer of the hypopharynx. Review of 101 operations. Head Neck Surg 1986;8:418–28.
7. Harrison DFN. Thyroid gland in the management of laryngopharyngeal cancer. Arch Otolaryngol 1973;97:301–2.
8. Lam KH, Wong J, Lim STK, Ong GB. Pharyngogastric anastomosis following pharyngolaryngoesophagectomy. Analysis of 157 cases. World J Surg 1981;5:509–16.
9. Price JC, Ridley MB. Hypocalcemia following pharyngoesophageal ablation and gastric pull-up reconstruction. Pathophysiology and management. Ann Otol Rhinol Laryngol 1988;97:521–6.
10. Buchanan G, West TET, Woodhead JS. Hypoparathyroidism following pharyngolaryngoesophagectomy. Clin Oncol 1975;1:89–96.

29

Replacement of Cervical Pharyngoesophageal Segment by Tubed Pectoralis Major Myocutaneous Flap

Kam Hing Lam, William I. Wei, Wai Fong Lau

The problem of pharyngoesophageal replacement has been addressed since the 1940s. Without the advantage of present-day understanding of flap circulation and technique of microvascular anastomosis, only local or adjacent tissues were used. There was, thus, enormous restriction on the pliability and maneuverability of the available flaps. The intervening decades have brought forth a plethora of reconstructive options for this and similar defects. Each has its advocates, and each has been reported to produce good results, although complications are not unknown. There are also accounts of use of a variety of methods in individual reported series, most often indicating the change of the surgeon's attitude with time. In the light of continued development and accumulation of experience, these changes are inevitable.

For more than a decade, our institution exclusively used the pharyngogastric anastomosis (gastric transposition) technique for replacing all types of pharyngeal defects.[1] This occasionally required resection of more than the necessary volume of uninvolved tissue to produce the appropriate defect. Although results improved as we gained experience,[2] mortality following the procedure was still considerable. In the meantime other reconstructive techniques became available. At present, the need to alter the defect to suit one single reconstruction method has largely disappeared. We have now adopted the philosophy of selection of the method of reconstruction with reference to the type of defect produced.[3]

The need to define types of pharyngoesophageal defects is apparent. Perhaps with future development, finer groupings may be necessary. At present, three types of defects can be classified[4] according to the amount of missing tissue and the shape of the required replacement:

1. Partial hypopharyngeal defect—a noncircumferential defect left after total laryngectomy and partial pharyngectomy.
2. Circumferential hypopharyngeal defect—a defect left after total pharyngectomy (hypopharynx only) and partial (limited) esophagectomy.
3. Pharyngoesophageal defect—a defect left after total pharyngectomy and total esophagectomy.

For each group of defects, a range of possible replacement methods is now available, affording a choice to the surgeon. For partial defects, only a "patch-on" flap is required. For circumferential defects, tubular replacement is necessary. The tubed pectoralis major myocutaneous flap, the subject of this chapter, is our choice. For the full pharyngoesophageal defect, a sufficiently long segment of some part of the gastrointestinal tract is needed.

INDICATIONS FOR USE OF TUBED PECTORALIS FLAP

Extensive laryngeal cancer may involve the pharyngeal wall by growth along the mucosa or by deep extension, so that, in addition to total laryngectomy, pharyngectomy of varying magnitude is required. Tumor creeping along the mucosa to involve the pharyngeal aspect of the aryepiglottic fold affects the upper part of the hypopharynx, which is wide, so that partial pharyngectomy is all that is required, and tubular tissue reconstruction is not needed. The more inferior parts of the hypopharynx may be affected by deep extension of the laryngeal cancer. Pyriform sinus mucosa can be involved by spread of tumor through the paraglottic space, whereas the postcricoid mucosa can be implicated by spread through the cricoarytenoid joint or the interarytenoid muscle. When the postcricoid region of the apex of the pyriform fossa is affected, a circumferential resection wil be required and the tubed pectoralis major flap used for repair.

In the occasional instance of involvement of esophagus by laryngeal tumor, we advocate total esophagectomy. This is based on our belief that, with adequate resection inferiorly, the level of transection of esophagus will be too low for safe anastomosis. Thus, the tubed pectoralis major flap is not indicated in such situations.

OPERATIVE TECHNIQUE

The anatomy and principles of the pectoralis major myocutaneous flap is well known and need not be repeated here. Details concerning the outline of the skin island and the anastomosis will be described.

The skin island required to produce a tubelike structure is either rectangular or trapezoid[5] in shape. The minimum width of the skin island required to produce an adequate lumen is 7 cm. The lower edge of the skin island may be 9 or 10 cm if interdigitation is not intended for the wide upper anastomosis with the oropharynx. For secondary reconstruction, interdigitation is essential and a rectangular island is used. The most suitable length of the skin island is equal to the span between the mucosal edges of the oropharynx and the esophagus. The length of the gap thus measured will be more than that of the resected tissue. The slight extra length of the skin tube will be taken up by the interdigitations at the anastomosis. A redundant flap should also be avoided.

Since the flap does not have to reach as high as required for oral cavity reconstruction, the skin island may be taken from the mid region rather than the most inferior portion of the chest wall. The outline of the island is placed between the third rib and the xiphisternum, with the long axis parallel to the border of the sternum. The nipple may be included in the skin island if necessary. The flap is raised in the usual manner. We prefer to divide the clavicular head of the muscle and isolate the pectoral vascular pedicle, so as to minimize bulk when delivered to the neck.

In order to reduce the chance of anastomotic stricture, the inferior anastomosis of tubular flap (upper edge of the skin island from the chest wall) to esophageal stump is constructed in a particular manner.[6] Three 2 cm longitudinal slits are made in the esophageal stump, one anteriorly and two posterolaterally; equidistant to each other (Fig. 29–1). Two such slits are made on the corresponding edge of the skin island (Fig. 29–2), through epidermis and dermis only (Fig. 29–3). The subcutaneous fat does not require incision in order to permit adequate separation of the cutaneous edges to accept the projections of the esophageal end. The arrangement of vertical defects and projections thus created will interdigitate as the anastomosis is made, producing a "staggered" suture line that will resist stricture formation (Fig. 29–4). Interrupted absorbable sutures of 000 polyglactin are used. A similar method may be employed, if necessary, for the superior anastomosis of skin tube to pharyngeal margin (Fig. 29–5).

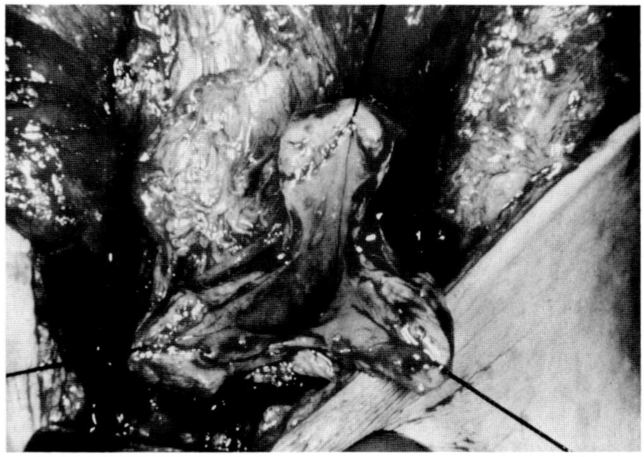

Figure 29–1. Three 2 cm slits are made on the esophageal stump. The three projections thus formed are held by stay sutures.

The vertical "tubing" line of sutures is placed last (Fig. 29–6). A nasogastric tube is inserted before its completion. Additional second layer sutures are not necessary and probably inadvisable along the anastomoses, but may be used to reinforce the vertical

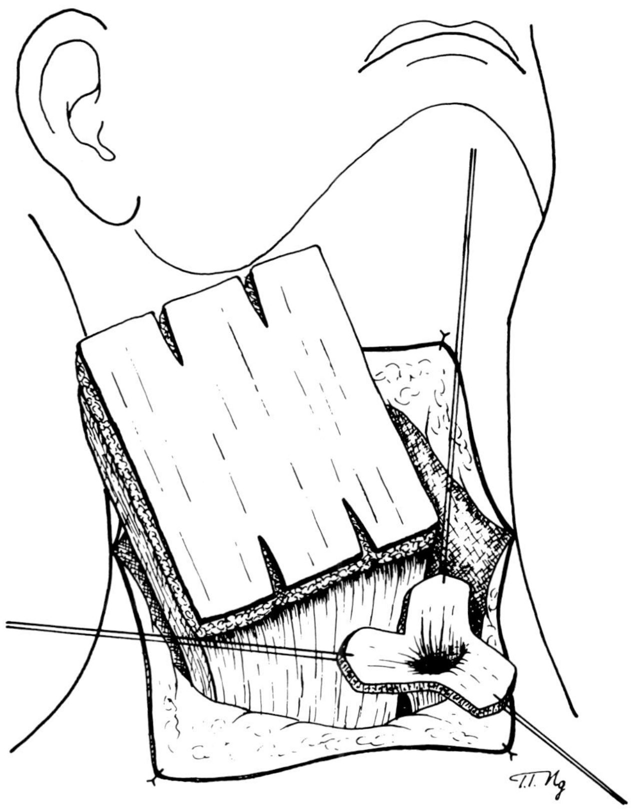

Figure 29–2. Two 2 cm slits are made on the anastomosing skin edge, which is about to be joined to the esophageal stump. Similar slits may be made on the skin edge for the upper anastomosis if intended.

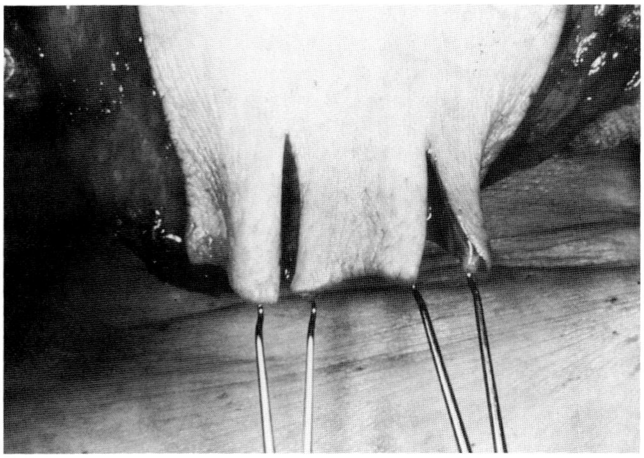

Figure 29–3. The slits on the skin edge are full thickness, carried through the epidermis and dermis. Subcutaneous fat is left intact.

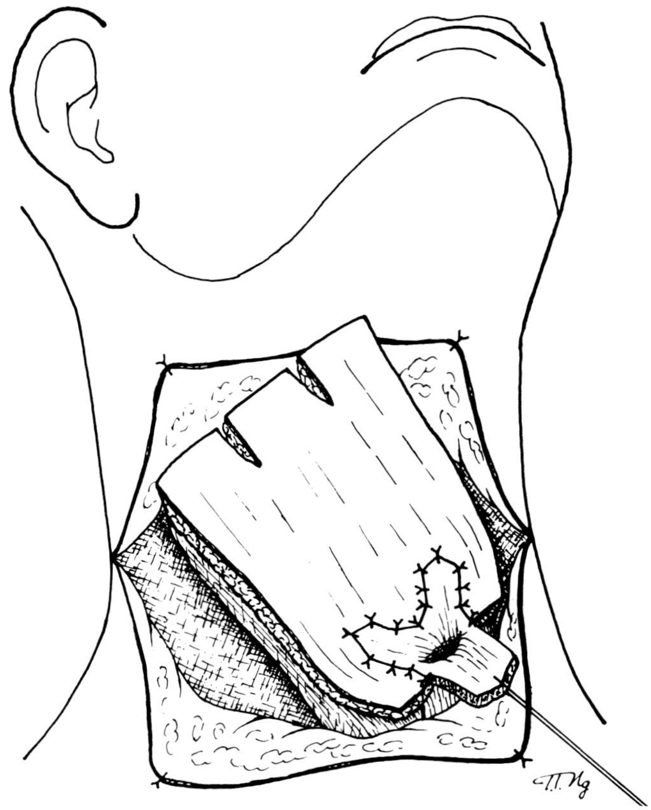

Figure 29–5. Before completion of inferior anastomosis, the upper anastomosis is started.

line. The neck and donor wounds are then closed in the usual manner.

If immediate tracheoesophageal puncture is intended, it can be fashioned after completion of the upper and lower anastomoses, before closure of the tubing suture line. A puncture is made through the posterior tracheal wall, 5 mm below the cut edge, and through the corresponding site on the anterior wall of the esophagus. The nasogastric feeding tube is passed through these two openings, as a stent, rather than transnasally. The tracheal and esophageal walls are "tacked" together to prevent extravasation of esophageal contents.

Feeding is maintained by nasogastric tube in the early postoperative period. Ten days after operation an esophagram is performed, to confirm integrity of the suture line prior to commencement of oral feeding (Fig. 29–7).

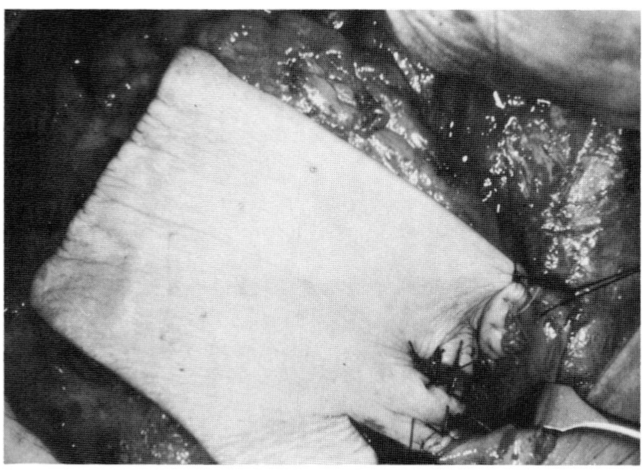

Figure 29–4. Inferior anastomosis in progress, projections being inserted into slits.

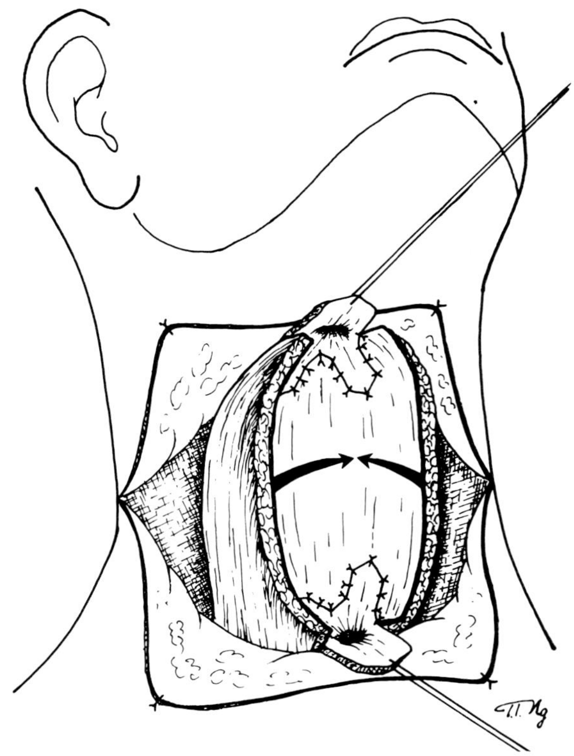

Figure 29–6. On completion of both anastomoses, the vertical tubing sutures are placed.

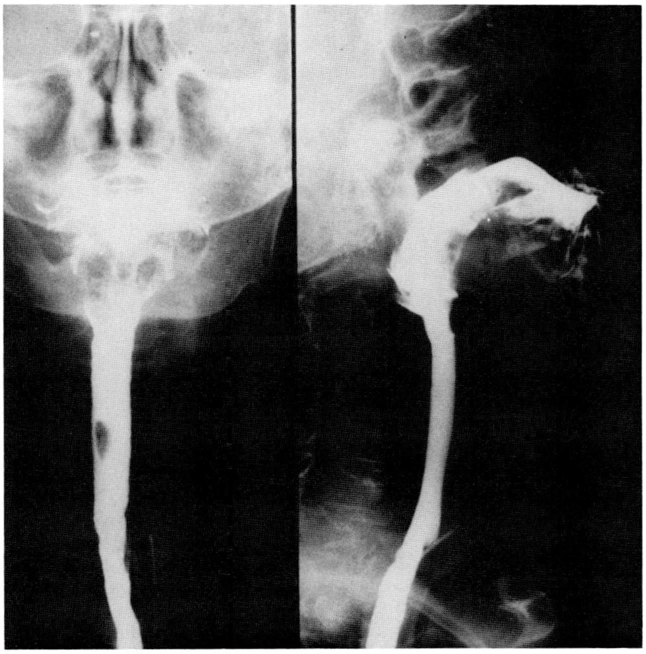

Figure 29–7. Postoperative contrast swallow showing straight, patent neopharynx and no leakage.

RESULTS

Ten years have elapsed since the pectoralis major myocutaneous flap was first used for head and neck reconstruction. As can be seen in Table 29–1, the number of reports on use of this flap for circumferential pharyngoesophageal defects is exceptionally small. The paucity of cases in each report indicates the infrequent need for circumferential replacement, whereas the paucity of reports indicates the general preference for other methods.

From the available data, it is evident that the pectoralis major flap remains a reliable source of tissue when used in this manner. There was only one flap loss among the several series. The occasional hospital mortality is related to extent of cancer and the resectional aspect of the operation, rather than the reconstructive technique.

Failure of this highly dependable flap to attract wide usage in circumferential pharyngoesophageal reconstruction is due to suggested technical difficulties and some reports of poor functional results. The latter may be averted by attention to details of operative technique. Although difficulty in forming a tube due to thickness of the subcutaneous fat has been reported,[7] most authors have not encountered this problem.[5,8–10]

Salivary fistula and stricture formation appear to be relatively frequent problems. Pharyngocutaneous fistula occurred in four of 18 patients in the early series of Baek et al.[11] This led the authors to adopt a practice of fashioning a temporary pharyngostoma, thus making the procedure two-staged. A subsequent report from the same center[9] reported an even higher incidence of salivary fistula; ten of 17 patients (59%). A literature review of 67 cases reported an overall fistula rate of 35.8%.[5] Most salivary fistulas healed without further operation.

The cause of frequent salivary fistula remains unidentifiable. Previous irradiation has been implicated.[5,10] Perhaps it is a specific problem of a mucocutaneous junction. It is not due to the interdigitation method of anastomosis, since the majority of fistulas that we have encountered are seen in the upper anastomosis, which is usually not interdigitated. Although the breakdown is often found on the contralateral aspect, which is furthest from the vascular pedicle, no evidence of necrosis has been found in any of the cases. Thus, vascular insufficiency would not seem to be the cause.

Anastomotic stricture is a more serious and difficult problem

Table 29–1. Reported Complications and Swallowing Function of Tubed Pectoralis Major Flap for Circumferential Pharyngeal Reconstruction

	YEAR	NO.	HOSPITAL DEATHS	FLAP LOSS	SALIVARY FISTULAS	ANASTOMOTIC STRICTURE	SWALLOWING ABILITY
Withers et al[12]	1981	2	0	0	1	0	1 good
Baek et al*[11]	1982	18	0	0	4	7	—
Murakami et al†[15]	1982	4	0	0	0	0	All good
Neifeld et al[8]	1983	5	1	0	3¶	—	—
Robertson and Robinson[7]	1984	3	0	0	1	2	—
Surkin et al‡[9]	1984	17	1	0	10	5	41% adequate
Stell§[10]	1984	22	4	1	6	3	—
Schuller‖[13]	1985	10	0	0	1	2	3 good 2 liquid 5 inadequate
Lam et al[4]	1989	18	1	0	7	1	71% normal 24% soft 5% liquid
Silver et al[14]	1989	10	2	0	4	1	80% good

*Eleven of 18, two-stage.
†Split-thickness skin graft on muscle flap.
‡Probably includes some cases reported by Baek et al.
§Skin island closed in spiral manner.
‖Anastomosis stented for several weeks.
¶One required a second flap repair.

to handle. It is, however, largely preventable, with the interdigitating method of anastomosis. Stenosis may or may not cause swallowing difficulties. The narrowed portion can be dealt with by dilation or surgical revision, and thus may not give rise to persistent problems.

Bolus retention may, on the other hand, occur in the absence of stricture. In the early report of Withers et al,[12] which included two cases of the operation under consideration, there were no strictures reported, but only one patient was able to swallow without difficulty. Robertson and Robinson[7] reported two strictures in three patients, but they did not indicate whether swallowing was affected. Surkin et al[9] reported five strictures in 16 cases (31%, excluding one hospital death); only 41% could swallow adequately. A similar stenosis rate was also reported by Stell[10] (three of 18, 17%), and Schuller[13] (two of ten, 20%). Schuller reported that only three of ten could eventually swallow satisfactorily. Only one of our patients developed an anastomotic stricture, and that was when conventional straight edge-to-edge suturing was initially used. Ninety-five percent of the patients eventually took a normal to soft diet and only one was restricted to liquids.[4] Silver and his group[5,14] also found stenosis not a problem, despite use of a simple circular anastomosis.

The cause of anastomotic stricture is the shortness of the edge of the esophagus and skin border. There is a natural tendency for any mucocutaneous suture line to contract excessively. It is surprising that Murakamei et al[15] found no stenosis even with split-thickness skin graft on bare muscle "anastomosed" to the esophagus. Dividing the esophagus obliquely, and stretching the esophageal wall before suturing, are inadequate methods of lengthening the suture line. Since we have adopted the interdigitating method of anastomosis, we have not encountered a stricture. This modification of anastomotic technique is recommended, not only for use with the pectoralis major flap, but also with other skin-lined flaps used in the same situation.

Inertia is assumed to be the cause of inability to swallow in the presence of an adequate passage. Obviously, the reconstructed pharynx has no peristalsis. Passage of food is dependent on gravity, assisted, in part, by the pharyngeal muscles. Thus, lubrication, softness of the bolus from chewing or special dietary preparation, and large lumenal size are extremely important. At the present time, it is uncertain whether there is any critical length beyond which inertial effect will overcome forces that promote deglutition.

CONCLUSIONS

We have found the tubed pectoralis major myocutaneous flap to be a simple and reliable source of tissue for reconstruction of circumferential pharyngoesophageal defects in the presence of an esophageal stump of adequate length. It does not require change of position or a separate surgical team, as for microvascular anastomosis, and can be accomplished in considerably less time. Frequent fistula formation may be an annoying complication, but fistulas usually heal spontaneously and do not interfere with long-term usefulness of reconstruction. Postoperative stricture formation and dysphagia are more serious problems, but may be prevented with appropriate surgical measures.

REFERENCES

1. Lam KH, Wong J, Lim STK, Ong GB. Pharyngogastric anastomosis following pharyngolaryngoesophagectomy—analysis of 157 cases. World J Surg 1981;5:509–16.
2. Lam KH, Choi TK, Wei WI, et al. Present status of pharyngogastric anastomosis following pharyngolaryngo-oesophagectomy. Br J Surg 1987;74:122–5.
3. Lau WF, Lam KH, Wei WI. Reconstruction of hypopharyngeal defects in cancer surgery: do we have a choice? Am J Surg 1987;154:374–80.
4. Lam KH, Ho CM, Lau WF, et al. Immediate reconstruction of pharyngoesophageal defects—preference or reference. Arch Otolaryngol Head Neck Surg 1989;115:608–12.
5. Cusumano RJ, Silver CE, Brauer RJ, Strauch B. Pectoralis myocutaneous flap for replacement of cervical esophagus. Head Neck 1989;11:450–6.
6. Lam KH, Wei WI, Lau WF. Avoiding stenosis in the tubed greater pectoral flap in pharyngeal repair. Arch Otolaryngol Head Neck Surg 1987;113:428–31.
7. Robertson MS, Robinson JM. Immediate pharyngoesophageal reconstruction—use of a quilted skin-grafted pectoralis major muscle flap. Arch Otolaryngol 1984;110:386–7.
8. Neifeld JP, Merritt WA, Theogaraj SD, Parker GA. Tubed pectoralis major musculocutaneous flaps for cervical esophageal replacement. Ann Plast Surg 1983;11:24–30.
9. Surkin MI, Lawson W, Biller HF. Analysis of the methods of pharyngoesophageal reconstruction. Head Neck Surg 1984;6:953–70.
10. Stell PM. Replacement of the pharynx after pharyngolaryngectomy. Ann R Coll Surg Engl 1984;66:388–90.
11. Baek SM, Lawson W, Biller HF. An analysis of 133 pectoralis major myocutaneous flaps. Plast Reconstr Surg 1982;69:460–7.
12. Withers EH, Franklin JD, Madden JJ, Lynch JB. Immediate reconstruction of the pharynx and cervical esophagus with the pectoralis major myocutaneous flap following laryngopharyngectomy. Plast Reconstr Surg 1981;68:898–904.
13. Schuller DE. Reconstructive options for pharyngeal and/or cervical esophageal defects. Arch Otolaryngol 1985;111:193–7.
14. Silver CE, Cusumano RJ, Fell SC, Strauch B. Replacement of upper esophagus: results with myocutaneous flap and with gastric transposition. Laryngoscope 1989;99:819–21.
15. Murakami Y, Saito S, Ikari T, et al. Esophageal reconstruction with a skin-grafted pectoralis major muscle flap. Arch Otolaryngol 1982; 108:719–22.

30

Replacement of the Cervical Esophagus by Free Jejunal Transplantation

Wilbur L. Baird, T. Roderick Hester, Jr.

Reconstruction of the cervical pharyngoesophageal segment following resection of aerodigestive tract tumors has long been a challenging problem. The complexity of the problem is attested to by the large number of procedures that have been tried and abandoned or retained. Early in surgical experience with these tumors, reconstruction was not even attempted, due to the poor prognosis of the disease. Subsequently, reconstruction was accomplished with skin grafts[1,2] or skin flaps;[3–5] however, the complication rate was high and multiple stages were often required. The results were greatly improved with the popularization of the axial deltopectoral flap by Bakamjian,[6] although two stages were still required. One stage reconstruction became more feasible and reliable with the development of musculocutaneous flaps[7–9] and pedicled flaps of intestinal segments.[10,11] A logical extension of these concepts has been the use of "free" jejunal transfer in the surgical rehabilitation of this difficult anatomic area.[12,13]

The feasibility of free tissue autotransplantation was demonstrated in the laboratory by Carrel[14,15] early in this century. This concept was confirmed by Longmire[16] in 1947, when he reported salvage of a pedicled jejunal transposition loop used for esophageal reconstruction by a mesenteric artery to internal mammary artery anastomosis. Seidenberg et al[17] in 1959 and Heibert and Cummings[18] in 1960 achieved replacement of the cervical esophagus with revascularized gastrointestinal segments. The procedures employed by these authors and others at the time were developed prior to the evolution and perfection of microvascular techniques.

The basic techniques of microvascular anastomosis were described in the 1960s.[19–21] The initial investigators and others then proceeded to develop the appropriate means for magnification, microinstrumentation, and microsuture. Reliable use of free tissue transfer in reconstructive surgery became relatively routine in the 1970s. These developments rekindled interest in using free tissue autotransplantation of bowel segments for reconstruction of the cervical pharyngoesophageal segment. By the 1980s, many authors reported experiences with large series of this type of reconstruction, with mortality and morbidity comparable to or better than previous reconstructive methods.[12,13,22]

In many centers free jejunal transfer has emerged as the procedure of choice for reconstruction of the cervical pharyngoesophageal segment, since the procedure can now be performed safely as a single stage reconstruction with acceptable morbidity. The primary reason for this is the excellent vascular supply of the flap and the fact that tissue similar to that removed is employed for replacement. In addition, the long vascular pedicle available is versatile in reaching various recipient vessels. The length of bowel that can be perfused by a single vascular pedicle is more than adequate to replace the segment extending from the base of the tongue to the thoracic inlet, and the attached mesentery may be used to cover exposed and/or irradiated vessels. Ths use of a bowel segment as a free flap also decreases the amount of dissection necessary to transfer the bowel to the neck; in contrast to pedicled flaps that require extensive intra-abdominal dissection and development of a pathway to the neck. Pedicled flaps, however, remain the procedure of choice in replacing the entire esophagus or longer segments than those usually encountered after resection for upper aerodigestive tract tumors.

SURGICAL TECHNIQUE

The surgical procedure is greatly facilitated by a two-team approach. This requires two separate sets of instruments and appropriate draping to ensure separation of the surgical fields. At a suitable time after the cervical portion of the procedure is begun, a laparotomy is performed to harvest the jejunal flap. The flap can then be inset and the microvascular anastomoses accomplished while the abdomen is closed.

The ablative phase of the procedure is performed in the usual fashion (Fig. 30–1). It is necessary, however, to consider possible recipient vessels for the jejunal transfer (Fig. 30–2). The external jugular vein should be divided as far cephalad as possible and then dissected caudad as far as possible on the side of the neck dissection. This maneuver is time consuming, but the length of vein is very helpful for the venous anastomosis. Vein grafting may be necessary if acceptable recipient veins cannot be saved in the course of the neck dissection. It is also helpful to preserve an adequate length of superior thyroid artery to use for anastomosis. Other commonly used recipient vessels are the facial artery and vein. If required, anastomosis can be accomplished end-to-side into the external carotid artery. Another alternative is use of the contralateral side of the neck for recipient vessels. In all cases, vein grafts should be used for either arterial or venous anastomoses if available pedicle length does not allow for tension-free union. Adequate exposure of the base of tongue area for proximal bowel anastomosis is usually achieved through the cervical incision, although mandibulotomy may occasionally be required for satisfactory access.

In the great majority of cases, the ablative portion of the procedure removes the larynx in addition to the pharyngoesophageal segment. On occasion, however, the larynx may remain in situ. This may cause problems with free jejunal transfer because it is difficult to position the jejunum appropriately with the larynx intact. In addition, aspiration may be a significant problem when the larynx has been preserved.

The abdominal portion of the procedure is performed through an upper midline incision. We employ preoperative bowel preparation routinely for this procedure. The ligament of Treitz is identified and the bowel is then traced distally to identify an acceptable bowel segment with a good vascular arcade. The length of bowel required is marked and dissection is begun in the mesentery. The bowel segment is isolated on a single artery and vein, which are traced as far proximally as possible. Branching of the vessels is encountered near the base of the mesentery and dissection is terminated at this point. The bowel segment is then divided with a stapling device and viability established with the segment isolated on its vascular pedicle. Bowel continuity is reestablished by end-to-end anastomosis while the isolated segment is left to perfuse in situ (Fig. 30-3). A feeding jejunostomy is created distal to the bowel anastomosis. At this point, the vascular pedicle is divided (Fig. 30–4) and the jejunal segment is delivered to the neck. The mesenteric defect is now sutured and the abdomen is closed in the usual manner.

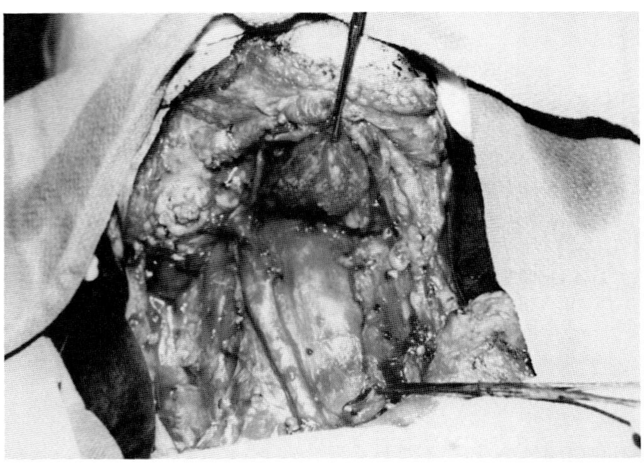

Figure 30–1. Defect following laryngopharyngectomy and right neck dissection. Proximal clamp is on the esophagus. Note absence of veins on neck dissection side. Vascular anastomoses were performed to the opposite neck vessels in this case.

The jejunal segment is positioned in the pharyngoesophageal defect in an isoperistaltic fashion. The proximal bowel anastomosis is performed first, using interrupted 000 absorbable sutures (Fig. 30–5). As previously mentioned, mandibulotomy may be necessary for adequate exposure of the base of tongue and oropharyngeal area. The jejunal segment often must be incised along the antimesenteric border to compensate for the discrepancy between the bowel lumen and the larger circumference of the oropharyx. Following completion of the proximal bowel anastomosis, the operating microscope is brought into the field and vessel preparation completed prior to the anastomoses. Arterial and venous microanastomoses are then performed between the jejunal and cervical vessels (Fig. 30–6). The artery is anastomosed, preferably, end-to-end to a branch of external carotid artery and the vein is anastomosed end-to-end to the external jugular, as previously discussed. Other alternatives available for vascular anastomoses are utilized as necessary. After blood flow has been reestablished, the bowel segment is shortened if necessary and the distal bowel anastomosis completed with absorbable sutures (Fig. 30–7). It is important to shorten the bowel, since any redundancy may produce kinking and obstruction with resultant swallowing problems. A nasogastric tube is placed through the bowel segment prior to completing the distal anastomosis. The cervical skin is then reapproximated, with closed wound suction drains sutured in place some distance from the vascular anastomoses. A small opening is left in the neck incision to allow visual monitoring of the transferred jejunum.

Postoperative care consists of frequent visual inspection of the flap to assess viability. The patients are usually kept heavily sedated for 2 to 3 days and sandbags are placed by the side of the head to avoid avulsion of the vessels with sudden movements. No circumferential neck dressings or tracheotomy tapes are used. Jejunostomy tube feedings are instituted as soon as feasible. Prophylactic antibiotics are routinely employed. The nasogastric tube is removed at approximately 7 days, at which time a barium swallow is performed (Fig. 30–8). If no leak is seen on barium swallow, oral liquid feeding may commence. If a leak is present, jejunostomy feeding may be continued after the patient has been discharged from the hospital, to permit time for the fistula to heal spontaneously. In many instances, however, secondary procedures are necessary to close the defect. It may be advisable to delay postoperative radiation therapy until any fistulas have resolved.

In addition to the standard operating procedure described, the jejunal segment may be opened entirely and used as a patch rather than as a circumferential replacement (Fig. 30–9). The procedure may also be used in the treatment of various postop-

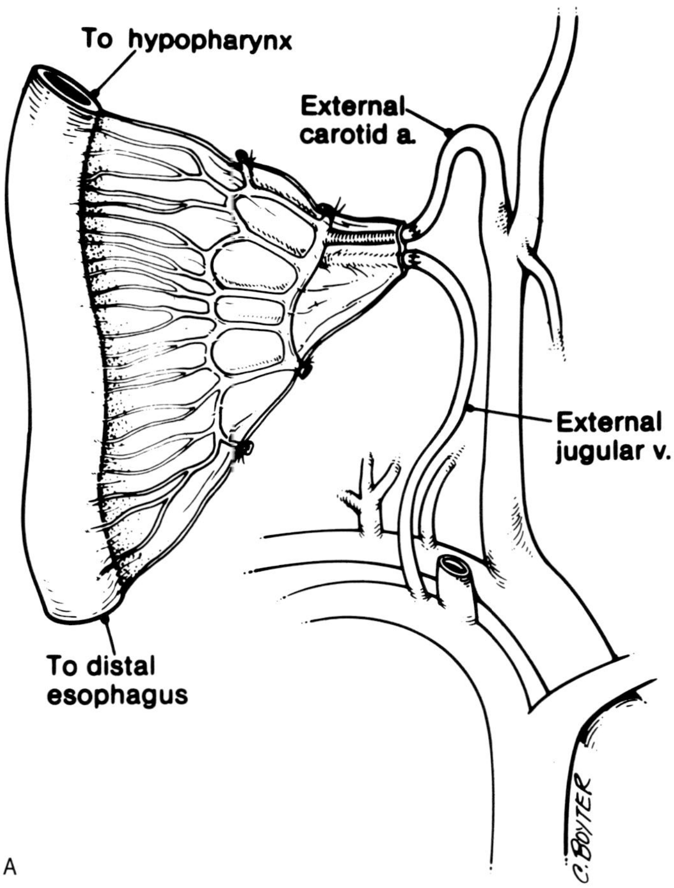

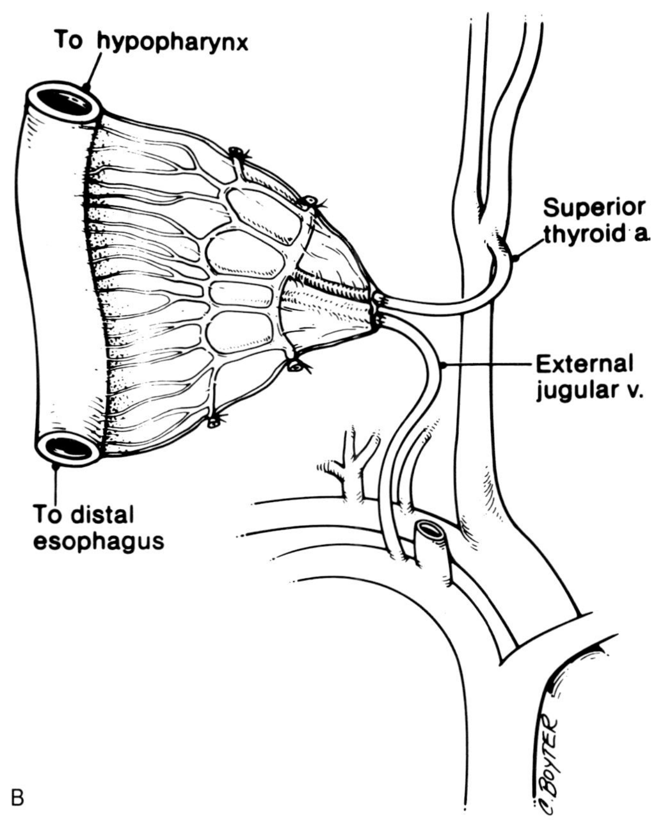

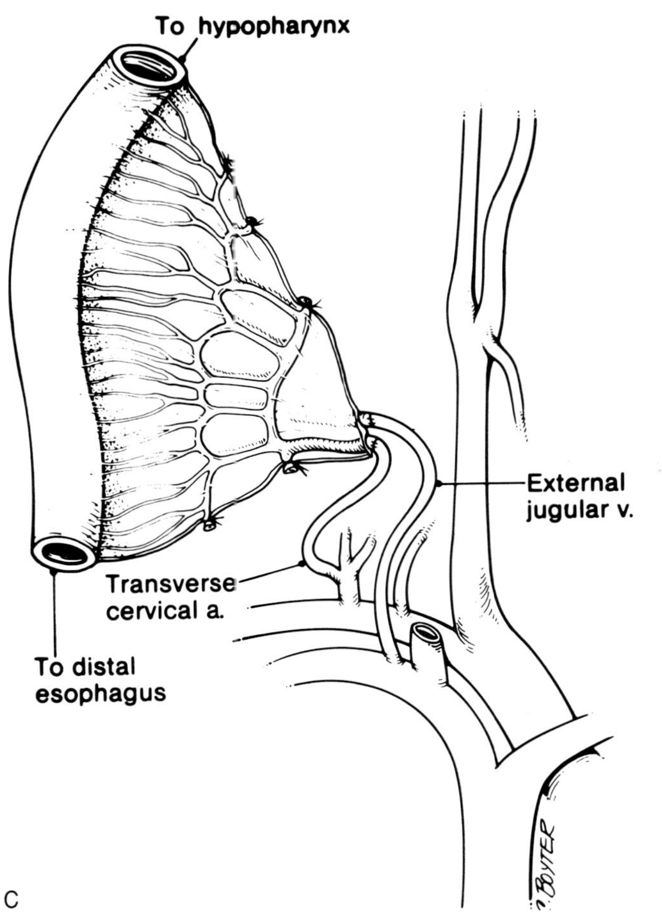

Figure 30–2. Possible recipient vessels in the neck. **A:** external carotid artery; **B:** superior thyroid artery; **C:** transverse cervical artery. The mesentery of the bowel may require asymmetrical preparation to accommodate recipient vessels.

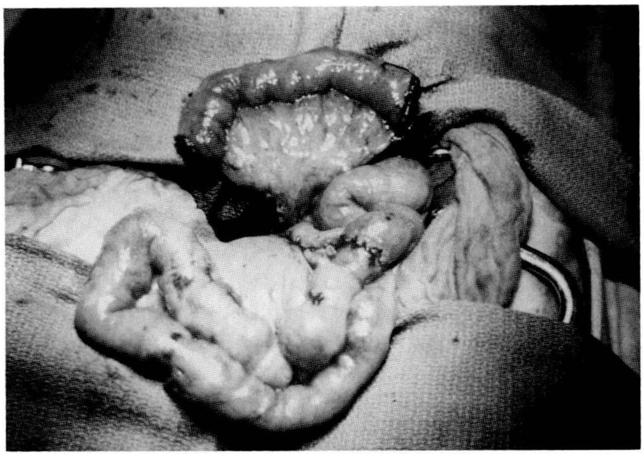

Figure 30–3. Jejunal segment isolated on vascular pedicle. Bowel continuity has been reestablished. The bowel is left to perfuse in situ until ready for transfer to the neck.

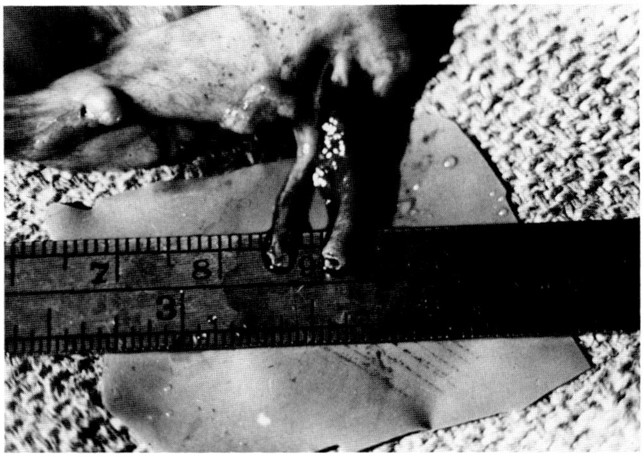

Figure 30–4. Magnified view of divided vascular pedicle. Vessels range in diameter from 2 to 4 mm.

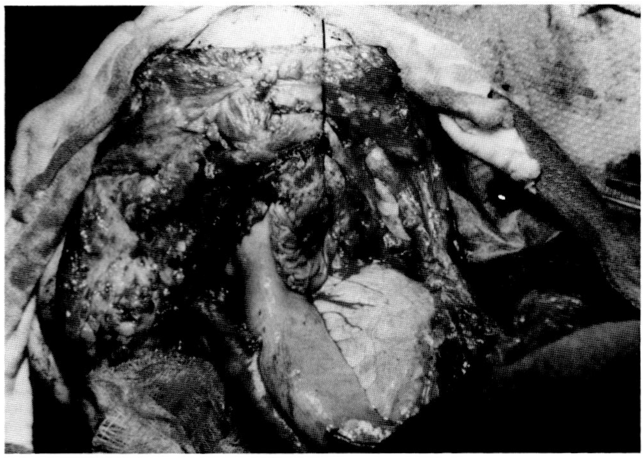

Figure 30–5. Proximal bowel anastomosis partially completed. The vascular pedicle is directed toward the contralateral side of the neck (see Fig. 30–1). The proximal bowel anastomosis is usually completed prior to vascular anastomoses. The bowel is oriented in an isoperistaltic fashion.

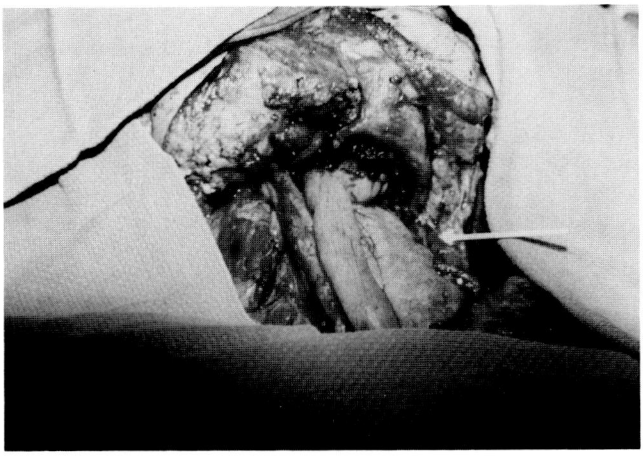

Figure 30–6. Vascular anastomoses completed: superior thyroid to jejunal artery, end-to-end; external jugular to jejunal vein, end-to-end. Although in this case anastomoses were performed on the contralateral side, in most cases adequate vessels will be available on the side of the neck dissection.

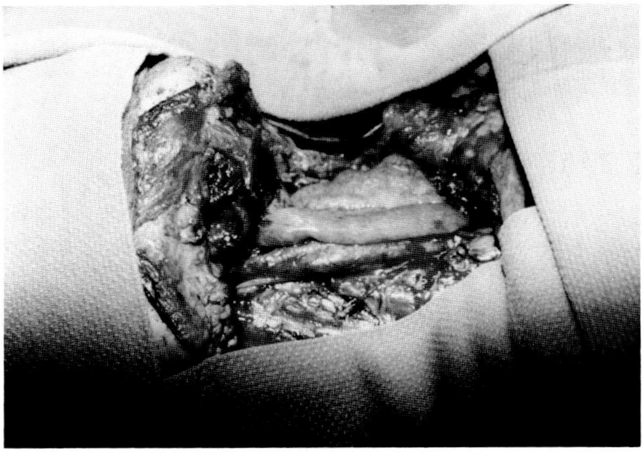

Figure 30–7. The bowel is shortened to alleviate any redundancy and the distal bowel anastomosis is completed.

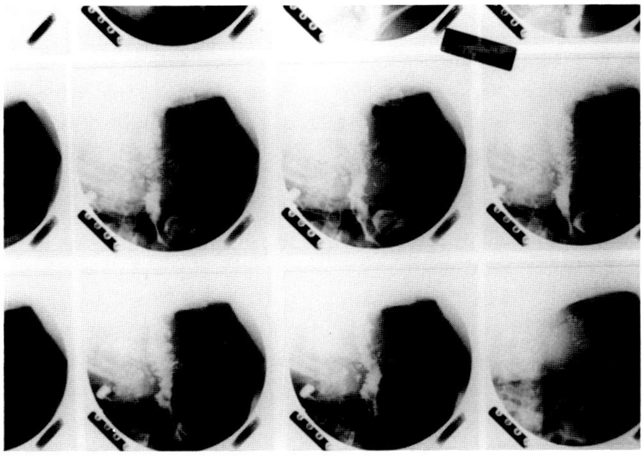

Figure 30–8. Postoperative barium swallow. There is a small amount of extravasation distally. This closed spontaneously within 3 weeks of the original surgery.

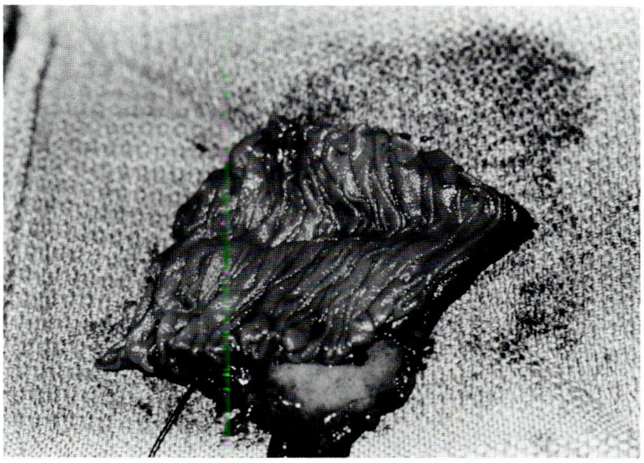

Figure 30–9. Jejunal segment opened along the antimesenteric border. The opened segment may then be used as a "patch" if the posterior pharyngeal wall remains after resection, or after a stricture has been opened longitudinally.

erative fistulas (Fig. 30–10), as well as for benign strictures of the pharyngoesophageal region.

RESULTS AND COMPLICATIONS

Coleman et al[13] recently reported results of 96 free jejunal transfers performed in 88 patients at Emory University Affiliated Hospitals. Seventy-nine of the 88 patients underwent operation for cancer, the remainder for various problems related to trauma or benign stricture. Initial operation was technically successful in 78 (89%) of the 88 patients. Second jejunal transfers were attempted in seven of the ten patients whose first operation failed; five were successful. Ultimately, repair of the defect by free jejunal autograft was achieved in 83 (94%) of the 88 patients.

At last reported follow-up, 34 of 79 patients with cancer died from recurrent disease. Ten died with no evidence of cancer, and 28 were alive and free of disease. There were five perioperative deaths, and two patients were lost to follow-up.

As would be anticipated with procedures of this complexity, the complication rate was significant. Postoperative morbidity occurred in the head and neck region as well as the abdomen. The most catastrophic complications were due to vascular compromise and subsequent graft failure, as already discussed. In most instances the best salvage procedure was another free jejunal transfer, although other methods, such as musculocutaneous flaps, were sometimes employed.

Other complications included fistulas, bowel anastomotic stenosis, redundant jejunum, infection, and hematoma. Anastomotic fistulas occurred in 28 patients; 16 healed with local wound care, and 12 required further surgery. Twenty-three of the 28 patients with fistulas regained satisfactory swallowing. Six patients developed stenosis of the suture lines of the jejunal graft. Two of these had healed fistulas. In three patients, stenosis was relieved by a single dilation. One required repeated dilation and two patients had persistent dysphagia despite attempts at operative correction of stenosis. Evaluation of ultimate swallowing function was possible in 68 patients and considered "good" in 52 (76%).

Eight patients required second operations to manage complications of laparotomy. Abdominal problems were a major contributory factor in the deaths of two patients.

CONCLUSIONS

Despite the possibility of significant postoperative morbidity, free jejunal transfer provides meaningful palliation and a high rate of restoration of function for a group of patients with difficult problems. This procedure is now preferred by many surgeons for replacement of the pharyngoesophageal segment following extirpative surgery for aerodigestive tract malignancies.

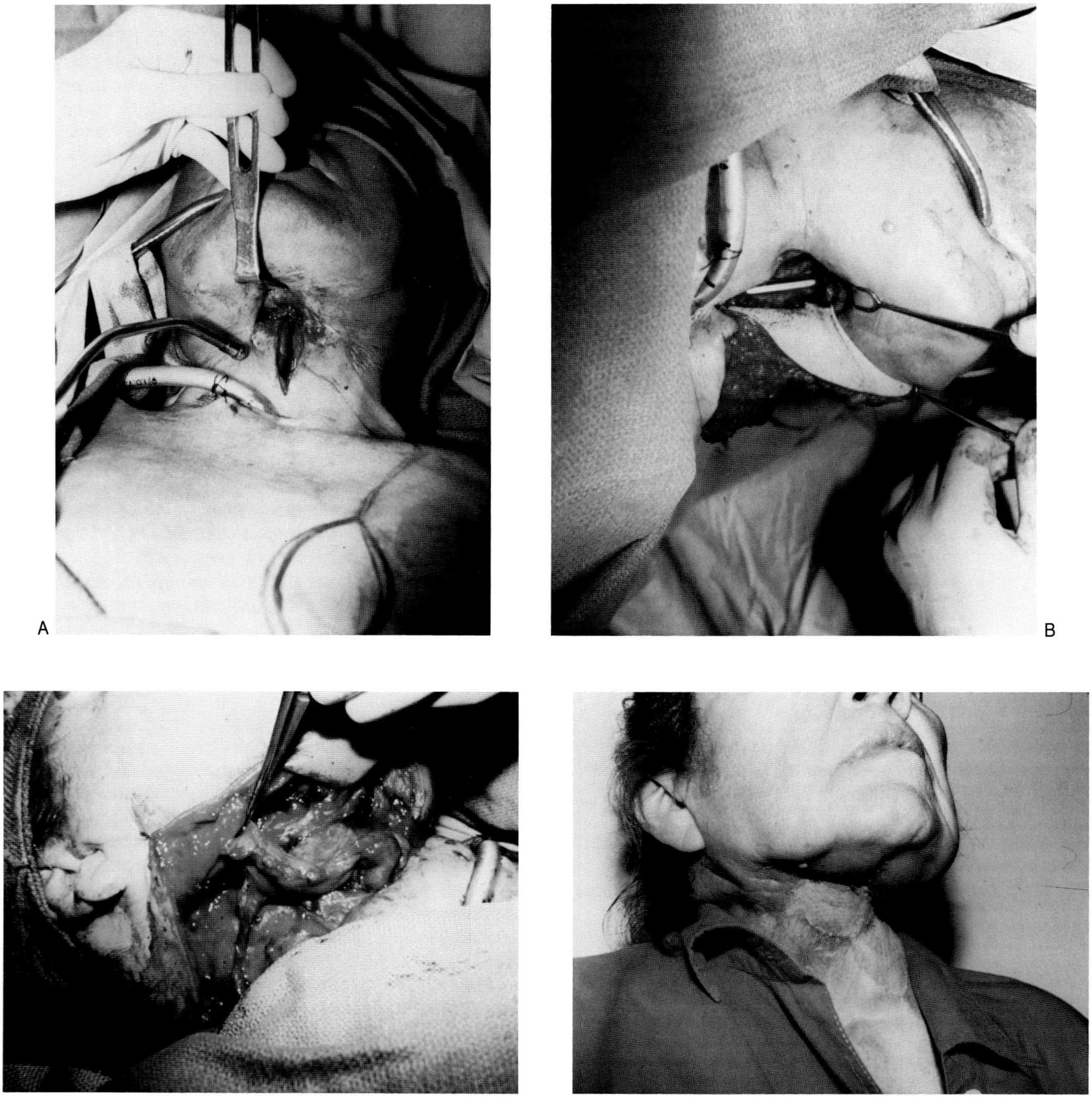

A B C D

Figure 30–10. Jejunal free flap used to repair pharyngeal fistula after failure of pectoralis major musculocutaneous flap. A: the fistula, with pectoralis major flap outlined; B: pectoralis major musculocutaneous flap partially inset to close fistula. External surface of muscle was skin grafted. C: jejunal free flap is used for salvage after pectoralis major flap has failed. D: healed orocutaneous fistula after free jejunal flap; the serosa of the jejunum has been skin grafted.

REFERENCES

1. Negus VE. Reconstruction of the pharynx after pharyngooesophagolaryngectomy. Br J Plast Surg 1953;6:99–101.
2. Edgerton MT. One-stage reconstruction of the cervical esophagus and trachea. Surgery 1932;31:239–50.
3. Lane WA. Excision of a cancerous segment of oesophagus by means of a skin flap. Br Med J 1911;1:16.
4. Trotter W. The Huntarian Lectures on the principles and technique of the operative treatment of malignant disease of the mouth and pharynx. Lancet 1913;1:1147.
5. Wookey H. Surgical treatment of carcinoma of pharynx and upper esophagus. Surg Gynecol Obstet 1947;75:499–506.
6. Bakamjian UY. A two-stage method for pharyngoesophageal reconstruction with a primary pectoral skin flap. Plast Reconstr Surg 1965;36:173–84.
7. McCraw JB, Dibbell DG, Carroway JH. Clinical definition of independent myocutaneous vascular territories. Plast Reconstr Surg 1977;60:341–52.
8. Ariyan S, Cuono CB. Myocutaneous flaps for head and neck reconstruction. Head Neck Surgery 1980;2:321–43.
9. Watson JS, Robertson J, Lendrum M, et al. Pharyngeal reconstruction using the latissimus dorsi myocutaneous flap. Br J Plast Surg 1982;35:401.
10. Ong CB, Lee TC. Pharyngogastric anastomosis after oesophagopharyngectomy for carcinoma of the hypopharynx and cervical oesophagus. Br J Surg 1961;48:193–200.
11. Goligher JC, Robin IG. Use of left colon for reconstruction of the pharynx and oesophagus after pharyngectomy. Br J Surg 1954;42:283–90.
12. Hester TR, McConnell FM, Nahai F, et al. Reconstruction of cervical esophagus, hypopharynx and oral cavity using free jejunal transfer. Am J Surg 1980;140:487–91.
13. Coleman JJ, Scarles JM, Hester TR, et al. Ten years' experience with the free jejunal autograft. Am J Surg 1987;154:394–8.
14. Carrel A. The surgery of blood vessels, etc. Johns Hopkins Hosp Bull 1907;190:18.
15. Carrel A. Results of the transplantation of blood vessels, organs, and limbs. JAMA, 1908;5:1662.
16. Longmire WP Jr. A modification of the Noux technique for antithoracic esophageal reconstruction-anastomosis of the mesenteric and internal mammary blood vessels. Surgery 1947;22:44.
17. Seidenberg B, Rosenak SS, Hurwitt ES, Som ML. Immediate reconstruction of the cervical esophagus by a revascularized isolated jejunal segment. Ann Surg 1959;149:162–71.
18. Heibert AC, Cummings GO. Successful replacement of the cervical esophagus by transplantation and revascularization of a free graft of gastric antrum. Ann Surg 1961;154:103–6.
19. Jacobson JH, Suarez EL. Microsurgery in anastomosis of small vessels. Surg Forum 1960;11:243.
20. Krizek TJ, Tesaburo T, Desprez JD, Kichn C. Experimental transplantation of composite grafts by microsurgical vascular anastomosis. Plast Reconstr Surg 1965;36:538.
21. Buncke HJ, Schulz WP. Total ear reimplantation in the rabbit utilizing microminiature vascular anastomosis. Br J Plast Surg 1966;19:15.

Appendix A

AJC* STAGING SYSTEM FOR LARYNX[1]

PRIMARY TUMOR (T)

T_x Primary tumor cannot be assessed
T_0 No evidence of primary tumor
T_{IS} Carcinoma in situ

SUPRAGLOTTIS

T_1 Tumor limited to one subsite of supraglottis with normal vocal cord mobility
T_2 Tumor invades more than one subsite of supraglottis or glottis, with normal vocal cord mobility
T_3 Tumor limited to larynx with vocal cord fixation and/or invades postcricoid area, medial wall of pyriform sinus, or preepiglottic tissues.
T_4 Tumor invades through thyroid cartilage, and/or extends to other tissues beyond the larynx (e.g., to oropharynx, soft tissues of neck)

GLOTTIS

T_1 Tumor limited to vocal cord(s) (may involve anterior or posterior commissures) with normal mobility
T_{1A} Tumor limited to one vocal cord
T_{1B} Tumor involves both vocal cords
T_2 Tumor extends to supraglottis and/or subglottis, and/or with impaired vocal cord mobility
T_3 Tumor limited to the larynx with vocal cord fixation
T_4 Tumor invades through thyroid cartilage and/or extends to other tissues beyond the larynx (e.g., oropharynx, soft tissues of neck)

SUBGLOTTIS

T_1 Tumor limited to the subglottis
T_2 Tumor extends to vocal cord(s) with normal or impaired mobility
T_3 Tumor limited to larynx with vocal cord fixation
T_4 Tumor invades through cricoid or thyroid cartilage and/or extends to other tissues beyond the larynx (e.g., oropharynx, soft tissues of neck)

REGIONAL LYMPH NODES (N)

N_x Regional lymph nodes cannot be assessed
N_0 No regional lymph node metastasis
N_1 Metastasis in a single ipsilateral lymph node, 3 cm or less in greatest dimension
N_2 Metastasis in a single ipsilateral lymph node, more than 3 cm but not more than 6 cm in greatest dimension, or multiple ipsilateral lymph nodes, none more than 6 cm in greatest dimension or bilateral or contralateral lymph nodes, none more than 6 cm in greatest dimension
N_{2A} Metastasis in a single ipsilateral lymph node more than 3 cm but not more than 6 cm in greatest dimension
N_{2B} Metastasis in multiple ipsilateral lymph nodes, none more than 6 cm in greatest dimension
N_{2C} Metastasis in bilateral or contralateral lymph nodes, none more than 6 cm in greatest dimension
N_3 Metastasis in a lymph node more than 6 cm in greatest dimension

DISTANT METASTASIS (M)

M_x Presence of distant metastasis cannot be assessed
M_0 No distant metastasis
M_1 Distant metastasis

STAGE GROUPING

Stage 0	T_{IS}	N_0	M_0
Stage 1	T_1	N_0	M_0
Stage II	T_2	N_0	M_0
Stage III	T_3	N_0	M_0
	T_1	N_1	M_0
	T_2	N_1	M_0
	T_3	N_1	M_0
Stage IV	T_4	N_0, N_1	M_0
	Any T	N_2, N_3	M_0
	Any T	Any N	M_1

*American Joint Committee on Cancer.

Appendix B

AJC** STAGING SYSTEM FOR HYPOPHARYNX[2]

PRIMARY TUMOR (T)

T_x Primary tumor cannot be assessed
T_0 No evidence of primary tumor
T_{IS} Carcinoma in situ
T_1 Tumor limited to 1 subsite of hypopharynx
T_2 Tumor invades more than one subsite of hypopharynx or an adjacent site, without fixation of hemilarynx
T_3 Tumor invades more than one subsite of hypopharynx or an adjacent site, with fixation of hemilarynx
T_4 Tumor invades adjacent structures (e.g., cartilage or soft tissues of neck)

LYMPH NODES (N)

N_x Regional lymph nodes cannot be assessed
N_0 No regional lymph node metastasis
N_1 Metastasis in a single ipsilateral lymph node 3 cm or less in greatest dimension
N_2 Metastasis in a single ipsilateral lymph node, more than 3 cm but less than 6 cm in greatest dimension, or in bilateral or contralateral lymph nodes, none more than 6 cm in greatest dimension
N_{2A} Metastasis in a single ipsilateral lymph node, more than 3 cm but less than 5 cm in greatest dimension
N_{2B} Metastasis in multiple ipsilateral lymph nodes, none more than 6 cm in greatest dimension
N_{2C} Metastasis in bilateral or contralateral lymph nodes, none more than 6 cm in greatest dimension
N_3 Metastasis in a lymph node more than 6 cm in greatest dimension

**American Joint Committee on Cancer.

DISTANT METASTASIS (M)

M_x Presence of distant metastasis cannot be assessed
M_0 No distant metastasis
M_1 Distant metastasis

STAGE GROUPING

Stage 0	T_{IS}	N_0	M_0
Stage 1	T_1	N_0	M_0
Stage II	T_2	N_0	M_0
Stage III	T_3	N_0	M_0
	T_1	N_1	M_0
	T_2	N_1	M_0
	T_3	N_1	M_0
Stage IV	T_4	N_0, N_1	M_0
	Any T	N_2, N_3	M_0
	Any T	Any N	M_1

REFERENCES

1. Beahrs OH, Henson DE, Hutter RVP, Myers MH, eds. *Manual for Staging of Cancer,* 3rd ed. Philadelphia: JB Lippincott, 1988:39–41.
2. Beahrs OH, Henson DE, Hutter RVP, Myers MH, eds. *Manual for Staging of Cancer,* 3rd ed. Philadelphia: JB Lippincott, 1988:34–35.

INDEX

(Italics indicate a figure or table)